A Colour Atlas and Textbook of the

Histopathology of Mycotic Diseases

Francis W. Chandler DVM, PhD
Chief, Histopathology Laboratory
Pathology Division, Bureau of Laboratories
Center for Disease Control, Atlanta

William Kaplan DVM, MPH
Chief, Developmental Mycology Branch
Mycology Division, Bureau of Laboratories
Center for Disease Control, Atlanta

Libero Ajello PhD
Director, Mycology Division
Bureau of Laboratories
Center for Disease Control, Atlanta

Wolfe Medical Publications Ltd

Published by Wolfe Medical Publications Ltd, 1980
Pictorial section printed by Royal Smeets Offset
b.v., Weert, Netherlands
Text section printed by Lochem Druk b.v., Lochem, Netherlands
ISBN 0 7234 0754 1 Cased edition
ISBN 0 7234 1606 0 Paperback edition

A CIP catalogue record for this book is available from the British Library.

Acknowledgements

The authors are indebted to investigators throughout the world, too numerous to cite individually, for supplying or lending histological preparations or tissue for study and photographic purposes. Without their interest and generosity we would not have been able to cover the subject matter as completely and as thoroughly as we desired. To them we extend our heartfelt thanks.

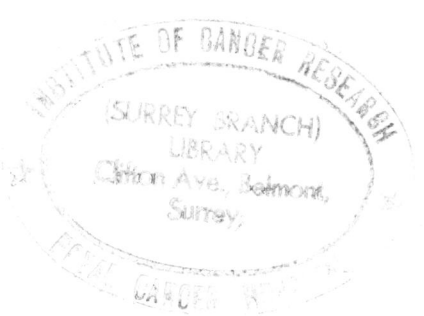

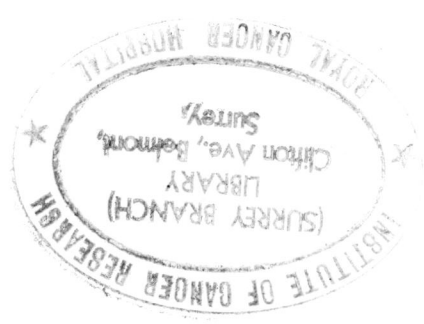

Contents

Text

Pictorial section

Foreword

Many worthwhile biomedical textbooks result from the cooperative efforts of experts who work in isolation at scattered campuses, laboratories, or institutions and who have to depend chiefly on correspondence, with only occasional brief personal contacts. However, *A Colour Atlas and Textbook of the Histopathology of Mycotic Diseases* is the culmination of almost daily joint effort by its authors over a period of several years in their busy laboratories at the Center for Disease Control, Atlanta, USA.

The authors' associated and separate bibliographies list more than 260 journal publications on mycological subjects and 20 chapters in texts or manuals. Their publications and frequent presentations at scientific conferences attest to their expertise in every aspect of medical mycology: pathology, cultural and diagnostic techniques, ecology, taxonomy, and treatment. Their cumulative experiences in this highly specialised area of microbiology and medicine total 68 years.

The authors have collected, over a number of years, extensive archives of histopathologic material as a result of their diagnostic services, travels, affiliations, and associations with fellow mycologists and pathologists throughout the world. Their frequent consultation in difficult or controversial cases has given the authors broad experience in the diagnosis of fungus diseases by histopathologic, cultural and immunofluorescence methods.

From a vast number of candidates, the photomicrographs selected for this atlas were the most representative of the respective lesions and the most photographically excellent. The illustrations and their captions stand alone, independent of the text, to facilitate the rapid review or differential diagnosis of an organism in tissue by pathologists while at the microscope.

Microbiologists will find the cultural, technical, and taxonomic discussions of extreme interest. Clinicians will appreciate the diagnostic dilemmas that fungus diseases may present to the pathologist and microbiologist, and may be guided to the most appropriate therapeutic decisions. Because of its comprehensive coverage of the subject, this book will be of value to all workers who have an interest in medical mycology.

Martin D. Hicklin, MD, MPH
Director, Pathology Division
Center for Disease Control
Atlanta, Georgia

Preface

The great number of infectious actinomycetes and fungi that cause human and animal disease pose a challenge to the entire medical community. The clinical signs of the actinomycoses and the mycoses are not pathognomonic in that they closely resemble those elicited by other microorganisms or those associated with other pathological conditions. Definitive diagnoses cannot be made unless actinomycetal and fungal elements are demonstrated in clinical materials and, ideally, unless an organism is isolated which is compatible with clinical and pathological findings.

Numerous textbooks are currently available in which the mycoses and actinomycoses are adequately described in terms of their clinical expressions and the in vitro characteristics of their aetiologic agents. However, too little emphasis has been placed on the value of histopathological findings in diagnosing the cutaneous, subcutaneous, and systemic mycoses and the actinomycotic diseases. All too frequently the only means of reaching a specific diagnosis is through the detection and identification of pathogenic actinomycetes and fungi in clinical materials and biopsied tissue. To a degree, at least, this situation exists because clinical and laboratory personnel are unfamiliar with appropriate methodology and interpretative techniques.

Often, diagnosticians must rely on their ability to identify actinomycetes and fungi in fixed tissue after using special staining procedures. Many of these organisms can be definitively identified in tissue when they are stained uniformly and when classical morphologic forms are present in sufficient numbers. However, when only immature or atypical forms are present, it may be difficult, if not impossible, to identify the organisms with conventional histological methods. In such instances, use of the fluorescent antibody technique on tissue sections often will lead to a specific diagnosis.

The morphologic variability of pathogenic actinomycetes and fungi in tissue and the range of tissue responses to these agents are neither generally appreciated by pathologists nor adequately illustrated in standard textbooks of medical mycology. For this reason, *A Colour Atlas and Textbook of the Histopathology of Mycotic Diseases* has been carefully and specifically designed to provide the information that pathologists, mycologists, and other diagnostic workers must have to identify actinomycotic and fungal elements in human and animal tissues. With its wealth of photomicrographs, and the basic information provided on each actinomycotic and fungal disease, the Atlas delineates the salient in vivo diagnostic features of the pathogens and the tissue reactions that they elicit in the host. A comprehensive glossary clarifies mycological and histopathological terminology, and carefully selected, pertinent references are provided at the end of each chapter and in a general reference section. Following the introductory chapters in which actinomycotic and mycotic diseases and their aetiologic agents are classified and histopathological and immunofluorescence procedures are discussed, the various diseases are treated in depth.

Dedicated to our wives,
Gloria, Margaret, and Gloria.

1 Introduction: Taxonomy of the fungi and classification of fungal and actinomycotic diseases

Basic to an understanding of the mycoses and their aetiologic agents is the use of logically developed and organised classification schemes. With respect to the names of the diseases, it is unfortunate that there are no rules or international agreements governing their creation and adoption. In the course of time, many names have been proposed for mycotic diseases. Some of these names were readily adopted and are still in use, while others fell by the wayside. The disease names that have presented the least difficulties, in respect to aptness and acceptability, have been those that were based on the genera of their aetiologic agents. Examples of such names are aspergillosis, candidiasis, coccidioidomycosis and rhinosporidiosis, which were derived respectively from *Aspergillus*, *Candida*, *Coccidioides* and *Rhinosporidium*. However, changes in the scientific names of the pathogenic fungi, stemming from new taxonomic studies, have raised havoc with some of the names that were formerly in wide use. Such was the fate of moniliasis and torulosis, when the genus *Monilia*, as used by medical mycologists, was replaced by *Candida*, and *Torula* by *Cryptococcus*.

Names based on geographical distribution have lost favour, because those diseases were found to be more widely distributed than at first believed. Thus, South American blastomycosis is now referred to as paracoccidioidomycosis, since it is endemic not only to South America but also Central America and Mexico. Similarly, the name North American blastomycosis has now been replaced by the nongeographically restrictive name blastomycosis, since this disease is now known to exist in Africa and the Middle East, as well as in the United States and Canada[1].

If a disease is of multiple aetiology, a name for the disease based on any one of the several genera of the fungi involved would be inappropriate. Accordingly, various descriptive terms have been devised and have come into common usage. Such names are adiaspiromycosis (for infections caused by *Chrysosporium parvum* var. *parvum* and *C. parvum* var. *crescens*), chromoblastomycosis, and the mycetomas. Other names originate from the vernacular and local names where the diseases flourish. Such is the origin of black and white piedra and tokelau.

Some disease names were created to end confusion caused by the indiscriminate lumping together of dissimilar diseases. This type of problem is well illustrated by the term chromomycosis, which unfortunately has come to be used by some as a common name for two distinct entities: chromoblastomycosis and phaeohyphomycosis[2].

In this Atlas, the names chosen for the diseases treated herein are based on common usage and contemporary knowledge regarding geographic distribution as well as the current taxonomic treatment of their aetiologic agents.

Traditionally, the mycotic diseases have been divided into four broad categories: superficial, cutaneous, subcutaneous, and systemic. We have chosen to follow that classification system in order to facilitate communication with our readers. The aetiologic agent or agents of each disease are also cited in this compilation.

I Superficial Mycoses

(Defined as those infections in which the invading pathogen is confined to the stratum corneum with little or no tissue reaction. In the case of hair infections (black and white piedra), growth is generally superficial with minimal damage to the hair and no host reaction).

A. Black Piedra
   1. *Piedraia hortai*
B. Tinea Nigra
   1. *Exophiala werneckii*, *Stenella araguata*
C. Tinea Versicolor
   1. *Malassezia furfur*
D. White Piedra
   1. *Trichosporon beigelii*

II Cutaneous Mycoses

(In the cutaneous mycoses all keratinised tissue, i.e., skin, hair, nail, feathers, are attacked. Although the pathogens are generally confined to the nonliving cornified layers of the skin and its appendages, destruction of these tissues is extensive and host immunological reactions may be severe.)

A. Cutaneous Candidiasis
   1. *Candida albicans*

B. Dermatomycoses
   1. *Hendersonula toruloidea*
   2. *Pyrenochaeta unguis-hominis*
   3. *Scopulariopsis brevicaulis*
   4. *Scytalidium hyalinum*

C. Dermatophytoses
   1. *Epidermophyton floccosum*
   2. *Microsporum* species
      a. *M. audouinii*
      b. *M. canis*
      c. *M. cookei*
      d. *M. distortum*
      e. *M. equinum*
      f. *M. ferrugineum*
      g. *M. fulvum*
      h. *M. gallinae*
      i. *M. gypseum*
      j. *M. nanum*
      k. *M. persicolor*
      l. *M. praecox*
      m. *M. racemosum*
      n. *M. vanbreuseghemii*
   3. Trichophyton species
      a. *T. concentricum*
      b. *T. equinum*
         (1) *T.e.* var. *equinum*
         (2) *T.e.* var. *autotrophicum*
      c. *T. gourvilii*
      d. *T. megninii*
      e. *T. mentagrophytes*
         (1) *T. m.* var. *erinacei*
         (2) *T. m.* var. *interdigitale*
         (3) *T. m.* var. *mentagrophytes*
         (4) *T. m.* var. *nodulare*
         (5) *T. m.* var. *quinckeanum*
      f. *T. rubrum*
      g. *T. schoenleinii*
      h. *T. simii*
      i. *T. soudanense*
      j. *T. tonsurans*
      k. *T. yaoundei*
      l. *T. violaceum*

D. Cutaneous Zygomycosis
   1. *Rhizopus rhizopodiformis*

III Subcutaneous Mycoses

(The subcutaneous mycoses constitute a heterogeneous group of diseases caused by a wide variety of fungi that invade the cutaneous and subcutaneous tissues after traumatic implantation. Some infections may remain localised, slowly spreading to contiguous tissues (i.e., chromoblastomycosis, mycetomas), while in others (i.e., sporotrichosis) lymphatic spread is frequent.)

A. Chromoblastomycosis
   1. *Cladosporium carrionii*
   2. *Fonsecaea compacta*
   3. *F. pedrosoi*
   4. *Phialophora verrucosa*
   5. *Rhinocladiella cerophilum*

B. Lobomycosis
   1. *Loboa loboi*

C. Mycetomas (Eumycotic)
   1. *Acremonium falciforme*
   2. *A. kiliense*
   3. *A. recifei*
   4. *Aspergillus nidulans*
   5. *Corynespora cassiicola*
   6. *Curvularia geniculata*
   7. *Exophiala jeanselmei*
   8. *Fusarium moniliforme*
   9. *Leptosphaeria senegalensis*
   10. *L. tompkinsii*
   11. *Madurella grisea*
   12. *M. mycetomatis*
   13. *Neotestudina rosatii*
   14. *Petriellidium boydii*
   15. *Pyrenochaeta mackinnonii*
   16. *Pyrenochaeta romeroi*

D. Subcutaneous Phaeohyphomycosis
   1. *Alternaria alternata*
   2. *Aureobasidium pullulans*
   3. *Drechslera rostrata*
   4. *D. spicifera*
   5. *Exophiala moniliae*
   6. *Phialophora parasiticia*
   7. *P. richardsiae*
   8. *P. spinifera*
   9. *Phoma hibernica*
   10. *Phoma* sp.
   11. *Wangiella dermatitidis*

E. Rhinosporidiosis
   1. *Rhinosporidium seeberi*

F. Sporotrichosis
   1. *Sporothrix schenckii*
      (1) *S.s.* var. *schenckii*
      (2) *S.s.* var. *luriei*

G. Subcutaneous Zygomycosis
   1. *Basidiobolus haptosporus*
   2. *Conidiobolus coronatus*

IV Systemic Mycoses

(These are basically pulmonary diseases in that the primary site of infection is almost invariably the lungs. Systemic mycoses, except in their subclinical, benign forms, may have grave consequences. All of the vital organs may be attacked and lesions may be extensive. Cutaneous and subcutaneous forms of these diseases do occur as the result of dissemination or as a consequence of direct inoculation following an injury.)

A. Adiaspiromycosis
  1. *Chrysosporium parvum*
    (a) *C.p.* var. *parvum*
    (b) *C.p.* var. *crescens*

B. Aspergillosis
  1. *Aspergillus fumigatus* group
  2. *A. flavus* group
  3. *A. nidulans* group
  4. *A. niger* group
  5. *A. oryzae* group
  6. *A. terreus* group

C. Blastomycosis
  1. *Blastomyces dermatitidis*

D. Systemic Candidiasis
  1. *Candida albicans*
  2. *C. glabrata*
  3. *C. guilliermondii*
  4. *C. krusei*
  5. *C. parapsilosis*
  6. *C. tropicalis*

E. Coccidioidomycosis
  1. *Coccidioides immitis*

F. Cryptococcosis
  1. *Cryptococcus neoformans*

G. Histoplasmosis Capsulati*
  1. *Histoplasma capsulatum* var. *capsulatum*

H. Histoplasmosis Duboisii
  1. *H. capsulatum* var. *duboisii*

I. Histoplasmosis Farciminosi*
  1. *H. farciminosum*

J. Paracoccidioidomycosis
  1. *Paracoccidioides brasiliensis*

K. Systemic Phaeohyphomycosis
  1. *Cladosporium bantianum* (trichoides)
  2. *C. cladosporioides*
  3. *Curvularia pallescens*
  4. *Dactylaria gallopava*
  5. *Drechslera hawaiiensis*
  6. *Exophiala pisciphila*
  7. *E. salmonis*
  8. *Scolecobasidium humicola*
  9. *S. tschawytschae*
  10. *Mycocentrospora acerina* (*Cercospora apii*)

L. Systemic Zygomycosis
  1. *Absidia corymbifera*
  2. *Cunninghamella bertholletiae*
  3. *Conidiobolus incongruus*
  4. *Mucor ramosissimus*
  5. *Mucor rouxianus*
  6. *Rhizomucor pusillus*
  7. *Rhizopus arrhizus*
  8. *R. microsporus*
  9. *R. oryzae*
  10. *R. rhizopodiformis*
  11. *Saksenaea vasiformis*

*In the interest of clarity, brevity and uniformity, we are coining the terms histoplasmosis capsulati and histoplasmosis farciminosi for infections caused by *H. capsulatum* var. *capsulatum* and *H. farciminosum* respectively. The precedent for this nomenclature was set in 1964 by Cockshott and Lucas[16], when they created the name histoplasmosis duboisii for infections by *H. capsulatum* var. *duboisii*.

The diseases caused by the anaerobic and aerobic actinomycetes are treated separately since these organisms are bacteria and not fungi. However, traditionally, the actinomycoses have been considered part of the province of medical mycology. Thus, they are dealt with in this Atlas.

I Actinomycosis

1. *Actinomyces bovis*
2. *A. israelii*
3. *A. naeslundii*
4. *A. odontolyticus*
5. *A. viscosus*
6. *Arachnia propionica*
7. *Rothia dentocariosa*

II Actinomycotic Mycetomas

1. *Actinomadura madurae*
2. *A. pelletieri*
3. *Nocardia asteroides*
4. *N. brasiliensis*
5. *N. caviae*
6. *Streptomyces somaliensis*

III Dermatophilosis

1. *Dermatophilus congolensis*

IV Nocardiosis

1. *Nocardia asteroides*
2. *N. brasiliensis*
3. *N. caviae*

V Streptomycosis

1. *Streptomyces griseus*

With respect to the classification of the pathogenic actinomycetes and fungi, most mycologists no longer accept the obsolete concept that all living things can be arbitrarily considered to be either animals or plants. The two-kingdom system has been found to be inadequate, and is being abandoned by most scientists. In its place, a five-kingdom system has evolved (Table 1), which is being used by most biologists[3-5]. The kingdoms Monera and Fungi contain the pathogenic actinomycetes and fungi, respectively.

Full details on the classification of the actinomycetes will be found in the 8th edition of *Bergey's Manual of Determinative Bacteriology*[6], and in the monograph on the filamentous bacteria by Slack and Gerencser[7].

The pathogenic fungi are classified in four of the six phyla of the Kingdom Fungi (Table 2): the Zygomycota, Ascomycota, Basidiomycota and Deuteromycota. The distinguishing features of these four phyla are presented in Table 3. In Tables 4–9, the pathogens in each of the four phyla are classified in their respective classes, orders, families and genera.

For a fuller treatment of the taxonomy of the fungi, the interested reader is urged to consult references 3 and 13–15.

Table 1 Five-kingdom classification of living things

Kingdoms	Salient features
I Monera	Prokaryotic (anucleate), DNA, no mitotic apparatus, direct cell division, primarily by binary fission. Nutrition ingestive, absorbtive, chemosynthetic, photoheterotrophic or photoautotrophic. Unicellular, filamentous or mycelial. Asexual reproduction. 14 Phyla: bacteria, myxobacteria, actinomycetes, blue-green algae.
II Protista	Eukaryotic (nucleate), DNA, RNA, ingestive, absorbtive or photoautotrophic nutrition, premitotic or mitotic division, diaminopimelic acid, lysine biosynthetic pathway, unicellular or multicellular. If motile, flagella or cilia composed of microtubules in the 9 + 2 pattern. 30 Phyla: protozoans, mycetozoans, brown algae, red algae, green algae, hyphochytrids, oomycetes.
III Fungi	Absorbtive nutrition, unicellular or mycelial. Cell walls with chitin-chitosan, chitin-B-glucan, mannan-B-glucan, chitin-mannan or galactosamine-galactose polymers. If flagellate, flagellum posteriorly uniflagellate of the whiplash type. Aminoadipic acid lysine biosynthetic pathway. 6 Phyla: chytrids, zygomycetes, ascomycetes, basidiomycetes, deuteromycetes, lichens.
IV Plantae	Autotrophic, highly differentiated, diploid phase. 9 Phyla: liverworts, mosses, ferns, conifers, seed plants, etc.
V Animalia	Heterotrophic, multicellular, diploid blastula. 32 Phyla: colenterates, flat worms, mollusks, insects, reptiles, birds, mammals, etc.

Table 2 The kingdom fungi

Phyla	Classes
I Chytridiomycota	Chytridiomycetes
II Zygomycota	Zygomycetes Trichomycetes
III Ascomycota	Hemiascomycetes Loculoascomycetes Plectomycetes Laboulbeniomycetes Pyrenomycetes Discomycetes
IV Basidiomycota	Teliomycetes Hymenomycetes Gasteromycetes
V Deuteromycota	Blastomycetes Hyphomycetes Coelomycetes
VI Mycophycophyta	Lichens: ascomycetes associated with algae basidiomycetes associated with algae deuteromycetes associated with algae

Table 3 Phyla with pathogenic fungi

Phyla	Basic characteristics
I Zygomycota	Moulds with sparsely septate mycelium. Asexual reproduction by means of spores borne in sporangia or as sporangiola. Sexual spores as zygospores. (Homothallic or heterothallic.)
II Ascomycota	Unicellular or filamentous, with septate mycelium. Asexual reproduction by means of conidia borne on a wide variety of conidiophores. Sexual reproduction by means of ascospores produced within asci.
III Basidiomycota	Unicellular or filamentous, with septate mycelium, with or without clamp connections. Asexual reproduction by conidia. Sexual reproduction by means of basidiospores borne typically on basidia.
IV Deuteromycota	Unicellular or filamentous with septate mycelium. Asexual reproduction used as the basis for their classification and identification; conidia produced. Some members sterile. Sexual reproduction usually absent, but when encountered, typical of the ascomycetes or basidiomycetes.

Table 4 Some genera and pathogenic species of the phylum Ascomycota

Class I Hemiascomycetes
- Order: Endomycetales
  - Family: Endomycetaceae
    - Genus: *Endomyces*
      - Species: *E. candidus*
        (*Geotrichum candidum*)*
  - Family: Saccharomycetaceae
    - Genus: *Issatchenkia*
      - Species: *I. orientalis*
        (*Candida krusei*)
    - Genus: *Kluyveromyces*
      - Species: *K. fragilis*
        (*Candida pseudotropicalis*)
    - Genus: *Pichia*
      - Species: *P. guilliermondii*

Class II Loculoascomycetes
- Order: Myriangiales
  - Family: Saccardinulaceae
    - Genus: *Piedraia*
      - Species: *P. hortae*
- Order: Pleosporales
  - Family: Pleosporaceae
    - Genus: *Cochliobolus*
      - Species: *C. spicifer*
    - Genus: *Leptosphaeria*
      - Species: *L. senegalensis*
        L. tomkinsii
  - Family: Zopfiaceae
    - Genus: *Zopfia*
      - Species: *Z. rosatii*[10]
  - Family: Microascaceae
    - Genus: *Petriellidium*
      - Species: *P. boydii*
        (*Scedosporium apiospermum*)

Class III Plectomycetes
- Order: Eurotiales
  - Family: Eurotiaceae
    - Genus: *Emericella*
      - Species: *E. nidulans*
        (*Aspergillus nidulans* group)
    - Genus: *Sartorya*
      - Species: *S. fumigata*
        (*Aspergillus fumigatus* group)
  - Family: Gymnoascacea
    - Genus: *Ajellomyces*
      - Species: *A. capsulatus*[11]
        (*Histoplasma capsulatum*)
        A. dermatitidis
        (*Blastomyces dermatitidis*)
    - Genus: *Arthroderma*
      - Species: *A. benhamiae*
        (*Trichophyton mentagrophytes*)
        A. ciferii
        (*T. georgiae*)
        A. flavescens
        (*T. flavescens*)
        A. gertlerii
        (*T. vanbreuseghemii*)
        A. gloriae
        (*T. gloriae*)
        A. insingulare
        (*T. terrestre*)
        A. lenticularum
        (*T. terrestre*)
        A. quadrifidum
        (*T. terrestre*)
        A. simii
        (*T. simii*)
        A. uncinatum
        (*T. ajelloi*)
        A. vanbreuseghemii
        (*T. mentagrophytes*)
    - Genus: *Nannizzia*
      - Species: *N. borellii*
        (*Microsporum amazonicum*)
        N. cajetanii
        (*M. cookei*)
        N. fulva
        (*M. fulvum*)
        N. grubyia
        (*M. vanbreuseghemii*)
        N. gypsea
        (*M. gypseum*)
        N. incurvata
        (*M. gypseum*)
        N. obtusa
        (*M. nanum*)
        N. otae
        (*M. canis*)
        N. persicolor
        (*M. persicolor*)
        N. racemosa
        (*M. racemosum*)

*Imperfect states in parentheses.

Table 5 Genera and pathogenic species of the phylum Zygomycota

Class: Zygomycetes	Genus: *Mortierella*
Order: Entomophthorales	Species: *M. wolfii*
Family: Entomophthoraceae	Genus: *Mucor*
Genus: *Basidiobolus*	Species: *M. ramosissimus*
Species: *B. haptosporus*	Genus: *Rhizomucor*
Genus: *Conidiobolus*	Species: *R. pusillus*[9]
Species: *C. coronatus*	Genus: *Rhizopus*
C. incorgruus	Species: *R. arrhizus*
	R. microsporus
Order: Mucorales	*R. oryzae*
Family: Mucoraceae	*R. rhizopodiformis*
Genus: *Absidia*	
Species: *A. corymbifera*	Family: Saksenaceae
Genus: *Cunninghamella*	Genus: *Saksenaea*
Species: *C. bertholletiae*[8]	Species: *S. vasiformis*

Table 6 Some genera and pathogenic species of the Basidiomycota

Class: Teliomycetes	Class: Hymenomycetes
Order: Ustilaginales	Subclass: Holobasidiomycetidae
Family: Filobasidiaceae	Order: Aphyllophorales
Genus: *Filobasidiella*	Family: *Schizophyllaceae*
Species: *F. neoformans*[12]	Genus: *Schizophyllum*
(*Cryptococcus neoformans*)*	Species: *S. commune*
	Order: Agaricales
	Family: Coprinaceae
	Genus: *Coprinus*
	Species: *C. cinereus*

*Imperfect state in parentheses.

Table 7 Genera and pathogenic species of the form class Blastomycetes of the Deuteromycota

Class: Blastomycetes	Genus: *Cryptococcus*
Family: Cryptococcaceae	Species: *C. neoformans*
Order:	Genus: *Malassezia*
Genus: *Candida*	Species: *M. furfur*
Species: *C. albicans*	*M. pachydermatis*
C. glabrata	Genus: *Trichosporon*
C. guilliermondii	Species: *T. beigelii*
C. krusei	
C. parapsilosis	
C. tropicalis	

Table 8 Common genera and pathogenic species of the form class Hyphomycetes of the Deuteromycota

- Genus: *Acremonium*
  - Species: *A. falciforme*
  - *A. kiliense*
  - *A. recifei*
- Genus: *Aspergillus*
  - Species: *A. flavus* group
  - *A. fumigatus* group
  - *A. nidulans* group
  - *A. niger* group
  - *A. oryzae* group
  - *A. terreus* group
- Genus: *Aureobasidium*
  - Species: *A. pullulans*
- Genus: *Blastomyces*
  - Species: *B. dermatitidis*
- Genus: *Chrysosporium*
  - Species: *C. parvum* var. *parvum*
  - *C. parvum* var. *crescens*
- Genus: *Cladosporium*
  - Species: *C. bantianum* (*trichoides*)
  - *C. carrionii*
- Genus: *Coccidioides*
  - Species: *C. immitis*
- Genus: *Corynespora*
  - Species: *C. cassiicola*
- Genus: *Curvularia*
  - Species: *C. geniculata*
  - *C. lunata*
  - *C. senegalensis*
- Genus: *Dactylaria*
  - Species: *D. gallopava*
- Genus: *Drechslera*
  - Species: *D. hawaiiensis*
  - *D. rostrata*
  - *D. spiciferum*
- Genus: *Exophiala*
  - Species: *E. jeanselmei*
  - *E. pisciphila*
  - *E. salmonis*
  - *E. werneckii*
- Genus: *Epidermophyton*
  - Species: *E. floccosum*
- Genus: *Fonsecaea*
  - Species: *F. compacta*
  - *F. pedrosoi*
- Genus: *Fusarium*
  - Species: *F. moniliforme*
  - *F. oxysporum*
  - *F. solani*
- Genus: *Geotrichum*
  - Species: *G. candidum*
- Genus: *Histoplasma*
  - Species: *H. capsulatum* var. *capsulatum*
  - *H. capsulatum* var. *duboisii*
  - *H. farciminosum*
- Genus: Loboa
  - Species: *L. loboi*
- Genus: *Madurella*
  - Species: *M. grisea*
  - *M. mycetomatis*
- Genus: *Microsporum*
  - Species: *M. audouinii*
  - *M. canis*
  - *M. cookei*
  - *M. distortum*
  - *M. equinum*
  - *M. ferrugineum*
  - *M. fulvum*
  - *M. gallinae*
  - *M. gypseum*
  - *M. nanum*
  - *M. persicolor*
  - *M. praecox*
  - *M. racemosum*
  - *M. vanbreuseghemii*
- Genus: *Mycocentrospora*
  - Species: *M. acerina*
- Genus: *Paracoccidioides*
  - Species: *P. brasiliensis*
- Genus: *Penicillium*
  - Species: *P. marneffei*
- Genus: *Phialophora*
  - Species: *P. mutabilis*
  - *P. parasitica*
  - *P. richardsiae*
  - *P. spicifera*
  - *P. verrucosa*
- Genus: *Prototheca**
  - Species: *P. wickerhamii*
  - *P. zopfii*
- Genus: *Rhinocladiella*
  - Species: *R. cerophilum*
- Genus: *Rhinosporidium*
  - Species: *R. seeberi*
- Genus: *Scedosporium*
  - Species: *S. apiospermum*
- Genus: *Scopulariopsis*
  - Species: *S. brevicaulis*
- Genus: *Sporothrix*
  - Species: *S. schenckii*
- Genus: *Trichophyton*
  - Species: *T. concentricum*
  - *T. equinum*
    - *T.e.* var. *equinum*
    - *T.e.* var. *autotrophicum*
  - *T. gourvilii*
  - *T. megninii*
  - *T. mentagrophytes* complex
    - *T. m.* var. *erinacei*
    - *T. m.* var. *interdigitale*
    - *T. m.* var. *mentagrophytes*
    - *T. m.* var. *nodulare*
    - *T. m.* var. *quinckeanum*
  - *T. rubrum*
  - *T. schoenleinii*
  - *T. simii*
  - *T. soudanense*
  - *T. tonsurans*
  - *T. yaoundei*
  - *T. violaceum*
- Genus: *Wangiella*
  - Species: *W. dermatitidis*

*Taxonomic status uncertain. Alga or fungus.

Table 9 Genera and pathogenic species of the form class Ceolomycetes of the Deuteromycota

- Order: Sphaeropsidales
  - Family
    - Genus: *Hendersonula*
      - Species: *H. toruloidea*
    - Genus: *Phoma*
      - Species: *P. hibernica*
    - Genus: *Pyrenochaeta*
      - Species: *P. romeroi*
      - *P. unguis-hominis*

References

1 Kuttin, E. S., Beemer, A. M., Levij, J., Ajello, L. and Kaplan, W. (1978). Occurrence of Blastomyces dermatitidis in Israel. First autochthonous Middle Eastern case. *Am. J. Trop. Med. Hyg.* **27**, 1203–1205.

2 Ajello, L. (1975). Phaeohyphomycosis: Definition and Etiology. In *Mycoses*. Proc. Third Int. Conf. on Mycoses: Scientific Publication No. 304, Pan American Health Organization, Washington, D.C. pp. 126–130.

3 Margulis, L. (1974). The classification and evolution of prokaryotes and eukaryotes. In *Handbook of Genetics*, vol. 1, pp. 1–41. R. C. King, ed. Plenum Pub. Corp., New York.

4 Ajello, L. (1977). Medically important infectious fungi. In *Contributions to Microbiology and Immunology*, vol. 3, pp. 7–19. Lindenmann, J. and Ramseier, H., eds. S. Karger, Basel.

5 Ajello, L. (1977). Taxonomy of the Dermatophytes: A review of their imperfect and perfect states. In *Recent Advances in Medical and Veterinary Mycology*, pp. 289–297. Iwata, K., ed. Univ. Tokyo Press, Tokyo.

6 Buchanan, R. E. and Gibbons, N. E., eds. (1974). *Bergey's Manual of Determinative Bacteriology*, 8th ed. Williams & Wilkins Co., Baltimore.

7 Slack, J. M. and Gerencser, M. A. (1975). *Actinomyces, Filamentous Bacteria, Biology and Pathogenicity*. Burgess Publishing Co., Minneapolis, Minnesota.

8 Weitzman, I. and Crist, M. Y. (1979). Studies with clinical isolates of Cunninghamella. I. Mating behavior. *Mycologia* **71**, 1024–1033.

9 Schipper, M. A. A. (1978). *On the genera Rhizomucor and Parasitella. Studies in Mycology No. 17*, pp. 53–71. Centraalbureau voor Schimmelcultures, Baarn, Netherlands.

10 Hawkesworth, D. L. and Booth, C. (1974). *A revision of the genus Zopfia Rabenh.* Mycological Papers No. 135, Commonwealth Mycological Institute, Kew, Surrey, England.

11 McGinnis, M. and Katz, B. (1979). Ajellomyces and its synonym Emmonsiella. *Mycotaxon* **8**, 157–164.

12 Kwon-Chung, K. J. (1975). Description of a new genus, Filobasidiella, the perfect state of Cryptococcus neoformans. *Mycologia* **67**, 1197–1200.

13 Ainsworth, G. C. and Sussman, A. S., eds. (1965–1973). *The Fungi. An advanced treatise*. 5 vols. Academic Press, New York.

14 Bartnicki-Garcia, S. (1970). Cell wall composition and other biochemical markers in fungal phylogeny. In *Phytochemical phylogeny*, pp. 81–103. J. B. Harborne, ed. Academic Press, New York.

15 Ragan, M. A. and Chapman, D. J. (1978). *A biochemical phylogeny of the protists*. Academic Press, New York.

16 Cockshott, W. P. and Lucas, A. O. (1964). Histoplasmosis duboisii. *Quart. J. Med.* **33**, 223–238.

2 Histopathological diagnosis

In the macroscopic evaluation of tissue specimens, mycotic infections are frequently mistaken for neoplasms or other diseases, and a mycosis often may not even be considered until the histopathologic examination is completed. By this time, only fixed tissues are usually available, and as a rule the pathologist must assume ultimate responsibility not only for the diagnosis but also for the tissues and how they are subsequently processed. At this stage it is too late for cultural examinations to be made, although it is always preferable that they be done in conjunction with histopathologic studies.

The situation is far from hopeless, however, because the histopathologic examination of biopsy and autopsy specimens is an excellent way to diagnose mycotic infections. Because of their size, characteristic morphology, and tinctorial properties, fungi can be studied very satisfactorily in tissue. For some diseases, e.g., lobomycosis and rhinosporidiosis, microscopic examination of histological material either in the form of sections or smears is the only way to establish a diagnosis, because the aetiologic agents of these diseases have not yet been grown in culture.

Histological studies make it possible to detect the presence of fungi and to confirm tissue invasion. (Such confirmation is of great value in diagnosing opportunistic fungal infections.) Histopathologic procedures are also rapid and relatively inexpensive, and often result in an immediate diagnosis or at least an immediate presumptive diagnosis of a mycotic infection. In most instances, the localisation and examination of fungal elements in stained tissue sections enables the laboratory worker to select the appropriate sites to be examined by fluorescent antibody (FA) tests in unstained replicate sections. Histologic examination of fungi also enables the microscopist to select the appropriate battery of FA reagents when they are needed (see Chapter 3).

The accuracy of a histopathologic diagnosis of a mycotic or actinomycotic disease depends upon a number of factors such as the agent involved, the adequacy of staining procedures, the use of proper stains and the expertise of the microscopist. The organisms that cause some mycoses have distinctive morphological characteristics in tissues. If these aetiologic agents are present in adequate numbers and if typical forms are seen, the organism can be identified and the disease diagnosed with a high degree of confidence. These diseases include: histoplasmosis capsulati, histoplasmosis duboisii, paracoccidioidomycosis, blastomycosis, lobomycosis, coccidioidomycosis, cryptococcosis, rhinosporidiosis and adiaspiromycosis.

Other mycotic diseases are caused by any one of several members of a genus. These agents may also have a distinctive morphology but can be identified or presumptively identified only to the genus level. However, the disease itself can be named. In this group are included such diseases as actinomycosis, nocardiosis, protothecosis, chlorellosis, candidiasis, and aspergillosis.

Still other mycoses are caused by any one of a number of fungi belonging to various genera. These fungi are similar if not identical in appearance in tissues, and even though the aetiologic agent cannot be identified, the disease can be named. In this group are such diseases as chromoblastomycosis, phaeohyphomycosis, zygomycosis and dermatophytosis.

Mycetomas constitute special cases. If the granules are studied in appropriately stained sections of infected tissue, it is easy to determine whether the aetiologic agent is an actinomycete or a eumycete, and if it is a eumycete, whether it is hyaline or dematiaceous. The size, shape, colour, and architecture of the granules in actinomycotic and eumycotic mycetomas are correlated with the aetiologic agent. Each species, with some exceptions, forms its own distinctive type of granule. Thus, the microscopic appearance of the granules provides an insight into the identity of the organisms involved. However, definitive identification of the aetiologic agents should be based, whenever possible, on their isolation and study in culture.

Lastly, in some cases, fungal elements can be detected in infected tissues but for various reasons it may be impossible to identify the fungus or even to name the disease. However, the microscopist can conclude that a fungal infection exists. A key for the morphologic identification of fungi in tissue sections is given in Appendix 1.

Using a battery of special staining procedures and immunofluorescence techniques, an experienced pathologist can accurately diagnose most of the common mycotic diseases if the aetiologic agent can be seen in histologic sections. Although certain types of tissue responses may suggest the presence of a mycotic agent, no specific inflammatory reaction is pathognomonic for infection by any particular fungus. The range of inflammatory responses to mycotic agents is as wide as or wider than that of any other group of infectious agents, and more than one type of tissue response may be elicited by a single fungus species. In addition, the type of inflammatory response often depends on which reproductive stage of a fungus is in contact with host tissues, e.g., in coccidioidomycosis (see Chapter 10). Even when a fungus is readily demonstrated, the possibility of coexistent diseases should never be overlooked, particularly in the immunosuppressed host where multiple infections with various fungi, bacteria, viruses, and protozoa may occur. Conversely, pathologists should diligently search for fungi whenever an inflammatory reaction is present without an obvious cause. Serial sections and special fungus stains may often be necessary to detect the fungi present.

Several histological stains can be used to demonstrate and study fungi in tissue sections. Those most commonly used are listed in the Table, together with their abbreviations as used in the figure legends of this atlas. The techniques of tissue processing and staining are described in many excellent texts[1-9] and manuals[10-13] and will not be presented here. Instead, we will briefly discuss our experiences with the stains that are of practical value to the pathologist, including the values and limitations of each (see Table). Immunofluorescence techniques will be covered in Chapter 3.

Haematoxylin and eosin (H&E) is a versatile stain that is useful for the histological diagnosis of fungal diseases. With this stain the tissue response can be visualised and a fungus can be characterised as hyaline or dematiaceous. Some fungi such as the aspergilli and zygomycetes stain well with H&E, but many fungal agents are not stained or stain poorly. Even in those instances, the outline of the unstained fungal cells can often be seen and the presence of a fungus infection can be established. In some cases, however, organisms are difficult to distinguish from tissue components, and fungi in small numbers may be overlooked with this stain.

Special fungus stains such as the Gomori methenamine silver (GMS)[14], the Gridley fungus (GF)[15], and the periodic acid-Schiff (PAS)[12] procedures are invaluable for delineating fungi and studying their morphology. These three stains are the ones we most commonly use in the histological study of mycotic diseases. Their staining reactions are based on the principle that in the presence of chromic or periodic acid, adjacent hydroxyl groups of the complex polysaccharides in fungal cell walls are oxidised to aldehydes. In the GMS procedure, the aldehydes reduce the methenamine silver nitrate complex, resulting in the brown-black staining of fungal cell walls due to the deposition of reduced silver wherever aldehydes are located. The depth of the colour produced depends on the amount of aldehyde present. In the GF and PAS procedures, the aldehydes react with Schiff's reagent, colouring fungi reddish-purple and pinkish-red, respectively. Most fungi stained by these methods are crisp and stand out in sharp contrast to the surrounding tissues that are lightly counterstained. The PAS procedure can be preceded by diastase digestion to remove glycogen. This will eliminate some of the nonspecific staining of normal tissue components and cellular debris and may result in greater contrast between the fungi and the background tissues.

We consider the GMS procedure to be the best of the special fungal stains for screening a tissue section because it provides better contrast and often stains fungal cells that are refractory to the GF and PAS procedures. As with most stains, the GMS staining time must be varied not only according to the control slide but also according to the aetiologic agent under consideration. Slides must periodically be removed from the silver nitrate bath and examined under the light microscope to determine when optimal staining has been achieved. However, the colour should never be so intense as to obscure the morphologic detail of a fungus. Staining time is usually prolonged when old and nonviable fungal elements, such as those of *Histoplasma capsulatum* var. *capsulatum* in fibrocaseous nodules, and filaments of the *Actinomyces* and *Nocardia* species are suspected. Precautions must also be taken to prevent overstaining of tissues with the GMS procedure, since erythrocytes and naked nuclei will stain and can mimic the appearance of yeast cells. This is especially important for *Pneumocystis spp*. (not fungi, but protozoans that may be confused with fungi) if crenated erythrocytes are present in alveolar spaces. Overstained blood vessels may mimic the appearance of the zygomycetes, particularly if the vessel is branched, within the same size range, and empty. Calcific bodies, whose appearance may mimic yeast cells, are dissolved by the chromic acid used in the GMS and GF procedures and are therefore unstained. However, these bodies do take the PAS stain.

Because the special fungus stains mask the natural colour of fungi, they are not useful in determining whether fungal clements are hyaline or dematiaceous, and such determinations are crucial in establishing a diagnosis of phaeohyphomycosis, chromoblastomycosis, and other diseases caused by dematiaceous fungi. Another limitation is that special fungus stains, in general, do not allow adequate study of the tissue response to fungal invasion. To circumvent this, we have used H&E as the counterstain for the GMS procedure with much success for many years. This combination of stains (GMS–H&E) was used for many of the illustrations in this book since it readily colours the fungus while staining the background tissue components and thus allows the fungus to be seen and the tissue response to be studied at the same time. When only a single unstained section from a fungal lesion is available, GMS–H&E is our stain of choice for attempting a diagnosis. Because of increased contrast of background tissues, the GMS–H&E stain is also ideal if black and white photomicrographs are needed.

For retrospective studies of unexplained inflammatory processes, tissue sections stained with H&E or the tissue Gram stains can be decolourised in acid alcohol and then restained with GMS and counterstained with H&E. This is very important because in many histopathology laboratories tissue blocks are discarded after two years, but the stained and mounted tissue sections are retained indefinitely. In our laboratory, we have decolourised tissue sections containing fungal elements that had been filed for as long as 20 years and have successfully restained them with the GMS–H&E procedure.

Mayer's mucicarmine procedure[12] stains the mucopolysaccharide capsular material of *Cryptococcus neoformans* a brilliant red. This staining reaction makes it possible to differentiate this fungus from most other fungi of similar size and appearance, but it is not specific for *C. neoformans* because *Rhinosporidium seeberi* and some cells of *Blastomyces dermatitidis* are also variably stained with Mayer's mucicarmine. However, the latter two fungi are so morphologically distinct that they ordinarily should not be mistaken for *C. neoformans*, and the mucicarmine stain is not required for their identification.

Tissue Gram stains such as the Brown and Brenn[16] and the Brown-Hopps[17] procedures are recommended for demonstrating the gram-positive filaments of the *Actinomyces*, *Nocardia* and *Streptomyces* species which appear bluish-black on a yellow background. The GMS and Giemsa procedures can also be used, but they may not stain the filaments uniformly. The GF, PAS, and H&E stains are not useful for demonstrating these microorganisms that are considered to be higher bacteria. (Actinomycotic granules stain well, but individual filaments do not.) Another use for tissue Gram stains is in the identification of those bacteria other than the actinomycetes which may coexist with a mycotic infection or, in the absence of fungal elements, may be the primary cause of disease.

Acid-fast stains are also of value in the histologic diagnosis of infections caused by the *Nocardia spp. Nocardia asteroides, N. brasiliensis*, and *N. caviae* are often, but not always, acid-fast in tissue sections stained with the modified Kinyoun or Fite-Faraco acid-fast staining procedures[12]. Because the nocardiae are weakly acid-fast, a weak decolourising agent such as 0.5–1.0% aqueous sulfuric acid must be used in these procedures instead of acid alcohol, the usual decolouriser used for acid-fast staining of the mycobacteria. The *Actinomyces spp.* and related species are not acid-fast.

Whenever possible, cultural studies should always complement histopathologic procedures. This becomes very important when tissue forms of a fungus cannot be demonstrated although clinical and histological evidence is suggestive of a mycotic infection, or when fungal elements are seen but cannot be identified. All too often, however, fixed tissue specimens are accessioned in laboratories without supportive cultural studies, and a logical approach must then be followed for obtaining the most accurate diagnosis possible. If a mycosis is suspected when the H&E-stained section is examined, we recommend that serial sections be treated with the following battery of special stains: Gomori methenamine silver, Brown and Brenn, and the modified Fite-Faraco acid-fast[12]. When needed, replicate sections that are deparaffinised and unstained should be submitted for specific mycological fluorescent antibody techniques (see Chapter 3). It is not necessary to retain frozen tissues for fluorescent antibody studies, because the mucopolysaccharide antigenic determinants of fungi are apparently not altered by formalin fixation[18]. In contrast, most protein antigens undergo rapid denaturation unless frozen sections, impression smears, or special fixatives are used.

Histological sections often contain normal and abnormal tissue components which, when coloured by certain stains, resemble fungi, e.g., Russell bodies, karyorrhectic debris, corpora amylaceae, calcific bodies, reticulin and elastic fibres, small blood vessels, and the structures seen in the phenomenon termed myospherulosis. Generally, an experienced pathologist can differentiate these structures or artifacts from fungi by using a battery of special stains. Use of tissue sections having artifacts or defects such as knife marks, chatter, folds, compressions, overthickness, alternating thick and thin areas, fixation artifacts, excess or insufficiency of mountant, incompleteness of dehydration or clearing, air bubbles, and extraneous pigments and structures should be avoided when possible. Artifacts found in the preparation of histologic sections are illustrated by Thompson and Luna[19].

Zugibe[6] has aptly stated, 'the fact that many conclusions have been reached, reported, and perpetuated without adequate controls on the original work is one of the major failures in science.' Histopathology is no exception. When special stains are used, quality control must be

Useful stains for the histopathologic diagnosis of mycotic and actinomycotic infections

Stain		Values	Limitations
Haematoxylin & Eosin (H&E)		Permits study of tissue response. Stains many fungi. Allows determination of innate colour of fungus. Demonstrates Splendore–Hoeppli material.	Some fungi are not stained; others are stained poorly.
Special Fungus Stains	Gomori Methenamine Silver (GMS) Gridley Fungus (GF) Periodic Acid-Schiff (PAS)	All three stains are excellent for delineating fungi. The GMS, in general, is better than the GF or PAS for screening. It stains old and nonviable fungal elements better than the other two, and demonstrates the filaments of *Actinomyces spp.*, *Nocardia spp.*, and other actinomycetes.	Do not allow determination of innate colour of a fungus (the GMS stains fungi black-brown, the GF and PAS stain fungi reddish, which may mask innate colour). Do not allow proper study of tissue responses. GMS may stain fungi intensely and obscure internal details.
Combined Gomori Methenamine Silver and Haematoxylin & Eosin (GMS–H&E)		Permits study of tissue responses and is excellent for delineating fungi and most actinomycetes. Very useful if black and white photomicrographs are to be made. The stain of choice if only one slide is available for histopathologic evaluation.	Does not allow determination of innate colour of fungus.
Mayer's Mucicarmine Alcian Blue		Permit differentiation of *Cryptococcus neoformans* from most other fungi of similar size and form.	Not specific for *Cryptococcus neoformans*; stains *Rhinosporidium seeberi* and some cells of *Blastomyces dermatitidis*.
Gram Stains	Brown & Brenn (B&B) Brown–Hopps (B–H) MacCallum–Goodpasture	Stain *Actinomyces* and *Nocardia spp.* and other actinomycetes well. Useful for detecting bacteria that may be causing a lesion under study or may be aggravating the fungus infection. Demonstrate agents of botryomycosis.	Do not selectively stain many fungi.
Acid-Fast Stains	Modified Kinyoun's Acid-Fast Modified Fite–Faraco Acid-Fast	Useful for detecting *Nocardia asteroides*, *N. brasiliensis*, and *N. caviae*. Valuable for detecting *Mycobacterium tuberculosis* and other mycobacteria that may be causing lesion under study.	*Nocardia asteroides*, *N. brasiliensis* and *N. caviae* in tissues are sometimes not acid-fast. Fungi are not acid-fast.

achieved by using appropriate positive tissue substrates[20]. For some procedures, certain components normally present in tissues that are available in any histopathology laboratory can be used as 'built-in' stain controls[21]. The histotechnologist must have sufficient knowledge of basic histology to identify such specific structures and their proper staining reaction. Because some kinds of control materials are difficult to obtain, including those for the special fungus stains, the Center for Disease Control* has made available for distribution the following control tissues that may be used in stain procedures for the identification of certain agents and structures: carminophilic and noncarminophilic fungi, gram-positive and gram-negative bacteria, acid-fast bacteria, spirochetes, iron, and amyloid. The Control Tissue Repository is maintained to assist technologists in determining whether the special stains are working properly. Such controls have been selected for the presence of large numbers of organisms or abnormal structural components. Many are obtained from experimentally induced lesions in animals. They are therefore not intended for teaching or reference. For the latter, we recommend that mycologists and pathologists either collect or obtain as complete a set of slides of the mycoses as possible. Replicate sections stained with H&E and the special fungus procedures should be included in the set.

Infectious materials, including pathogenic fungi, and toxic reagents require special methods of disposal. Personnel in the histopathology laboratory should be knowledgeable in these methods and should develop an emergency plan to be followed when accidents involving infectious agents or dangerous chemicals occur. Excellent references are: 'Inspection Check List, Section VIII', *Anatomic Pathology and Cytology*, published by the Inspection and Accreditation Commission of the College of American Pathologists, and *Lab Safety at the Center for Disease Control*, DHEW Publication No. CDC 76-8118.

In the histopathology laboratory, the instrument most likely to be contaminated by infectious agents is the cryostat. (Because mycotic lesions on gross examination may be mistaken for cancer, frozen sections are often prepared and read by the pathologist near the operating room to confirm or refute a diagnosis of malignancy.) The microtome knife in the cryostat can be decontaminated of fungal pathogens by 10 minutes' immersion in undiluted formalin (40 per cent formaldehyde solution). Then it should be rinsed and thoroughly wiped to prevent corrosion. The cryostat chamber is then decontaminated by disconnecting it from the electrical outlet, placing a beaker containing 250 to 500 ml of undiluted formalin in it, closing the cover tightly, and letting the chamber defrost overnight while being continuously exposed to formalin fumes. The next morning, the beaker of formalin should be removed and the cryostat chamber cleaned, drained, and dried. All movable parts should then be reoiled before the instrument is used again.

*Center for Disease Control, Attn: Control Tissue Repository, Pathology Division, Building 1/2301, Atlanta, GA 30333, USA.

References

1 Davenport, H. A. (1960). *Histological and Histochemical Technics*. W. B. Saunders Co., Philadelphia.
2 Lillie, R. D. (1965). *Histopathologic Technic and Practical Histochemistry*, 3rd ed. McGraw-Hill, New York.
3 Humanson, G. L. (1967). *Animal Tissue Techniques*, 2nd ed. W. H. Freeman and Co., San Francisco.
4 Mallory, F. B. (1968). *Pathological Technique*. Hafner Publishing Co., Inc., New York.
5 Conn, H. J. (1969). *Biological Stains*, 8th ed. Lillie, R. D., ed. Biotech Publications, New York.
6 Zugibe, F. T. (1970). *Diagnostic Histochemistry*. C. V. Mosby, St Louis.
7 Pearse, A. G. E. (1972). *Histochemistry, Theoretical and Applied*, 3rd ed. Churchill Livingstone, London.
8 Smith A. and Bruton, J. (1977). *A Colour Atlas of Histological Staining Techniques*. Wolfe Medical Publications Ltd, London.
9 Kennedy, A. (1977). *Basic Techniques in Diagnostic Histopathology*. Churchill Livingstone, London.
10 Wells, G. G. (1966). *Manual of Histologic Techniques*, 3rd ed. University of Tennessee, Center Health Services, 800 Madison Ave., Memphis.
11 Bowling, M. C. (1967). *Histopathology Laboratory Procedures of the Pathologic Anatomy Branch of the National Cancer Institute*. Government Printing Office, Washington, D.C.
12 Luna, L. G. (1968). *Manual of Histologic Staining Methods of the Armed Forces Institute of Pathology*, 3rd ed. McGraw-Hill, New York.
13 Putt, F. A. (1972). *Manual of Histopathological Staining Methods*. John Wiley and Sons, Inc., New York.
14 Grocott, R. G. (1955). A stain for fungi in tissue sections and smears using Gomori's methenamine-silver nitrate technic. *Am. J. Clin. Pathol.* **25**, 975–979.
15 Gridley, M. F. (1953). A stain for fungi in tissue sections. *Am. J. Clin. Pathol.* **23**, 303–307.
16 Brown, J. H. and Brenn, L. (1931). A method for the differential staining of gram-positive and gram-negative bacteria in tissue sections. *Bull. Johns Hopkins Hospital* **48**, 69–73.
17 Brown, R. C. and Hopps, H. C. (1973). Staining of bacteria in tissue sections: a reliable Gram stain method. *Am. J. Clin. Pathol.* **60**, 234–240.
18 Kaplan, W. and Kraft, D. E. (1969). Demonstration of pathogenic fungi in formalin-fixed tissues by immunofluorescence. *Am. J. Clin. Pathol.* **52**, 420–432.
19 Thompson, S. W. and Luna, L. G. (1978). *An Atlas of Artifacts Encountered in the Preparation of Microscopic Tissue Sections*. Charles C. Thomas, Springfield, Ill.
20 Wright, E. A. (1975). Quality control in histopathology. *Proc. Roy. Soc. Med.* **68**, 619–622.
21 Luna, L. G., ed. (1976). *Histo-Logic*, vol. VI, no. 1, p. 77.

3 Immunofluorescence diagnosis – current status

The usefulness of the fluorescent antibody (FA) technique as a diagnostic and research tool in medical mycology has been firmly established. It can be used for the rapid detection and identification of both viable and nonviable fungi in cultures and in most types of clinical materials, including paraffin sections of formalin-fixed tissue. Immunofluorescence can also be used for detecting and measuring antibodies in sera and in other body fluids.

Basically, the FA technique is an immunochemical staining procedure in which a fluorochrome or fluorescent dye is coupled with antibody so that the antigen-antibody reaction can be observed under the microscope. The fluorochrome-antibody complex, often referred to as labelled antibody or conjugate, fluoresces when examined under a fluorescence microscope.

There are two general types of fluorescence microscopes: (1) the earlier type which involves transmitted fluorescence excitation light and (2) the more recently developed type which involves incident excitation light[1]. The components of the transmitted light instruments are a standard microscope, generally fitted with a darkfield condenser of the cardioid type; a very bright light source that yields a powerful flow of energy, especially in the short wave length region of the light spectrum; and selective filters for the control of the fluorescence excitation and the emission radiation. With the incident type of fluorescence microscope, the exciting radiation is directed at the specimen from above through the microscope's objective. The full aperture of the objective is utilised for excitation. Such incident excitation results in high fluorescence intensities because no light is lost through scattering or through primary absorption in the specimen, which is possible with transmitted light excitation. In addition to providing brighter fluorescence intensities, the incident excitation type of fluorescence microscope has other advantages such as not requiring the use of oil on a darkfield condenser and allowing fluorescence microscopy to be carried out on opaque specimens.

The commonly used fluorochromes are derivatives of fluorescein, a dye that fluoresces with a yellow-green colour. Fluorochromes of other colours such as rhodamine and its derivatives, which fluoresce with a reddish colour, have also been used as labelling compounds.

The simplest FA procedure, termed the direct FA technique, involves the application of solutions of labelled antibody on smears of cultures or clinical materials, or sections of tissue. After an appropriate period of incubation (generally 30–40 minutes at 37°C), the preparation is rinsed, mounted (generally with buffered glycerol saline, pH 7.8) and examined for stained organisms (or antigen).

A commonly used modification of this basic procedure is the indirect FA method. In this system a conjugate directed against globulins of the animal species producing the initial antibody is used to make the antigen-antibody reaction visible. This is a two-stage system. In the first stage, unlabelled antibody serves as antibody; in the second stage it plays the role of antigen. The indirect FA method can be used for detecting and identifying organisms (or antigens) or it can be used for detecting and measuring antibodies.

Another modification of the basic FA technique is the FA inhibition procedure. It involves blocking the reaction between antigen and conjugate by saturating antigenic sites with homologous unlabelled antibody. It can be carried out in either one or two steps. The FA inhibition procedure is mainly used for the detection of antibodies.

We prefer to use the basic direct FA method for detecting fungi in culture and in clinical materials, primarily because this method is simple and easy to perform.

A mycotic infection can be diagnosed with confidence by conventional direct microscopy if the aetiologic agent produces diagnostically distinct forms in tissue and if it is present in its typical form. If such is not the case, the diagnosis is only presumptive. Under such circumstances, use of the FA technique as an adjunctive diagnostic procedure, with its added dimension of serologic specificity, increases the accuracy of direct examinations. The FA technique can also be the initial procedure used to examine specimens for the presence of fungi.

Before being tested by FA, the various types of specimens must be prepared in a manner appropriate to the particular specimen. Smears can be fixed by heat or other fixatives. Paraffin can be removed from tissue sections by treating them twice with xylol, and then with alcoholic solutions of graded concentrations, and finally with buffered saline, pH 7.2. The direct application of FA reagents to deparaffinised tissue sections is usually satisfactory if the sections have been cut thin (4–6 μm or less), if fungal elements are numerous, and if the tissue is not dense. When such desirable conditions do not exist, better results are obtained if deparaffinised sections are digested in a 1.0% trypsin solution (pH 8.0) for 1 hour at 37°C before the FA reagents are applied[2].

At times, sections of tissue need to be decalcified before the FA tests for fungi can be performed properly. They can be decalcified by treating them for 2 hours with a reagent prepared as follows: 1 part formic acid, 1 part 10% buffered formalin, and 40 parts H_2O. The sections so treated are then washed twice in H_2O for a total of 5 minutes, air-dried, digested in a 1.0% trypsin solution if necessary, and tested by FA.

The FA technique is useful in detecting and identifying fungi in histologic sections previously stained with H&E, or by the Giemsa, Brown and Brenn, Brown–Hopps, or Wright methods. For FA staining of fungi in such previously stained sections, coverslips are removed by gently heating the slides to soften the adhesive and immersing them in xylol to remove the coverslips and residual adhesive. The preparations are then rinsed in phosphate-buffered saline (pH 7.2) and, if required, are digested in 1.0% trypsin (pH 8.0) as are unstained, deparaffinised sections. Fungi in sections previously stained by the PAS, Gridley, or Gomori methenamine-silver procedures cannot as a rule be stained by the FA procedure. Apparently, the oxidation of polysaccharides in the walls of the fungi alters the antigenicity of the organisms so they do not react with the labelled antibodies[2].

Prolonged storage of formalin-fixed tissues, either wet or in paraffin blocks, does not seem to affect the antigenicity of fungi. Therefore, in addition to being useful in diagnosing a current infection, the FA procedure can be used to diagnose a mycotic infection in retrospect. The antigenic stability of fungi makes it possible to ship smears, as well as fixed tissues, to distant central laboratories for FA examinations.

Sensitive and specific reagents have been developed for detecting and identifying *Cryptococcus neoformans* (**Figure 1**) and the tissue form of *Blastomyces dermatitidis* (**Figure 2**), *Coccidioides immitis* (**Figures 3, 4**), and *Sporothrix schenckii* (**Figure 5**) by means of the direct FA method[3]. A conjugate at first thought to be useful for the specific staining of the tissue form of *Histoplasma capsulatum* var. *capsulatum* was produced by adsorbing fluorescein-labelled *H. capsulatum* var. *capsulatum* antiglobulins with the yeast-form cells of *B. dermatitidis*. Extensive evaluation disclosed, however, that this adsorbed reagent did not stain a number of *H. capsulatum* var. *capsulatum* isolates, or stained them poorly. Most of these belonged to one of the five recognised serotypes of *H. capsulatum* var. *capsulatum* designated type 1,4. This deficiency severely limits this reagent's value for diagnostic purposes. A partially specific reagent prepared by adsorbing fluorescein-labelled *H. capsulatum* var. *capsulatum* antiglobulins with *Candida albicans* cells is preferable for diagnostic work[4]. This *C. albicans*-adsorbed reagent stains the yeast form of all known serotypes of *H. capsulatum* var. *capsulatum*, and, with the exception of *B. dermatitidis* and *H. capsulatum* var. *duboisii*, apparently does not cross-stain other pathogenic fungi. Despite the presence of cross-reacting antibodies, this *C. albicans*-adsorbed product is very useful for diagnostic purposes. In most cases, the tissue form of *H. capsulatum* var. *capsulatum* can be differentiated from that of *B. dermatitidis* on the basis of morphology. However, when required, these two fungi can be differentiated by FA procedures in which a conjugate specific for the tissue form of *B. dermatitidis* is used. The tissue form of *H. capsulatum* var. *capsulatum* can be differentiated from that of the *duboisii* variety by conventional methods[4]. It is noteworthy that FA reagents for *H. capsulatum* var. *capsulatum* regularly stain this fungus in sections of fixed tissue in which active disease is present. Thus, FA is a valuable aid in the histological diagnosis of active histoplasmosis (**Figure 6**). *H. capsulatum* var. *capsulatum* in healed, calcified lesions or fibrocaseous nodules is not regularly stained by FA, however[5]. This unpredictability limits the value of FA for detecting *H. capsulatum* var. *capsulatum* in such foci. Reagents for demonstrating the tissue form of *Paracoccidioides brasiliensis* have also been developed; however, they need further evaluation.

In contrast to progress in developing specific FA reagents for the tissue forms of the dimorphic fungi, relatively little progress has been made in producing specific reagents for their mycelial forms. Such reagents are not available. A number of investigators have attempted, without success, to produce specific reagents for the *Candida* species of medical importance. Some of the *Candida* species may be identified, however, by using a combination of adsorbed FA reagents[6]. Furthermore, sensitive conjugates can be produced for differentiating members of the genus *Candida* (**Figure 7**) of medical importance from morphologically similar heterologous organisms in clinical materials. Genus-specific conjugates for differentiating in tissue the aspergilli from morphologically similar fungi belonging to other genera have been produced. FA reagents, however, have not been developed for the differential identification of the *Aspergillus* species[3]. Conjugates have also been developed for demonstrating *Petriellidium*

Fungi and actinomycetes that are currently identified by the fluorescent antibody technique

Actinomyces israelii	*Cryptococcus neoformans*
A. naeslundii	*Histoplasma capsulatum* (tissue forms of both varieties)
A. viscosus	*Petriellidium boydii*
Arachnia propionica	*Prototheca wickerhamii*
Aspergillus sp. (to genus)	*P. zopfii*
Blastomyces dermatitidis (tissue form)	*Sporothrix schenckii* (tissue form)
Candida sp. (to genus)	
Coccidioides immitis (tissue form)	

(*Allescheria*) *boydii* (**Figures 8, 9**) and *Rhizopus sp.* (**Figure 10**) in clinical materials.

Although protothecosis in man usually involves the skin, this disease usually appears in a systemic form in animals. Specific FA reagents have also been developed for detecting and identifying the *Prototheca* species in culture (**Figure 11**) and in formalin-fixed tissues[7].

The FA technique is valuable for detecting and identifying the principal aetiologic agents of actinomycosis in man. FA reagents have been developed for the specific staining of *Actinomyces israelii* (the three recognised serotypes), *A. naeslundii* (the three recognised serotypes), and *A. viscosus* (the two recognised serotypes)[8]. These conjugates can be effectively used for the specific detection of these actinomycetes in culture and in smears of clinical materials[9]. In addition, fluorescein-labelled antiglobulins have been prepared for the specific staining of *Arachnia* (*Actinomyces*) *propionica* in culture and in smears of clinical materials (**Figure 12**)[10]. Considerable difficulties have been encountered in attempts to apply the FA procedure to the detection and identification of these actinomycetes in deparaffinised sections of fixed tissue. Hence, at present, this technique is not recommended for this purpose.

A broad battery of FA reagents has been developed for the detection and identification of fungi in clinical materials, and further studies will undoubtedly enlarge this list of diagnostic products. The organisms that are currently identified by FA are listed in the Table. The FA technique is now in routine use in several medical mycological diagnostic centres, and the overall results have been satisfactory. Still, immunofluorescence has not received the widespread application that it merits. This situation is due in large part to the fact that FA reagents for the identification of fungi are currently not available commercially. Thus, those who wish to use the procedure for the identification of fungi must prepare their own conjugates. Production of these products is not difficult, and publications dealing with preparation of antisera and labelling of antibodies are listed in the reference section at the end of this chapter.

Another deterrent to the more extensive use of FA in medical mycology is the shortage of personnel trained to perform FA examinations. A recently published manual[11] which provides laboratorians with detailed instructions on performing FA tests in medical mycology could be useful in alleviating this problem. Courses on the principles and diagnostic applications of FA in microbiology are presented at the Center for Disease Control in Atlanta, Georgia. Such courses also help to fill the need for trained personnel.

References

1 Jones, G. L., Hebert, G. A. and Cherry, W. B. (1978). *Fluorescent Antibody Techniques and Bacterial Applications.* DHEW Publication (CDC) No. 78-8364. Center for Disease Control, Atlanta.

2 Kaplan, W. and Kraft, D. E. (1969). Demonstration of pathogenic fungi in formalin-fixed tissues by immunofluorescence. *Am. J. Clin. Pathol.* **52**, 420–437.

3 Kaplan, W. (1975). Practical application of fluorescent antibody procedures in medical mycology. In *Mycoses*, pp. 178–185. Scientific Publication No. 304, Pan American Health Organization, Washington, D.C.

4 Kaufman, L. and Blumer, S. (1968). Development and use of a polyvalent conjugate to differentiate Histoplasma capsulatum and Histoplasma duboisii from other pathogens. *J. Bacteriol.* **95**, 1243–1246.

5 Hotchi, M., Schwarz, J. and Kaplan, W. (1972). Limitations of fluorescent antibody staining of Histoplasma capsulatum in tissue sections. *Sabouraudia* **10**, 157–163.

6 Gordon, M. A., Elliott, J. D. and Hawkins, T. W. (1967). Identification of Candida albicans, other Candida species and Torulopsis glabrata by means of immunofluorescence. *Sabouraudia* **5**, 323–328.

7 Sudman, M. S. and Kaplan, W. (1973). Identification of the Prototheca species by immunofluorescence. *Appl. Microbiol* **25**, 981–990.

8 Lambert, F. W., Brown, J. M. and Georg, L. K. (1967). Identification of Actinomyces israelii and Actinomyces naeslundii by fluorescent antibody and agar gel diffusion techniques. *J. Bacteriol.* **94**, 1287–1295.

9 Blank, C. H. and Georg, L. K. (1968). The use of fluorescent antibody methods for the detection and identification of Actinomyces species in clinical material. *J. Lab. Clin. Med.* **71**, 283–293.

10 Gerencser, M. A. and Slack, J. M. (1967). Isolation and characterization of Actinomyces propionicus. *J. Bacteriol.* **94**, 109–115.

11 Palmer, D. F., Kaufman, L., Kaplan, W. and Cavallaro, J. J. (1977). *Serodiagnosis of Mycotic Diseases.* Publication No. 1000, American Lecture Series. Charles C. Thomas, Springfield, Illinois.

4 Actinomycosis

Aetiologic agents:

The principal agents are *Actinomyces bovis, A. israelii, A. naeslundii, A. odontolyticus, A. viscosus, Arachnia propionica* and *Rothia dentocariosa*.

Definition and background information

Actinomycosis is a chronic, suppurative disease of man and lower animals characterised by extensive fibrosis, multiple abscesses, and the formation of sinus tracts that drain the suppurative lesions. The aetiologic agent, which is usually found in the centre of an abscess or in purulent exudate, consists of a few branched filaments 1 μm or less in diameter or a well-developed granule which may be compact or loosely formed. Clubs of irregular length or width frequently are found on the surface of a granule. Clubs may, however, be absent[1].

By tradition, actinomycosis falls within the province of medical mycology. However, its aetiologic agents are bacteria, not fungi. The causative agents belong to a group of microorganisms classified in the Order Actinomycetales and commonly referred to as actinomycetes.

The agents of actinomycosis are anaerobic, microaerophilic, or facultatively anaerobic, depending upon the species. All of the species grow best at 37°C and require enriched media for good growth. Some isolates are aerophilic; all are inhibited by the commonly used antibacterial antibiotics. None will grow on simple mycological media such as Sabouraud dextrose agar. Their colonies are small, raised, discrete, and whitish. Like many other bacteria, these organisms have two basic growth forms that are usually described as rough or smooth. The differences in appearance reflect the degree of filamentation that the isolate develops. The colonies are composed of gram-positive, nonacid-fast, branching filaments that are 1 μm or less in diameter[2].

The identification of the organisms that cause actinomycosis is based upon studies of their morphological, physiological, and biochemical characteristics[2]. Immunofluorescence is also useful for their identification[3, 4].

The principal agent of actinomycosis in man is *Actinomyces israelii*. Other agents of the disease in man are *A. naeslundii*, *A. viscosus*, *Arachnia propionica*, and, rarely, *A. odontolyticus* and *Rothia dentocariosa*. The principal aetiologic agent of the disease in lower animals is *A. bovis*. *A. viscosus* has also been implicated as a cause of actinomycosis in dogs. *A. israelii* has only rarely been found to cause disease in lower animals.

On the basis of the anatomical site of the lesions, most human infections can be classified as cervicofacial, thoracic, or abdominal types[1, 5]. Additional manifestations of the disease that do not fall into these categories are also recognised.

Human infections most commonly involve the cervicofacial area. The disease may develop without any known antecedent injury to the oral mucosa. Frequently, however, it follows a dental extraction. Sometimes it is a sequel to dental caries, periodontal disease, or an accidental injury to the mucosa of the mouth. The infection usually develops in the submucous tissue of the gums; in other cases it may start in the tonsillar crypts. From these initial sites, the infection may spread slowly to adjacent tissues. The onset is insidious and is characterised by swelling of the infected tissues. The swollen tissues may feel firm and elastic, or they may be hard. As the disease progresses, abscesses form and draining sinus tracts appear. In most cases the disease remains localised in the facial or neck regions. However, if untreated, the infection may extend upward to involve the sinuses, the orbit, or the cranial bones. The infection may also extend downward to the thorax and then eventually disseminate to other parts of the body.

Thoracic actinomycosis may follow aspiration of infectious material or develop as a result of the extension of cervicofacial infections. All of the tissues of the thoracic cavity are susceptible to infection. When the lungs are involved, early symptoms include cough, low-grade fever, purulent sputum, night sweats, and weight loss. The infection tends to spread extensively and may involve the pleura, pericardium, and chest wall. The development of abscesses and draining sinus tracts that break through the chest wall is not uncommon.

Abdominal actinomycosis may develop by direct extension of a thoracic infection or may result from penetration of the aetiologic agent through the wall of the stomach or intestines. Spread of the infection within the abdomen may involve the liver, the kidneys, and other retroperitoneal structures, including the vertebral column. The signs and symptoms induced by abdominal infections vary, depending upon the structure involved and the extensiveness of the infection.

Once the infection becomes established in the thoracic or abdominal cavities, it may spread to other organs of the body including the bones, central nervous system, and skin, either by direct extension or via the blood stream and lymphatics.

In addition to occurring in the cervicofacial, thoracic, and abdominal regions, primary actinomycotic infections have been reported in other body sites such as the lacrymal glands, the extremities following human bites[5], and the female pelvic organs in association with intrauterine contraceptive devices[6, 7].

Actinomycosis in lower animals is similar to the disease in man[8]. Most lower animal infections are of the cervicofacial type, and the bovine is the most commonly affected species. Cervicofacial actinomycosis in bovines often appears first as a circumscribed, hard, immovable protuberance of the mandible or maxilla. The infection destroys bone and at the same time stimulates the formation of new bony tissue, resulting in a proliferative osteitis. This syndrome is commonly called 'lumpy jaw'. Along with bone involvement, there is often infection and extensive fibrosis of adjacent soft tissues. Abscess formation is characteristic of the infection, and as the disease progresses, draining sinus tracts develop[9]. The disease usually remains localised, but in rare cases may become systemic. Cervicofacial actinomycosis in the bovine must be differentiated from actinobacillosis, which is caused by a gram-negative bacillus, *Actinobacillus lignieresi*, and which also forms granules in infected tissues (see Botryomycosis, Chapter 17).

Cervicofacial and systemic actinomycosis have been recognised in many different lower animals, including domesticated and wild species.

Actinomycosis in man and lower animals is a sporadic disease of world-wide distribution. Its causative agents have never been isolated from soil, plants, or any natural habitats outside of the body. The agents of actinomycosis occur as commensals in the mouth, around teeth, and in the tonsillar crypts of many apparently normal people. These organisms are opportunists that have the capacity to invade injured oral tissues and other tissues under conditions of reduced resistance. It can be assumed that agents of actinomycosis also occur as commensals in the oral cavity of lower animals. Actinomycosis is an endogenously acquired disease. It is not contagious.

Penicillin is the drug of choice for treating actinomycosis. Prolonged treatment (6 to 18 months) is generally required because relapse is common with short courses. Other antibiotics, including erythromycin, tetracycline, lincomycin, and also sulfonamides can be effectively used to treat patients who are allergic to penicillin. Adjunctive surgery, when indicated, is also important in the treatment of this disease[5].

Histopathology (Figures 13–31)

Because actinomycosis is an endogenous disease, it is not included with the mycetomas (Chapter 17) despite the fact that its aetiologic agents very often develop in the form of granules in tissue.

The most common tissue reaction in active lesions of actinomycosis is suppuration with the formation of abscesses that contain one or more actinomycotic granules (organised aggregates of filaments) and are encapsulated by fibrosing granulation tissue[1, 8–12]. Large granules can be seen with the naked eye when a stained tissue section is held up to the light or when 'sulphur granules' are present in the pus that drains or is expressed from a lesion. Sinus tracts filled with purulent exudate often interconnect abscesses or open to a surface or into a body cavity. Abscesses vary in size, and they may be solitary or multiple. When very large, they are frequently multilocular, and the locules are separated from each other by cords of granulation tissue that extend into the abscess from its periphery. Generally, the abscesses contain abundant neutrophils that intimately envelop a granule and are either intact or necrotic and poorly stained. Multinucleated giant cells or palisading epithelioid cells are sometimes apposed to the external surface of a granule, but eosinophils are rarely seen. The purulent centre of an abscess is enclosed by a zone of macrophages, occasional Langhans' or foreign body giant cells, and an irregular but well-developed outer layer of granulation tissue containing various numbers and types of inflammatory cells. Often, particularly in chronic lesions, lymphocytes and plasma cells, which are either scattered or in large clusters, are seen in the areas of granulation. The macrophages that form the innermost wall of an abscess may be numerous and have a foamy cytoplasm because of their lipid content (lipophages, 'foam cells'). In patients with actinomycosis, fibrosis is common and may be severe, whereas in those with nocardiosis (Chapter 19) it is uncommon and usually mild[1, 5, 11].

The granules of the actinomycetes usually appear as round, oval, or scalloped masses that are solid and characteristically bordered by a radial corona of eosinophilic, club-like Splendore–Hoeppli material[1, 11, 13, 14]. The entire granule is basophilic or amphophilic and is easily detected in H&E-stained sections, but individual filaments within the granule are not visible. In our experience, granules may range from 30 to 3,000 μm or more in maximum diameter. Extremely large granules often appear to be made up of smaller confluent ones. In addition, small satellite granules composed of loose aggregates of actinomycete filaments may occasionally be seen near a large granule. However, only rarely are individual filaments free in neutrophilic exudate not contiguous to a granule.

We have seen only a few actinomycete granules in which a finely serrate or club-like border of eosinophilic Splendore–Hoeppli material was completely absent. More commonly, when distinct clubs are not apparent, Splendore–Hoeppli material is present but not pronounced. In a comprehensive study involving 181 patients with actinomycosis[11], Brown reported that a radial arrangement of eosinophilic, parallel clubs was present on the surface of granules in 85% of the cases. Prominent clubbing is most often seen around densely aggregated granules. When granules are loosely aggregated, Splendore–Hoeppli material is less prominent and may not occur along their entire border. Clubs range from 1.0 to 15.0 μm in width and up to 100 μm in length. Large clubs may have fine serrated borders or secondary projections. Most clubs are brightly eosinophilic when stained by H&E. They are refractile and homogeneous, have round ends, and are either clearly separated from each other or fused. Neutrophils are often seen in intimate contact with the exterior surface of Splendore–Hoeppli material, and some of these cells interdigitate and even appear to be embedded in the material.

Most actinomycete granules contain numerous delicate (≤ 1 μm), branched filaments that are gram-positive, nonacid-fast, and sometimes beaded[11, 15]. Beading is seen less frequently with the *Actinomyces spp.* than with the *Nocardia spp.* This results from alternating gram-positive and gram-negative regions within a filament. Compact aggregates of filaments are either arranged in an orderly parallel fashion at the periphery of a granule or are haphazardly arranged throughout a granule. Peripheral filaments frequently project out into and interdigitate with the clubs of Splendore–Hoeppli material; some filaments even appear to be embedded in this material. If examined closely under oil immersion, advancing filaments can be seen extending into the surrounding zone of neutrophils in most cases.

Actinomycete filaments are coloured deep bluish-purple and are well demonstrated with the tissue Gram stains. They are also well delineated with the GMS and Giemsa stains, but are not stained by H&E, GF, and PAS. The filaments are nonacid-fast with the modified acid-fast procedures used for the nocardiae and with the regular acid-fast methods used for the mycobacteria. In general, the matrix of an actinomycete granule and the peripheral clubs of Splendore–Hoeppli material are gram-negative, PAS and GF variable, and are coloured faintly brown or not at all by GMS. H&E is the best stain for demonstrating the peripheral eosinophilic clubs. The morphologic and tinctorial features of the *Actinomyces spp.* and *Nocardia spp.* are reviewed by Robboy and Vickery[15] and Brown[11].

Occasionally, the actinomycete filaments within a granule may be mixed with gram-positive or gram-negative nonfilamentous bacteria, particularly staphylococci, streptococci, enteric gram-negative rods and *Actinobacillus sp.*[5]. These organisms may also be found outside of a granule and may contribute to the pathogenesis of the disease. Short gram-positive rods may also represent fragments of degenerated actinomycete filaments.

Actinomycosis should be suspected whenever a compact granule within an abscess contains gram-positive, nonacid-fast, branched filaments and is surrounded by eosinophilic clubs. However, a definitive diagnosis cannot be based on these observations alone. Peripheral eosinophilic clubbing is neither specific nor diagnostic for actinomycosis. *Nocardia spp.* may form granules that are morphologically indistinguishable from those seen in actinomycosis. Furthermore, one cannot rely on the acid-fastness of the nocardiae within an organised granule to differentiate these organisms from those of the *Actinomyces* and related genera because *Nocardia spp.* are not invariably acid-fast. For these reasons, cultural studies must be done to accurately diagnose the disease and to identify the aetiologic agent.

In some instances, the characteristic granules of actinomycosis may not be formed in purulent lesions. Instead, small aggregates of filaments may be present. At other times, granules may be present in such small numbers that a needle biopsy will not include any of them[16]. Even when a biopsy includes an abscess, the granule located in its centre may be missed unless serial or step sections are carefully examined. An actinomycete granule is occasionally folded or even displaced from the centre of an abscess by the drag of the microtome knife. When the latter occurs, a narrow zone of neutrophils and cellular debris will often adhere to the periphery of the displaced granule.

The granules of the *Actinomyces spp.* and members of the related genera must also be differentiated from the granules of the eumycotic mycetomas and botryomycosis (Chapter 17) because each of these diseases is managed differently. The granules of the eumycotic mycetomas contain broad hyphae and chlamydospores, while the granules in botryomycosis contain aggregates of either gram-negative or gram-positive nonfilamentous bacteria. The three different types of granules can easily be differentiated from each other if appropriate histologic stains are used.

References

1 Guidry, D. J. (1970). Actinomycosis. In *The Pathologic Anatomy of Mycoses. Human Infection with Fungi, Actinomycetes, and Algae,* pp. 1019–1058. R. D. Baker, ed. Springer-Verlag, Berlin.

2 Georg, L. K. (1970). Diagnostic procedures for the isolation and identification of the etiologic agents of actinomycosis. In *Proceedings – International Symposium on Mycoses*, pp. 71–81. Scientific Publication No. 205, Pan American Health Organization, Washington, D.C.

3 Lambert, F. W., Brown, J. M. and Georg, L. K. (1967). Identification of Actinomyces israelii and Actinomyces naeslundii by fluorescent antibody and agar-gel diffusion techniques. *J. Bacteriol.* **94**, 1287–1295.

4 Holmberg, K. and Forsum, U. (1973). Identification of Actinomyces, Arachnia, Bacterionema, Rothia and Propionibacterium species by defined immunofluorescence. *Appl. Microbiol.* **25**, 834–843.

5 Causey, W. A. (1978). Actinomycosis. In *Handbook of Clinical Neurology*, vol. 35. *Infections of the Nervous System*, part III, pp. 383–394. North Holland Publishing Company, Amsterdam.

6 Henderson, S. R. (1973). Pelvic actinomycosis associated with an intrauterine device. *Obstet. et Gynecol.* **41**, 726–732.

7 Schiffer, M. A., Elguezabal, A., Sultana, M. and Allen, A. C. (1975). Actinomycosis infections associated with intrauterine contraceptive devices. *Obstet. Gynecol.* **45**, 67–72.

8 Aman, E. B. (1954). Actinomycosis (Actinomycosis in Animals). *Southwest Veterinarian* **7**, 356–362.

9 Jungerman, P. F. and Schwartzman, R. M. (1972). *Veterinary Medical Mycology*, pp. 159–170. Lea & Febiger, Philadelphia.

10 Menges, R. W., Larsh, H. W. and Habermann, R. T. (1953). Canine actinomycosis. *J. Am. Vet. Med. Assoc.* **122**, 73–78.

11 Brown, J. R. (1973). Human actinomycosis: A study of 181 subjects. *Human Pathol.* **4**, 319–330.

12 Weed, L. A. and Baggenstoss, A. H. (1949). Actinomycosis. A pathologic and bacteriologic study of twenty-one fatal cases. *Am. J. Clin. Pathol.* **19**, 201–216.

13 Hotchi, M. and Schwarz, J. (1972). Characterization of actinomycotic granules by architecture and staining methods. *Arch. Pathol.* **93**, 392–400.

14 Moore, M. (1946). Radiate formation on pathogenic fungi in human tissue. *Arch. Pathol.* **22**, 113–153.

15 Robboy, S. J. and Vickery, A. L. (1970). Tinctorial and morphologic properties distinguishing actinomycosis and nocardiosis. *N. Engl. J. Med.* **282**, 593–596.

16 Moncure, A. C. and Proppe, K. H. (1978). Case records of the Massachusetts General Hospital. Enlarging pulmonary lesion with pleural involvement in an elderly man. *N. Engl. J. Med.* **299**, 85–92.

5 Adiaspiromycosis

(Haplomycosis, adiaspirosis)

Aetiologic agents:

1 *Chrysosporium parvum* var. *parvum*
Synonyms: *Haplosporangium parvum*
Emmonsia parva
2 *C. parvum* var. *crescens*
Synonym: *Emmonsia crescens*

Definition and background information

Adiaspiromycosis is primarily a disease of lower animals and rarely of humans. The portal of entry of the infectious spores of the aetiologic agent is the respiratory tract. The disease remains confined to the lungs since the infectious spores do not multiply in host tissue, a phenomenon unique among the pathogenic fungi. The inhaled conidia produced by *C. parvum* in nature simply enlarge in lung tissue, achieving diameters of 40 μm in infections caused by the parvum variety and 400 μm in those caused by the crescens variety.

Spores that grow in size without replicating are known as adiaspores. Thus the name of the disease was derived from the nature of the spores that develop in pulmonary tissue.

Numerous animal infections caused by *C. parvum* have been diagnosed in Africa, Asia, Europe, New Zealand, North America, and South America among an extremely wide range of mammals[1-3] and a bird[4].

Relatively few human infections have been reported. The first such case was diagnosed in France[5]. Subsequent cases have been recorded in Czechoslovakia[6], France[7, 8], Guatemala[9], Honduras[10], Union of Soviet Socialist Republics[11] and Venezuela[12].

Adiaspiromycosis is not a contagious disease. All victims are infected by the spores produced in soil by a single species of *Chrysosporium – C. parvum*. *C. parvum* exists in two forms or variations: *C. parvum* var. *parvum* and *C. parvum* var. *crescens*. This fungus has been isolated from natural sites in the United States[13] and the Union of Soviet Socialist Republics[14]. Two other species implicated as disease agents, *Emmonsia brasiliensis* and *E. cifferina*, were found to be identifiable with the saprophytic mould *C. pruinosum*. This species produces adiaspores at high temperatures in vitro[20, 24].

In humans, adiaspiromycosis is generally a self-limited, benign infection with few, if any, symptoms. Such infections have been discovered incidentally in the course of histopathological study of pulmonary tissues for other causes[7, 12, 15]. The diagnosis in such cases rested upon the discovery of adiaspores in various stages of development and degeneration. The size of the adiaspores seen was dependent not only on the variety of *C. parvum* that caused the infection, but also upon the plane in which the spores had been cut by the microtome and the developmental stage of the adiaspore. In one well-documented case the adiaspores, at their equatorial plane, averaged 245 μm in diameter. The thickness of the cell walls averaged 24 μm[9]. So far, all human infections have been attributed to *C. parvum* var. *crescens*. The only described symptomatic case was diagnosed in Czechoslovakia[16, 17]. The clinical manifestations in the 11-year-old male patient were dyspnea, fatigue, cough, night sweats, stabbing chest pains, and mild fever. Radiographic examination revealed an image suggestive of miliary tuberculosis. The diagnosis of adiaspiromycosis was established only when biopsy tissue from the left lower lobe was examined histologically and the striking adiaspores of *C. parvum* var. *crescens* were found to be numerous and widely disseminated in the lung tissue. The adiaspores were as large as 250 μm in diameter with a cell wall 20–70 μm thick. The aetiologic agent was not isolated.

Diagnosis of adiaspiromycosis in wild animals has been based either on the histological examination of lung tissue or on isolation of *C. parvum* var. *crescens* and var. *parvum* from tissue[1]. The two varieties are distinguished from each other on the basis of the relative sizes of their adiaspores and by the fact that these spores remain uninucleate in the *parvum* variety, but become multinucleate in the *crescens* variety when the adiaspore begins its phenomenal increase in volume by a factor estimated to be 10^6 [18].

Although Emmons and Jellison[19] stressed nuclear number as one of the criteria for considering the *crescens* variety to merit species rank, Carmichael[20] did not accept this concept. We have chosen to follow Carmichael in this matter, since in culture at 25° or 30°C, the two varieties are indistinguishable from each other.

The concept suggested by Jellison[21] that Korean haemorrhagic fever was caused by *C. parvum* was disproved in 1978 by the isolation of the viral aetiologic agent from patients with that disease[22, 23].

C. parvum grows well on most media. However, the isolates vary considerably in gross appearance. Young colonies are generally glabrous and colourless. In older colonies, white aerial mycelium develops in tufts or covers the colony. Surface growth ranges from downy to floccose or even granular. A glabrous periphery may persist, or the colony may remain glabrous. Surface colorations range from white to cream or even shades of brown. The growth rate at 25°C is fairly rapid. The reverse of the colonies ranges from white to yellow to brown among isolates.

The hyaline, septate mycelium produces conidia at the tips of hyphal filaments, but typical conidia are produced on short peg-like conidiophores. Some conidiophores develop secondary spores on short branches. The conidia are unicellular and are subglobose to pyriform, with a smooth or delicately spiny surface. They are borne singly or in chains of two. They measure 2×4 to $2.5 \times 4.5\ \mu m$.

The two varieties of *C. parvum* cannot be distinguished unless they are grown at temperatures higher than 25°C on enriched media. At 37°C on brain heart infusion blood agar, the conidia of *C. parvum* var. *crescens* enlarge to become adiaspores that attain diameters of 25–400 μm with cell walls that may be up to 70 μm thick. At 37°C, *C. parvum* var. *parvum* does not produce adiaspores. However, at 40°C on rich media, this variety does produce adiaspores, but they only attain diameters of 10–25 μm with cell walls that are 2 μm thick.

Reports of budding and endosporulation by the adiaspores of *C. parvum* are believed to be erroneous[18].

Histopathology (Figures 32–51)

The histopathologic changes seen in adiaspiromycosis are similar in both humans and lower animals[1, 3, 9, 18, 25]. To our knowledge, the lung is the only organ involved in natural infections. In each case of pulmonary adiaspiromycosis, the histologic features of the discrete lesions (adiaspiromas) are monotonously similar from field to field in a lung section. Apparently, a granuloma is formed around each adiaspore after large numbers of conidia are inhaled and lodge in the lung. The adiaspores do not multiply or disseminate. Adiaspiromycosis is therefore not a progressive disease. The lung contains solitary or multiple nonnecrotic granulomas (adiaspiromas), each of which contains a single adiaspore. Grossly, the granulomas appear as single or multiple, greyish-white nodules on the exterior or cut surfaces of the lung, 0.5–2.0 mm in diameter. Although lesions are typically discrete, a single coalescent granuloma may contain two or more adiaspores in a single plane of section. Granulomas may be located in a peribronchiolar position where they encroach on the tunica muscularis or compress the smaller bronchioles.

The inflammatory reaction elicited by both varieties of *Chrysosporium* is confined to a narrow zone immediately surrounding each adiaspore. Lesions resemble typical foreign body or tuberculoid granulomas except that necrosis or caseation is almost never seen. Large adiaspores are intimately surrounded by foreign body and Langhans' giant cells. Huge giant cells are usually in direct contact with the external spore wall, and several of these cells may be seen attempting to ingest an intact or degenerating spore. Giant cells may also be seen within a fragmented adiaspore, having migrated inside from the periphery. Portions of the fragmented spore wall can often be seen within huge giant cells. A layer of epithelioid cells usually encloses the giant cells, and these in turn are surrounded by thick, concentric layers of fibrous connective tissue containing variable numbers of lymphocytes, plasma cells, macrophages, and fibroblasts. Polymorphonuclear leucocytes, especially eosinophils, may also be seen in some lesions, particularly those containing smaller immature adiaspores. Occasionally, there may be little or no host response to the adiaspores of either variety of *Chrysosporium* regardless of the immunocompetence of the host or the age of the lesions. Old 'burned-out' granulomas appear as masses of dense collagenous connective tissue with little or no caseation. Because necrosis is not common, calcification is rarely observed.

In adiaspiromycosis, the intervening pulmonary tissues are usually unaltered except for the compressive effects of adjacent adiaspores[9]. Typically, alveolar septa are stretched and compressed around the periphery of the granulomas. Alveolar septa are not thickened and do not usually contain inflammatory cells. However, in a few cases, adjacent alveolar spaces may contain edematous fluid and macrophages. The visceral pleura may be thickened by dense, sparcely cellular, fibrous tissue, especially when adiaspores rest just beneath the pleura.

Large thick-walled adiaspores, especially of the *crescens* variety, often appear as empty rings that can be easily seen with the naked eye when a tissue section is held up to the light. The spores are symmetrical and are round to oval. Because of their large size, they are sectioned in many different planes and show a corresponding variation in size and mural structure. Because of this variation, measurements should be obtained only from those spores that are sectioned in or near the equatorial plane. Small spores with extremely thick walls apparently represent lateral sections of large mature spores rather than smaller developing or degenerating ones. When sectioned tangentially, adiaspores usually appear solid in H&E-stained sections. They are much smaller than adjacent spores that are sectioned near their equatorial plane. Degenerating and apparently dead adiaspores are often granular, attenuated, fragmented, folded, or separated into distinct layers. Entire spores may be displaced because of the drag on the microtome knife during sectioning.

In experimentally infected mice, Emmons reported that adiaspores of *C. parvum* var. *parvum* reached a diameter of 40 μm[18]. Their walls were 2–4 μm thick. In samples that we have examined from animals with spontaneous infections, adiaspores of the *parvum* variety ranged from 23.4–46.0 μm in diameter. Mature adiaspores of *C. parvum* var. *crescens* can reach a diameter of 200–400 μm. This represents a volume increase by a factor of 10^6 approximately[18]. Their walls range from 10–80 μm in width. It is reported that the mature spore of the *crescens* variety may contain hundreds of nuclei, whereas adiaspores of the *parvum* variety remain uninucleate regardless of their age or size[18]. In sections from subjects with spontaneous adiaspiromycosis, we have observed what apparently represents a single large amphophilic nucleus in the *parvum* variety and many small basophilic or amphophilic nuclei in the *crescens* variety. Usually, however, most adiaspores of the latter appear empty in sections from naturally infected lungs. When internal contents are seen, their appearance is variable. Occasionally, spherical, refractile, eosinophilic or unstained granules of uniform size fill the adiaspore or line the internal portion of its wall and cluster in its centre[9]. The nature of these granules is unknown.

Distinct zones can be seen in the adiaspore wall of *C. parvum* var. *crescens* depending on which histological stain is used[9]. When stained with H&E, the wall of the mature adiaspore appears to be composed of two zones: a thick, deeply eosinophilic outer zone containing a fenestrated, non-staining circumferential layer, and a thick inner zone that is homogeneous and faintly eosinophilic or unstained. Although only two zones are seen in the walls of the H&E-stained spores, the GF and GMS stains reveal three zones. With the GF procedure, an outer zone measuring 1–2 μm in width stains intensely. A middle zone 7–9 μm wide is unstained, but contains a circumferential fenestrated layer that stains positively. This layer has previously been interpreted as a 'honeycomb-like structure'[16] or a 'network-like structure'[26] in the middle layer. The inner zone is very wide, measuring 13–18 μm. It is moderately stained in its outer portion and deeply stained in its inner portion. When stained by GMS, the entire adiaspore wall is silver-positive but there are zonal differences in staining intensity which correspond to the three layers demonstrated with the GF stain. The trilaminar mural substructure seen when the *crescens* variety of *Chrysosporium* is stained by the GF and GMS procedures is similar to the three layers described in the wall of this variety by Zdarska and Slais[26].

When lateral or tangential sections of the spore wall are seen, the fenestrated layer lining the inner aspect of the middle zone, as described above, appears as a broad fibrillar layer containing cribriform perforations. These perforations are best demonstrated with the GMS and GF stains[9].

Budding or endosporulation has never been observed in any of the adiaspores that we have examined. Occasionally, dense and deeply eosinophilic material intimately surrounds a portion of or an entire adiaspore. These focal eosinophilic aggregates or protrusions, which may be irregular or stellate, probably represent Splendore–Hoeppli material[27]. In two reports, focal aggregates of similar material were interpreted as buds[28, 29].

Adiaspores have a distinctive appearance, and there is no reason to confuse them with the spores of other fungi.

References

1 Jellison, W. L. (1969). *Adiaspiromycosis*. Mountain Press, Missoula, Montana.

2 Dvorak, J., Otcenasek, M. and Propopic, J. (1965). The distribution of adiaspiromycosis. *J. Hyg. Epidemiol. Microbiol. Immunol.* **9**, 510–514.

3 Smith, J. M. B. and Lancaster, M. C. (1965). Adiaspiromycosis in the brush opossum, Trichosurus vulpecula, in New Zealand. *Sabouraudia* **4**, 146–147.

4 Sharapov, V. M. (1975). Is possible adiaspiromycosis of birds. *Reports Siberian Div. Acad. Sci. U.S.S.R. Biol. Sci. Series* **1**, 68–71.

5 Doby-Dubois, M., Chevrel, M. L., Doby, J. M. and Louvet, M. (1964). Premier cas humain d'adiaspiromycose par Emmonsia crescens Emmons et Jellison, 1960. *Bull. Soc. Pathol. Exot.* **57**, 240–244.

6 Kodousek, R., Sery, Z. and Votjek, V., eds. (1972). Proc. Second Symposium on Adiaspiromycosis. *Acta Univer. Palackianae Olomucensis* **63**, 1–111.

7 Vermeil, C., Gordeeff, A. and Geffrioud, M. (1975). Pulmonary and human adiaspiromycosis in Brittany: a new observation. *Mycopathologia* **56**, 109–111.

8 Quilici, M., Lebreuil, G., Dumon, H., Perrimond, G. and Orsini, A. (1976). A propos d'un nouveau cas humain d'adiaspiromycose. *Bull. Soc. Fr. Mycol. Med.* **5**, 195–199.

9 Watts, J. C., Callaway, C. S., Chandler, F. W. and Kaplan, W. (1975). Human pulmonary adiaspiromycosis. *Arch. Pathol.* **99**, 11–15.

10 Adan Cueva, J. and Little, M. D. (1971). Emmonsia crescens infection (adiaspiromycosis) in man in Honduras. *Am. J. Trop. Med. Hyg.* **20**, 282–287.

11 Leshchenko, V. M. and Sheklavok, N. D. (1974). Adiaspiromycosis. *Vest. Derm. Syphil.* **6**, 46–51.

12 Salfelder, K. and Viloria, H. J. E. (1975). Tercer caso de adiaspiromycosis en Merida. *Rev. Col. Med. (Merida)* **34**, 21–22.

13 Orr, G. F. and Kuehn, H. H. (1972). Notes on Gymnoascaceae. II. Some Gymnoascaceae and keratinophilic fungi from Utah. *Mycologia* **64**, 55–72.

14 Sharapov, V. M. (1972). On the natural focality of adiaspiromycosis. (In Russian.) *News Siberian Division Acad. Sci. U.S.S.R. Series of Biol. Sci. No. 2*, 45–50.

15 Slais, J., Dvorak, J. and Otcenasek, M. (1970). The morphology of solitary adiaspores of Emmonsia crescens from the lung of man. *Folia Parasitol.* **17**, 177–182.

16 Kodousek, R., Vortel, V., Fingerland, A., Vojtek, V., Sery, Z., Hajek, V. and Kucera, K. (1971). Pulmonary adiaspiromycosis in man caused by Emmonsia crescens: Report of a unique case. *Am. J. Clin. Pathol.* **56**, 394–399.

17 Vojtek, V., Sery, Z. and Berkova, I. (1970). Klinika a terapie adiaspiromykozy. *Studia Pneumol. Phtiseolog. Cechoslovaca* **30**, 295–309.

18 Emmons, C. W., Binford, C. H., Utz, J. P. and Kwon-Chung, K. J. (1977). *Medical Mycology*, 3rd ed. Lea & Febiger, Philadelphia.

19 Emmons, C. W. and Jellison, W. J. (1960). Emmonsia crescens sp. n. and adiaspiromycosis (haplomycosis) in mammals. *Ann. N.Y. Acad. Sci.* **89**, 91–101.

20 Carmichael, J. W. (1962). Chrysosporium and some other aleuriosporic hyphomycetes. *Can. J. Bot.* **40**, 1137–1173.

21 Jellison, W. L. (1971). *Korean Hemorrhagic Fever and Related Diseases. A Critical Review and Hypothesis.* Mountain Press Publishing Co., Missoula, Montana.

22 Lee, H. W., Lee, P. W. and Johnson, K. M. (1978). Isolation of the etiologic agent of Korean hemorrhagic fever. *J. Infect. Dis.* **137**, 298–308.

23 Traub, R. and Wisseman, C. L., Jr. (1978). Korean hemorrhagic fever. *J. Infect. Dis.* **138**, 267–272.

24 Padhye, A. A. and Carmichael, J. W. (1968). Emmonsia brasiliensis and Emmonsia ciferrina are Chrysosporium pruinosum. *Mycologia* **60**, 445–447.

25 Schwarz, J. (1978). Adiaspiromycosis. *Pathology Annual*, vol. 16, pp. 41–53. S. C. Sommers and P. P. Rosen, eds. Appleton-Century-Crofts, New York.

26 Zdarska, Z. and Slais, J. (1972). Morphology and histochemistry of the differentiated adiaspore of Emmonsia crescens. In *Proc. Second Symposium on Adiaspiromycosis*, vol. 63, pp. 73–79. Olomouc, Czechoslovakia, Palacky University.

27 Liber, A. F. and Ho-Soon Hahn Choi (1973). Splendore–Hoeppli phenomenon about silk sutures. *Arch. Pathol.* **95**, 217–220.

28 Fingerland, A. and Vortel, V. (1972). The accidental finding of adiaspiromycosis caused by Emmonsia crescens in a case of lung tuberculosis. In *Proc. Second Symposium on Adiaspiromycosis*, vol. 63, pp. 19–22. Olomouc, Czechoslovakia, Palacky University.

29 Fingerland, A. (1972). Some histological similarities and differences between adiaspiromycosis, rhinosporidiosis and other related mycoses. In *Proc. Second Symposium on Adiaspiromycosis*, vol. 63, pp. 59–66. Olomouc, Czechoslovakia, Palacky University.

6 Aspergillosis

Aetiologic agents:

Aspergillus fumigatus group, *A. flavus* group, *A. niger* group, *A. terreus* group, and others

Definition and background information

Aspergillosis refers to a variety of diseases of man and lower animals caused by several species of *Aspergillus*. The diseases vary in severity and clinical course, depending upon the organs affected, the host, and the form of the disorder. Most cases of aspergillosis are caused by members of the *A. fumigatus* group. However, several other species belonging to other *Aspergillus* groups, particularly, *A. flavus*, *A. niger*, and *A. terreus*, can also cause aspergillosis[1, 2].

Aspergilli are abundant in the environment. They live in soil as saprophytes, deriving nutrients from dead plant and animal matter. Their spores are produced in great abundance and are readily disseminated into the air by wind currents. In most instances infections are contracted via the respiratory route. All of the species have a cosmopolitan distribution, and aspergillosis occurs throughout the world. Aspergillosis is not communicable from one host to another.

The genus *Aspergillus* is characterised by the formation of a distinctive conidiophore. This conidiophore consists of a stalk that arises from a specialised cell of the mycelium called a foot cell. The stalk is enlarged at its uppermost point to form a globose, hemispherical, flask-shaped or clavate structure called the vesicle. From fertile areas of the vesicle arise peg-like, conidium-producing cells termed sterigmata. The sterigmata may be formed in a single layer (uniseriate), or they may be arranged in two layers (biseriate) with the second row arising from the first. The sterigmata form unbranched chains of conidia from their distal ends.

More than 130 species of *Aspergillus* are recognised. The species have been put in groups of one or more species having a series of common characteristics. Two keys to the separation of the groups are provided in the excellent monograph 'The Genus Aspergillus'[1]. One key is based primarily on morphologic criteria; the other is based primarily upon the colour of the conidial heads. Group keys for separating individual species are also provided in this monograph.

The most common forms of aspergillosis in man are pulmonic. Several clinical forms of pulmonary aspergillosis are recognised, and they may be classified as follows:

1 Primary invasive
2 Secondary invasive
3 Secondary noninvasive
4 Primary allergic bronchopulmonary.

1 *Primary invasive form*. An individual with apparently normal defense mechanisms may be infected with this form of aspergillosis, most commonly by a member of the *A. fumigatus* group. As a rule, the infection results from repeated and prolonged exposure to overwhelming numbers of fungus cells. The normal body defenses are apparently unable to cope with the massive challenge. Usually the disease occurs as a fulminating pneumonic process with a progressive downhill course and is fatal. Characteristically, there is dissemination of the infection from the lungs to other parts of the body. A chronic form of primary invasive aspergillosis that resembles tuberculosis has also been described. Primary invasive pulmonary aspergillosis is a rare disorder, because exposure *per se* is much less important in the development of aspergillosis than is abnormal susceptibility.

2 *Secondary invasive form*. This type occurs in individuals whose resistance is lowered as a result of a severe debilitating disease such as leukaemia or lymphoma and in individuals receiving immunosuppressive drugs, broad spectrum antibiotics, corticosteroids, or a combination of these medicaments[3, 4]. It has been recognised with increasing frequency in recent years. Members of the *A. fumigatus* group are most frequently involved in secondary invasive aspergillosis. Members of the *A. flavus* group rank next in importance. Clinically, patients with this form of aspergillosis are chronically ill and debilitated and usually develop nonproductive cough, dyspnea, and fever. Dissemination of the infection to other parts of the body may also occur. The most common sites for the disseminated lesions are the brain, kidney, gastrointestinal tract, and myocardium.

3 *Secondary noninvasive form*. In this form the fungus colonises a pre-existing cavity in the lungs such as an ectatic bronchus, a tuberculous cavity,

or a lung cyst[5, 6]. The fungus grows to form a compact mass of mycelium called a 'fungus ball', or 'aspergilloma'. These ball-like masses may lie free in the cavity, but more often are attached to the cavity wall by a fibrinous exudate. The lesion is usually single, but may be multiple. Sometimes the fungus colony does not develop as a mobile fungus ball. It may appear as a solid mass in an area of lung that has been previously damaged by some other disease process. In most instances the fungus does not invade surrounding tissue and spread to other parts of the body. Members of the *A. niger* and *A. fumigatus* groups are most often involved in this form of aspergillosis. Clinically, secondary noninvasive aspergillosis may be asymptomatic. Symptoms are often noted, however, and they include haemoptysis of varying degree of severity and chronic productive cough. The haemoptysis may on occasion be sufficiently severe to warrant surgical resection. If surgery is not indicated, other treatment may not be necessary.

4 *Primary allergic bronchopulmonary aspergillosis*. This allergic disease is being recognised with increasing frequency[7, 8]. It occurs in previously sensitised persons who are exposed to the spores of an *Aspergillus* sp. Members of the *A. fumigatus* group are the usual aetiologic agents. In allergic bronchopulmonary aspergillosis, recurrent febrile episodes are associated with severe cough, wheezing, and production of purulent sputum containing eosinophils and bronchial plugs harbouring mycelial elements of the fungus. This syndrome is associated with pulmonary consolidation and peripheral blood eosinophilia.

In addition to the various pulmonic forms of aspergillosis, clinical syndromes involving other organs are also recognised. Otomycosis is one such disorder. Members of the *A. niger* group are the principal aspergilli involved in this type of ear infection[9]. The fungus grows on cerumen, epithelial scales, and debris in the external ear canal. The resulting mass of mycelium and debris causes irritation, pruritus, and impairment of hearing. Some superficial erosion of membranes may occur, but usually the tympanic membrane is not seriously damaged. This disorder is benign, but often chronic and recurrent.

Aspergillosis of the paranasal sinuses is another interesting entity[10, 11]. This condition can occur in two forms:

1 a noninvasive form that can clinically mimic nonspecific chronic sinusitis, and
2 an invasive form in which the sinuses and adjacent tissue are involved. This form can simulate neoplastic disease.

Paranasal aspergillosis occurs without known predisposing systemic disease and is caused by members of the *A. fumigatus* and *A. flavus* groups.

Traumatic corneal ulcers may become infected with aspergilli, especially if they are treated with corticosteroids. Invasion of nail tissue by aspergilli has also been reported.

Aspergillosis has been recorded in a wide variety of domesticated and wild animals. Birds, in particular, are susceptible to infection by aspergilli[12]. Almost any organ of the avian body may be affected; therefore the signs of the disease in birds are extremely varied. The signs may be respiratory, digestive, or nervous. Avian aspergillosis may be acute or chronic. Acute aspergillosis usually occurs in young birds and is often fatal. Clinical signs include loss of condition, anorexia, rapid breathing, diarrhea, elevated body temperature, and listlessness. Chronic aspergillosis is the form usually seen in adult birds. Affected birds usually manifest, to a lesser degree, the signs of the acute form of aspergillosis. The onset is insidious, and affected birds may survive for relatively long periods of time in a gradually declining state.

Aspergillosis occurs in many mammalian species. The lungs are the primary site of infection with dissemination, not infrequently, to other parts of the body. The clinical signs of infection are essentially similar to those described for pneumonia due to other causes. The *Aspergillus* species may also infect the paranasal sinuses of dogs, and the placentas of cattle, sheep and horses, causing abortion. They may also infect the intestinal tract of cats, horses, and other animals.

Serologic tests are of great value for the diagnosis of the various forms of aspergillosis. The most widely used procedure for these disorders is the immunodiffusion test. Demonstration of one or more precipitins in a patient's serum may denote infection, colonisation of preexisting cavities, or allergy to *Aspergillus* antigens. The test is also useful in diagnosing invasive aspergillosis when the patient is not receiving extensive immunosuppressive therapy. Sera from patients with invasive aspergillosis, who are receiving immunosuppressants, are often negative. The indirect fluorescent antibody procedure is also considered by some workers to be very useful for the diagnosis of aspergillosis.

The treatment and management of aspergillosis depends upon the form of the disease. Amphotericin B has been reported to be of some value in treating invasive aspergillosis[13], if the diagnosis is made early enough. Secondary noninvasive aspergillosis may not require treatment unless haemoptysis is severe; then surgery is indicated[14]. Primary allergic bronchopulmonary aspergillosis responds to corticosteroid therapy[15]. Otomycosis is treated by removing the fungal growth and keeping the ear canal dry.

Histopathology (Figures 52–101)

In primary and secondary invasive aspergillosis the tissue response is generally that of a mixed purulent and necrotising inflammatory reaction[1, 12, 15, 16]. Necrosis may be extensive and is probably attributable to both vascular obstruction and toxin production by the invading organism. In the early stages of infection the fungus develops small or large aggregates of mycelium formed by radiating hyphae or sheets of compact hyphae usually growing in one direction. The peripheral hyphae are usually surrounded by polymorphonuclear leucocytes. Alternation of rapid and slow growth phases of the fungus may give a striped appearance to the mycelial aggregates because of differences in the density of the fungal elements and in affinity for the stain. This is often referred to as zonation of hyphal growth.

Chronic lesions of invasive pulmonary aspergillosis are usually focal and granulomatous and contain scattered giant cells, neutrophils, and eosinophils. Fibrosis is progressive and may be severe. Isolated lesions, which become walled off by a granulomatous reaction, contain Langhans' giant cells similar to those seen in tuberculosis. The centre of a granuloma may become necrotic and caseous or may liquefy, forming a cavity. When a cavity becomes contiguous with a bronchiole, some of the necrotic material along with fungal elements may be coughed up in the sputum. If the cavity is well aerated, conidiophores (fruiting bodies or conidial heads) may develop. These structures may be formed within any cavity or on any surface exposed to air such as the pleura, nasal mucosa, and the air-sacs of birds. In some cases of invasive aspergillosis, epithelioid and giant cells completely destroy the mycelium, and the lesion heals. However, in other cases, the mycelium proliferates further and forms a radiating ('sun burst') pattern known as the actinomycetoid form of the fungus. This form is usually embedded in necrotic tissue and is restricted to actively disseminating stages of the disease.

Rapid dissemination to other organs is common because of the propensity of the mycelium to invade blood vessels[17]. The primary lesion in invasive aspergillosis is almost always pulmonary, and the spread is haematogenous. Hyphae growing in the same direction appear to penetrate walls of blood vessels directly, even those of the large muscular arteries. Thrombosis may lead to haemorrhage, infarction, and death. Thrombosis of the carotid artery has been reported[18]. Granulomatous lesions and abscesses may occur in many organs, especially the brain, meninges, and endocardium[16, 17, 19, 20, 21].

Secondary noninvasive pulmonary aspergillosis is characterised by the presence of a so-called 'fungus ball' or 'aspergilloma'[15, 22]. This structure consists of a tangled mycelial mass usually located within a preformed pulmonary cavity, e.g., tuberculous or bronchiectatic, or necrotic tissue cavity. Clinically, the 'aspergilloma' may be mistaken for a neoplasm. When a pulmonary cavity becomes infected with an *Aspergillus sp.*, the 'fungus ball' progressively enlarges because of growth of mycelium at the periphery of a nidus of necrotic tissue, mucus, etc. Rarely does the fungus ball develop *de novo*. The mycelium usually does not invade surrounding parenchyma. Rather, it is surrounded by a thin fibrotic capsule that contains few inflammatory cells. 'Fungus balls' may become coated with an irregular layer of Splendore–Hoeppli material. At times, zonal growth of mycelial elements within an 'aspergilloma' occurs.

Allergic bronchopulmonary aspergillosis[23–25] is thought to be caused by a combined asthmatic and Arthus-type of reaction in a hypersensitised host. Smaller bronchi are typically dilated and filled with viscid mucus containing cellular debris, eosinophils, and hyphal fragments of an *Aspergillus sp.* that are usually scarce and difficult to identify as those of an *Aspergillus*. The walls of bronchi are infiltrated with a prominent component of eosinophils and fewer lymphocytes and plasma cells. In many patients with advanced cases, necrotising bronchiolitis with bronchiolitis obliterans and granulation tissue formation are seen. Alveolitis and angiitis may also occur. Typically, a necrotic bronchus is effaced by an intense acute purulent infiltrate containing many intact and degranulating eosinophils ('eosinophil abscess'). The abscess is surrounded by one or more layers of palisading epithelioid cells and occasional giant cells, some of which contain brightly eosinophilic Charcot–Leyden crystals and granular material from necrotic, degranulating eosinophils. Fungal elements are almost never seen in H&E-stained sections but are usually delineated with the special fungus stains, especially GMS. When typical forms of aspergilli cannot be found, specific fluorescent antibody techniques are invaluable for identifying the fungal elements.

An interesting form of chronic aspergillosis is that of the paranasal sinuses[1, 10, 11, 26]. Here, the infection can be invasive or noninvasive. In the latter type, 'fungus balls' usually occupy a portion of the sinus cavity. They are only partially embedded in the mucosa and are associated with a minimal inflammatory response. In the invasive form, short, fragmented, and distorted hyphae with bulbous dilatations are usually seen with the special fungus stains. A similar picture is rarely observed in lesions of the orbit and central nervous system[1, 16, 27]. In H&E-stained sections, hyphae are not usually seen because generally they do not stain. Even when revealed with special fungus stains, hyphal fragments may be scarce, and when seen, usually lack branches or septations. Conidiophores or conidia are not generally produced. The inflammatory response in aspergillosis of the paranasal sinuses involves the submucosa. It is granulomatous with large bizarre giant cells of both types containing hyphal fragments. Almost all of the hyphal fragments are intracellular, usually within the giant cells which may be elongated and irregular in shape, apparently in an attempt to accommodate the fungus. Splendore–Hoeppli material sometimes coats both intracellular and extracellular hyphal fragments. Neutrophils and eosinophils may be scattered among the giant cells, and stromal fibrosis with formation of dense collagenous connective tissue is common.

In acute invasive lesions, the septate hyphae of the aspergilli usually have dichotomous branches at acute (45°) angles and are of relatively uniform width (3–6 μm). In chronic lesions, short, globose and distorted hyphae up to 12 μm wide may also be seen. Most hyphae stain with H&E if the tissue is properly fixed, is not necrotic, and is not understained with haematoxylin. They appear basophilic to amphophilic, but when embedded in necrotic tissue, hyphae are pale and eosinophilic. Fungal elements of the *Aspergillus sp.* are best revealed with the special fungus stains, especially the GMS. When typical mycelial forms are present, a presumptive diagnosis of aspergillosis can be made. However, the species involved cannot be determined. If conidial heads are seen, their morphology and pigmentation (clearly seen only in H&E-stained or unstained sections) may be characteristic for a certain group of *Aspergillus sp.*, e.g., *A. niger*, and an identification may be made. Nevertheless, cultural studies are almost always required for a definitive identification of the fungus as to species.

Extensive local deposition of calcium oxalate crystals in association with the *Aspergillus* species occasionally occurs in humans[28, 29] and in animals[30]. These crystals are birefringent and are easily seen under polarised light. They presumably are formed from oxalic acid produced by the fungus. Calcium oxalate crystals are seen only in areas in which either hyphae or fruiting bodies, or both, are associated with necrotic tissue. The presence of such crystals, however, is not differentially associated with *Aspergillus* species.

On occasion, the *Aspergillus* species may be confused with other fungi that form hyphae in tissues, particularly the zygomycetes and the species of *Candida*. Individual hyphae in disseminated infections due to *Petriellidium boydii* may also be mistaken for those of an *Aspergillus*. The hyphae of the zygomycetes are broader (up to 15μm) and infrequently septate, have nonparallel walls, and often appear collapsed and acutely twisted. The branching of the *Aspergillus sp.* hyphae is more acute than that of the zygomycetes, is typically dichotomous, and frequently is oriented in the same direction. Generally, the zygomycetes do not take the special fungus stains as uniformly or as intensely as do members of the *Aspergillus* groups. The *Candida* species usually can be separated from the *Aspergillus* species since, in addition to hyphae, they form pseudohyphae and budding yeast cells. The disseminated hyphae of *P. boydii* are narrower and usually branch at less acute angles.

The spores from the conidial heads of the *Aspergillus* species, that on occasion develop in tissue, become detached and lie free in tissues or tissue cavities. If only spores are seen in GMS-stained sections, they can be mistaken for small yeast cells and, when in alveolar or other pulmonary spaces, for cyst forms of *Pneumocystis carinii*[31, 32]. The *Aspergillus* spores may appear indented, crescent-shaped, and unevenly stained. However, most intact yeast cells are smoothly contoured, stain uniformly with GMS, and may be budding. When only the transected hyphae of an *Aspergillus sp.* are present, they may be mistaken for empty yeast form cells of several fungi or even for the rounded spores of certain *Aspergillus* species. Replicate sections should be examined for longitudinally sectioned hyphae. Sporulation by the *Aspergillus* species rarely occurs in solid intact tissues.

References

1 Raper, K. B. and Fennell, D. I. (1965). *The Genus Aspergillus*. Williams and Wilkins Company, Baltimore.

2 Young, R. C., Jennings, A. and Bennett, J. E. (1972). Species identification of invasive aspergillosis in man. *Am. J. Clin. Pathol.* **58**, 554–557.

3 Meyer, R. D., Young, L. S., Armstrong, D. and Yu, B. (1973). Aspergillosis complicating neoplastic disease. *Am. J. Med.* **54**, 6–15.

4 Young, R. C., Bennett, J. E., Vogel, C. L., Carbone, P. P. and DeVista, V. T. (1970). Aspergillosis: The spectrum of the disease in 98 patients. *Medicine* **49**, 147–173.

5 Aslam, P. A., Eastridge, C. E. and Hughes, F. A. (1971). Aspergillosis of the lung – an eighteen-year experience. *Chest* **59**, 28–32.

6 Orie, N. G. M., de Vries, G. A. and Kikstra, A. (1960). Growth of Aspergillus in the human lung. Aspergilloma and aspergillosis. *Am. Rev. Resp. Dis.* **82**, 649–662.

7 Hoehne, J. H., Reed, C. E. and Dickie, H. A. (1973). Allergic bronchopulmonary aspergillosis is not rare. With a note on preparation of antigen for immunologic tests. *Chest* **63**, 177–181.

8 Jordan, C., Bierman, C. W. and Van Arsdel, P. O. (1971). Allergic bronchopulmonary aspergillosis. *Arch. Intern. Med.* **128**, 576–581.

9 Emmons, C. W., Binford, C. H., Utz, J. P. and Kwon-Chung, K. J. (1977). *Medical Mycology,* 3rd ed. Lea & Febiger, Philadelphia.
10 Hora, J. F. (1965). Primary aspergillosis of the paranasal sinuses and associated areas. *Laryngoscope* **75**, 768–773.
11 Guntz, A. A. and Page, L. R. (1977). Aspergillosis of the maxillary sinus. Review of the literature and report of a case. *Oral. Surg.* **43**, 350–356.
12 Ainsworth, G. C. and Austwick, P. K. C. (1973). *Fungal Disease of Animals.* Commonwealth Agricultural Bureaux, Farnham Royal, Slough, England.
13 Burton, J. R., Zachery, J. B., Bessin, R., Rathbun, H. K., Greenough, W. B., Stenoff, S., Wright, J. R., Slaven, R. E. and Williams, G. M. (1972). Aspergillosis in four renal transplant recipients. Diagnosis and effective treatment with amphotericin B. *Ann. Intern. Med.* **77**, 383–388.
14 Craddock, D. R. and Donald, D. J. (1972). Pulmonary mycetoma and its surgical management. *Med. J. Austral.* **2**, 1477–1480.
15 Symmers, W. S. (1974). Histopathology of aspergillosis of the respiratory system. In *Aspergillosis and Farmer's Lung in Man and Animal*, pp. 75–87. Bern, Huber.
16 Schwarz, J. (1973). Aspergillosis. *Pathol. Annu.* S. C. Sommers, ed. **8**, 81–107. Appleton-Century-Crofts, New York.
17 Khoo, T. K., Sugai, K. and Leong, T. K. (1966). Disseminated aspergillosis: case report and review of the world literature. *Am. J. Clin. Pathol.* **45**, 697–703.
18 MacCormick, W. F., Schochet, S. S., Jr., Weaver, P. R. and McCrary, J. A., III. (1975). Disseminated aspergillosis. Aspergillus endophthalmitis, optic nerve infarction, and carotid artery thrombosis. *Arch. Pathol.* **99**, 353–359.
19 Kammer, R. B. and Utz, J. P. (1974). Aspergillus species endocarditis. The new face of a not so rare disease. *Am. J. Med.* **56**, 506–521.
20 Kirschstein, R. L. and Sidransky, H. (1956). Mycotic endocarditis of the tricuspid valve due to Aspergillus flavus: report of a case. *Arch. Pathol.* (Chicago) **62**, 103–106.
21 Tveten, L. (1965). Cerebral mycosis: a clinicopathologic report of four cases. *Acta Neurol. Scand.* **41**, 19–33.
22 Ikemoto, H. (1964). Pulmonary aspergilloma or intracavitary fungus ball: report of 5 cases. *Sabouraudia* **3**, 167–174.
23 Spencer, H. (1977). *Pathology of the Lung,* 3rd ed. pp. 708–712. W. B. Saunders, Philadelphia.
24 Warnock, M. L., Fennessy, J. and Rippon, J. (1974). Chronic eosinophilic pneumonia, a manifestation of allergic aspergillosis. *Am. J. Clin. Pathol.* **62**, 73–81.
25 Riley, D. J., MacKenzie, J. W., Uhlman, W. E. and Edelman, N. H. (1975). Allergic bronchopulmonary aspergillosis: evidence of limited tissue invasion. *Am. Rev. Resp. Dis.* **111**, 232–236.
26 Pena, C. E. (1975). Aspergillus intranasal fungus ball. Report of a case. *Am. J. Clin. Pathol.* **64**, 343–344.
27 Green, W. R., Font, R. L. and Zimmerman, L. E. (1969). Aspergillosis of the orbit. *Arch. Ophthalmol.* **82**, 302.
28 Kurrein, F., Greer, G. H. and Rowles, S. L. (1975). Localised deposition of calcium oxalate around a pulmonary *Aspergillus niger* fungus ball. *Am. J. Clin. Pathol.* **64**, 556–563.
29 Nime, F. A. and Hutchins, G. M. (1973). Oxalosis caused by Aspergillus infection. *Johns Hopkins Med. J.* **133**, 183–194.
30 Kaplan, W., Arnstein, P., Ajello, L., Chandler, F. W. and Watts, J. (1975). Fatal aspergillosis in imported parrots. *Mycopathologia* **56**, 25–29.
31 Reinhardt, D., Kaplan, W. and Chandler, F. W. (1977). Morphologic resemblance of zygomycete spores to Pneumocystis carinii cysts in tissue. *Am. Rev. Resp. Dis.* **115**, 170–172.
32 Chandler, F. W., Frenkel, J. K. and Campbell, W. G., Jr. (1979). Animal model of human disease. Pneumocystis carinii pneumonia in the immunosuppressed rat. *Am. J. Pathol.* **95**, 571–574.

7 Blastomycosis

(North American blastomycosis, Gilchrist's disease)

Aetiologic agent:

Blastomyces dermatitidis (Perfect state: *Ajellomyces dermatitidis*)

Definition and background information

Blastomycosis is a chronic granulomatous and suppurative disease of humans and lower animals caused by the fungus, *Blastomyces dermatitidis*. Although this disease was long thought to be restricted to the North American continent, in recent years autochthonous cases have been diagnosed in a number of African countries[1] and Israel.

B. dermatitidis is a dimorphic fungus. It grows as a yeast in mammalian tissues and also in vitro at 37°C. Typical yeast-form cells are spherical, 8–15 μm in diameter, and have thick walls. They reproduce by a budding process in which the buds are attached to their mother cells by a broad base. Generally, only one bud is produced. The occasional occurrence in tissues of small forms of *B. dermatitidis* (2–4 μm in diameter) has been reported[2,3], but they have always been present as part of a continuous series of sizes ranging from the unusually small to the normal. When grown at room temperature, *B. dermatitidis* develops in a mycelial form with colonies that are white to tan and downy to fluffy. The mycelium bears smooth, round to oval conidia, 3–5 μm in diameter on the sides of hyphae and on the ends of simple conidiophores.

All available clinical and epidemiological evidence indicates that humans and lower animals contract blastomycosis from some source in nature. However, the natural habitat of *B. dermatitidis* has not as yet been discovered, despite recent reports of its recovery from soils in Kentucky and Georgia[4,5]. Lungs and skin were both once thought to be the common portals of entry for *B. dermatitidis*. The current consensus is that most blastomycosis infections result from inhalation of the spores of the fungus growing as a saprophyte in nature and that the primary lesion occurs in the lungs[3,6,7].

Clinically apparent human blastomycosis can be either systemic or cutaneous. The systemic form is primarily a pulmonary disease. The infection may be confined to the lungs or may spread to other organs and tissues of the body. Pulmonary blastomycosis generally begins as a mild respiratory infection that progresses gradually, causing fever, loss of weight, malaise, and productive cough. Dissemination to bones, joints, prostate gland, and the testes is not uncommon. Signs and symptoms vary, depending upon the extent of involvement and the degree of interference with normal function. When the fungus spreads to the skin, it produces ulcerated or verrucous, granulomatous lesions. Untreated systemic blastomycosis is a serious and often fatal disease. By contrast, the general health of the patient with lesions confined to the skin and without apparent visceral involvement is not impaired. Skin lesions generally occur on exposed body surfaces and may start as a subcutaneous nodule, or first appear as a papule or pustule that ulcerates. Lesions slowly become larger and more severe, and characteristically develop into ulcerated, verrucous granulomata with serpiginous borders. The course of the disease is chronic and is marked by remissions and exacerbations with gradually enlarging lesions[3,6]. The recognised cases in lower animals have generally been systemic in form, characterised by extensive pulmonary involvement and dissemination to the skin, bones, and other organs[8].

Serological tests are very useful in the diagnosis of blastomycosis. They are rapid and provide presumptive evidence of infection. Serological determinations also have prognostic value and can be used to monitor patients' responses to therapy. The most widely used tests are the complement fixation and immunodiffusion tests[9]. The exoantigen test is of great value for the rapid identification of mycelial-form cultures of *B. dermatitidis*[10].

Amphotericin B is the drug of choice for treating blastomycosis in humans and animals[8,11], but 2-hydroxystilbamidine has also been successfully used to treat humans[12,13].

Histopathology (Figures 102–135)

In both localised and systemic blastomycosis, the fungus characteristically incites a mixed granulomatous and purulent inflammatory reaction – either may predominate, depending on the site and age of the lesion[14–18]. In newly formed lesions, the reaction is usually purulent, with infiltration of neutrophils and abscess formation. Older ones appear as focal and confluent epithelioid cell granulomas, some of which have central abscessation or caseation, or both. Unless the yeast-form cells of *B. dermatitidis* are demonstrated, it is often difficult to distinguish these lesions from those of chronic active tuberculosis or, at times, from those of histoplasmosis[19, 20].

In subjects with primary pulmonary blastomycosis there is usually disseminated involvement of both lungs. Pyemia may occur and lead to systemic disease. The tissue reaction ranges from acute purulent to chronic granulomatous pneumonia, in which the regional lymph nodes may be involved[3, 17]. Focal and diffuse fibrosis is common in long-standing infections. *B. dermatitidis* cells are either extracellular and intimately surrounded by neutrophils in central abscesses or are within epithelioid and multinucleated giant cells at the periphery of abscesses. Occasionally, giant cells that contain fungus cells are present in the central abscess. Pleuritis is reported to be common when the pneumonia is severe, and lesions may penetrate the chest wall to form subcutaneous abscesses that drain externally. In very old lung lesions, focal scarring may follow the healing of primary lesions. However, fibrocaseous nodules, commonly seen with histoplasmosis, and pulmonary cavitation are rarely sequelae of blastomycosis.

In patients with systemic blastomycosis, the organs most commonly involved are the lungs, skin, bone, prostate, epididymis, seminal vesicles, urinary bladder, brain, and spinal cord[21–24]. Subcutaneous abscesses or sinuses that drain through the skin may occur, especially in patients with granulomatous osteomyelitis. Usually, the fungus cells are far more numerous in the systemic lesions than in the cutaneous ones. Miliary lesions are histologically identical to those previously described in the lung.

Although cutaneous blastomycosis usually develops hematogenously from a primary lung infection, occasional cases result from the direct inoculation of the fungus into the skin. Such infections usually do not become systemic. Microabscesses in the dermis and subcutis are commonly found in early skin lesions. They may contain moderate numbers of fungus cells. In older lesions, abscessation progresses to granuloma formation with mild fibrosis. Frequently, because few organisms are present, many serial sections must be examined with special fungus stains before a single yeast cell is found and identified. Typical budding forms may never be found. Pseudoepitheliomatous hyperplasia of the epidermis can be particularly striking as a secondary manifestation of the underlying chronic inflammatory reaction incited by *B. dermatitidis*. Clinically, and on gross pathological examination, hyperplastic lesions of the skin are often thought to be neoplastic. However, microscopic examination of tissue sections stained with H&E and special fungus stains can be used to rule out neoplasia and help establish a correct diagnosis of blastomycosis. Downward growth of well-differentiated epidermis may extend to and surround dermal abscesses or their draining sinuses, thus creating intraepithelial abscesses. Such abscesses in skin sections with chronic granulomatous dermatitis are highly suggestive of blastomycosis. However, a definitive diagnosis can only be made by demonstrating typical fungal cells in tissue sections stained with H&E and special fungus stains, or with specific fluorescent antibody conjugates. Regional lymph nodes which drain skin lesions usually show focal or diffuse granulomatous lymphadenitis. Yeast forms of the fungus may be present within epithelioid and giant cells.

With care and experience, the microscopist can usually detect *B. dermatitidis* cells in H&E-stained tissue sections. The fungal cells appear as round or oval yeasts with thick, sharply defined, refractile cell walls. The yeast cells generally range from 6–15 μm in diameter, but we have seen yeast forms as small as 2–4 μm and as large as 20–30 μm. With H&E, the protoplasm readily stains basophilic or amphophilic and is usually separated from the rigid, unstained cell wall by a clear space. In other instances however, the protoplasm is contiguous to the cell wall. Several nuclei may be visible in the protoplasm[25, 26], but in our experience, nuclei are very difficult to detect even with optimal fixation and H&E staining. Typically, these cells reproduce by single budding. The bud is attached to the parent cell by a very wide base, which is distinctive for this fungus. Budding cells of *B. dermatitidis* are less often seen than those, for example, of *Cryptococcus neoformans*. In lesions containing few organisms, budding forms are infrequently found. *B. dermatitidis* usually exists only as a yeast in tissues. Rarely are germ tubes and hyphae formed[27].

Special fungus stains are much more effective than H&E for demonstrating intact and degenerating *B. dermatitidis* cells, and are a must when only a few tissue-form cells are present. With the GMS, PAS, and GF procedures, both the cell wall and the contents of the yeast cell are readily stained. Some cells may have a small amount of weakly carminophilic capsular-like material, but never as much as do typical *C. neoformans* cells.

When typical budding forms with a broad base are found in tissue sections, *B. dermatitidis* can be identified with confidence. If such forms are not seen, this fungus may be confused with others. For example, lightly encapsulated, nonbudding cells of *C. neoformans* may be mistaken for *B. dermatitidis*. In such instances, Mayer's mucicarmine stain should be used to demonstrate the mucopolysaccharide capsule of the former. Budding forms of *C. neoformans* can be differentiated from those of *B. dermatitidis* because the former are attached to the parent cells by a narrow base. Single cells of *B. dermatitidis* which are empty or have poorly stained inner contents may be mistaken for immature or empty spherules of *Coccidioides immitis*. In such a case, serial sections must be carefully examined to demonstrate intact or broken spherules that contain endospores. *Paracoccidioides brasiliensis* tissue-form cells with only one bud may be mistaken for *B. dermatitidis*. Here again, sections must be carefully examined to find the characteristic multiple budding or 'spoke wheel' forms of the former. *P. brasiliensis* buds are also attached to parent cells by a narrow base. Tissue form cells of *Histoplasma capsulatum* var. *duboisii* (aetiologic agent of histoplasmosis duboisii) are comparable in size to those of *B. dermatitidis*, but the two can be differentiated because the former bud with a narrow base and have a typical 'hour-glass' shape. They are also uninucleate and often have a vacuolated cytoplasm. The small intracellular forms of *B. dermatitidis* may be confused with *H. capsulatum* var. *capsulatum*[2]. In the former, several nuclei may be seen in H&E-stained sections, the budding is by a much broader base, and other cells usually are present that vary in size ranging up to that of typical *B. dermatitidis* cells. When attempts to identify *B. dermatitidis* with all available histochemical procedures and morphological criteria fail, specific immunofluorescence is a useful diagnostic tool.

References

1 Ajello, L. (1967). Comparative ecology of respiratory mycotic disease agents. *Bacteriol Rev.* **31**, 6–14.

2 Tuttle, J. G., Lichtwardt, H. E. and Altshuler, C. H. (1953). Systemic North American blastomycosis. Report of a case with small forms of blastomycetes. *Am. J. Clin. Pathol.* **23**, 890–897.

3 Schwarz, J. and Baum, G. L. (1951). Blastomycosis. *Am. J. Clin. Pathol.* **21**, 999–1029.

4 Denton, J. F., McDonough, E. S., Ajello, L. and Ausherman, R. J. (1961). Isolation of Blastomyces dermatitidis from soil. *Science* **133**, 1126–1127.

5 Denton, J. F. and DiSalvo, A. F. (1964). Isolation of Blastomyces dermatitidis from natural sites at Augusta, Georgia. *Am. J. Trop. Med. Hyg.* **13**, 848–861.

6 Baum, G. L. and Schwarz, J. (1959). North American blastomycosis. *Am. J. Med. Sci.* **238**, 661–683.

7 Wilson, J. W., Cawley, E. P., Weidman, F. D. and Gilmer, W. S. (1955). Primary cutaneous North American blastomycosis. *Arch. Dermatol.* **71**, 39–45.

8 Jungerman, P. F. and Schwartzman, R. M. (1972). *Veterinary Medical Mycology*, pp. 124–138. Lea & Febiger, Philadelphia.

9 Kaufman, L. (1970). Serodiagnosis of fungal diseases. In *Manual of Clinical Microbiology*, pp. 386–394. Blair, J. E., Lennette, E. H. and Truant, J. P., eds. American Society for Microbiology, Bethesda, Maryland.

10 Kaufman, L. and Standard, P. (1978). Immunoidentification of cultures of fungi pathogenic to man. *Curr. Microbiol.* **1**, 135–140.

11 Turner, D. J. and Koenig, M. G. (1970). The treatment of blastomycosis with amphotericin B. *Ped. Clin. North Am.* **17**, 437–447.

12 Lockwood, W. R., Busey, J. F., Batson, B. E. and Allison, F. (1962). Experiences in the treatment of North American blastomycosis with 2-hydroxystilbamidine. *Ann. Intern. Med.* **57**, 553–562.

13 Lockwood, W. R., Allison, F., Blair, B. E. and Busey, J. F. (1969). The treatment of North American blastomycosis. Ten years' experience. *Am. Rev. Resp. Dis.* **100**, 314–320.

14 Busey, J. F., ed. (1964). Blastomycosis: 1. A review of 198 collected cases in the Veterans' Administration Hospitals. *Am. Rev. Resp. Dis.* **89**, 659–672.

15 Duttera, M. J., Jr. and Osterhout, S. (1969). North American blastomycosis. A survey of 63 cases. *South. Med. J.* **62**, 295–301.

16 Kunkel, W. M., Jr., Weed, L. A., McDonald, J. R. and Clagett, O. T. (1954). Collective review: North American blastomycosis-Gilchrist's disease. Clinicopathologic study of 90 cases. *Int. Abstr. Surg.* **99**, 1–26.

17 Vanek, J., Schwarz, J. and Haken, S. (1970). North American blastomycosis. *Am. J. Clin. Pathol.* **54**, 385–400.

18 Witorach, P. and Utz, J. P. (1968). North American blastomycosis. A study of 40 patients. *Medicine* **47**, 169–200.

19 Allison, F., Jr., Lancaster, M. G., Whitehead, A. E. and Woodbridge, H. B., Jr. (1962). Simultaneous infection in man by Histoplasma capsulatum and Blastomyces dermatitidis. *Am. J. Med.* **32**, 476–489.

20 Brandsberg, J. W., Tosh, F. E. and Furcolow, M. L. (1964). Concurrent infection with Histoplasma capsulatum and Blastomyces dermatitidis. *N. Engl. J. Med.* **270**, 874–877.

21 Schwenzfeier, C. W. (1976). Pathologic quiz case 2. North American blastomycosis. *Arch. Otolaryngol.* **102**, 710–712.

22 Friedman, L. L. and Signorelli, J. J. (1946). Blastomycosis: Brief review of literature and a report of a case involving the meninges. *Ann. Intern. Med.* **24**, 385–400.

23 Rippon, J. W., Zvetina, J. R. and Reyes, C. (1977). Case report: Miliary blastomycosis with cerebral involvement. *Mycopathologia* **60**, 121–125.

24 Wilson, R. W., van Dreumel, A. A. and Henry, J. N. R. (1973). Urogenital and ocular lesions in canine blastomycosis. *Vet. Pathol.* **10**, 1–11.

25 Bakerspigel, A. (1957). The structure and mode of division of the nuclei of Blastomyces dermatitidis. *Can. J. Microbiol.* **3**, 923–936.

26 Emmons, C. W. (1959). Fungus nuclei in the diagnosis of mycoses. *Mycologia* **51**, 227–236.

27 Collins, D. N. and Edwards, M. R. (1970). Filamentous forms of Blastomyces dermatitidis in mouse lung. *Sabouraudia* **7**, 237–240.

8 Candidiasis*

(Moniliasis, candidosis, thrush)

Aetiologic agents:

Candida albicans (*Monilia albicans*)
C. glabrata (*Torulopsis glabrata*)
C. guilliermondii (*M. guilliermondii*)
C. krusei (*M. krusei*)
C. parapsilosis (*M. parapsilosis, C. parakrusei*)
C. pseudotropicalis (*M. pseudotropicalis*)
C. stellatoidea†
C. tropicalis (*M. tropicalis*)

Perfect states:

C. guilliermondii = *Pichia guilliermondii*
C. krusei = *P. kudriauzevii*
C. parapsilosis = *Loderomyces parapsilosis*
C. pseudotropicalis = *Kluyveromyces fragilis*

Definition and background information

Candidiasis is undoubtedly one of the most widespread and prevalent of the mycotic diseases of man. This is especially true of the infections caused by the endogenous species, *C. albicans*. This yeast is one of the components of the body's natural flora. Most, if not all, humans acquire this fungus at birth during passage through the birth canal[4]. Ordinarily *C. albicans* lives in balance with the other microorganisms in the body and merely exists there as a colonist. But various factors can upset this balance and lead to the development of active, progressive symptomatic disease.

The other species of *Candida* involved in candidiasis are opportunistic, basically saprophytic yeasts that are found in nature on many substrates[5]. They reach the body from these exogenous sources and develop and cause disease under conditions which make it possible for them to overwhelm the host's natural defense mechanisms.

The clinical forms of candidiasis can be divided into three broad categories: mucocutaneous, cutaneous, and systemic.

A. Mucocutaneous Candidiasis
In this form of candidiasis the oral and vaginal mucosa are the most commonly involved tissues. In oral candidiasis or thrush, whitish, creamy plaques composed of yeast cells and mycelium develop on the tongue, gums, and buccal mucosa. Thrush commonly develops in infants within a few weeks after birth.

Diagnosis is based on noting the presence of round or oval, hyaline budding yeast cells 3–4 μm D and hyaline septate mycelium or pseudomycelium 3–5 μm D in the mucoid plaques scraped from the infected sites. Definitive identification of the aetiologic agent rests upon its isolation and identification on the basis of morphology and biochemical reactions[5]. *C. albicans* is the usual causative agent in this form of candidiasis.

Thrush does develop in adults, but this generally occurs in individuals with hormonal or immunological problems. However, the administration of antibiotics, immunosuppressive drugs, and other medications, such as steroids, can lead to the development of secondary candidiasis in the form of chelitis, perleche, and anal pruritus in patients of all ages.

Vaginitis, again almost exclusively due to *C. albicans,* frequently develops during pregnancy when vaginal pH is low. Diabetes and drug therapy for primary bacterial and other diseases may also induce the development of vaginal candidiasis. Conjugal infections do occur and may lead to candidal balanitis.

B. Cutaneous Candidiasis
Chronic mucocutaneous candidiasis is one of the most dramatic and devastating forms of the disease. The victims of this disease are individuals with a variety of underlying genetic defects, i.e., endocrinological, haematological, immunological, and metabolic[6,7]. The disease occurs most often in children, and *C. albicans* again is the aetiological agent. It frequently involves the skin of the entire body, nails, and mucous membranes, with marked

*The disease formerly known as torulopsosis is included in this chapter since its aetiologic yeast, *Torulopsis glabrata*, has been reclassified in the genus *Candida*, as *C. glabrata*[1]. However, this transfer may not stand the test of time.

†This species is not treated here as a separate and valid species since it is considered to be a variant of *C. albicans*[2,3].

hyperkeratosis and a chronic granulomatous inflammatory reaction in the underlying tissues. Diagnosis is based on the demonstration of yeast cells and mycelial elements in skin and nail scrapings and by isolation of *C. albicans*.

Milder but persistent forms of cutaneous candidiasis occur that involve the intertriginous areas of the skin such as the interdigital areas of the hands, inframammary folds, groin, and the axillae. Typically, the lesions are erythematous, scaly, and moist. Pustules and vesicles may develop in the centre of the affected areas. Pruritus is a common complaint.

Intertriginous candidiasis frequently is an occupational disease among individuals whose work involves prolonged immersion of their hands in water. Bartenders, cannery workers, and housewives thus are among those whose macerated skin becomes infected by the *C. albicans* harbored in their bodies. Other factors predisposing to this form of candidiasis are diabetes, obesity, and tropical climates.

Paronychial candidiasis is also encountered among individuals whose hands are frequently immersed in water. Clinically this type of candidiasis is characterised by inflammation and swelling of the paronychial tissue around one or more of the nails. Secondary bacterial infections are frequent and present diagnostic and therapeutic problems.

C. Systemic Candidiasis

The various *Candida spp.* can and do invade most organ systems of the body. Pulmonary candidiasis, endocarditis, fungemia, and nephritis are examples of systemic infections. In these forms of the disease, the most frequent culprits, aside from *C. albicans,* are *C. glabrata*[8, 9], *C. guilliermondii*[10, 11], *C. krusei*[12], *C. parapsilosis*[10, 13], and *C. tropicalis*[14].

Primary pulmonary candidiasis is rare, but secondary lung infections frequently occur in individuals with another primary disease, i.e., tuberculosis, other bacterial and viral infections, as well as neoplasms. The symptoms of pulmonary candidiasis resemble those of other respiratory diseases. Patients develop cough, dyspnea, night sweats, fever, and weight loss. The sputum produced is mucoid and sanguinous. Radiography will reveal pulmonary densities and hilar and peribronchial lymphadenopathy. Pulmonary candidiasis can be caused by any of several species of *Candida*. All, with the exception of *C. glabrata*, form both budding yeast cells and mycelium in tissue. *C. glabrata*, however, only produces yeast cells that are ovate and 2–3 μm in diameter.

Lower animals, especially birds, are also subject to candidiasis. Avian infections generally involve the upper digestive tract, especially the crop. As with humans, the clinical signs are not specific. Some of the signs are poor growth, listlessness, rough feathers, and loss of appetite. The most severe lesions usually are found in the crop, but they may also occur in other sites. Commonly, the curd-like, greyish-white lesions are loosely adherent to the mucous membranes. In birds with chronic infections, the wall of the crop thickens and its membranes become coated with a wrinkled mass of yellowish-white necrotic material.

In mammals, candidiasis may involve the digestive tract, various internal organs, and the skin. Cattle and swine are common victims. In calves the disease most often involves the digestive tract. Such infections lead to watery diarrhea, melena, anorexia, dehydration, prostration, and even death. Several *Candida sp.* have been incriminated as causal agents of bovine mastitis, and systemic infections have occurred in feed-lot cattle that were given antibiotics in their feed. Candidiasis in swine generally involves the digestive tract, especially in young animals. In piglets, the signs of infection include diarrhea, emaciation, and vomiting.

In clinical materials and histological sections, the cells of *C. glabrata* resemble those of *Histoplasma capsulatum* var. *capsulatum,* especially when groups of them are present in macrophages[15]. Differentiation of *C. glabrata* infections from cases of histoplasmosis capsulati is dependent upon the use of specific fluorescent antibody (FA) conjugates for *H. capsulatum* var. *capsulatum,* serological tests for candidiasis and histoplasmosis capsulati, and cultural studies. *C. glabrata* cells and sera from patients with candidiasis glabrata do not react with the histoplasmosis FA conjugates or in serological tests for histoplasmosis. Sera from patients with *C. glabrata* infection, however, readily cross-react in the serological tests for candidiasis caused by *C. albicans*[16]. In culture, *C. glabrata* is differentiated from the other *Candida* species by its failure to form mycelium on any medium, on the basis of fermentation and assimilation reactions against a battery of sugars, and by its failure to utilise KNO_3[5].

Serological tests for candidiasis are highly useful in diagnosing the disease and in monitoring the effect of therapy[17, 18]. A number of serodiagnostic tests have been developed for this disease. They include immunodiffusion, counterimmunoelectrophoresis, tube and latex agglutination, and indirect fluorescent antibody tests. Since many noninfected individuals have serum antibodies to *Candida* antigens, because members of this genus are common inhabitants of the mucous membranes and gastrointestinal tract, the results of serodiagnostic tests may be difficult to interpret. The latex agglutination, immunodiffusion, and counterelectrophoresis tests demonstrate fewer reactions with sera from normal individuals than do the tube agglutination and indirect fluorescent antibody tests, and they are therefore considered by many workers to be more specific indicators of *Candida* infections.

Candidiasis presents formidable challenges to the therapist. Infections in the form of chronic mucocutaneous candidiasis, pulmonary candidiasis, endocarditis, and fungemia, unless diagnosed early and treated promptly, are fatal. Amphotericin B and 5-fluorocytosine are effective in systemic infections[19]. Vaginitis responds to treatment with various antibiotics such as nystatin and miconazole[20]. Cutaneous, oral, and intestinal infections are treated with nystatin and miconazole as well as a number of other compounds[21, 22, 23].

Histopathology (Figures 136–174)

In mucocutaneous candidiasis, masses of branching, septate hyphae, pseudohyphae and round to oval budding yeast cells (blastospores) measuring 3–5 μm in diameter are seen on the surface of and within the epithelium[23–27]. Generally, blastospores are most numerous on the surface of mucocutaneous lesions, whereas the hyphae and pseudohyphae occupy deeper zones. The infection is usually limited to the epithelial layers, and in patients with the ordinary form of mucocutaneous candidiasis, inflammation in the underlying tissues is mild to moderate.

Although usually intraepithelial in mucocutaneous lesions, proliferating hyphae and pseudohyphae of *Candida* occasionally penetrate the epithelial basement membrane and extend into the lamina propria and submucosa or dermis. Fungal elements may even invade the deeper skeletal muscle in severely compromised individuals[12]. The underlying tissues may be heavily infiltrated with mixed inflammatory cells, predominantly neutrophils and lymphocytes. On the other hand, some preterminal infections of the skin and mucous membranes (e.g., in the esophagus and stomach) may be associated with little or no cellular reaction, even when the mycelium penetrates the epithelium and extends well into the underlying tissues.

Chronic mucocutaneous candidiasis is a distinct variety of this disease. It is usually found in infants and children with defects in cellular immunity or a variety of endocrinopathies[7, 28]. The oral mucosa, the fingernails and paronychial tissues, and the skin of the face and scalp are the sites most often involved. Microscopically, there is marked hyperkeratosis, acanthosis, and pseudoepitheliomatous hyperplasia of the epidermis, and dense collections of lymphocytes, plasma cells, polymorphonuclear leucocytes, macrophages, and foreign body giant cells in the dermis. This granulomatous reaction in the dermis is not seen in the ordinary types of mucocutaneous candidiasis. Inflammation may extend into the subcutaneous tissues, and it has been reported to be perifollicular and periglandular in some cases[28]. *Candida* elements are characteristically abundant and are located in the superficial layers of the epidermis; rarely do they invade the dermis. The mycelium consists of greatly elongated hyphae and very few blastospores.

Systemic *Candida* infections may not be diagnosed until necropsy. Here, the exclusive presence or predomination of a *Candida sp.* in lesions assumes, in general, a pathological significance. Although any organ may be affected, the kidneys and lungs are most frequently involved[29–31]. For unknown reasons, *Candida spp.* have a predilection for the kidneys, and these organs may be so heavily infected that they cease to function. Pyelonephritis is a frequent complication, and large numbers of *Candida* elements often fill the renal pelvis and tubules. Valvular endocarditis with large mycotic vegetations containing numerous *Candida sp.* is sometimes seen in patients who have had heart surgery or who have some other underlying heart disease[9, 13, 32]. This lesion frequently leads to large vessel embolism, and fungal elements may penetrate the contiguous myocardium and pericardium. Candidal meningitis may also occur.

Lesions in patients with systemic candidiasis are generally acute and are characterised by suppuration and necrosis[29–31, 33]. Microscopically, sections show multifocal abscesses or microabscesses containing abundant neutrophils mixed with numerous pseudohyphae, hyphae, and blastospores of *Candida*. Fibrin and erythrocytes may also be components of the lesion. Either all or any combination of these fungal elements can be seen in the suppurative lesions, and radiating colonies of *Candida* are sometimes present. The usual abscesses may not be present during the early stage of infection because of lack of sufficient time for their formation, and they may not be present in severely immunosuppressed hosts because of marked depression of the cellular response. Instead, areas of haemorrhagic necrosis containing proliferating hyphae are usually seen.

Chronic lesions are occasionally seen in patients with candidiasis. They usually consist of multiple abscesses rimmed by epithelioid cells, giant cells, and fibroblasts. *Candida* elements are also occasionally seen in solid granulomas. In these lesions, the fungus cells may not be visible when stained by H&E, especially if they are few in number and are within giant cells. However, when stained by PAS or GF, hyphal fragments, pseudohyphae, and fewer blastospores can be clearly seen in large Langhans' and foreign body giant cells. Some giant cells may be elongated and distorted, apparently in an attempt to accommodate the hyphae.

Although aspergilli and zygomycetes have a greater tendency to invade the walls of blood vessels, *Candida spp.* may at times also show this property. As with the former fungi, angioinvasion by *Candida spp.* may lead to thrombosis, infarction, and disseminated infection.

The presence of blastospores mixed with characteristic pseudohyphae or hyphae in tissues enables the microscopist to identify a fungus as a species of *Candida* and to make a diagnosis of candidiasis. However, the particular species that is present cannot be identified by histologic examination. For this reason, cultural studies should also be done when possible. It should be emphasized that demonstrating tissue invasion is important in diagnosing this disease since the *Candida spp.* are part of the normal flora of the skin and of the gastrointestinal and upper respiratory tracts. Cultural studies alone may therefore not be sufficient for making a diagnosis.

Because the *Candida spp.* are so poorly stained by H&E, they may be overlooked when a tissue section is scanned. However, all candidal elements are coloured intensely with any of the special fungus stains, particularly PAS and GF. The GMS stain is also satisfactory for demonstrating *Candida,* and when combined with H&E, it is the stain of choice when only one tissue section is available for study.

If only blastospores of *Candida* are seen, they may be confused with morphologically similar yeast forms in tissue, such as those of *H. capsulatum* var. *capsulatum, Blastomyces dermatitidis* and poorly encapsulated *Cryptococcus neoformans.* In these instances, serial sections should be carefully searched for the presence of typical pseudohyphae and hyphae of the *Candida spp.* Immunofluorescence is also very useful for differentiating *Candida* from other morphologically similar fungi.

In tissue, the moniliform hyphae of some dematiaceous fungi (Chapter 21) may be mistaken for pseudohyphae and hyphae of the *Candida spp.* However, a careful search will usually reveal that some or all of these pigmented fungi are dematiaceous in H&E-stained sections.

Hyphae of *Candida spp.* may at times resemble aspergilli and other filamentous fungi in tissues. In such instances, cultural and direct fluorescent antibody examinations are required for a differential identification to be made.

In candidiasis due to *C.* (*Torulopsis*) *glabrata,* the lungs, kidneys, heart, and central nervous system are the sites most frequently involved[8, 9, 34–37]. Like the other *Candida spp., C. glabrata* is usually an opportunist. The inflammation it causes can range from little or no cellular response to a necrotising purulent or granulomatous reaction that is similar to that caused by other *Candida spp.* Minimal inflammation is commonly seen in preterminal infections where varying numbers of yeast cells fill alveolar spaces or renal tubules. In H&E-stained sections, *C. glabrata* cells are lightly basophilic or amphophilic, and they may not be completely stained. The organisms are better delineated with GMS (our stain of choice for this *Candida sp.*) and usually appear as individual or clustered, round to oval yeasts that are 2–5 μm in diameter and bud by a relatively narrow basal attachment to the parent cell. In contrast to other *Candida spp., C. glabrata* does not produce hyphae.

Because of similarity in size and appearance, *C. glabrata* cells may be mistaken for those of *Histoplasma capsulatum* var. *capsulatum,* especially when the former are clustered in macrophages. However, there are subtle differences between the two. In general, yeast cells of *C. glabrata* bud more frequently and are slightly larger. *C. glabrata* cells are also more often extracellular. When histological studies are equivocal, *C. glabrata* can be differentiated from *H. capsulatum* var. *capsulatum* by the use of fluorescent antibody tests and by cultural studies.

References

1 Yarrow, D. and Meyer, S. A. (1978). Proposal for amendment of the diagnosis of the genus Candida Berkhout nom. cons. *Int. J. Systematic Bacteriol.* **28**, 611–615.

2 Hasenclever, H. F. and Mitchell, W. O. (1961). Antigenic studies of Candida. III. Comparative pathogenicity of Candida albicans Group A, Group B, and Candida stellatoidea. *J. Bacteriol.* **82**, 578–581.

3 Ahearn, D. Personal communication.

4 Kozinn, P. J. and Taschdjian, C. L. (1963). Pathogenesis, epidemiology and prevention of neonatal oral thrush. *Pediatrics Digest* **5**, unnumbered pp. (Reprint).

5 Lodder, J., ed. (1970). *The Yeasts.* A taxonomic study, 2nd ed. North-Holland Publishing Co., Amsterdam.

6 Kirkpatrick, C. H. (1971). Chronic mucocutaneous candidiasis: model building in cellular immunity. *Ann. Intern. Med.* **74**, 955–978.

7 Matsumoto, T. (1977). Chronic mucocutaneous candidiasis. *Trans. Mycol. Soc. Jpn.* **17**, 515–531.

8 Block, C. S., Young, C. N. and Myers, R. A. M. (1977). Torulopsis glabrata fungaemia. *S. Afr. Med. J.* **51**, 632–636.

9 Heffner, D. K. and Franklin, W. A. (1978). Endocarditis caused by Torulopsis glabrata. *Am. J. Clin. Pathol.* **70**, 420–423.

10 Kay, J. H., Bernstein, S., Tsuji, H. K., Redington, J. V., Milgram, M. and Brem, T. (1968). Surgical treatment of Candida endocarditis. *J. Am. Med. Assoc.* **203**, 621–626.

11 Ratzman, G. W. (1977). The problem of Candida meningitis in newborn babies and infants and its therapy with miconazole. *Z. Aerztl. Fortbild.* **71**, 657–661.

12 Diggs, C. H., Eskenasey, G. M., Sutherland, J. C. and Wiernik, P. H. (1976). Fungal infection of muscle in acute leukemia. *Cancer* **38**, 1771–1772.
13 Robboy, S. J. and Kaiser, J. (1975). Pathogenesis of fungal infection on heart valve prostheses. *Human Pathol.* **6**, 711–715.
14 Rosner, R. (1966). Isolation of Candida protoplasts from a case of Candida endocarditis. *J. Bacteriol.* **91**, 1320–1326.
15 Minkowitz, S., Koffler, D. and Zar, F. G. (1963). Torulopsis glabrata septicemia. *Am. J. Med.* **34**, 252–255.
16 Stickle, D., Kaufman, L., Blumer, S. and McLaughlin, D. W. (1972). Comparison of a newly developed latex agglutination test and an immunodiffusion test in the diagnosis of candidiasis. *Appl. Microbiol.* **23**, 490–499.
17 Merz, W. G., Evans, G. L., Shadomy, S., Anderson, S., Kaufman, L., Kozinn, P. J., Mackenzie, D. W., Protzman, W. P. and Remington, J. S. (1978). Laboratory evaluation of serologic tests for systemic candidiasis: a cooperative study. *J. Clin. Microbiol.* **5**, 596–603.
18 Gentry, L. O., McNitt, J. R. and Kaufman, L. (1978). Use and value of serologic tests for the diagnosis of systemic candidiasis in cancer patients: a prospective study of 146 patients. *Current Microbiol.* **1**, 239–242.
19 Chesney, P. J., Justman, R. A. and Bogdanowicz, W. M. (1978). Candida meningitis in newborn infants: a review and report of combined amphotericin B and fluorocytosine therapy. *Johns Hopkins Med. J.* **142**, 155–160.
20 Clayton, Y. M. (1977). Antifungal drugs in current use: a review. *Proc. Roy. Soc. Med.*, Supplement No. 4. **71**, 15–17.
21 Fischer, T. J., Klein, R. B., Keishnar, H. E. Borut, T. C. and Stiehn, E. R. (1977). Miconazole in the treatment of chronic mucocutaneous candidiasis: a preliminary report. *J. Ped.* **91**, 815–819.
22 Kirkpatrick, C. W. and Alling, D. W. (1978). Treatment of chronic oral candidiasis with clothrimazole troches. *N. Engl. J. Med.* **299**, 1201–1203.
23 Odds, F. (1979). *Candida and Candidosis.* University Park Press, Baltimore, Md.
24 Urdaneta, E., Pinto, V. B. and Gaveller, B. (1961). Candidiasis. *Mycopathologia* **15**, 317–342.
25 Kral, F. and Uscavage, J. P. (1960). Cutaneous candidiasis in a dog. *J. Am. Vet. Med. Assoc.* **136**, 612–615.
26 Reynolds, I. M., Miner, P. W. and Smith, R. E. (1968). Cutaneous candidiasis in swine. *J. Am. Vet. Med. Assoc.* **152**, 182–186.
27 Kaufman, A. F. and Quist, K. D. (1969). Thrush in a rhesus monkey: report of a case. *Lab. Anim. Care* **19**, 526–527.
28 Aronson, I. K. and Soltani, K. (1976). Chronic mucocutaneous candidoses: a review. *Mycopathologia* **60**, 17–25.
29 Louria, D. B., Stiff, D. P. and Bennett, B. (1962). Disseminated moniliasis in the adult. *Medicine* (*Balt.*) **41**, 307–337.
30 Myerowitz, R. L., Pazin, G. J. and Allen, C. M. (1977). Disseminated candidiasis. Changes in incidence, underlying diseases, and pathology. *Am. J. Clin. Pathol.* **68**, 29–38.
31 Gruhn, J. G. and Sanson, J. (1963). Mycotic infections in leukemic patients at autopsy. *Cancer* **16**, 61–73.
32 Hyun, B. H. and Collier, F. C. (1961). Mycotic endocarditis following intracardiac operations. *N. Engl. J. Med.* **263**, 1339–1341.
33 Mills, J. H. L. and Hirth, R. S. (1967). Systemic candidiasis in calves on prolonged antibiotic therapy. *J. Am. Vet. Med. Assoc.* **150**, 862–870.
34 Grimley, P. M., Wright, L. D. and Jennings, A. E. (1965). Torulopsis glabrata infection in man. *Am. J. Clin. Pathol.* **43**, 216–223.
35 Minkowitz, S., Koffler, D. and Zak, F. G. (1963). Torulopsis glabrata septicemia. *Am. J. Med.* **34**, 252–255.
36 Newman, D. M. and Hogg, J. M. (1969). Torulopsis glabrata pyelonephritis. *J. Urol.* **102**, 547–548.
37 Oldfield, F. S. J., Kapica, L. and Pirozynski, W. J. (1968). Pulmonary infection due to Torulopsis glabrata. *Can. Med. Assoc. J.* **98**, 165–168.

9 Chromoblastomycosis

(Chromomycosis (in part), Dermatitis verrucosa, Dermatite verrucosa chromoparasitaria).

Aetiologic agents:

Cladosporium carrionii, Fonsecaea compacta, F. pedrosoi, Phialophora verrucosa, Rhinocladiella cerophilum

Definition and background information

Chromoblastomycosis is a cosmopolitan, chronic, disease of the skin and subcutaneous tissues caused by any one of five species of dematiaceous fungi that live as saprophytes in soil or organic matter in nature. Infections result from the inoculation (through some traumatic incident) of exposed parts of the body with matter containing these fungi.

Clinically the disease manifests itself by the development of verrucous, cutaneous lesions that develop slowly but inexorably to form striking papillomatous vegetations that frequently ulcerate. The infection spreads by way of the lymphatic ducts to establish satellite lesions. The most commonly afflicted areas are the legs and arms, but infections may develop on other parts of the body, such as the hands, face, and thorax. At the traumatic site, the primary lesion begins as a small pinkish papule. With time the papule enlarges and becomes a protuberant, verrucous nodule.

Chromoblastomycosis is a disease of humans. Authenticated cases have not been reported in other mammals. A mycotic disease of amphibians has been diagnosed as chromoblastomycosis by some investigators, but the identity of its aetiologic agent(s) remains unclear[1,2].

In its primary stages, chromoblastomycosis is best treated by surgical excision. In advanced cases, promising results have been obtained through the combined administration of amphotericin B and 5-fluorocytosine[3].

The aetiologic agents are dimorphic black moulds. Regardless of the genus and species of mould involved, the tissue form of the invading fungus seen in the body is in the nature of large (6–12 μm), thick-walled, dark brown muriform cells, commonly referred to as sclerotic bodies. These multiply through the separation of cells after septations have developed along longitudinal and horizontal planes. They do not bud. Dematiaceous mycelium is occasionally produced, especially in the superficial crusts of lesions, but the diagnostic, mycologic hallmark of chromoblastomycosis is the dark, thick-walled muriform cells that develop in tissue.

All of the fungi that cause chromoblastomycosis form slow-growing velvety colonies that are dark brown to greenish black on Sabouraud's dextrose agar. The genera and species of the causative agents are distinguished from each other and identified on the basis of the morphology of their conidiophores and the mode by which their unicellular conidia are produced.

Aetiologic agents: *Rhinocladiella cerophilum* is a newly described agent of chromoblastomycosis[4,5]. The two known cases originated in Brazil and Mexico. This fungus produces only a sympodial type of conidiophore. Its single-celled conidia are borne on the tips and sides of the conidiophore. The spores measure 4.5–7.5 × 1.5–2.4 μm. Hoog[6] equates *A. aquaspersa* with *Ramichloridium cerophilum.*

Cladosporium carrionii has a single type of conidiophore that produces branched chains of conidia. The simple conidiophores are erect and branched at the top, producing conidia in short, branching chains. The conidiophore is dark walled. The spores are smooth and measure 1.5–3.0 × 2.5–7.5 μm.

Phialophora verrucosa also has one kind of conidiophore, a phialide. This is a flask-shaped structure with a cup-like tip from within which conidia are extruded. The conidia tend to aggregate in a compact mass around the conidiophore.

The species of the genus *Fonsecaea* are characterised by the production of three types of conidiophores with varying degrees of frequency. In addition to the cladosporium and phialide types, the so-called acrotheca type of conidiophore is produced. In the latter type, unicellular spores are produced both at the tip and sides of the conidiophore stalk. The primary conidia produce secondary conidia.

Chromoblastomycosis is a cosmopolitan disease, but most cases occur in the tropical areas of Latin America and Africa. *F. pedrosoi* is the most prevalent of the five aetiologic agents, with *P. verrucosa*, *C. carrionii*, *F. compacta*, and *R.*

cerophilum, occurring in descending order of frequency.

Detailed clinical descriptions of the disease, its therapy, and the diagnostic features of the fungi are found elsewhere[7-11].

Chromoblastomycosis is a clear-cut disease entity with distinctive clinical, histopathological, and aetiological features. It should not be confused with phaeohyphomycosis (see Chapter 21).

Histopathology (Figures 175–185)

The agents of chromoblastomycosis incite a mixed purulent and granulomatous inflammatory reaction[12, 13]. This type of tissue response is not specific for this mycosis, but is also seen in skin lesions caused by certain other mycoses, particularly blastomycosis, coccidioidomycosis, paracoccidioidomycosis and sporotrichosis. In chromoblastomycosis, lesions are almost always confined to the skin and subcutaneous tissues. Direct extension into underlying tissues seldom occurs. As in sporotrichosis, lymphatic spread may lead to multiple skin lesions. Local spread has also been noted after biopsy of skin lesions to assess treatment[14]. Haematogenous dissemination from a primary skin lesion is extremely rare. When it does occur, the brain and meninges are usually involved[15, 16, 17]. Here, many small abscesses that contain either dematiaceous spherical fungal cells or branched hyphae or both are usually surrounded by epithelioid cells, giant cells, and granulation tissue. In some disseminated lesions there has been little or no inflammatory reaction associated with these fungi.

Skin sections from subjects with chromoblastomycosis characteristically contain small, irregularly circumscribed and often confluent granulomatous nodules in the dermis. The subcutaneous tissues are less frequently involved. These nodules consist of epithelioid cells and large multinucleated giant cells of both the Langhans' and foreign body types. Granulomas may be solid or may contain central microabscesses consisting of neutrophils and necrotic debris. The dematiaceous round to polyhedral fungal cells of chromoblastomycosis are found singly or in compact clusters within giant cells. Clusters of these muriform cells may also be seen extracellularly, usually within microabscesses in the dermis and epidermis. In some cases, typical forms are readily found; in others, careful search may be required to observe them. Rarely will examination of serial sections be necessary to demonstrate the typical fungal bodies. The surrounding stroma contains proliferating granulation tissue infiltrated with lymphocytes, plasma cells, macrophages, and polymorphonuclear leucocytes. Thickening of the dermis and subcutaneous tissues may be striking because of marked fibrosis. The overlying epidermis shows either variable acanthosis or pseudoepitheliomatous hyperplasia, or both. Hyperkeratosis and keratinolytic microabscesses are also seen. When the epidermis is ulcerated, secondary bacterial infection is common and the dermis may be heavily infiltrated with polymorphonuclear leucocytes. Because of the epithelial changes, cutaneous chromoblastomycosis is often mistaken clinically for a squamous cell carcinoma.

Recent histologic studies indicate that the phenomenon of transepithelial elimination is an important mechanism in the pathophysiology of cutaneous chromoblastomycosis[18]. Transepithelial elimination is a spontaneously occurring dermo-epidermal phenomenon in certain skin diseases in which damaged connective tissue, foreign materials and certain microbes in the dermis are expelled through the epidermis in an apparent attempt at healing. It appears to be responsible for the histogenesis of the epidermal changes in chromoblastomycosis and in certain other cutaneous mycoses.

In H&E-stained tissue sections, a diagnosis of chromoblastomycosis can readily be made by demonstrating the brown, round to polyhedral, thick-walled fungal (muriform) cells that measure 5–12 μm in diameter. Occasional organisms may be crescent-shaped. Because of their thick walls, these organisms have been referred to as 'sclerotic' cells or bodies. Some but not all of the fungal cells will be septate. Septations are formed along one or two planes, the latter giving rise to a tetrad of daughter cells. When septations are newly formed, the apposing surfaces of the daughter cells may be flattened. The natural pigmentation plus reproduction by septation or equatorial splitting along one or two planes and not by budding are the salient identifying features of the agents of chromoblastomycosis. Occasionally, brown, branched and septate hyphae can be found in the superficial layers of the epidermis, usually within keratinolytic or other intraepidermal abscesses. Because the tissue forms of the several aetiologic agents are morphologically similar, the exact genus and species can only be determined by cultural studies.

Special fungus stains are not indicated unless the agents of chromoblastomycosis are sparse. However, special stains can be used to improve contrast for purposes of illustration. If used for routine diagnosis, these stains will mask the distinct brown colour of the fungus.

References

1 Velasquez, L. F. and Restrepo, A. (1975). Chromoblastomycosis in the toad (Bufo marinus) and a comparison of the aetiologic agent with fungi causing human chromoblastomycosis. *Sabouraudia* **13**, 1–9.

2 Beneke, E. S. (1978). Dematiaceous fungi in laboratory-housed frogs. In *The Black and White Yeasts*. Scientific Publication No. 356, pp. 101–108. Pan American Health Organization, Washington, D.C.

3 Bopp, C. (1978). New method for the treatment of chromoblastomycosis. In *The Black and White Yeasts*. Scientific Publication No. 356, pp. 33–34. Pan American Health Organization, Washington, D.C.

4 Borelli, D. (1972). Acrotheca aquaspersa nova species agente de cromomicosis. *Acta. Cient. Venez.* **23**, 193–196.

5 Borelli, D., Marcano, C. and Feo, M. (1974). Informe sobre las actividades de la seccion de micologia medica durante el ano de 1972. *Gac. Med. de Caracas* **82**, 133–149.

6 Hoog, G. S. de. (1977). *The Black Yeasts and Allied Hyphomycetes*. Studies in Mycology, No. 15. Centraalbureau voor Schimmelcultures, Baarn, Netherlands.

7 Carrion, A. L. (1942). Chromoblastomycosis. *Mycologia* **34**, 424–441.

8 Putkonen, T. (1966). Die Chromomykose in Finnland. *Der Hautarzt.* **17**, 507–509.

9 Silva, D. (1972). Cromomicose. *Ann. Brasil Dermatol.* **47**, 265–272.

10 Zaias, N. and Rebell, G. (1973). A simple and accurate diagnostic method in chromoblastomycosis. *Arch. Dermatol.* **108**, 545–546.

11 Londero, A. T. and Ramos, C. D. (1976). Chromomycosis: A clinical and mycologic study of thirty-five cases observed in the hinterland of Rio Grande du Sul, Brazil. *Am. J. Trop. Med. Hyg.* **25**, 132–135.

12 Cameron, H. M., Gatei, D. and Bremner, A. D. (1973). The deep mycoses in Kenya: a histopathological study. 3. Chromomycosis. *East Afr. Med. J.* **50**, 406–412.

13 Vollum, D. I. (1977). Chromomycosis: a review. *Br. J. Dermatol.* **96**, 454–458.

14 Bayles, M. A. H. (1971). Chromomycosis: treatment with thiabendazole. *Arch. Dermatol.* **104**, 476–485.

15 Kajikawa, K., Izumi, H. and Izaki, K. (1960). An autopsy case of brain abscess due to Hormodendrum sp. *Acta. Pathol. Jpn.* **10**, 525–529.

16 Duque, O. (1961). Meningo-encephalitis and brain abscess caused by Cladosporium and Fonsecaea: review of the literature, report of two cases, and experimental studies. *Am. J. Clin. Pathol.* **36**, 505–517.

17 Shimazono, Y., Isaki, K., Torii, H. and Otsuka, R. (1963). Brain abscess due to Hormodendrum dermatitidis (Kano) Conant, 1953: report of a case and review of the literature. *Folia Psychiatr. Neurol. Jpn.* **17**, 80–96.

18 Batres, E., Wolf, J. E., Jr., Rudolph, A. H. and Knox, J. M. (1978). Transepithelial elimination of cutaneous chromomycosis. *Arch. Dermatol.* **114**, 1231–1232.

10 Coccidioidomycosis

(Valley fever, Desert rheumatism, Coccidioidal granuloma, San Joaquin fever, Posada-Wernicke's disease)

Aetiologic agent:

Coccidioides immitis

Definition and background information

Coccidioidomycosis is an acute, generally mild, self-limiting respiratory disease that rarely becomes chronic or generalised. The disease is endemic in certain desert-like areas in the Southwestern United States, Mexico, and Central and South America. Occasional cases are diagnosed in individuals outside the endemic areas. Such infections prove to have been contracted during visits to endemic areas or by contact with fomites imported from the endemic areas[1].

Coccidioides immitis is a dimorphic fungus. Cultures grown on routine laboratory media and incubated at room temperature or at 37°C grow in a mycelial form. Young colonies are typically white and cottony but tend to darken with age. Microscopically, colonies are seen to be composed of hyaline, septate hyphae, 2–4 μm in diameter. Most isolates produce abundant rectangular or barrel-shaped arthroconidia that usually measure 2.5×4 to $3 \times 6\,\mu$m. They are formed by the close septation of hyphae, and they characteristically alternate with smaller empty cells. The empty cells rupture easily to free the arthroconidia, leaving on the latter remnants of their thin cell walls. Atypical isolates are not uncommon. They vary considerably in colour, texture, growth rate, and sporulation[2].

In mammalian tissues and also under special culture conditions[3], *C. immitis* ceases to be mycelial and develops endosporulating spherules that are thick-walled, rounded structures ranging in size from 20–200 μm. As they mature, their cytoplasm undergoes a process of progressive cleavage to form small spores 2–5 μm in diameter. These endospores may be distributed peripherally or throughout the spherule. At maturity, the spherules rupture and release their endospores, which gradually enlarge and become spherules that in turn form and discharge endospores. When endospores or spherules are inoculated on routine laboratory media, the mycelial form develops.

C. immitis grows in the mycelial form in soil in the endemic areas. There, arthroconidia are produced in abundance. They are raised by air currents to contaminate the air. In most instances, man and lower animals become infected by inhaling the arthroconidia, although infections may be contracted by the accidental inoculation of the infectious elements of *C. immitis* into the skin.

Coccidioidomycosis in man manifests itself in four basic forms: (a) Pulmonary – asymptomatic or symptomatic, (b) Disseminated, (c) Residual pulmonary, and (d) Primary cutaneous.

The pulmonary form, which is the most common, results from the inhalation of arthroconidia. It is estimated that 60% of the victims of pulmonary infections remain asymptomatic, whereas the other 40% have symptoms that range from those characteristic of a mild acute upper respiratory disease to those of a severe one. Early clinical signs in self-limiting symptomatic pulmonary coccidioidomycosis include cough, pleuritic pain, loss of appetite, malaise, and fatigue. An estimated 0.2% of individuals with pulmonary coccidioidomycosis develop the disseminated form of the disease. Such patients may continue to have the previously described symptoms, but they may also develop lesions in cutaneous and subcutaneous tissues, bones, visceral organs, and the meninges. Disseminated coccidioidomycosis is a serious disease and, if untreated, may be fatal. Negroes and Filipinos are more apt to develop disseminated coccidioidomycosis than are people in other racial groups. Residual pulmonary coccidioidomycosis is usually diagnosed by the radiographic finding of thin-walled cavities in the lungs. Some patients may have chest pains, cough, and haemoptysis. Primary cutaneous coccidioidomycosis is very rare and results from the direct inoculation of the fungus into the skin. In such instances, the ulcer or chancre which develops at the point of inoculation is often accompanied by regional lymphadenopathy[4].

Coccidioidomycosis has been recognised in a wide variety of lower animals[5]. Naturally occurring infections have been reported in nearly all species of domestic animals, various species of desert rodents, and various captive wild animals. Among domestic animals, the dog is the most seriously affected by *C. immitis*. Canine infections range from subclinical to acute. Disseminated disease may be fatal. Signs of clinically apparent canine coccidioidomycosis are cough, diarrhea, loss of weight, and fever. Radiographic studies frequently show pulmonary and skeletal lesions. Cattle and sheep are commonly infected by *C. immitis*, but the disease is generally benign, with lesions confined to the lungs and lymph nodes of the thorax. The disease in other animals may be similar to that described in dogs.

Coccidioidomycosis is not communicable from man to man or from animals to man.

Serological tests are valuable aids to the diagnosis of coccidioidomycosis. These tests are rapid and provide presumptive evidence of infection. The most widely used serodiagnostic tests for this disease are complement fixation and immunodiffusion. Both procedures are very useful for the diagnosis of localised and disseminated coccidioidomycosis. Both have prognostic value and can be used to monitor patients' responses to therapy. Tube precipitin and latex agglutination tests are also used and are of value for the diagnosis of early primary infections.

The exoantigen test is of great value for the identification of mycelial-form cultures of *C. immitis*.

At present, amphotericin B is the drug of choice for the treatment of coccidioidomycosis[6].

Histopathology (Figures 186–213)

In the pulmonary, disseminated, and primary cutaneous forms of coccidioidomycosis, the inflammatory response is typically of the mixed granulomatous and purulent type and is very similar to that associated with disseminated blastomycosis[7, 8, 9, 10]. The relative predominance of each inflammatory component depends on the form of the disease and on which reproductive stage (or part) of the fungus is in direct contact with host tissues. A severe, localised, purulent reaction occurs when a mature spherule of *C. immitis* ruptures and releases endospores. As each freed endospore matures, the surrounding polymorphonuclear leucocytes are gradually replaced by lymphocytes, plasma cells, epithelioid cells, and variable numbers of Langhans' or foreign body-type giant cells. When the enlarging spherule reaches maturity, it may be intimately surrounded by or within epithelioid cells and multinucleated giant cells. When the mature spherule ruptures, the entire inflammatory cycle is repeated, with immediate infiltration of polymorphonuclear leucocytes into the centre of the granuloma. Because the entire reproductive cycle of *C. immitis* may be completed in a few days, a single microscopic field may contain spherules in all stages of development. Thus, a very acute reaction where polymorphonuclear leucocytes predominate may be found contiguous to a chronic granulomatous reaction where epithelioid cells predominate.

The similarity of coccidioidal and tuberculous lesions was noted by early workers[4, 7]. The characteristic feature of both is the tubercle. However, in both diseases, granulomatous and purulent reactions occur, and as is true in tuberculosis, the balance between purulent and granulomatous components seems to determine the outcome. If host resistance is good, granuloma formation is followed by fibrosis, scarring, and occasional calcification. If resistance is poor, as in rapidly progressing cases, the purulent reaction predominates[11, 12]. Primary pulmonary coccidioidomycosis is preponderantly granulomatous; secondary disseminated coccidioidomycosis tends to be purulent.

The histologic diagnosis of active coccidioidomycosis is established by demonstrating spherules of *C. immitis* measuring 20–200 μm in diameter. Mature ones contain many uninucleate endospores 2–5 μm in diameter. Spherules in various stages of development are found in tissue:

1 small immature and maturing spherules,
2 mature spherules with endospores, and
3 collapsed spherules without endospores.

Immature spherules occur as round cells with or without homogeneous contents. The developing spherule may show peripherally placed cytoplasm. It is round or oval and has a thick, refractile wall that becomes progressively thinner as the spherule enlarges and forms endospores. The routine H&E procedure usually stains both endospores and the cell wall of spherules deeply basophilic, and is usually adequate for demonstrating intact spherules in tissue. Special fungus stains increase the contrast between the fungus and background tissue and allow one to study morphology in greater detail. Generally, the PAS procedure stains endospores but not the cell walls of spherules. We prefer the GF and GMS procedures because they readily stain the walls of both endospores and spherules.

In primary coccidioidal pneumonia, peribronchial, peritracheal, hilar, and mediastinal lymph nodes commonly contain metastatic lesions very early in the course of the disease[7]. Nodal lesions may lead to dissemination. Fibrinous or granulomatous pleuritis has been reported to occur over areas of severe pneumonia[4, 8].

The residual pulmonary form of coccidioidomycosis is characterised by the presence of solitary or multiple fibrocaseous granulomas (coccidioidomas) with thin fibrotic capsules. These lesions may be several centimeters in diameter and are usually found incidentally at autopsy or in lung biopsies performed to rule out neoplasia[4, 13, 14]. As in chronic tuberculosis and some of the other deep mycoses, viable organisms may remain in old caseous lesions for years. If the immune competence of the host is altered, these smoldering foci of infection may again become active and disseminate throughout the lung as well as to other parts of the body. Unlike fibrocaseous granulomas due to *Histoplasma capsulatum* var. *capsulatum*, there is usually little or no calcification in the caseous centres of coccidioidomas. With special fungus stains, *C. immitis* cells may be readily found in the central caseous material and occasionally within epithelioid and giant cells at the periphery. Even in old lesions, intact spherules with typical endospores may be seen. However, in our experience, empty and fragmented spherules are more commonly seen, but a few endospores and immature spherules may still be present. Giant cells may be found in and around these empty spherules, which are sometimes calcified. Although adequate for demonstrating intact spherules, the H&E stain is of little value for detecting small numbers of empty organisms. For this purpose, the GMS procedure is our stain of choice.

Hyphae can occasionally be found in the walls of pulmonary cavities and rarely within the caseous centres of fibrocaseous nodules in the lung and other organs[15]. Hyphae are usually mixed with typical round forms, but a spherule with characteristic endospores must be identified before coccidioidomycosis can be definitively diagnosed histologically.

Primary cutaneous coccidioidomycosis is rare and results from direct inoculation of the skin[16]. (Cutaneous lesions usually are a result of haematogenous dissemination.) Typically, there is a mixed purulent and granulomatous reaction in the dermis and subcutis. As is true for cutaneous blastomycosis, infection is usually associated with pronounced pseudoepitheliomatous hyperplasia of the overlying epidermis.

Empty spherules of *C. immitis* may be mistaken for large single cells of *B. dermatitidis* whose inner contents are absent or poorly stained. Serial sections must be carefully examined to demonstrate intact or ruptured spherules containing endospores. If typical spherules are not found, specific immunofluorescence can be a useful diagnostic tool. Because of similarity in size, the free endospores of *C. immitis* may also be confused with cells of *H. capsulatum* var. *capsulatum* and of *C. neoformans*. Again, sections should be examined for spherules of *C. immitis* containing endospores or for budding forms typical of the latter two fungi. In addition, Mayer's mucicarmine stain will readily demonstrate the mucopolysaccharide capsule of *C. neoformans*.

The novice may confuse the mature spherules of *C. immitis* with the sporangia of *Rhinosporidium seeberi*, with the endosporulating cells of the *Prototheca sp.*, or perhaps with the 'membrane-enclosed' spherical bodies in the phenomenon known as myospherulosis[17]. The mature sporangium of *R. seeberi* is much larger than the mature *C. immitis* spherule. The endospores of *R. seeberi* vary in size, stain entirely, contain globular bodies, and are usually smaller and flattened near the periphery. The endospores of *C. immitis* are round, and only their walls stain. The mature spherule of *C. immitis* is larger than that of the *Prototheca spp.*, and the endospores of the latter are less numerous, usually polyhedral instead of round, and larger.

The spherule-like structures ('myospherules') in the phenomenon termed 'myospherulosis' should not be confused with the spherules of *C. immitis*. The former are composed of round to polyhedral 'endobodies', 5–7 μm in diameter, within a membrane-like structure or 'parent body', 20–120 μm in overall diameter. Until recently, the nature of the 'myospherules', first described in cystic lesions in skeletal muscle of six Africans[18], was not definitely determined. However, in a recent study using histochemical and experimental methods[17], Rosai proved that the 'myospherules' are altered erythrocytes. These structures are reddish-brown when stained with H&E, but they are refractory to the GMS stain. This observation alone should readily differentiate 'myospherules' from the spherules and sporangia of the endosporulating fungi. 'Myospherules' are also positive with the various stains for haemoglobin.

References

1. Ajello, L. (1967). Comparative ecology of respiratory mycotic disease agents. *Bacteriol. Rev.* **31**, 6–24.
2. Huppert, M., Jung, H. S. and Bailey, J. W. (1967). Natural variability in Coccidioides immitis. In *Coccidioidomycosis*, pp. 323–328. Ajello, L., ed. University of Arizona Press, Tucson.
3. Sun, S. H., Huppert, M. and Vukovich, K. R. (1976). Rapid in vitro conversion and identification of Coccidioides immitis. *J. Clin. Microbiol.* **3**, 186–190.
4. Fiese, M. J. (1958). *Coccidioidomycosis.* Charles C. Thomas, Springfield, Illinois.
5. Kaplan, W. (1973). Epidemiology of the principal systemic mycoses of man and lower animals and the ecology of their etiologic agents. *J. Am. Vet. Med. Assoc.* **163**, 1043–1047.
6. Utz, J. P. (1967). Recent experience in the chemotherapy of the systemic mycoses. In *Coccidioidomycosis*, pp. 113–117. Ajello, L., ed. University of Arizona Press, Tucson.
7. Forbes, W. D. and Bestebreurtje, A. M. (1946). Coccidioidomycosis: A study of 95 cases of the disseminated type with special reference to the pathogenesis of the disease. *Milit. Surg.* **99**, 653–719.

8 Huppert, M. (1968). Recent developments in coccidioidomycosis. *Rev. Med. Vet. Mycol.* **6**, 279–294.
9 Maddy, K. T. (1960). Coccidioidomycosis. *Adv. Vet. Sci.* **6**, 251–286.
10 Straub, M., Trautman, R. J., Reed, R. E. and Schwarz, J. (1961). Canine coccidioidomycosis in Arizona. *Arch. Pathol.* **72**, 674–687.
11 Castellot, J. J., Creveling, R. L. and Pitts, F. W. (1960). Fatal miliary coccidioidomycosis complicating prolonged prednisone therapy in a patient with myelofibrosis. *Ann. Intern. Med.* **52**, 254–258.
12 Wilson, J. W. (1962). Factors which may increase the severity of coccidioidomycosis. *Lab. Invest.* **11**, 1146–1150.
13 Drutz, D. J. and Catanzaro, A. (1978). Coccidioidomycosis. Part I. *Am. Rev. Respir. Dis.* **117**, 559–585.
14 Drutz, D. J. and Catanzaro, A. (1978). Coccidioidomycosis. Part II. *Am. Rev. Respir. Dis.* **117**, 727–771.
15 Puckett, T. F. (1954). Hyphae of Coccidioides immitis in tissues of the human host. *Am. Rev. Tuberc.* **70**, 320–327.
16 Wilson, J. W., Smith, C. E. and Pluckett, D. A. (1953). Primary cutaneous coccidioidomycosis: The criteria for diagnosis and report of a case. *Calif. Med.* **79**, 233–239.
17 Rosai, J. (1978). The nature of myospherulosis of the upper respiratory tract. *Am. J. Clin. Pathol.* **69**, 475–481.
18 McClatchie, S., Warambo, M. W. and Bremner, A. D. (1969). Myospherulosis. A previously unreported disease? *Am. J. Clin. Pathol.* **51**, 699–704.

11 Cryptococcosis

(Torulosis, European blastomycosis, Busse-Buschke's disease)

Aetiologic agent:

Cryptococcus neoformans
Synonyms: *Saccharomyces neoformans, Cryptococcus hominis, Torula neoformans, Torula histolytica, Blastomyces neoformans*
(Perfect state: *Filobasidiella neoformans*)

Definition and background information

Basically cryptococcosis is a pulmonary disease of humans and lower animals caused by the soil-inhabiting basidiomycetous yeast, *Cryptococcus neoformans*[1, 2]. Clinically, the disease manifests itself in two basic forms: pulmonary cryptococcosis and, by dissemination, cerebral cryptococcosis. However, cutaneous, mucocutaneous, osseous, and visceral forms of the disease do develop through dissemination from the primary pulmonary focus.

A benign, asymptomatic form of cryptococcosis undoubtedly exists. But the absence of a sensitive, specific skin test antigen has prevented verification of its occurrence.

In tissues, *C. neoformans* develops as a budding yeast-like fungus whose unicellular cells are generally surrounded by a large capsule. Thus, when capsules are obvious, it can be readily distinguished from other fungi with a yeast-like tissue form, since they are not encapsulated; the unencapsulated fungi include *Blastomyces dermatitidis, Candida albicans, C. glabrata, Histoplasma capsulatum, H. farciminosum, Loboa loboi, Paracoccidioides brasiliensis* and *Sporothrix schenckii.*

Unencapsulated *C. neoformans* cells or those with small capsules produced by the so-called dry form can be identified by doing appropriate culture studies if the aetiologic agent is isolated, or by applying specific fluorescent antibody procedures to tissue sections or culture smears[3].

Symptomatic lung infections by *C. neoformans* do not have any pathognomonic features. The clinical manifestations include such signs as cough, malaise, weight loss, the raising of scant mucoid or bloody sputum, and pleuritic pain. Lung infections may be bilateral or unilateral. Radiography may reveal discrete, isolated areas of infiltration. In heavy infections the areas of infiltration are more diffuse or there may be marked peribronchial infiltrates. Cavitation, caseation, and calcification develop only rarely.

Because the symptomatology and roentgenological findings vary, a diagnosis of pulmonary cryptococcosis must be based on the demonstration of the yeast cells of *C. neoformans* in sputum or biopsied lung tissue. Their identity must be confirmed, whenever possible, by using appropriate cultural and biochemical tests or by the use of specific fluorescent antibody conjugates on smears and tissue sections[4, 5].

For reasons that are not understood, *C. neoformans* has a predilection for the central nervous system (CNS) and frequently metastasizes to the CNS from apparent or inapparent primary pulmonary infections. Headaches are the most frequent and dominating early symptoms of cerebral cryptococcosis. These may be intermittent or continuous with increasing degrees of severity. Vertigo and vomiting are other signs of CNS infection. Another common symptom is nuchal rigidity with associated tenderness of the skull and neck. Ocular disorders may develop as the result of increased cerebrospinal fluid pressure. These are expressed as anisocoria, diplopia, nystagmus and strabismus. Anorexia also is one of the consequences of CNS cryptococcosis. Loss of weight and strength may be so severe that intravenous feeding may be required.

Roentgenographic study of the skull may reveal a picture of an expanding intracranial lesion. Duration of the disease varies from a few days to 20 years or more. The course, however, is usually quite rapid and is characterised by increasing deterioration of the patient's condition. If untreated, CNS cryptococcosis is almost invariably fatal.

Definitive diagnosis of central nervous system cryptococcosis is based on demonstration of the cells of *C. neoformans* in spinal fluid or in biopsied or autopsied tissue and, whenever possible, by the isolation of *C. neoformans*[2].

Serological tests are of great value for the diagnosis of cryptococcosis. Those most commonly used are the latex agglutination test for cryptococcal polysaccharide antigen and the tube agglutination and indirect fluorescent antibody tests for *C. neoformans* antibodies. The latex agglutination test is the most specific of the three procedures and the most useful for detecting cryptococcal meningitis. This test has prognostic value since changes in titer are indicative of progression or regression of the disease during therapy. For maximum diagnostic coverage, the three tests should be used concurrently[6, 7].

Aside from the two basic types of cryptococcosis, cases with cutaneous manifestations also occur, generally in patients with disseminated pulmonary infections. The skin lesions are in the form of papules, pustules, or subcutaneous abscesses that have erupted through the skin. Since such lesions closely resemble those caused by other microorganisms, or other pathological conditions, diagnosis of cutaneous cryptococcosis must be based either on demonstration of cryptococcal cells in lesion exudate or biopsied tissue, or isolation of *C. neoformans*, or both.

Osseous and visceral involvement by *C. neoformans* occurs, and the disease must be differentiated from other pathological conditions.

Cryptococcosis has been recorded in a great diversity of lower animal species. With the exception of cattle, most of the affected lower animals have had a generalised form of the disease, which was fatal. Many of the animals also had CNS involvement. The vast majority of the bovine cases involved the mammary tissue and adjacent lymph nodes.

In the therapy of cryptococcosis, amphotericin B is the drug of choice, although 5-flurocytosine is effective in some patients with the disease.

In tissues, *C. neoformans* occurs in the form of large unicellular cells that vary in size from case to case, but diameters of 4–10 μm are the most commonly encountered. Typically, a clear spherical zone represents the yeast's capsule, which may have a diameter up to five times that of the yeast cell it surrounds.

Small lightly encapsulated strains of *C. neoformans* may present diagnostic problems since their cells may be confused with the tissue-form cells of *Histoplasma capsulatum* var. *capsulatum*, but careful search of a section may reveal capsulated forms. If they cannot be found, specific fluorescent antibody conjugates can be used to differentiate the unencapsulated cells of *C. neoformans* from morphologically similar yeast-like cells.

Isolation of *C. neoformans* from clinical materials generally is not difficult. It should be remembered, however, that this yeast is extremely sensitive to cycloheximide and that this antibiotic should not be used in isolation media when cryptococcus is suspected.

On Sabouraud dextrose agar, *C. neoformans* grows rapidly and develops a moist, mucoid white to pale yellow colony. Microscopic examination reveals that the colony is made up of spherical cells, 4–20 μm in diameter, that multiply by budding. One or more buds may be produced by the mother cell. Each cell is surrounded by a capsule that varies in size from isolate to isolate. It is best visualised by examining the cells in an India ink preparation[4]. Since the colonies and cells of *C. neoformans* cannot be distinguished from those of the saprophytic species of *Cryptococcus* and other yeasts on a morphological basis, specific identification must be based on appropriate biochemical and physiological tests[4] or by FA.

Mating studies by Kwon-Chung[1, 2] have shown that *C. neoformans* is a species whose sexual state reveals it to be a basidiomycete. The perfect state discovered was placed in the new genus *Filobasidiella* as *F. neoformans*. It is heterothallic.

Cryptococcus neoformans is widespread in nature throughout the world. It is most abundant in pigeon habitats and has been shown by surveys of pigeon nests to be present in both rural and urban areas[8, 10, 11]. Cryptococcosis is not a contagious disease. It is generally acquired by the inhalation of the infectious cells of *C. neoformans* that are produced in nature.

Histopathology (Figures 214–246)

In H&E-stained tissue sections, the yeast cells of *C. neoformans* stain pale blue to pink and range from 2–20 μm in diameter. They have relatively thin walls and are very pleomorphic, appearing round, oval, elliptical and crescent- or cup-shaped. Cells of many shapes and sizes often are present in a single microscopic field, and their internal details cannot be seen in such sections. Fungal cell walls may be fragmented, especially in granulomatous lesions where the cryptococci are predominantly intracellular. The mucopolysaccharide capsule, when obvious, appears as a smoothly contoured, clear, unstained space or 'halo' that surrounds the fungus cell. It does not stain with H&E. The capsules, when evident, vary from 2–10 μm or more in width. They may not be seen when the fungus cells are lightly encapsulated. The clear space in heavily encapsulated cryptococci is striking when fungal cells are seen within histiocytes and giant cells. The clear capsular zone clearly and uniformly separates the fungus cell from the host cell's cytoplasm.

When cryptococci with well-developed capsules are stained with Mayer's mucicarmine, the capsule is uniformly coloured a bright carmine red whereas the background tissue elements are stained blue or yellow, depending on the counterstain used. (The alcian blue procedure can also be used to stain the capsule). The stained capsule may have a spinous or scalloped appearance as the result of the irregular contraction of the capsular material during formalin fixation. Cryptococci are also well demonstrated with the special fungus stains that colour the entire fungal cell. In active lesions containing abundant fungus cells, budding is frequent. Single budding is common, but multiple budding may also be observed. Germ tubes and pseudohyphae are occasionally seen. However, mycelium has not been reported in tissue.

In humans and lower animals, *C. neoformans* may produce mucinous (hypo-reactive) or granulomatous lesions in the lungs, brain, spinal cord, meninges, adrenal glands, lymph nodes, mammary glands, bones, and other organs[12-19]. The number and distribution of fungal cells and the tissue response that they elicit vary from case to case. Underlying disease and immunosuppression may affect the type and degree of inflammation; disseminated miliary cryptococcosis may develop as a terminal infection in subjects with certain types of neoplasia[13]. However, disseminated lesions of cryptococcosis are also seen in the noncompromised or apparently normal host.

Primary lesions of cryptococcosis are most commonly found in the lungs as solid granulomatous or mucinous nodules. These nodular lesions range from 1–8 cm diameter. They are usually subpleural, solitary, and nonencapsulated[20]. When multiple, they may involve one or all lung lobes. Central necrosis and, at times, pulmonary cavitation may occur, but unlike the pulmonary nodules seen with histoplasmosis capsulati (Chapter 13), these lesions rarely calcify[12, 21-23].

Although any organ can be affected, disseminated cryptococcosis most commonly involves the brain and spinal cord, including the meninges[12, 24]. Lesions in the CNS may also be found without readily detectable lesions in the lungs or elsewhere in the body. Cutaneous and subcutaneous cryptococcosis may be primary or secondary and is usually seen as ulcerative gummatous lesions. If there is minimal inflammation in large tumourous masses of cryptococci in the subcutaneous tissues, the lesion may resemble a myxoma when sectioned and examined grossly.

The tissue reaction of the host to *C. neoformans* is very broad and may vary from little or no inflammation to a purely granulomatous reaction with varying degrees of necrosis. Often, it may be difficult to detect any tissue response at all. In these instances, the yeast cells of *C. neoformans* multiply profusely. They then displace the normal tissues and form a 'cystic' lesion filled with myriads of closely packed fungal cells whose wide mucoid capsules give the lesion a glistening appearance and slimy consistency on gross examination. This appearance is particularly striking in some cases of cryptococcal meningitis in which large masses of fungi in the leptomeninges displace the underlying brain parenchyma. Perivascular spaces in the brain may also be markedly distended by densely packed cryptococci. Inflammation within and surrounding the masses of cryptococci is usually minimal and consists of endothelial swelling, moderate perivascular cuffing with mononuclear cells, and small focal collections of mixed inflammatory cells. Irregular areas of haemorrhage and necrosis may also be seen in the brain parenchyma. In the lungs, the normal histologic architecture is often effaced by clusters of densely packed organisms that fill and compress alveoli[12, 20, 25]. The yeast cells are both free and contained within large alveolar macrophages or giant cells.

In other cases of cryptococcosis, there is either a purely granulomatous or a mixed purulent and granulomatous reaction with varying degrees of necrosis. In these lesions, most yeast cells are within multinucleated giant cells. Generally, poorly encapsulated intracellular cryptococci stimulate a granulomatous inflammatory reaction[26]. Cryptococcal granulomas are composed of varying numbers of histiocytes, giant cells, lymphocytes, plasma cells, neutrophils and fibroblasts. Although neutrophils may be present, they are not numerous, and the tissue response to cryptococci is typically nonsuppurative. Necrosis is not a common feature of the granulomas; when present, it is usually seen in fibrocaseous nodules or in conjunction with rapid proliferation of cryptococci. Huge foreign body and Langhans' giant cells may contain many fungal cells in a single plane of section. Histiocytes and giant cells often contain so many proliferating cryptococci that it is difficult to recognise the type of tissue response. Typically, the microscopic appearance is that of myriads of poorly stained cryptococci within phagocytes supported by a delicate stroma. Shields reported that at least some cryptococcal granulomas can mimic the epithelioid nodular lesions of sarcoidosis in humans[27].

Extensive necrosis, which is usually in the form of fibrocaseous pulmonary nodules, is sometimes seen in cryptococcosis and may be accompanied by varying degrees of inflammation and fibrosis. Cryptococci may be scarce and they are either diffusely scattered or clustered within the caseous material.

Baker[28] recently reported that a cryptococcal primary pulmonary lymph node complex representing first-infection cryptococcosis exists in approximately 1% of humans with this mycosis. He examined lungs and hilar lymph nodes at autopsy or after thoracotomy. In the normal or immunocompetent host, the complex consisted of a small granulomatous cryptococcoma in the lung and a focal granulomatous lymphadenitis. In the compromised host, he found a diffuse cryptococcal pneumonia and a diffuse cryptococcal lymphadenitis. Although the complex appears to be rare, it is now well-documented[29]. Its pathogenesis is very similar to that of first-infection tuberculosis.

Because *C. neoformans* varies greatly in size and shape, and its encapsulated forms are not always prominent, cryptococcosis should be considered in the histologic differential diagnosis of virtually any yeast infection. In most mucinous or 'cystic' lesions, encapsulated cryptococci are readily visible and can be identified in sections stained with H&E. However, their morphology can be studied in greater detail when the special fungus stains are used. Of these, we prefer the GMS or GMS-H&E procedures.

In solid cryptococcal granulomas, most of the yeast cells are intracellular and they may be small and scarce. Because of this, they may not be detected in H&E-stained sections and a diagnosis of a fungus infection will not be made. Very small, poorly encapsulated cryptococci ('dry' variants) are usually found in granulomatous lesions. In rare cases when the capsules of uniformly small 'dry' variants do not stain with mucicarmine, it may be very difficult to differentiate them from the yeast cells of *Histoplasma capsulatum* var. *capsulatum*[30], *Candida* (*Torulopsis*) *glabrata* and small forms of *Blastomyces dermatitidis*, even when the special fungus stains are used. In most instances, however, at least some cryptococci will have capsules that are histochemically detectable with the mucicarmine stain. This stain colours the capsular material a bright carmine red, and the cryptococci can therefore be differentiated from most other fungi that may morphologically resemble *C. neoformans*. *H. capsulatum* var. *capsulatum* is not carminophilic, and the walls of *B. dermatitidis* yeast cells are usually unstained or only faintly stained with mucicarmine.

Rarely, free endospores of *Rhinosporidium seeberi*, which are variably carminophilic, may be confused with cryptococcal cells. This is particularly true when typical sporangia of the former are not seen. When this occurs, serial sections should be examined for typical spherules of *R. seeberi* or for budding cells of *C. neoformans*. The endospores of *R. seeberi* do not bud and are not encapsulated. Because the morphology of the spherule of *R. seeberi* is so distinct, it is unlikely to be confused with *C. neoformans*.

C. neoformans, like *H. capsulatum* var. *capsulatum* and *Coccidioides immitis*, may form solitary or multiple fibrocaseous granulomas in the lungs. These lesions are often found incidentally at autopsy or are suspected of being neoplasms and are resected for histopathological evaluation. In fibrocaseous lesions, old distorted and degenerated cells of *C. neoformans* may stain poorly or not at all with the special fungus stains. In addition, the capsules of these cells may not be carminophilic. Fluorescent antibody tests are indicated when the carminophilic reaction is equivocal.

Smoothly contoured and spherical calcific bodies may occasionally be mistaken for cryptococci, especially when found in fibrocaseous pulmonary nodules and necrotic or granulomatous lesions in the central nervous system. The concentrically laminated lines in the outer portions of some calcific bodies may give the false appearance of a capsule or of 'doubly contoured' cell walls, and when these bodies appose each other they may be mistaken for budding yeast cells. Calcific bodies are variably stained with the H&E and PAS procedures but are usually refractory to the GMS stain. These bodies are also very pleomorphic and may contain multiple concentric rings that give them a 'bulls-eye' appearance. They usually stain deeply basophilic or amphophilic with H&E.

Corpora amylaceae are spherical bodies that are commonly seen in the central nervous system, primarily in the grey matter close to the pia mater or around blood vessels in the white matter of the brain and spinal cord. They should not be mistaken for cryptococci or other fungal cells. Corpora amylaceae have an average diameter of 15 μm and usually stain lightly basophilic with H&E. They are variably stained with the special fungus procedures, including GMS. Usually, corpora amylaceae contain a deeply basophilic and distinct central core as seen by H&E, and they are metachromatic with toluidine blue.

A diagnosis of cryptococcosis cannot always be based solely on the demonstration of budding yeast-form cells that appear to be surrounded by a clear zone in H&E-stained tissue sections. On occasion, we have seen adipose tissue (especially brown fat), vacuolated inflammatory cells, and even 'clear' cell neoplasms mistaken for mucinous lesions of cryptococcosis. Special fungus stains should always be used on replicate sections. Even though cryptococci are well-demonstrated with these stains, further studies with the Mayer's mucicarmine procedure may be warranted. This procedure will usually confirm the morphologic identification of yeast-like cells suspected of being *C. neoformans* in H&E-stained sections. When the capsule stains intensely with mucicarmine, a diagnosis of cryptococcosis can be made with confidence. It should be remembered that the amount of mucopolysaccharide capsular material and therefore the thickness of the capsule varies. In some cases, poorly encapsulated or 'dry' variants of *C. neoformans* may lack a histochemically detectable capsule, or the staining reaction may be so faint that it is equivocal. When budding yeast cells morphologically compatible with *C. neoformans* do not stain with mucicarmine, specific fluorescent antibody tests are indicated. These tests are the only means of making a definitive diagnosis in the absence of cultures.

References

1 Kwon-Chung, K. J. (1975). A new genus Filobasidiella, the perfect state of Cryptococcus neoformans. *Mycologia* **67**, 1197–1200.

2 Kwon-Chung, K. J. (1976). A new species of Filobasidiella, the sexual state of Cryptococcus neoformans B and C serotypes. *Mycologia* **68**, 942–946.

3 Kaplan, W. and Kraft, D. E. (1969). Demonstration of pathogenic fungi in formalin-fixed tissues by immunofluorescence. *Am. J. Clin. Pathol.* **52**, 420–432.

4 Silva-Hutner, M. and Cooper, B. H. (1974). Medically important yeasts. In *Manual of Clinical Microbiology,* 2nd ed. pp. 491–507. E. H. Lennette, E. H. Spaulding and J. P. Truant, eds. *Amer. Soc. Microbiol.*, Washington, D.C.

5 Kaplan, W. (1973). Direct fluorescent antibody tests for the diagnosis of mycotic diseases. *Ann. Clin. Lab. Sci.* **3**, 25–29.

6 Kaufman, L. and Blumer, S. (1978). Cryptococcosis: the awakening giant. In *The Black and White Yeasts,* pp. 176–182. Scientific Publication No. 356. Pan American Health Organization, Washington, D.C.

7 Palmer, D. F., Kaufman, L., Kaplan, W. and Cavallaro, J. J. (1977). *Serodiagnosis of Mycotic Diseases.* Charles C. Thomas, Springfield, Ill.

8 Ajello, L. (1967). Comparative ecology of respiratory mycotic disease agents. *Bacteriol. Rev.* **31**, 6–24.

9 Innes, J. R. M., Seibold, H. R. and Arentzen, W. P. (1952). The pathology of bovine mastitis caused by Cryptococcus neoformans. *Am. J. Vet. Res.* **13**, 469–475.

10 Hubalek, Z. (1975). Distribution of Cryptococcus neoformans in a pigeon habitat. *Folia Parasitol.* **22**, 73–79.

11 Ajello, L., Mantovani, A. and Mazzoni, A. (1967). La criptococcosi nell'uomo. *Parasitologia* **9**, 1–67.

12 Baker, R. D. and Haugh, R. K. (1955). Tissue changes and tissue diagnosis in cryptococcosis. A study of twenty-six cases. *Am. J. Clin. Pathol.* **25**, 14–24.

13 Lurie, H. I. and Duma, R. J. (1970). Opportunistic infections of the lungs. *Human Pathol.* **1**, 233–257.

14 Littman, M. L. and Walter, J. E. (1968). Cryptococcosis: current status. *Am. J. Med.* **45**, 922–932.

15 Barron, C. N. (1955). Cryptococcosis in animals. *J. Am. Vet. Med. Assoc.* **127**, 125–132.

16 Wagner, J. L., Pick, J. R. and Kirgman, M. R. (1968). Cryptococcus neoformans infection in a dog. *J. Am. Vet. Med. Assoc.* **153**, 945–949.

17 Garner, F. M., Ford, D. F. and Ross, M. A. (1969). Systemic cryptococcosis in two monkeys. *J. Am. Vet. Med. Assoc.* **155**, 1163–1168.

18 Olander, H. J., Reed, H. and Pier, A. C. (1963). Feline cryptococcosis. *J. Am. Vet. Med. Assoc.* **142**, 138–143.

19 Rubin, L. F. and Craig, P. H. (1965). Intraocular cryptococcosis in a dog. *J. Am. Vet. Med. Assoc.* **147**, 27–32.

20 Haugh, R. K. and Baker, R. D. (1954). The pulmonary lesions in cryptococcosis with special reference to subpleural nodules. *Am. J. Clin. Pathol.* **24**, 1381–1390.

21 Hawkins, J. A. (1961). Cavitary pulmonary cryptococcosis. *Am. Rev. Resp. Dis.* **84**, 579–581.

22 Cohen, A. A., Davis, W. and Finegold, S. M. (1965). Chronic pulmonary cryptococcosis. *Am. Rev Resp. Dis.* **91**, 414–423.

23 Tynes, B., Mason, K. N., Jennings, A. E. and Bennett, J. E. (1968). Variant forms of pulmonary cryptococcosis. *Ann. Intern. Med.* **69**, 1117–1125.

24 Katz, R. I., Birnbaum, H. and Eckmann, B. H. (1961). Resection of pulmonary cr ptococcosis associated with meningitis. *Am. Rev. Resp. Dis.* **84**, 725–729.

25 Kent, T. H. and Layton, J. M. (1962). Massive pulmonary cryptococcosis. *Am. J. Clin. Pathol.* **38**, 596–604.

26 Farmer, S. G. and Komorowski, R. A. (1973). Histologic response to capsule-deficient Cryptococcus neoformans. *Arch. Pathol.* **96**, 383–387.

27 Shields, L. H. (1959). Disseminated cryptococcosis producing a sarcoid type reaction. The report of a case treated with amphotericin B. *Arch. Intern. Med.* **104**, 763–770.

28 Baker, R. D. (1976). The primary pulmonary lymph node complex of cryptococcosis. *Am. J. Clin. Pathol.* **65**, 83–92.

29 Salyer, W. R., Salyer, D. C. and Baker, R. D. (1974). Primary complex of Cryptococcus and pulmonary lymph nodes. *J. Infect Dis.* **130**, 74–77.

30 Gutierrez, F., Fu, Y. S. and Lurie, H. I. (1975). Cryptococcus histologically resembling histoplasmosis. *Arch. Pathol.* **99**, 347–352.

12 Dermatophilosis

(Cutaneous streptothricosis, mycotic dermatitis, lumpy wool, strawberry foot rot)

Aetiologic agent:

Dermatophilus congolensis

Definition and background information

Dermatophilosis is a skin disease of lower animals and man caused by *Dermatophilus congolensis,* an actinomycete that produces motile spores called zoospores[1]. This disease is cosmopolitan in distribution.

D. congolensis is a facultative anaerobe that requires a rich medium for growth. On solid media, growth is apparent within 24–48 hours, depending upon the temperature of incubation. Growth is more rapid at 37°C than at room temperature. After one week at 37°C, colonies may attain a diameter of up to 4–6 mm depending upon the isolate and conditions of growth. Colonies vary in appearance. They may be rough or smooth with a shiny or dull surface. Colonies are usually greyish-white at first, becoming yellowish or orange with age. Microscopic examination of 24- to 48-hour-old colonies reveals the presence of branched, septate filaments, 0.5–1.5 μm in diameter. By the third day, or earlier, the filaments increase in diameter (3.0–5.0 μm wide) and divide transversely into narrow segments and then divide longitudinally two or more times, forming packets of coccoid spores that are up to 8 cells wide. The mature filaments break up, releasing the flagellated, motile coccoid zoospores. These spores germinate and form filaments that, when mature, produce zoospores as described. The microscopic morphology of *D. congolensis* in tissue is the same as that observed in culture. *D. congolensis* is gram-positive and is not acid-fast.

Dermatophilosis is a zoonotic disease. It may occur in man as a result of direct contact with infected animals[2,3]. The disease affects the skin, and self-limited lesions appear as nonpainful pustules containing a serous or whitish-yellow exudate. When expressed, this exudate leaves a reddish, shallow ulcer. Lesions remain active for a period of up to 14 days and then heal spontaneously. The incubation period can be as short as 2 days. In one unusual case, *D. congolensis* was incriminated as the agent of a chronic subcutaneous nodular disease in an 8-year-old boy[4].

Some investigators believe that *D. congolensis* is a cause of pitted keratolysis[5,6]. Pitted keratolysis[7] is a multifocal superficial erosion of the stratum corneum, usually limited to the heels and soles of the feet. Lesions appear in the form of pits that may coalesce and form irregularly shaped areas of superficial erosions. Pitted keratolysis occurs worldwide. Cases are more frequently encountered and are more severe in humid tropical and subtropical regions where rainfall is abundant and inhabitants habitually walk barefooted. Histological examination of affected skin shows that lesions are punched-out craters of the stratum corneum. In some pitted keratolysis cases, microorganisms closely resembling *D. congolensis* are observed within the pits and also invading the margins of the pits[5,6]. Attempts to recover *D. congolensis* from such lesions have been unsuccessful. In the absence of proof by culture, it may be premature to consider *D. congolensis* an agent of pitted keratolysis.

D. congolensis has a remarkably broad host range. Although it is most commonly found in cattle, sheep, and horses, it has been reported in goats, donkeys, dogs, domestic cats, deer, antelopes, zebras, swine, monkeys, raccoons, and a wide variety of other wild animal species. Except in the cats, the disease in lower animals characteristically appears as an exudative dermatitis, followed by the formation of scabs and crusts. Hairs or wool fibres are matted by the exudate and their bases are embedded in the crusts. As healing takes place, crusts and scabs separate from the underlying epithelium. They may then remain attached to the hair or wool fibres or fall away, leaving patches of alopecia. This disease is of economic importance in some countries where raising livestock is an important industry. Monetary losses are due principally to damage to hides, skins, and wool of infected animals. Loss in condition of affected animals, reduction in milk production, and fatalities further contribute to its economic importance[8].

Four feline cases have been recorded, and in each instance the infection involved tissues other than skin[9]. One case involved glossal muscle; another, the serosal surface of the urinary bladder; a third, the tongue; and a fourth, a popliteal lymph node. Diagnosis of the first three cases was based on the demonstration of the organism in sections of fixed tissue. The fourth case was diagnosed on histological grounds along with the recovery of *D. congolensis* in culture.

D. congolensis has to date been isolated only from clinical materials from infected animals and man. Attempts to recover the organism from environmental samples have been unsuccessful. Thus, available knowledge indicates that in most cases an infected animal serves as a source of infection for others. However, there is little information on methods of transmission of the infectious agent from one host to another. It has been found that humans can contract the disease by handling an infected animal. Whether direct contact is the mode of spread from animal to animal remains to be determined. That ticks or other arthropod vectors might play a role in spread of the disease has been postulated. Although the mode of spread remains to be fully established, some of the factors that predispose humans and animals to development of the disease have been determined. They include damage to the skin by prolonged wetting by rain, mechanical injuries such as scratches by thorns and abrasions by shearing instruments, and tick bites[8].

The usual approach to the treatment and control of dermatophilosis has been to apply topical medicaments either directly to the lesions or to the entire body in the form of dips or sprays. Although externally applied medicaments are often helpful in individual cases, none have been fully satisfactory for treatment and control of this disease. This failure is apparently due to inability of the medicaments to reach the organisms in crusts, scabs and other sites. It has been reported that injection of streptomycin and procaine penicillin together intramuscularly is effective for treating *D. congolensis* infections in domestic animals[10, 11].

Histopathology (Figures 247–261)

In dermatophilosis, infection is usually limited to the epidermis and hair follicles. Any portion of the body may be affected, and regional lymphadenitis is frequently seen. In general, the histopathologic features of cutaneous infections are similar in the various species of animals in which the disease has been documented[12–18]. For this reason, they will be described together.

Microscopically, sections of skin infected with *D. congolensis* reveal varying degrees of hyperkeratosis, parakeratosis, and acanthosis of the epidermis and hair follicles. Other epidermal changes that may be observed include intercellular edema, exocytosis, spongiosis, and ballooning degeneration that occasionally lead to the formation of intraepidermal abscesses and vesicles. Typically, the epidermis is covered by a thick scab composed of one to several alternating layers of cornified epithelial cells and inflammatory cell debris. In the early stages of infection, filaments of *D. congolensis* penetrate the epidermis. Roberts[15, 16] reported that such penetration was by mechanical force and that approximately 24 hours was required for filaments to penetrate perpendicularly as far as the dermal-epidermal junction. The epidermis is then separated from the underlying dermis by a layer of inflammatory exudate containing neutrophils, cellular debris, and amorphous proteinaceous material. Organisms do not usually penetrate the layer of exudate separating the infected epidermis from the dermis[12, 14]. In an attempt to regenerate, a new epidermal layer forms under the exudate while the overlying infected and detached epidermis cornifies and lyses. As soon as the new layer of regenerated epidermis is formed, it may be penetrated by peripheral growth of filaments of *D. congolensis* usually extending from adjacent infected hair follicles[12, 14–16]. The recently infected and regenerated epidermis is quickly separated from the dermis because of another inflammatory infiltrate, and a third epidermal layer is soon regenerated. This cycle of epidermal regeneration and reinfection may be repeated many times and may result in the formation of a very thick scab with alternating layers of inflammatory exudate and degenerated keratin. Such layers often can be seen with the naked eye when a tissue section is held up to the light.

Filaments of *D. congolensis* can invade and proliferate within all layers of the epidermis, but they are most numerous in the cornified layers. The septate filaments are branched, stain weakly basophilic with H&E, and divide in a characteristic multidimensional fashion, creating a 'stacked coin' appearance. Clusters of coccoid forms (zoospores) may also be seen. The detailed microscopic morphology of *D. congolensis* in culture as well as in tissue is given in the Definition and Background Information section of this chapter.

The dermal reaction to the presence of *D. congolensis* in the epidermis varies according to the stage of infection[13]. In the early stages, neutrophils usually predominate, with fewer lymphocytes and macrophages also being present. As the disease progresses, the neutrophils are gradually replaced by mononuclear cells and there may be some fibrosis. Some authors have reported a granulomatous response in the dermis where numerous epithelioid and multinucleated giant cells were seen in the absence of dermal invasion by *D. congolensis*[13]. In the specimens that we have examined, a granulomatous dermatitis was not observed.

In a large study involving 100 skin specimens taken by biopsy from 23 cattle with advanced dermatophilosis, Amakiri[12] found that organisms were located predominantly in the epidermis, especially in the stratum corneum, but on occasion were also observed in the papillary dermis. In many specimens, filaments often penetrated to the basement membrane of the epidermis (dermo-epidermal interface) and infiltrated hair follicles and sebaceous glands. The affected sebaceous glands were usually contiguous to heavily infected hair follicles whose walls were frequently ruptured. From the rupture sites, organisms were seen invading the papillary dermis. This mechanism of dermal invasion was also reported by Roberts[15,16] and Jubb and Kennedy[14]. Organisms were also seen in the papillary layer of the dermis in focal areas where the basement membrane of the epidermis was destroyed. In these instances, organisms were very close to the disintegrated basement membrane, and the overlying epidermis was usually eroded. Little or no inflammatory reaction was associated with the presence of *D. congolensis* in the dermis. Mycelium was never seen in the dermis when the overlying basement membrane was intact. From these studies, it is apparent that the epidermal basement membrane serves as a barrier to the downward growth of *D. congolensis* into the papillary dermis. No ducts or bodies of sweat glands, blood vessels, or lymphatics were found to be invaded by *D. congolensis*.

Organisms morphologically and tinctorially identical to *D. congolensis* were reported in granulomatous lesions of 4 cats in sites other than the skin[9,19,20]. (See Definition and Background Information). In one culturally confirmed case, lesions were observed in a lymph node and consisted of irregularly circumscribed areas of necrosis, each of which contained a tangled mass of gram-positive, branched filaments morphologically compatible with *D. congolensis*. The necrotic areas were surrounded by neutrophils and fewer mononuclear inflammatory cells. Epithelioid or multinucleated giant cells were not seen. In the other 3 cats, lesions consisted of granulomas surrounded by concentric layers of dense fibrous tissue. The granulomas were composed of a central necrotic zone surrounded by degenerating neutrophils which were in turn enclosed by epithelioid cells and lymphocytes. Masses of filamentous organisms morphologically compatible with *D. congolensis* were confined exclusively to the necrotic centres of the granulomas.

A diagnosis of dermatophilosis can be made by demonstrating typical branched, septate filaments of *D. congolensis* undergoing multidimensional division. In H&E-stained tissue sections, organisms are weakly basophilic and can usually be seen and identified if diligently searched for and if well stained with haematoxylin. However, filaments and coccoid forms are best demonstrated with the Gram and Giemsa stains. With these procedures, organisms stain uniformly and contrast sharply against a pale background. They are predominantly gram-positive (rarely, coccoid forms or zoospores are gram-negative) and appear as chains of flattened organisms ('stacked coins', coccoid forms); the characteristic multidimensional division is clearly delineated. In our experience, Wolbach's Giemsa stain has been most useful for demonstrating *D. congolensis*. Whenever possible, histologic studies should be complemented by cultural isolation.

Pitted keratolysis, originally called 'keratoma plantare sulcatum'[21] is a disease of humans in which there is focal erosion of the stratum corneum, usually on the soles and heels of the feet[6,7,22,23]. This condition is caused by superficial infection with organisms that in many cases may be morphologically and tinctorially similar to *D. congolensis*. Histologic examination of the focal erosions or pits under low magnification reveal that they are punched-out craters with sharply defined vertical walls[24]. Usually, the pits do not penetrate beyond the stratum corneum. Individual pits range from 0.5–3.0 mm in diameter when sectioned in their equatorial plane. However, if the lesions are severe, they may coalesce and form large irregularly shaped areas of superficial erosions. At higher magnification, branched, septate, filaments which are 0.5–1.5 μm in diameter and which stain basophilic with H&E can be seen embedded within the keratin lining the bottom and vertical walls of the pit. The filaments are predominantly gram-positive, are non acid-fast, and divide both transversely and longitudinally to form coccoid bodies. Masses of coccoid bodies not associated with filaments may be observed near or on the surface of the pit. Such bodies may on occasion form delicate germ tubes. In some pits that we have examined, an irregular and granular layer of brownish opaque material that probably represented soil was present on the surface of the keratin.

In H&E-stained skin sections, a diagnosis of pitted keratolysis can be made by demonstrating typical forms of *D. congolensis*-like organisms invading the margins of pits as described above. The organisms stain well with the Giemsa and tissue Gram stains, and we recommend that these procedures be used for studying the filaments and coccoid bodies in detail. Organisms are also variably stained with the GMS procedure. However, they are refractory to the PAS and GF procedures.

References

1 Gordon, M. A. (1964). The genus Dermatophilus. *J. Bacteriol.* **88**, 509–522.

2 Dean, D. J., Gordon, M. A., Severinghaus, C. W., Kroll, E. T. and Reilly, J. R. (1961). Streptothricosis: A new zoonotic disease. *N.Y. State J. Med.* **61**, 1283–1287.

3 Kaminski, G. W. and Suter, I. J. (1976). Human infection with Dermatophilus congolensis. *Med. J. Aust.* **1**, 443–447.

4 Albrecht, R., Horowitz, S., Gilvert, E., Hong, R., Richard, J. and Connor, D. H. (1974). Dermatophilus congolensis chronic nodular disease in man. *Pediatrics* **53**, 907–912.

5 Rubel, L. R. (1972). Pitted keratolysis and Dermatophilus congolensis. *Arch. Dermatol.* **105**, 584–586.

6 Gordon, H. H. (1975). Pitted keratolysis, forme fruste: A review and new therapies. *Cutis.* **15**, 54–58.

7 Zaias, N., Taplin, D. and Rebell, G. (1965). Pitted keratolysis. *Arch. Dermatol.* **92**, 151–154.

8 Ainsworth, G. C. and Austwick, P. K. C. (1973). *Fungal Diseases of Animals,* 2nd ed. Review Series No. 6, pp. 135–144. Commonwealth Agricultural Bureau, Farnham, Slough, England.

9 Jones, R. T. (1976). Subcutaneous infection with Dermatophilus congolensis in a cat. *J. Comp. Pathol.* **86**, 415–421.

10 Roberts, D. S. (1967). Chemotherapy of epidermal infection with Dermatophilus congolensis. *J. Comp. Pathol.* **77**, 129–136.

11 Le Roux, J. D. (1968). The treatment of "lumpy wool", Dermatophilus congolensis infection on Merino sheep with streptomycin and penicillin. *J. S. Afr. Vet. Med. Assoc.* **39**, 87–88.

12 Amakiri, S. F. (1976). Anatomical location of Dermatophilus congolensis in bovine cutaneous streptothricosis. In *Dermatophilus Infection in Animals and Man,* pp. 163–171. D. H. Lloyd and K. C. Sellers, eds. Academic Press, New York.

13 Oduye, O. O. (1976). Histopathological changes in natural and experimental Dermatophilus congolensis infection of the bovine skin. In *Dermatophilus Infection in Animals and Man,* pp. 172–181. D. H. Lloyd and K. C. Sellers, eds. Academic Press, New York.

14 Jubb, K. V. F. and Kennedy, P. C. (1970). *Pathology of Domestic Animals,* vol. 2, pp. 606–607. Academic Press, New York.

15 Roberts, D. S. (1965). The histopathology of epidermal infection with the actinomycete Dermatophilus congolensis. *J. Pathol. Bacteriol.* **90**, 213–216.

16 Roberts, D. S. (1967). Dermatophilus infection. *Vet. Bull.* **37**, 513–521.

17 Bridges, C. H. and Romane, W. M. (1961). Cutaneous streptothricosis in cattle. *J. Am. Vet. Med. Assoc.* **138**, 153–157.

18 Bentinck-Smith, J., Fox, F. H. and Baker, D. W. (1961). Equine dermatitis (cutaneous streptothricosis) infection with Dermatophilus in the U.S. *Cornell Vet.* **51**, 334–349.

19 O'Hara, P. J. and Cordes, D. O. (1963). Granulomata caused by Dermatophilus in two cats. *N.Z. Vet. J.* **11**, 151–154.

20 Baker, G. J., Breeze, R. G. and Dawson, C. O. (1972). Oral dermatophilosis in a cat. *J. Small Anim. Practice* **13**, 649–653.

21 Castellani, A. (1910). Keratoma plantare sulcatum. *J. Ceylon Brit. Med. Assoc.* **7**, 10.

22 Gill, K. A., Jr. (1968). Pitted keratolysis. *Arch. Dermatol.* **98**, 7–11.

23 Lamberg, S. I. (1969). Symptomatic pitted keratolysis. *Arch. Dermatol.* **100**, 10–11.

24 Connor, D. H. and Neafie, R. C. (1976). Pitted keratolysis. In *Pathology of Tropical and Extraordinary Diseases, An Atlas*, vol. 2, pp. 678–680. C. H. Binford and D. H. Connor, eds. Armed Forces Institute of Pathology, Washington, D.C.

13 Histoplasmosis capsulati†

(Classical histoplasmosis, Small-form histoplasmosis, Darling's disease, Tingo Maria fever)

Aetiologic agent:

Histoplasma capsulatum var. *capsulatum*
(Perfect state: *Ajellomyces capsulatus*, Syn. *Emmonsiella capsulata*)

Definition and background information

Histoplasmosis, a systemic mycotic disease of man and lower animals, occurs as: (a) the classic or small-celled* type with a global distribution and (b) the large-celled* type, apparently confined to the African continent and frequently referred to as African histoplasmosis. The classical type is caused by the *capsulatum* variety of *Histoplasma,* and the large-celled form is caused by the variety *duboisii.* Because these two forms of the disease are distinct clinical and histological entities, they are assigned separate chapters in this Atlas (see 'Histoplasmosis Duboisii'). The equine disease caused by *H. farciminosum* is described in the chapter entitled 'Histoplasmosis Farciminosi'.

Basically, histoplasmosis capsulati is a respiratory disease contracted by inhaling airborne infectious spores of *H. capsulatum* var. *capsulatum* originating in soil. The primary sources of almost all such infections are avian and chiropteran habitats that favour the growth and multiplication of this fungus[1]. The most common and widespread types of histoplasmosis capsulati can be characterised in four clinical categories[2]:

1 Asymptomatic Form
Epidemiologists have estimated that 90–95% of all histoplasmosis capsulati infections are of this type. Victims have no overt symptoms, do not feel ill, and hence do not seek or require medical attention. However, they do react positively in skin tests with histoplasmin, and in time develop multiple lung calcifications.

2 Acute Pulmonary Form
Individuals in this category develop flu-like pulmonary symptoms including fever, malaise, chest pains, cough, myalgia, chills, and weight loss. The severity and duration of this form of histoplasmosis depend upon host resistance and the number of fungus spores inhaled. X-ray studies reveal diffuse nodular densities in the lungs. Most cases of acute histoplasmosis occur in individuals exposed to aerosols of *H. capsulatum* var. *capsulatum* spores from disturbed blackbird roosts, chicken coops, or other avian habitats, or areas such as caves and attics where bat guano has accumulated. The incubation period is about 15 days. Most cases of acute histoplasmosis resolve with bed rest and other supportive therapy, but specific therapy with amphotericin B is sometimes required.

3 Disseminated Form
In a minority of the patients with acute pulmonary histoplasmosis, infections do not remain localised but disseminate throughout the body by way of the reticuloendothelial system and set up foci of infection in various vital organs. As expected, symptoms associated with infections of this third category are more severe than those associated with the two already discussed. In addition to the symptoms described for acute histoplasmosis, patients may develop leukopenia, anemia, progressive hepatomegaly and splenomegaly. The fatality rate is potentially great for patients with disseminated histoplasmosis, and treatment with amphotericin B is imperative. Before the advent of amphotericin B, mortality was high and the duration of the disease ranged from 1–30 months[3].

4 Chronic Pulmonary Form
This is a disease primarily of adults between the ages of 26 and 70 years. It may immediately follow the acute form of the disease or become clinically apparent after long dormancy. The symptoms most often associated with the development of

---

†In the interest of clarity, brevity and uniformity, we are coining the terms histoplasmosis capsulati and histoplasmosis farciminosi for infections caused by *H. capsulatum* var. *capsulatum* and *H. farciminosum* respectively. The precedent for this nomenclature was set in 1964 by Cockshott and Lucas[26], when they created the name histoplasmosis duboisii for infections by *H. capsulatum* var. *duboisii.*

*The terms 'small form' and 'large form' refer to the relative sizes of the yeast-like cells of the two fungus varieties in host tissue.

chronic, pulmonary histoplasmosis are cough, weight loss, dyspnea, fever, chest pain, and haemoptysis. Patients frequently develop unilateral cavities in the apex or subapical region of the lungs[3].

The diagnosis of histoplasmosis capsulati is based on demonstration of the unicellular (2–4 μm D) yeast-like form of the fungus in tissue with histological and fluorescent-antibody procedures, on results of appropriate serological tests on sera, and ideally on the isolation and identification of *H. capsulatum* var. *capsulatum*[4–5].

Colonies of *H. capsulatum* var. *capsulatum* are downy in texture and are white to golden-brown. Two types of asexual conidia are produced: macroconidia and microconidia. The diagnostic macroconidia are large (8–14 μm D), thick-walled, and covered with digitate protuberances that vary in length and diameter. These macroconidia are sometimes mistakenly referred to as chlamydospores. As the name implies, the smooth-surfaced microconidia are small, ranging in size from 2–4 μm.

H. capsulatum var. *capsulatum* is a dimorphic fungus that can be altered from mycelial to yeast form in vitro or in experimental animals. The unicellular organisms, produced at 37°C on rich media, are similar in form and size to those found in infected tissue. Attempts to transform the mycelial growth to the yeast form in vitro may require repeated trials or may continue to be unsuccessful. Such isolates, or atypical ones, may be identified with a serological procedure developed to identify fungus cultures[6].

Sexual reproduction has also been reported for this fungus[7]. It has been found to be a heterothallic ascomycete. The perfect stage was originally named *Emmonsiella capsulata* but was transferred to the genus *Ajellomyces* as *A. capsulatus* by McGinnes and Katz in 1979[8].

Lower animals of many genera and species are victims of *H. capsulatum* var. *capsulatum*. Dogs are among the most susceptible of the domestic animals, but cases have also been recorded among cats, cattle, horses, and swine. The list of wild or captive animal species that have contracted this type of histoplasmosis includes various rodents, badgers, bats, foxes, raccoons, skunks, and a kodiak bear in a zoo[9, 10]. No infections among amphibians, reptiles, or birds have been reported. There is no evidence that the disease is contagious. All victims, animal or human, are infected by the spores of *H. capsulatum* var. *capsulatum* that originate in soil.

Histopathology (Figures 262–294)

After the spores of *H. capsulatum* var. *capsulatum* have been inhaled, the primary active lesion begins as a patchy bronchopneumonia in which clusters of yeast-laden macrophages and giant cells fill the alveolar spaces[11, 12]. In the later stages of the disease various tissue responses may develop. These may be characterised by marked proliferation of histiocytes or by the development of epithelioid and giant cell granulomas with or without central caseation. Cavitary lesions may also develop[13]. In all of these lesions, yeast-form cells of *H. capsulatum* var. *capsulatum* occur both intracellularly and extracellularly. Many small lesions resolve completely or heal by fibrosis. However, in the characteristic method of healing, the larger granulomas become fibrocaseous nodules which frequently calcify and remain indefinitely (discussed later in chapter).

In both the asymptomatic and acute pulmonary forms of histoplasmosis capsulati, granulomas with or without necrotic centres usually develop in the immune host. These granulomas commonly contain Langhans' giant cells and cannot be differentiated from those of active tuberculosis in H&E-stained tissue sections. There are, however, some important differences in the two diseases. Histoplasmosis capsulati commonly begins as widely disseminated lung lesions accompanied by massive involvement of the hilar lymph nodes. This picture is only rarely seen in tuberculosis. Another difference is the greater tendency of the lesions of histoplasmosis capsulati to become calcified. In the latter, there is frequently a greater incidence of multiple lesions in the spleen. Noncaseous granulomas in histoplasmosis capsulati may also be confused with those seen in sarcoidosis unless special fungus stains are used to demonstrate the organisms[14, 15].

In disseminated histoplasmosis capsulati, the most severe and life-threatening form, all tissues of the body except cartilage and cortical bone can be affected. Most commonly involved are the lungs, lymph nodes, spleen, liver, bone marrow, gastrointestinal tract, and adrenals – organs with abundant reticuloendothelial (RE) cells[11, 12, 16]. Microscopically, the tissue-form cells of *H. capsulatum* var. *capsulatum* are almost always seen within the cytoplasm of large RE cells (fixed and wandering macrophages) – hence the designation 'histiocytomycotic' or 'reticuloendothelial cytomycotic' disease[11]. Other yeast cells are probably released from ruptured RE cells. (In peripheral blood smears, yeast cells may rarely be seen in monocytes[17]). Marked infiltration and proliferation of histiocytes in many organs often obliterates normal architecture. Bland necrosis, resembling that seen in some neoplasms, may occur in any organ. For example, necrosis of the adrenals due to histiocytic proliferation commonly causes symptoms of Addison's disease[18]. There is little tendency for encapsulation of lesions, and clusters of yeast-laden histiocytes can be seen without any other inflammatory response. Lymphocytes and plasma cells may be present, but polymorphonuclear leucocytes are rare. In general, cells of *H. capsulatum* var. *capsulatum* grow within masses of histiocytes in the immunologically compromised or nonimmune host, whereas the fungus elicits an epithelioid and giant cell granulomatous reaction with or without caseous necrosis in the immune host.

A diagnosis of histoplasmosis capsulati can usually be made when large histiocytes packed with yeast cells are demonstrated in H&E-stained sections. Each yeast cell appears as a central, spherical, lightly basophilic body surrounded by a clear zone or 'halo' which, in turn, is encircled by a thin, poorly stained cell wall. (Many have interpreted the clear zone as a nonstaining capsule, but the tissue form of *H. capsulatum* var. *capsulatum* is not encapsulated.) With the H&E stain, each yeast cell appears much smaller than when stained with the special fungus procedures because the cell wall is not delineated and the readily stained cytoplasm is retracted to give the appearance of a capsule. The cell wall of *H. capsulatum* var. *capsulatum* is readily stained with the GMS, PAS, and GF procedures, and the fungi appear as small, round or oval, yeast-like cells 2–5 μm in diameter. They produce single buds that are attached to the parent cell by a narrow base. With these stains, the 'halo' is not evident. In Giemsa- or Wright-stained preparations, a pale, light blue ring, which indicates the fungus cell wall, surrounds the darker blue of the cell protoplasm. A clear space is usually seen between the protoplasmic mass and the cell wall. Darker violet staining chromatin material appears as an oval, half-moon to crescent-shaped mass within the protoplasm.

Most patients with active *H. capsulatum* var. *capsulatum* lesions usually recover without the disease having been recognised until old 'healed' necrotic lesions are noted as an incidental finding at autopsy or at biopsy to rule out malignancy. These lesions have been variously termed 'tuberculomas', histoplasmomas, fibrocaseous nodules, and burned-out granulomas[11, 19, 22]. They are usually located in the lungs just beneath the pleura and are less frequently found in the spleen, liver, lymph nodes, and other organs. Microscopically, the nodule consists of a caseous, often irregularly calcified centre surrounded by a thick fibrotic capsule that may contain scattered mononuclear and multinucleated giant cells. If present, fungal cells are within the caseous material as extracellular forms; they appear singly or in clusters, the latter due to their intracellular confinement before death of their host cells. The yeast-form cells are almost impossible to demonstrate with the H&E stain. However, a careful search in the central caseous material stained with the GMS procedure usually reveals small numbers of yeast cells that are generally distorted and poorly stained ('ghost' forms). Fragments of yeast cells may be seen, as may large, bizarrely shaped fungus cells and short hyphal forms. (Hyphal forms are also rarely found in pulmonary cavities and thrombi of heart valves[11, 23].) Not every fibrocaseous nodule will contain fungus cells, and serial sections may be necessary to search for them thoroughly. We prefer the GMS method for demonstrating these presumably dead organisms because it provides excellent contrast, often stains the entire yeast cell, and does not stain calcified debris that may mimic fungus cells. The PAS and GF stains are less dependable because they do not stain the internal portions of the yeast cells. With these stains, organisms usually appear as empty rings, or they may not be visible at all. The PAS procedure readily stains calcified debris that may mimic yeast forms.

Lightly encapsulated, small *Cryptococcus neoformans* cells, growing within histiocytes, epithelioid cells, or giant cells, mimic the intracellular forms of *H. capsulatum* var. *capsulatum* and present a diagnostic challenge to the pathologist[24]. It is possible for the mucicarmine stain to be completely negative for certain poorly encapsulated cells of *C. neoformans*. In those instances, the direct FA procedure is invaluable for establishing a diagnosis. The tissue form cells of *H. capsulatum* var. *capsulatum* must also be differentiated from those of *Sporothrix schenckii,* which are usually intracellular and have similar staining and morphological features. Here, specific FA conjugates are also needed to establish a diagnosis. Yeast cells of *S. schenckii* are generally sparsely distributed. Small tissue forms of *Blastomyces dermatitidis* may be confused with the tissue form cells of *H. capsulatum* var. *capsulatum,* but the former are usually larger, bud on a broader base, and are often mixed with *B. dermatitidis* cells of normal size. In tissue, *Candida* (*Torulopsis*) *glabrata* cells may be easily confused with those of *H. capsulatum* var. *capsulatum* because they are comparable in size and both may occur intracellularly. *C. glabrata* cells often are slightly larger than those of *H. capsulatum* var. *capsulatum,* oval to elongated yeast forms of *C. glabrata* are common, budding occurs with greater frequency, and buds are usually attached by a broader base. Released endospores of *Coccidioides immitis* can be confused with the yeast cells of *H. capsulatum* var. *capsulatum,* but the tissue response to the endospores is usually suppurative. One must search for spherules or remnants of spherules in order to identify *C. immitis* positively.

Although intracellular *H. capsulatum* var. *capsulatum* yeast cells can be seen in H&E-stained sections viewed under medium power, definitive identification should be made under the oil immersion objective. For example, intracellular forms of the protozoan *Leishmania donovani* appear similar to the tissue-form cells of *H. capsulatum* var. *capsulatum,* and only under oil immersion can the bar-shaped kinetoplast be seen in the *L. donovani* cells. The *H. capsulatum* yeast cells have no such structure. The cysts of *Toxoplasma gondii* may mimic intracellular tissue-form cells of *H. capsulatum* var. *capsulatum*, but under oil immersion the *T. gondii* cells are slightly smaller and lack a clear zone around each organism. The special fungus stains do not stain the cells of these two protozoans.

In equines, the tissue-form cells of *H. farciminosum*, the aetiologic agent of histoplasmosis farciminosi (epizootic lymphangitis; see Chapter 15), cannot be differentiated from those of *H. capsulatum* var. *capsulatum* in sections[25]. Therefore, a differential diagnosis must be based on results of cultural studies.

References

1 Ajello, L. (1967). Comparative ecology of respiratory mycotic disease agents. *Bacteriol. Rev.* **31**, 6–24.

2 Vanek, J. and Schwarz, J. (1971). The gamut of histoplasmosis. *Am. J. Med.* **50**, 89–104.

3 Reddy, P., Gorelick, D. F., Brasher, C. A. and Larsh, H. (1970). Progressive disseminated histoplasmosis as seen in adults. *Am. J. Med.* **48**, 629–635.

4 Ajello, L., Georg, L. K., Kaplan, W. and Kaufman, L. (1970). Mycotic infections. In *Diagnostic Procedures for Bacterial, Mycotic and Parasitic Infections,* 5th ed. H. L. Bodily, E. L. Updyke and J. O. Mason, eds. *Am. Public Health Assoc.* New York.

5 Palmer, D., Kaufman, L., Kaplan, W. and Cavallero, J. (1978). *Serodiagnosis of Mycotic Diseases.* Charles C. Thomas, Springfield.

6 Standard, P. G. and Kaufman, L. (1976). Specific immunological test for the rapid identification of members of the genus Histoplasma. *J. Clin. Microbiol.* **3**, 191–199.

7 Kwon-Chung, K. J. (1972). Emmonsiella capsulata: Perfect state of Histoplasma capsulatum. *Science* **177**, 368–369.

8 McGinnis, M. R. and Katz, B. (1979). Ajellomyces and its synonym Emmonsiella. *Mycotaxon* **8**, 157–164.

9 Menges, R. W., Habermann, R. T., Selby, L. A., Ellis, H. R., Behlow, R. F. and Smith, C. D. (1963). A review and recent findings on histoplasmosis in animals. *Vet. Med.* **58**, 331–338.

10 Menges, R. W., Furcolow, M. L., Habermann, R. T. and Weeks, R. J. (1967). Epidemiologic studies on histoplasmosis in wildlife. *Environ. Res.* **1**, 129–144.

11 Binford, C. H. (1955). Histoplasmosis: Tissue reactions and morphologic variations of the fungus. *Am. J. Clin. Pathol.* **25**, 25–36.

12 Rowley, D. A., Haberman, R. T. and Emmons, C. W. (1954). Histoplasmosis: Pathologic studies of fifty cats and fifty dogs from Loudoun County, Virginia. *J. Infect. Dis.* **95**, 98–108.

13 Chick, W. E., Dillon, M. L. and Tahanasab, A. (1977). Acute cavitary histoplasmosis. *Chest* **71**, 674–676.

14 Pinkerton, H. and Iverson, L. (1952). Histoplasmosis: Three fatal cases with disseminated sarcoid-like lesions. *Arch. Intern. Med. (Chicago)* **90**, 456–467.

15 Walker, J. V., Baran, D., Yakub, N. and Freeman, R. B. (1977). Histoplasmosis with hypercalcemia, renal failure, and papillary necrosis. Confusion with sarcoidosis. *J. Am. Med. Assoc.* **237**, 1350–1352.

16 Sarosi, G. A., Voth, D. W., Dahl, B. A., Doto, I. L. and Tosh, F. E. (1971). Disseminated histoplasmosis: Results of long-term follow-up. *Ann. Intern. Med.* **75**, 511–516.

17 Girard, D. E., Fred, H. L., Bradshaw, M. W., Blakely, R. W. and Ettlinger, R. (1977). Disseminated histoplasmosis diagnosed from peripheral blood film. *South. Med. J.* **70**, 65–66.

18 Crispell, K. R., Parson, W., Hamlin, J. and Hollifield, G. (1956). Addison's disease associated with histoplasmosis: Report of four cases and review of the literature. *Am. J. Med.* **20**, 23–29.

19 Baker, R. D. (1964). Histoplasmosis in routine autopsies. *Am. J. Clin. Pathol.* **41**, 457–470.

20 Goodwin, R. A., Jr. and Snell, J. D. (1969). The enlarging histoplasmoma. *Am. Rev. Resp. Dis.* **100**, 1–12.

21 Goodwin, R. A., Jr., Owens, F. T., Snell, J. D., Hubbard, W. W., Buchanan, R. D., Terry, R. T. and Des Prez, R. M. (1976). Chronic pulmonary histoplasmosis. *Medicine (Baltimore)* **55**, 413–452.

22 Puckett, T. K. (1953). Pulmonary histoplasmosis; A study of twenty-two cases with the identification of Histoplasma capsulatum in resected tissues. *Am. Rev. Tuberc.* **67**, 453–476.

23 Canlas, M. S. and Dillon, M. L., Jr. (1977). Histoplasma capsulatum endocarditis: Report of a case following heart surgery. *Angiology* **28**, 454–463.

24 Gutierrez, F., Fu, Y. S. and Lurie, H. I. (1975). Cryptococcosis histologically resembling histoplasmosis. A light and electron microscopical study. *Arch. Pathol.* **99**, 347–352.

25 Panciera, R. J. (1969). Histoplasmic (Histoplasma capsulatum) infection in a horse. *Cornell Vet.* **59**, 306–312.

26 Cockshott, W. P. and Lucas, A. O. (1964). Histoplasmosis duboisii. *Quart. J. Med.* **33**, 223–238.

14 Histoplasmosis duboisii

(African histoplasmosis, Large-form histoplasmosis)

Aetiologic agent:

Histoplasma capsulatum var. *duboisii*
(Common synonym: *Histoplasma duboisii*)
(Perfect state: *Ajellomyces capsulatus,* Syn. *Emmonsiella capsulata*)

Definition and background information

As stated in the previous chapter on histoplasmosis capsulati, the duboisii form of histoplasmosis is essentially confined to the African continent. As of 1976, 162 cases of histoplasmosis duboisii had been described and published[1]. Human and simian cases (*Papio cynocephalus* and *P. papio*) have been confirmed in 20 of the 50 African republics (Angola, Benin, Cameroon, Chad, Congo, Gambia, Ghana, Guinea, Guinea Bissau, Ivory Coast, Malawi, Mali, Niger, Nigeria, Senegal, Tanzania, Uganda, Upper Volta and Zaire[2–10]. One autochthonous case of histoplasmosis duboisii, however, was reported from Japan[11].

Histoplasmosis duboisii* must be considered to be basically a pulmonary disease with a marked tropism for the bones and skin[12]. Clark and Greenwood[14] described two patients with pulmonary involvement and cited ten other cases from the literature with evidence of pulmonary lesions. Chest X-rays of the two patients showed diffuse changes in both lung fields. At autopsy, granulomas with caseous centres were present in the lungs. Schwarz[12] points out that 'pulmonary lesions can be found in subjects with African histoplasmosis if searched for with proper knowledge and open mind'. Nevertheless, pulmonary lesions continue to be rarely reported.

The cardinal signs of the disease, as summarised by Renoirte et al.[13], are lymphadenopathy and skin and bone lesions. Most patients are found to have one or more of these conditions when diagnosed. Cervical, axillary, and inguinal lymph nodes become swollen and evolve into cold abscesses that may drain. Skin lesions manifest themselves as papules that abscess and eventually ulcerate. Osteolytic bone lesions may be insidious, for they may remain silent. Almost any bone may be affected by *H. capsulatum* var. *duboisii,* but the most frequently attacked are the ribs, the long bones of the legs and arms, and the cranium. The fungus may also disseminate, presumably from the lungs, to such parts of the body as the liver, spleen, and intestines. Chronic forms of the disease have been reported in which the infection persisted for several decades[14].

Histoplasmosis duboisii is distinguished from histoplasmosis capsulati on the basis of the size of the aetiologic agent's cells in tissue. The diagnostic, yeast-like tissue-form cells of *H. capsulatum* var. *duboisii* are large, moderately thick-walled and measure 8–15 μm D. In contrast, those of *H. capsulatum* var. *capsulatum* are 2–4 μm D. Both types of cells divide by a budding process.

In cultures grown at 25°C, both macroscopically and microscopically, the mycelial forms of the two varieties of *H. capsulatum* cannot be distinguished from each other. The in vitro yeast forms of the two varieties are also morphologically identical. The serologic test developed by Standard and Kaufman[15] to identify cultures of *H. capsulatum* is only genus specific and does not separate the two varieties of that species and *H. farciminosum* from each other. Cultures of the two varieties can be identified with certainty only by infecting laboratory animals, such as guinea pigs, hamsters and mice, and determining the size of the tissue forms that the isolates produce.

The perfect or sexual state of the two varieties of *H. capsulatum* is *Ajellomyces capsulatus*[16].

Amphotericin B is the medication of choice in treating the disseminated and osseous types of histoplasmosis duboisii. Surgery has been used successfully to excise isolated lesions of the fixed type.

Histopathology (Figures 295–307)

Unlike *H. capsulatum* var. *capsulatum, H. capsulatum* var. *duboisii* does not cause readily detectable pulmonary lesions[12, 14]. Instead, lesions of the skin, subcutaneous tissues, lymph nodes, spleen, and bones are common. In both humans and animals, the tissue reactions to all forms of the disease are similar[12, 14, 17, 18]. The fungus

*This name for the disease caused by *H. capsulatum* var. *duboisii* was first used by Cockshott and Lucas in 1964[5].

characteristically incites a granulomatous inflammatory reaction with great numbers of yeast cells within the cytoplasm of histiocytes and numerous multinucleated giant cells of both the foreign body and Langhans' type. In chronic lesions, this granulomatous response is often accompanied by fibrosis. Almost every phagocyte will contain yeast cells, and it is not unusual to see enormous giant cells up to 150 μm in diameter containing 20 or more organisms in a single plane of section. Although most yeast cells are intracellular, small numbers may be extracellular either singly or in clusters. Occasionally, neutrophils, lymphocytes, and plasma cells are scattered among the giant cells. Neutrophils do not contain organisms and, in our experience, are only a minor component of the inflammatory reaction. A pure epithelioid granulomatous reaction rarely occurs. In some instances, we have seen foci of caseous necrosis with or without neutrophilic infiltration. These necrotic areas usually contained intact fungal cells, and unlike caseous lesions caused by *H. capsulatum* var. *capsulatum*, calcification was not observed.

In tissue sections, the yeast cells of *H. capsulatum* var. *duboisii* are round to oval, are 8–15 μm in diameter, have moderately thick ('doubly contoured') refractile cell walls, and bud by a relatively narrow base. A very broad-based bud may occasionally be seen. When budding, the daughter cell may enlarge until it is approximately equal in size to the parent cell while still attached by a narrow isthmus, thus creating typical 'hourglass', 'double cell', or 'figure eight' forms. With H&E, the internal contents of *H. capsulatum* var. *duboisii* cells usually stain basophilic to amphophilic, but the cell walls do not stain and appear translucent in tissue sections. The special fungus stains, particularly the GMS procedure, colour the cell walls uniformly and intensely, but staining of the inner contents of the fungus varies.

Because of their similarity in size and shape, the tissue forms of *H. capsulatum* var. *duboisii* and *Blastomyces dermatitidis* may be mistaken for each other. However, the former usually buds by a narrower base with typical 'hour glass' forms. The typical budding form of *B. dermatitidis* is broad based. When stained with H&E, each cell of *H. capsulatum* var. *duboisii* is usually uninucleate, whereas *B. dermatitidis* cells contain multiple nuclei[19]. In our experience, these nuclei may be difficult to detect, even when tissues are properly fixed and optimally stained. Yeast cells of *H. capsulatum* var. *duboisii* are easily distinguished from typical yeast cells of *H. capsulatum* var. *capsulatum*. The former are much larger, usually bud more frequently with classical 'hour glass' forms, and are predominantly within huge foreign body giant cells instead of histiocytes. The large atypical forms of *H. capsulatum* var. *capsulatum*, for example, those occasionally described in thrombi of cardiac valves, are also morphologically different from the yeast cells of histoplasmosis duboisii. The former have very thin cell walls, are extracellular, and usually appear empty; their internal contents are poorly stained. In addition, large atypical forms of *H. capsulatum* var. *capsulatum* may be mixed with smaller typical forms.

Natural infection due to *H. capsulatum* var. *duboisii* is only known to occur in humans and nonhuman primates from Africa.* In these hosts, the lesions generally contain the large form of the fungus but small cells of the variety *capsulatum* type may also occur[20]. In early stages of experimental infection in animals, many small forms morphologically similar to the yeast cells of *H. capsulatum* var. *capsulatum* are usually found along with the typical large forms[21]. When such small forms predominate, an erroneous diagnosis of histoplasmosis capsulati could result.

References

1 Vanbreuseghem, R. (1976). Etude clinique, mycologique et histopathologique de l'histoplasmose africaine. *Bruxelles-Medical* **56**, 85–95.

2 Ajello, L., Manson-Bahr, P. E. C. and Moore, J. C. (1960). Amboni caves, Tanganyika, a new endemic area for Histoplasma capsulatum. *Am. J. Trop. Med. Hyg.* **9**, 633–638.

3 Almeida, M. G. (1974). Dois novos casos de histoplasmose africana. *Rev. Med.* Angola **64**, 1–6.

4 Cruz Ferreira, F. S., Cunha, C. C. L., Rocha, R. M. and Re, R. F. (1963). Um novo caso de histoplmose africana osteo-cutanea. *J. Soc. Cien. Med.* Lisboa **126**, 295–313.

5 Cockshott, W. P. and Lucas, A. O. (1964). Histoplasmosis duboisii. *Quart. J. Med.* **33**, 223–238.

6 Cole, A. C. E., Ridley, D. S. and Wolfe, H. R. I. (1965). Bowel infections with Histoplasma duboisii. *J. Trop. Med. Hyg.* **68**, 92–96.

7 Piloux, Y., Thevenot, P. and Robert, H. (1965). L'histoplasmose. *Med. Trop.* **25**, 439–456.

8 Walker, J. and Spooner, E. T. C. (1960). Natural infection of the African baboon (Papio papio) with the large cell form of histoplasmosis. *J. Pathol. Bacteriol.* **8**, 436–439.

9 Lunn, H. F. (1960). A case of histoplasmosis of bone in East Africa. *J. Trop. Med. Hyg.* **63**, 175–180.

10 Picq, J. J., Ricosse, J. H., Albert, J. P. and Drouhet, E. (1968). Deux cas d'histoplasmose africaine en Haute-Volta. *Med. Trop.* **28**, 67–74.

11 Yamato, H., Hitomi, H., Maekawa, S. and Mimura, K. (1957). A case of histoplasmosis. *Acta Med.* Okayama **11**, 347–364.

*With the exception of one reported case from Japan[11].

12 Schwarz, J. (1971). African histoplasmosis (Part 2). In *The Pathologic Anatomy of Mycoses,* pp. 139–146. R. D. Baker, ed. Springer-Verlag, Berlin.
13 Renoirte, R., Michaux, J. L., Gatti, F. and Vanbreuseghem, R. (1967). Nouveaux cas d'histoplasmose africaine et de cryptococcose observes en Republique Democratique du Congo. *Bull. Acad. R. Med. Belg.* **7**, 465–526.
14 Clark, B. M. and Greenwood, B. B. (1968). Pulmonary lesions in African histoplasmosis. *J. Trop. Med. Hyg.* **71**, 4–10.
15 Standard, P. G. and Kaufman, L. (1976). Specific immunological tests for the rapid identification of members of the genus Histoplasma. *J. Clin. Microbiol.* **3**, 191–199.
16 McGinnis, M. R. and Katz, B. (1979). Ajellomyces and its synonym Emmonsiella. *Mycotaxon* **8**, 157–164.
17 Lanceley, J. L., Lunn, N. F. and Wilson, A. M. A. (1961). Histoplasmosis in an African child. *J. Ped.* **59**, 756–764.
18 Williams, A. O., Lawson, E. A. and Lucas, A. O. (1971). African histoplasmosis due to Histoplasma duboisii. *Arch. Pathol.* **92**, 306–318.
19 Emmons, C. W. (1959). Fungus nuclei in the diagnosis of mycoses. *Mycologia* **51**, 227–236.
20 Devreese, A., Donkers, J., Ninane, G. and Vanbreuseghem, R. (1961). Histoplasmose africaine a formes capsulatum causée par Histoplasma duboisii Vanbreusęghem 1952. *Ann. Soc. Belg. Med. Trop.* **5**, 403–414.
21 Okudaira, M. and Schwarz, J. (1961). Infection with Histoplasma duboisii in different experimental animals. *Mycologia* **53**, 53–63.

15 Histoplasmosis farciminosi*

(Epizootic lymphangitis, African farcy, Japanese farcy, pseudo-glanders)

Aetiologic agent:

Histoplasma farciminosum

Synonym:

Cryptococcus farciminosus

Definition and background information

Histoplasmosis farciminosi is a chronic disease of horses and related animals that generally involves the subcutaneous lymph nodes and lymphatics of the neck and legs. However, primary pulmonary infections with a fatal outcome have been reported in Sudanese horses[1,2].

In the equidae (horses, mules, donkeys) the subcutaneous involvement of the lymph nodes and their connecting vessels gives rise to a clinical picture that may closely resemble that associated with sporotrichosis.

According to Bullen[3], the primary nodule develops insidiously and remains undetected until it breaks down and drains. In the meantime, the infection spreads along the lymphatic vessels that drain the afflicted area. These superficial vessels enlarge, and a linear series of nodules that tend to break down will then develop. The disease spreads along the lymphatic ducts. Muscles are only rarely involved and then generally through the rupture of subcutaneous abscesses.

The lesions develop and regress over a period of 2–3 months. When several contiguous lymph nodes are affected, the abscesses tend to coalesce and form large protrusions projecting 5–7 centimetres above the surface of the skin.

Pus aspirated from subcutaneous abscesses or picked up from those that have surfaced and opened contains yeast-like cells that are globose to ovoid and 2.5–3.5 μm long by 2–3 μm wide. They are readily demonstrated with the Giemsa stain as well as with the special fungus stains. Most of the tissue-form cells of *H. farciminosum* are intracellular within phagocytes. They are indistinguishable from those produced by *Histoplasma capsulatum* var. *capsulatum* on the basis of size, morphology, and tinctorial properties.

Because of the extreme similarity of the tissue forms of *H. capsulatum* var. *capsulatum* and *H. farciminosum,* a specific diagnosis of histoplasmosis farciminosi cannot be made solely on the basis of the yeast cells found in tissue. However, the tissue-form cells of *H. farciminosum* are readily distinguished from those of *Sporothrix schenckii,* and these two diseases should not be mistaken for each other despite their clinical similarity.

Histoplasmosis farciminosi is now known to exist with certainty only in Africa, especially in Egypt and the Sudan; Asia; and Eastern Europe, notably in Poland and the Union of Soviet Socialist Republics[4,5]. Formerly it was endemic in Western Europe – in Denmark, Finland, Great Britain, Germany, Italy, and Sweden. A slaughter policy eradicated the disease in Great Britain, and presumably similar control measures eliminated the disease in the other countries in Western Europe. However, an equine case of histoplasmosis farciminosi was diagnosed as recently as 1966 in Sweden[5].

Histoplasmosis farciminosi never entered the New World. Reports of the disease in Latin America and the United States have proved to be cases of sporotrichosis[5].

H. farciminosum infections in humans apparently are rare. An accidentally acquired infection was described in 1911 from Algeria in a veterinarian who contaminated an open wound on his thumb with pus from a horse with histoplasmosis farciminosi[6]. A deep abscess developed at the primary site, and the lymphatic ducts up to his axilla developed nodules that abscessed and openly discharged pus. The abscesses healed and repeatedly broke down until the patient was treated with a single injection of '606'. During the 2-month course of the disease, the patient developed a spiking fever of 40°C and experienced pain when the enlarged lymphatic ducts and nodes were palpated.

A consistently effective treatment for equines

---

*In the interest of clarity, brevity and uniformity, we are coining the terms histoplasmosis capsulati and histoplasmosis farciminosi for infections caused by *H. capsulatum* var. *capsulatum* and *H. farciminosum* respectively. The precedent for this nomenclature was set in 1964 by Cockshott and Lucas[19], when they created the name histoplasmosis duboisii for infections by *H. capsulatum* var. *duboisii*.

with the disease has yet to be developed. Surgical excision of early lesions has been reported after injection of mercuric chloride. Intravenous injection of diluted formol has also been used for therapy[7]. Woloszyn suggested that amphotericin B may be useful also[4].

In 1960, vaccines were reported to be effective in the treatment of horses in the Union of Soviet Socialist Republics[8].

Investigators have found it difficult to isolate *H. farciminosum* from clinical materials. Bullen[9] achieved greatest success with Hartley's blood agar incubated at 37°C, but Woloszyn of Poland reported Sabouraud dextrose agar with cycloheximide, penicillin, and streptomycin to be highly effective[4].

On Sabouraud agar, growth is slow. Colonies are glabrous, raised, and wrinkled in the early stages of growth but later are covered with white, downy mycelium. Microscopically, the mycelium is hyaline, septate and 2–4 μm in diameter. Growth is usually sterile, but large, smooth spores 10–12 μm in diameter occasionally are produced. These resemble the smooth, thick-walled macroconidia produced by some isolates of the two varieties of *H. capsulatum*. Production of microconidia has been reported. Such isolates are identified as a species of *Histoplasma* by converting the mycelial form to its yeast form. This is done by inoculating the mycelial growth on rich media, such as Francis cystine blood agar, and incubating the culture tubes at 37°C. Serial passage is usually required to convert most isolates. The yeast cells produced in vitro are similar to those produced in tissue and are indistinguishable from the yeast-form cells of *H. capsulatum* var. *capsulatum*.

Until better methods are developed, a diagnosis of histoplasmosis farciminosi must be based on the clinical expression of the disease in equidae, the demonstration of *H. capsulatum* var. *capsulatum*-type yeast cells in pus or tissue, and the gross and microscopic characteristics of isolates.

Antigenically, *H. farciminosum* is remarkably similar to *H. capsulatum*. For that reason, a specific immunological test that would distinguish this fungus from *H. capsulatum* could not be developed[10,11]. In time, perhaps, *H. farciminosum* will be found to be another variety of *H. capsulatum*.

Histopathology (Figures 308–313)

Infection with *H. farciminosum* is characterised by the formation of chronic granulomatous and suppurative nodules that are most frequently located in the skin, superficial lymphatics, and either the subcutaneous or regional lymph nodes or both[3,7,12–15]. Such nodules usually occur on the lower limbs, chest, neck, and shoulders of solipeds (e.g., horses, mules, and donkeys). Sites less commonly involved include the conjunctiva, nictitating membrane, cornea, external nares, nasal mucosa, nasal sinuses, pharynx, larynx, trachea, bronchi, lungs, and vaginal mucosa. Dissemination to internal organs may occur, but is extremely rare.

The pathogenesis of histoplasmosis farciminosi has been studied but is still not fully understood[3,15,16]. Bullen[3,9] reported that spread via the superficial lymphatics occurs after a primary cutaneous infection. The primary infection may wax and wane for weeks before complete healing takes place. He found that many intradermal nodules (1–2 cm in diameter), which developed along the course of enlarged and tortuous lymphatics draining a primary skin lesion, originated from small subcutaneous lymph nodes. Like the primary lesion, these secondary nodules often ulcerated and discharged pus. In time, an entire lymph node was reported to be transformed into a large abscess surrounded by a thick fibrotic capsule. When sectioned, the abscess was found to contain viscid, creamy material.

In our experience, the tissue response in epizootic lymphangitis is similar to that seen in primary active lesions of histoplasmosis capsulati. In cutaneous lesions, ulceration and marked pseudoepitheliomatous hyperplasia of the epidermis may be observed. The yeast cells of *H. farciminosum* stimulate a chronic granulomatous inflammatory response characterised by diffuse or nodular accumulations of densely packed histiocytes and occasional multinucleated giant cells in the dermis and subcutaneous tissues. Fewer lymphocytes, plasma cells, and neutrophils are also usually present. In general, the inflammatory reaction is purely granulomatous in the early stages of infection. In advanced lesions, scattered neutrophils or abscesses may be seen which probably result from secondary bacterial infection of ulcerated skin lesions. Prominent granulation tissue may be formed, but the infection usually does not extend into deeper tissues such as skeletal muscle and bone. Sinus tracts lined by histiocytes mixed with neutrophils and cellular debris are sometimes seen. The cytoplasm of almost every histiocyte and giant cell is distended with the yeast cells of *H. farciminosum;* rarely are fungal cells seen in neutrophils. Some of them may be extracellular, probably having been released from ruptured histiocytes.

Regardless of the anatomic location, the tissue response to *H. farciminosum* in active lesions is similar to that described above. Fawi[2] isolated *H. farciminosum* from granulomatous lesions in the lungs of two horses. The lung pathology in each case was not associated with skin lesions. Microscopically, the granulomas were seen to be of various sizes and to consist of macrophages and multinucleated giant cells containing abundant yeast cells. Fewer lymphocytes, plasma cells, and neutrophils were also present. Lesions were not found in the regional lymph nodes.

H. farciminosum exists in tissues in the form of small, round to oval yeast cells, no larger than 2–5 μm in diameter[5, 9, 17]. These cells produce single buds that are attached to the parent cell by a narrow base. Large, bizarre, elongated yeast forms or short hyphae are observed rarely[18], especially near or within draining sinus tracts in the dermis and subcutaneous tissues. Yeast cells of *H. farciminosum* are morphologically and tinctorially indistinguishable from those of *H. capsulatum* var. *capsulatum* in tissue sections. Like the latter, they are primarily intracellular parasites. However, *H. farciminosum* has, with rare exceptions[6], been reported only in solipeds.

The appearance of *H. farciminosum* cells in tissue varies according to the staining method employed. In H&E-stained tissue sections, *H. farciminosum* stains poorly. Usually, only a central, slightly basophilic protoplasmic mass surrounded by a clear space or 'halo' is observed. There is no differentiation in the protoplasm, and only if a tissue section is overstained with haematoxylin can the outline of the thin cell wall be seen. The so-called 'halo' effect is considered to be an artifact resulting from shrinkage of the protoplasm within the cell wall during fixation. It is also noticeable in organisms stained with the Giemsa and Wright techniques. With the special fungus stains, the cell wall of *H. farciminosum* is usually stained intensely.

In active lesions of histoplasmosis farciminosi, yeast-form cells are abundant and have a typical morphology. However, in old healing lesions, organisms may be sparse, and atypical degenerated forms may be seen. The GMS stain is superior to the PAS and GF procedures for demonstrating these latter forms. In our experience, calcification does not occur in healed lesions of histoplasmosis farciminosi involving the skin.

In equidae, a presumptive diagnosis of histoplasmosis farciminosi can be made by demonstrating abundant and typical yeast cells in granulomatous lesions that are clinically compatible with the disease. Because *H. capsulatum* var. *capsulatum* is morphologically and tinctorially indistinguishable from *H. farciminosum* in tissues, the criteria for differentiating the former organism from other yeast-like fungi of similar size in tissues also apply to *H. farciminosum*. The reader is referred to the end of Chapter 13 for these criteria. Most importantly, it should be reemphasised that the tissue-form cells of *H. farciminosum* cannot be differentiated from those of *H. capsulatum* var. *capsulatum* in various lesions of solipeds, including the skin. However, the diseases produced by these two organisms are distinct, and the clinical picture may provide a clue as to which of the two organisms one is dealing with. Their definitive differential identification would require cultural studies.

References

1 Bennett, S. C. J. (1931). Cryptococcus pneumonia in equidae. *J. Comp. Pathol.* **44**, 85–105.

2 Fawi, M. T. (1971). Histoplasma farciminosum, the aetiological agent of equine cryptococcal pneumonia. *Sabouraudia* **9**, 123–125.

3 Bullen, J. J. (1951). Epizootic lymphangitis: Clinical symptoms. *J. R. Army Vet. Corps* **22**, 8–11.

4 Woloszyn, S. (1968). Investigations in the properties and antigenic structure of Histoplasma farciminosum. I. Culture and Morphology. II. Biochemical properties. III. Spectrophotometric and chromatographic analysis. IV. Evaluation of sensitivity to some antimycotic substances (In Polish). *Medycyn. Wet.* **24**, 134–140; 140–143; 207–212; 212–214.

5 Ajello, L. (1968). Comparative morphology and immunology of members of the genus Histoplasma. *Mykosen* **11**, 507–514.

6 Negre, L. and Bridrê, J. (1911). Un cas de lymphangite epizootique chez l'homme. Traitement et guerison par le "606". *Bull. Soc. Pathol. Exot.* **4**, 384–386.

7 Ainsworth, G. C. and Austwick, P. R. C. (1973). *Fungal Disease of Animals.* Commonwealth Agricultural Bureaux, Farnham Royal, Slough, England.

8 Noskov, A. I. (1960). Immunity to epizootic lymphangitis and the efficacy of vaccines (In Russian). *Tr. Vsesoyuz. Inst. Vet. Sanit.* **16**, 368–372.

9 Bullen, J. J. (1949). The yeast-like form of Cryptococcus farciminosus (Rivolta): (Histoplasma farciminosum). *J. Pathol. Bacteriol.* **61**, 117–120.

10 Standard, P. and Kaufman, L. (1976). Specific immunological test for the rapid identification of members of the genus Histoplasma. *J. Clin. Microbiol.* **3**, 191–199.

11 Kaufman, L. and Standard, P. (1978). Improved version of the exoantigen test for identification of Coccidioides immitis and Histoplasma capsulatum cultures. *J. Clin. Microbiol.* **8**, 42–45.

12 Bennett, S. C. J. (1944). Cryptococcus infection in equidae. *J. Army Vet. Corps* **16**, 108–118.

13 Plunkett, J. J. (1949). Epizootic lymphangitis. *J. Army Vet. Corps.* **20**, 94–99.

14 Singh, S. (1956). Equine cryptococcosis (epizootic lymphangitis). *Indian Vet. J.* **32**, 260–270.

15 Singh, T. (1965). Studies on epizootic lymphangitis. I. Modes of infection and transmission of equine histoplasmosis (epizootic lymphangitis). *Indian J. Vet. Sci.* **35**, 102–110.

16 Singh, T., Varmani, B. M. L. and Bhalla, N. P. (1965). Studies on epizootic lymphangitis. II. Pathogenesis and histopathology of equine histoplasmosis. *Indian J. Vet. Sci.* **35**, 111–120.

17 Singh, T. and Varmani, B. M. L. (1967). Some observations on experimental infection with Histoplasma farciminosum (Rivolta) and the morphology of the organism. *Indian J. Vet. Sci.* **37**, 47–57.

18 Bennett, S. C. J. (1932). Epizootic lymphangitis: mycelial forms of the parasite in a natural case. *J. Comp. Pathol.* **45**, 158–160.

19 Cockshott, W. P. and Lucas, A. O. (1964). Histoplasmosis duboisii. *Quart. J. Med.* **33**, 223–238.

16 Lobomycosis

(Keloidal blastomycosis, Lobo's disease)

Aetiologic agent:

Loboa loboi

Common synonyms:

Glenosporella loboi, Glenosporopsis amazonica, Paracoccidioides loboi, Blastomyces loboi.

Definition and background information

Lobomycosis is a New World disease currently known to afflict only man and dolphins. It is a chronic, indolent disease that generally afflicts the exposed parts of the body. The lesions that develop, presumably after some traumatic incident, involve the skin and subcutaneous tissues. They are characteristically nodular and keloidal in appearance. In early stages of the infection the free-moving nodules are sharply delimited from the normal skin areas that surround them. The infection gradually spreads by peripheral extension, and large verrucose, nodular plaques are formed. However, satellite lesions may, in time, appear at sites distant from the primary infection, probably as a result of autoinoculation rather than of haematogenous or lymphatic spread.

Diagnosis is based on demonstrating the presence of spherical, thick-walled yeast-like cells ranging from 5–12 μm in diameter in lesion exudate or tissue sections. The fungus multiplies by budding, and thus mother cells with single buds are often encountered. However, characteristically sequential budding leads to the production of chains of cells that are linked to each other by a tubular connection or isthmus. Budding may occur at more than one point on a cell, giving rise to branched or radiating chains of cells.

The thick-walled hyaline, spherical cells with chains of cells interconnected by tubular isthmuses are the basis on which a diagnosis of lobomycosis rests. They are readily observed in tissue smears or exudate mounted in 10% KOH or in histological sections.

Less than 200 cases of lobomycosis in humans have been recorded in Central and South America: Brazil, Colombia, Costa Rica, French Guiana, Panama, Peru, Surinam and Venezuela[1,2].

In addition, inexplicable infections by *L. loboi* have been recorded in dolphins captured or observed off the east and west coasts of Florida (*Tursiops truncatus*) and in the estuary of the Surinam River in Surinam (*Sotalia guianensis*)[1,3].

Loboa loboi, the aetiological agent of lobomycosis, has yet to be isolated and grown *in vitro*; therefore, nothing is known of its basic cultural characteristics and growth requirements.

Material from infected humans has been successfully used to transmit infection to other humans[1,4]. Florida dolphin infections have been passed through three generations of mice inoculated in their foot pads (unpublished data). In Brazil a human infection was successfully transferred to the six-banded armadillo[5].

Surgical excision of infected tissue is the only known effective treatment for this disease.

Histopathology (Figures 314–326)

Generally, lesions caused by *L. loboi* are confined to the skin. However, there are a few reports of subcutaneous lesions and of lymphatic involvement with dissemination to regional lymph nodes[6–8]. We know of no case in which visceral organs were involved. The organism apparently prefers the coolest sites of the body. Secondary skin lesions may occur and probably result from autoinoculation[6].

The histopathologic features of lobomycosis in humans[6, 8–10] and dolphins[1, 3, 11] are characteristic and are remarkably similar from case to case and specimen to specimen. They will therefore be described together. In skin lesions, the epidermis that covers the typical, smooth, keloid-like nodules, is usually of normal thickness or atrophic. In older (usually >2 years) verrucous and crusted skin lesions, hyperkeratosis and acanthosis may be seen. Ulceration may also occur. The dermis, including the adnexa, is replaced by a dense granulomatous inflammatory reaction of the nodular type. As a rule the reaction is purely granulomatous, and it extends from just beneath the epidermis downward to, but usually not including, the subcutaneous tissues. The granulomatous tissue consists of densely packed histiocytes and foreign body and Langhans' giant cells which in most cases contain abundant fungal cells. Occasionally, foci of lymphocytes may also be present, but foci of necrosis or of other inflammatory cells are uncommon. Stromal fibrosis with collagen deposition is ordinarily minimal, even in long-standing lesions. Instead, special stains most often reveal an intricate network of reticular fibres that support the giant cells and histiocytes. Occasionally, Masson's trichrome stain will reveal that the dermal granuloma is clearly separated from the epidermis by a narrow and irregular zone of collagen fibres. Delicate streaks of these fibres may extend deep into the granulomatous nodule.

In H&E-stained tissue sections, the cells of *L. loboi* are usually evident but stain poorly. Often, only their outlines are visible. When stained, their internal contents are homogeneous and appear faintly basophilic to amphophilic. The thick translucent cell wall does not stain with H&E. With the special fungus stains, the organisms usually stain intensely and are readily demonstrated. Fungi stained by these procedures appear even more abundant than when studied in replicate sections stained with H&E. Individual fungal cells are usually round to oval and of relatively uniform size, measuring 5–12 μm in diameter (average of 9 μm). The cells reproduce by single or multiple budding with short 'bridges' or tube-like structures connecting one cell to another. The connected cells form characteristic chains of 2–5 cells each, and it is not uncommon to see 6–8 cells linked together. When the yeast cells of *L. loboi* form multiple buds, as many as three separately attached daughter cells can be seen in a single plane of section, in addition to those attached within the chain. Occasionally, secondary budding is seen where daughter cells in turn have formed one or more buds.

In our experience, the GF procedure is superior to the GMS and PAS procedures for demonstrating internal details of this fungus. With this stain, the fungal cell wall and its contents are well delineated. The protoplasm often is seen to contain vacuoles and is retracted and separated from the cell wall, leaving a clear space. This clear space is similar to that seen in *Blastomyces dermatitidis* and certain other yeasts stained by various methods. It apparently represents a fixation artifact. The GMS procedure usually stains entire cells of *L. loboi* intensely. At times, however, such cells will appear empty. GF- and PAS-positive granular material may be seen within the cytoplasm of giant cells, apparently resulting from death and fragmentation of phagocytised fungal cells. Distorted, fragmented, and poorly stained fungal cells that are apparently dead are usually seen in the vicinity of the phagocytised granular material. The cell wall of *L. loboi* is microporus when studied by electron microscopy[12], a feature that permits macrophage pseudopods to be introduced into the interior of the fungal cell.

A number of investigators, as well as ourselves, have observed eosinophilic and homogeneous material that irregularly or uniformly coats some but not all of the *L. loboi* cells in tissue sections stained with H&E. The tinctorial features of this material are not unlike those of the Splendore–Hoeppli reaction (see Chapter 25). What may be the same eosinophilic material seen in H&E-stained sections is also apparent when fungal cells are stained with the GF and PAS procedures. With these stains, the irregular or 'ragged' granular-like material that surrounds the outer cell wall is well delineated. This extracellular material does not usually stain with the GMS procedure. However, we have seen wide unstained spaces that uniformly outline the contour of GMS-stained fungal cells, and these spaces probably represent unstained material.

A diagnosis of lobomycosis can be made by demonstrating typical chains of organisms in tissue sections stained with the special fungus procedures. In most cases, typical forms are present in great abundance and a diagnosis can be made without difficulty. In rare instances, when typical forms are not seen[8, 13], *L. loboi* cells may be confused with those of *Paracoccidioides brasiliensis*, which also reproduce by single and multiple budding. This is particularly true when a central mother cell of *L. loboi* produces several buds oriented in different directions. However, *P. brasiliensis* does not normally form cells in chains with connecting tubes. When budding forms are seen, the daughter cells of *P. brasiliensis* are often much smaller than the mother cell. Bud scars may also be seen on parent cells of *P. brasiliensis*. *Cryptococcus neoformans* cells may occasionally show multiple budding. However, such cells are not connected by distinct tube-like structures as are *L. loboi* cells, and the former usually have a mucicarmine-positive capsule. *Blastomyces dermatitidis* should not be confused with *L. loboi* because the former shows budding by a very broad base and rarely forms chains. It should also be remembered that the inflammatory response to *L. loboi* is purely granulomatous. There are no microabscesses like those usually seen in skin lesions of blastomycosis, paracoccidioidomycosis, chromoblastomycosis, and sporotrichosis.

References

1 Caldwell, D. K., Caldwell, M. C., Woodard, J. C., Ajello, L., Kaplan, W. and McClure, H. M. (1975). Lobomycosis as a disease of the Atlantic bottle-nosed dolphin (Tursiops truncatus Montagu, 1821). *Am. J. Trop. Med. Hyg.* **24**, 105–114.

2 Rivas, O. R. (1972). Enfermedad de Jorge Lobo (Blastomicosis queloidiana). Primer caso diagnosticado en el Peru. *Arch. Peruanos Patol. Clin.* **26**, 63–86.

3 De Vries, G. A. and Laarman, J. J. (1973). A case of Lobo's disease in the dolphin Sotalia guianensis. *Aquatic Mammals* **1**, 26–33.

4 Borelli, D. (1962). Lobomycosis experimental. *Dermatol. Venez.* **3**, 72–82.

5 Sampaio, M. M. and Braga-Dias, L. (1977). The armadillo Euphractus sexcinctus as a suitable animal for experimental studies of Jorge Lobo's disease. *Rev. Inst. Med. Trop.* Sao Paulo **19**, 215–220.

6 Jaramillo, D., Cortes, A., Restrepo, A., Builes, M. and Robledo, M. (1976). Lobomycosis. Report of the eighth Colombian case and review of the literature. *J. Cutan. Pathol.* **3**, 180–189.

7 Azulay, R. D., Carneiro, J. A., Cunha, M. G. S. and Reis, L. T. (1976). Keloidal blastomycosis (Lobo's disease) with lymphatic involvement: a case report. *Int. J. Dermatol.* **15**, 40–42.

8 Wieserma, J. P. (1971). Lobo's disease (keloidal blastomycosis). In *The Pathologic Anatomy of Mycoses, Human Infections with Fungi, Actinomycetes and Algae*. R. D. Baker, ed. Springer-Verlag, Berlin. pp. 577–588.

9 Azulay, R. D., Carneiro, J. A. and Andrade, L. C. (1970). Blastomicose de Jorge Lobo. *Anais Brasileiros de Dermatologia* **45**, 47–66.

10 Wieserma, J. P. and Niemel, P. L. A. (1965). Lobo's disease in Surinam patients. *Trop. Geograph. Med.* **17**, 89–111.

11 Migaki, G., Valeiro, M. G., Irvine, G. and Garner, F. M. (1971). Lobo's disease in an Atlantic Bottle-nosed dolphin. *J. Am. Vet. Med. Assoc.* **159**, 578–582.

12 Woodward, J. C. (1972). Electron microscopic study of lobomycosis (*Loboa loboi*). *Lab. Invest.* **27**, 606–612.

13 Diaz, L. B., Sampao, M. M. and Silva, D. (1970). Jorge Lobo's disease. Observations on its epidemiology and some unusual morphological features of the fungus. *Rev. do Inst. Med. Trop.* Sao Paulo **12**, 8–15.

17 Mycetomas

(Madura foot, maduromycosis)

Aetiologic agents:

Mycetomas are caused by two different types of microorganisms: actinomycetes and fungi. The principal aetiologic agents of the actinomycotic and eumycotic mycetomas are listed in Tables 1 and 2 respectively.

Table 1 Aetiologic agents of the actinomycotic mycetomas

Actinomadura madurae	*N. brasiliensis*
A. pelletieri	*N. caviae*
Nocardia asteroides	*Streptomyces somaliensis*

Table 2 Aetiologic agents of the eumycotic mycetomas

Acremonium falciforme	*Leptosphaeria senegalensis*
A. kiliensis	*L. tompkinsii*
A. recifei	*Madurella grisea*
*Aspergillus nidulans**	*M. mycetomatis*
Curvularia geniculata	*Neotestudina rosatii*
C. lunata	*Petriellidium boydii*†
Exophiala jeanselmei	*Pyrenochaeta romeroi*
Fusarium moniliforme	

*Imperfect state of *Emericella nidulans*
†Perfect state of *Scedosporium* (*Monosporium*) *apiospermum*[1].

Definition and background information

Mycetomas are granulomatous tumours of the subcutaneous tissues that eventually may involve bone. They are caused by a wide variety of free-living or exogenous, geophilic actinomycetes and fungi. These microorganisms are introduced into some part of the body, usually a foot or hand, as the result of a traumatic incident. Once the offending agent begins to develop in tissue, its mycelium proliferates and becomes organised into aggregates known as granules or grains. These granules, the hallmark of the mycetomas, are of various sizes, colours, and degrees of hardness depending on the species causing the mycetoma. As the mycetoma develops, the affected area enlarges as a result of the interaction of the host and parasite and the formation of fibrotic tissue. Abscesses develop and multiple draining sinus tracts eventually emerge. These tracts discharge serosanguinous fluid containing the tell-tale granules.

Basically there are two distinct groups of mycetomas: the actinomycotic mycetomas and the eumycotic mycetomas. In the actinomycotic mycetomas the granules are characterised and identified by the presence of mycelial filaments that are 1 μm or less in diameter. In contrast, the granules of the eumycotic mycetomas are composed of septate mycelial filaments that are at least 2–4 μm in diameter. The mycelium in the eumycotic granules is frequently distorted and bizarre in form and size. Chlamydospores are frequently present, especially at the periphery of the granule. In both types of mycetomas, the mycelium of the granules may or may not be embedded in a cement-like substance, depending upon the species involved[2]. Frequently the granules elicit an immunological response, the so-called Splendore–Hoeppli reaction[3]. This reaction is manifested histologically by a deposit of an eosinophilic material around the granule.

Each species or group of species of the aetiologic agents of mycetoma is characterised by the development of a specific type of granule. With experience, investigators can correlate the colour, shape, size, and internal configuration of a granule with a specific aetiologic agent or a group of actinomycetes and fungi. In Tables 3 and 4 the diagnostic characteristics of the actinomycotic and eumycotic granules are described.

Although the gross and microscopic characteristics of the granules provide an insight into the identity of the aetiologic agent or of a particular group in which it belongs, definitive identification is dependent upon the isolation and identification of the organism involved.

The incubation period of the mycetomas is generally considered to be long because of the time needed for the invading organism to become adapted to the internal environment of the host's tissues. The infections are insidious since discomfort is minimal. The subcutaneous nodule that initially develops and erupts to the surface may be mistaken for a bacterial infection. Unlike most superficial bacterial infections, the infection persists and fistulae develop from which granules are discharged. The subcutaneous tumour slowly enlarges and penetrates deeper to the muscles and enters between the laminae of the muscles. Suppurative and fibrotic reactions take place and lead to abnormal swelling of the infected area. Abscesses are formed, and their fistulisation and emergence to the surface give rise to the classical picture of a mycetoma. The infection eventually reaches the bone and frequently causes extensive bone destruction. X-rays are useful to determine the occurrence and extent of osteolytic activity. Mycetomas are basically localised infections. They spread to the adjacent tissues through dissemination of mycelial elements or granules and their fragments. Lymphatic spread from the primary subcutaneous locus has been reported on rare occasions[4, 5]. A thorough description of the clinical aspects of the mycetomas will be found in references 6–8.

Authenticated cases of mycetomas in nonhumans have been rare. The dog has been the prime victim[9, 10] and *Curvularia geniculata* the principal aetiologic agent. Many cases of phaeohyphomycosis, especially those caused by *Drechslera rostrata* and *D. spicifera* (see Chapter 21), have been erroneously diagnosed as mycetomas[11, 12].

The mycetomas are not contagious infections. All victims are infected from sources in nature.

Treatment of the eumycotic mycetomas is primarily limited to surgical methods. Chemotherapy with drugs has not proven to be effective[6]. In contrast, if the actinomycotic mycetomas are treated early and vigorously for an extended period of time, they respond to dapsone plus streptomycin sulphate or sulfamethoxazole-trimethoprim plus streptomycin[13].

In most instances the granules present in clinical materials are visible to the naked eye, especially when the pus is spread thinly over the bottom of a sterile petri dish. The picked granules should be repeatedly washed in several changes of sterile physiological saline to remove contaminating bacterial and mould cells. Several of the washed granules should be examined directly and others inoculated onto appropriate isolation media[7]. Special procedures are required to identify the actinomycotic and eumycotic mycetoma agents. The reader is referred to references 7 and 8 for taxonomic information.

A word needs to be said regarding the nomenclature adopted in this Atlas for designating the aetiologic agents of the mycetomas. Changes in generic concepts and study of their interrelationships have led to the creation of new genera to accommodate some of these agents or have necessitated their transfer to other genera. The synonyms of these renamed organisms are as follows:

Actinomadura madurae
- Synonyms:
  - *Nocardia madurae*
  - *Streptomyces madurae*

A. pelletieri
- Synonym:
  - *Streptomyces pelletieri*

Acremonium falciforme
- Synonym:
  - *Cephalosporium falciforme*

A. kiliensis
- Synonyms:
  - *Cephalosporium madurae*
  - *Cephalosporium infestans*

A. recifei
- Synonym:
  - *Cephalosporium recifei*

Exophiala jeanselmei
- Synonyms:
  - *Phialophora gougerotii*
  - *P. jeanselmei*
  - *Torula bergeri*
  - *T. jeanselmei*

Neotestudina rosatii
- Synonym:
  - *Zopfia rosatii*

Petriellidium boydii
- Synonym:
  - *Allescheria boydii*

Table 3 Diagnostic characteristics of the actinomycotic granules

SPECIES	COLOUR	SIZE RANGE	CEMENT	TEXTURE	TINCTORIAL PROPERTIES
Actinomadura madurae	White	0.5–5 mm	—	Soft	Non acid-fast mycelium. Periphery is intensely stained by haematoxylin
A. pelletieri	Red	0.3–0.5 mm	—	Soft to hard	Non acid-fast. Uniformly stained by haematoxylin
Nocardia asteroides†	White	15–200 μm	—	Soft	Acid-fast. Variable staining with H&E
N. brasiliensis†	,,	,,	—	,,	,, ,, ,,
N. caviae†			—		,, ,, ,,
Streptomyces somaliensis	Yellow	0.5–2 mm	+	Hard	Non acid-fast. Homogeneous, very light staining with eosin

†Granules of these three species are indistinguishable from each other.

Table 4 Diagnostic characteristics of the eumycotic granules

SPECIES	COLOUR	SIZE RANGE	CEMENT	TEXTURE	HISTOLOGICAL FEATURES*
Acremonium falciforme	White	0.5–1 mm	—	Soft	Eosinophilic border darker than interior. Intricate network of hyaline mycelium and chlamydospores
A. kiliensii	,,	,,	—	,,	,, ,, ,,
A. recifei	,,		—		,, ,,
Aspergillus nidulans	,,	0.5–4 mm	—	,,	Eosinophilic with light and dark zones. Dense network of mycelium with extremely large chlamydospores, 10–40 μm D
Curvularia geniculata	Black	0.5–>1 mm	+	Hard	Lobulated; dark periphery with loose network of mycelium and large chlamydospores in cemented periphery (similar to granules of *L. senegalensis* and *L. tompkinsii*)
C. lunata	,,	1–2 mm	+	,,	,, ,, ,,

Exophiala jeanselmei	,,	0.2–0.3 mm	—	Soft	Irregularly shaped (round, oval to crescent shaped); dark periphery made up of mycelium and chlamydospores
Fusarium moniliforme	White	0.5–1.0 mm	—	Soft	Eosinophilic, entire or lobed granules composed of a tangled mass of mycelium. Hyphae in peripheral zone swollen and distorted
Leptosphaeria senegalensis	Black	0.5–2 mm	+ in periphery	Hard	See description of *C. geniculata* and *C. lunata* granules
L. tompkinsii	,,	,,	,,	,,	,, ,, ,,
Madurella grisea	,,	0.3–0.6 mm	Variable	,,	Dark peripheral zone, variably shaped. Dense internal network of mycelium with chlamydospores
M. mycetomatis	,,	0.5–4 mm	+	,,	Two basic types of granules 1. Compact, filamentous type of variable size and form; may be lobulated; cement throughout granule stained uniformly brown 2. Vesicular type that is more irregular in size and form than compact type; cement only in periphery, stained dark brown; Mycelium in periphery with chlamydospores. Central zone lightly stained. Both types of development may be found in a single granule
Neotestudina rosatii	Brownish white	0.5–1 mm	+ in periphery	,,	Irregular in form, eosinophilic border. Central zone with disintegrated mycelium and chlamydospores
Petriellidium boydii	White	0.5–1 mm	—	Soft	Eosinophilic border, rest of granule lightly coloured. Made up of dense network of hyaline interwoven mycelium with prominent chlamydospores
Pyrenochaeta romeroi	Black	0.3–0.6 mm	Variable	Soft	Dark peripheral zone, variably shaped. Internal dense network of mycelium without chlamydospores

*Haematoxylin & Eosin Stain.

Histopathology (Figures 327–392)

Biopsy tissue should first be examined grossly for the presence of granules which are variable in shape and size (2.5 μm to 2 mm). They may be embedded in either solid lesions or abscesses. Sinus or fistulous tracts that contain granules may be discharging a serosanguinous or purulent exudate. Granules are either white, yellow, pinkish-red, brown, or black. When black, they contrast sharply with the surrounding tissue, which is usually greyish white. Curettings and the exudate from draining sinuses should also be examined for granules. If found, the granules should be washed repeatedly in normal saline solution and then examined in a drop of 10% KOH. After the colour, size, shape, and texture of the granules are noted, they should be pressed out under a coverslip or between two slides, if hard, and examined microscopically. They may also be processed by standard histologic procedures. Granules vary in texture from very soft and friable to extremely hard and brittle. They also vary in colour and microscopic architecture. These characteristics can serve as a basis for their specific identification (see Tables 3 and 4).

Microscopically, the salient feature of a mycetoma is the presence of one or more spherical, subspherical, or lobular granules in a tumourous mass of chronically inflamed tissue[14-20]. A granule consists of an organised mass of fungal hyphae or actinomycete filaments which may or may not be embedded in a cement-like substance and may or may not be naturally pigmented. Discrete zones may be apparent in some granules stained with H&E. Amorphous, deeply eosinophilic, radially arranged or smoothly contoured Splendore–Hoeppli material[3] intimately surrounds a portion of or usually the entire granule of some mycetomas, and may interdigitate with mycelial elements. (Individual or small groups of fungal elements embedded in or surrounded by Splendore–Hoeppli material are not true granules). Sometimes foreign materials such as thorns are seen near the granules and are presumed to have been the vehicle of infection.

A mycetoma infection often may extend directly into contiguous tissues and may involve an entire limb. Extensive tissue invasion often results in bone and muscle destruction, osteomyelitis, tendinitis, arthritis, and ulceration of the overlying epidermis. Haematogenous dissemination or lymphatic spread rarely occurs, especially in the eumycotic mycetomas[4, 8, 16]. When dissemination is seen, it usually occurs during the early stages of a mycetoma.

All mycetomas, eumycotic and actinomycotic, are associated with a similar tissue response regardless of the causative organism. The dermis and subcutaneous tissues contain localised abscesses of varying sizes, each of which usually contains a discrete mycotic granule or a cluster of granules in its centre. Dense accumulations of intact neutrophils, which may be mixed with necrotic debris, are in direct apposition with the granules. Around this central abscess there is a chronic inflammatory reaction that often consists of palisading epithelioid cells and multinucleated giant cells mixed with smaller numbers of plasma cells and lymphocytes. At times, an epithelioid and giant cell granulomatous reaction will intimately surround a granule with little or no neutrophilic response. Diameters of granules may range from 0.1 mm to several mm depending on the aetiologic agent and the specimen examined. Granules are sometimes displaced to one side of an abscess and may even be removed from the entire section because of the drag on the microtome knife during sectioning. Some granules are also easily fragmented when sectioned, e.g. those caused by *Streptomyces somaliensis*.

In the stroma, between abscesses, there is dense granulation tissue that may be highly vascular and heavily infiltrated by mature plasma cells, lymphocytes, and macrophages. The latter cells may have a foamy cytoplasm (lipophages or 'foam cells'). Epithelioid and giant cells may also be seen lying in the reactive stroma. Fibrosis around granules, particularly in long-standing infections, is often severe. As the result of extensive fibrosis, tumefaction and deformity are such characteristic features of the mycetomas that they may be mistaken for neoplasms.

The predominance of each inflammatory component associated with a mycetoma will vary from case to case and specimen to specimen. Since the tissue reaction is not specific, one must demonstrate granules before a diagnosis of mycetoma can be made. Serial sections may be necessary to find granules. To further define a granule as being actinomycotic or eumycotic, special stains for bacteria and fungi are needed. With the latter, granules of the eumycotic mycetomas can be seen to contain broad (2–6 μm) hyphae. In addition, a large number of chlamydospores may be found in the mycelium of the eumycotic mycetomas (see Table 4), but not of actinomycotic mycetomas.

When the special fungus stains fail to demonstrate broad hyphae within a granule and the tissue Gram stains reveal gram-positive branched filaments $\leq$ 1.0 μm in width, a diagnosis of an actinomycotic mycetoma can be made. These filaments also stain well with the GMS and Giemsa procedures, but they are refractory to the PAS, GF, and H&E stains. When a pure population of nonfilamentous bacteria (bacilli, cocci, or coccobacilli) is seen to compose the granule, a diagnosis of botryomycosis should be made (covered later in this chapter).

Rarely, nonfilamentous bacteria are found within eumycotic or actinomycotic granules that are intimately associated with the hyphae or filaments, respectively. Winslow[14, 16] has used the term 'mixed mycetoma' for such granules. The intragranular nonfilamentous bacteria in a 'mixed mycetoma' should not be confused with those found scattered about in the reactive stroma and in draining sinus tracts due to secondary bacterial infection of ulcerated skin lesions.

The delicate, gram-positive, branched filaments within actinomycotic granules may be beaded and are most prominent at the periphery of a granule. Filaments of the *Nocardia* species may be partially acid-fast, but a negative staining reaction does not rule out their presence. Cultures are needed for definitive identification of the causative agents. Because actinomycosis is an endogenous disease, it is not included in this chapter on mycetomas despite the fact that its aetiologic agents (*Actinomyces bovis*, *A. israelii*, *A. naeslundii* and others) usually appear in the form of granules in tissue. The *Nocardia* species can produce localised or systemic infections without the formation of granules. Such infections are covered in Chapter 19, entitled 'Nocardiosis'.

Since actinomycotic mycetomas respond to treatment with currently available antibiotics and eumycotic mycetomas do not, the microscopic distinction between granules formed by actinomycetes and fungi is very important. With experience and a battery of appropriate stains, the pathologist should easily be able to differentiate them. When cultures are not available, accurate histologic differentiation is crucial in determining the form of treatment and the prognosis. When only a single unstained section is available for histologic studies, the GMS with H&E counterstain is recommended.

The salient features of the granules of the actinomycotic and eumycotic mycetomas in tissues are presented in Tables 3 and 4. These tables and the illustrations in this chapter are included as guides in making a presumptive identification of the aetiologic agents responsible for mycetomas. Most granules have a characteristic architecture, and this feature together with the presence or absence of natural pigments enables the microscopist to presumptively identify the causative agents. However, specific identification of the aetiologic agents generally requires correlation of histological and cultural findings.

Botryomycosis (Figures 393–398)

Although botryomycosis ('bacterial pseudomycosis') is an infection caused by nonfilamentous bacteria (Eubacteriales), we include it here because botryomycotic granules may be mistaken for those of the actinomycotic and eumycotic mycetomas. Conversely, we have seen mycetomas mistaken for botryomycosis in H&E-stained tissue sections. In order to be classified as botryomycosis, a bacterial colony must appear as a granule.

Botryomycosis is usually a chronic, localised bacterial infection of the skin and subcutaneous tissues in humans and animals[21, 22]. Dissemination with visceral involvement can also occur[23], but it is not common. The disease is characterised by the presence of one or more granules in the centre of localised abscesses which are surrounded by fibrous tissue. As in the mycetomas, fibrosis may be severe. Botryomycotic granules are composed of compact bacterial colonies that are almost always surrounded by an amorphous, deeply eosinophilic zone of radially or irregularly arranged Splendore–Hoeppli material[3]. Projections from the radial corona of Splendore–Hoeppli material are often referred to as 'clubs' (see Actinomycosis, Chapter 4). The bacteria most commonly implicated in botryomycosis are *Pseudomonas aeruginosa*, *Actinobacillus lignieresi*, *Staphylococcus aureus*, *Streptococcus*, *Proteus*, and *Escherichia* species. Rarely is more than one species of bacterium found in a granule.

In H&E-stained tissue sections, botryomycotic granules may be indistinguishable from those of the actinomycotic mycetomas because the bacteria that occur in these granules are not clearly seen. Special stains are therefore mandatory for a differential diagnosis. Individual coccoid and bacillary bacteria within a granule are best seen when stained with the tissue Gram stains such as the Brown and Brenn or Brown–Hopps procedures, and when viewed with the oil immersion objective. In our experience, the latter stain is superior for demonstrating gram-negative bacteria. The GMS and Giemsa procedures may also stain some bacteria, but the PAS and GF procedures do not.

References

1 Arx, J. A. von. (1973). The genera Petriellidium and Pithoascus (Microascaceae). *Persoonia* **7**, 367–375.

2 Findlay, G. H. and Vismer, H. F. (1974). Black grain mycetoma. A study of the chemistry, formation and significance of the tissue grain in Madurella mycetomi infection. *Br. J. Dermatol.* **91**, 297–303.

3 Liber, A. F. and Ho-Soon Hahn Choi. (1973). Splendore–Hoeppli phenomenon about silk sutures. *Arch. Pathol.* **95**, 217–220.

4 El Hassan, A. M. and Mahgoub, E. S. (1972). Lymph node involvement in mycetoma. *Trans. Roy. Soc. Trop. Med. Hyg.* **66**, 165–169.

5 Oyston, J. K. (1961). Madura foot. A study of twenty cases. *J. Bone Joint Surg.* **43B**, 259–267.

6 Mahgoub, E. S. and Murray, I. G. (1973). *Mycetoma.* William Heinemann, Medical Books Limited, London.

7 Ajello, L., Georg, L. K., Kaplan, W. and Kaufman, L. (1970). Mycotic Infections. In *Diagnostic Procedures for Bacterial, Mycotic and Parasitic Infections,* 5th ed. H. L. Bodily, E. L. Updyke and J. O. Mason, eds. *Am. Public Health Assoc.,* New York.

8 Mariat, F., Destombes, P. and Segretain, F. (1977). The mycetomas: clinical features, pathology, etiology and epidemiology. In *Host-Parasite Relationships in Systemic Mycosis.* Vol. 4, Part II: Specific Diseases and Therapy, pp. 1–39. A. M. Beemer, A. Ben-David, M. A. Klinberg and E. S. Kuttin, eds. S. Karger, Basel.

9 Brodey, R. S., Shryver, H. F., Deubler, M. J., Kaplan, W. and Ajello, L. (1967). Mycetoma in a dog. *J. Am. Vet. Med. Assoc.* **151**, 442–451.

10 Bridges, C. H. (1957). Maduromycotic mycetomas in animals. *Am. J. Pathol.* **33**, 411–427.

11 Muller, G. H., Kaplan, W., Ajello, L. and Padhye, A. A. (1975). Phaeohyphomycosis caused by Drechslera spicifera in a cat. *J. Am. Vet. Med. Assoc.* **166**, 150–154.

12 Pritchard, D., Chick, B. F. and Connole, M. D. (1977). Eumycotic mycetoma due to Drechslera rostrata. *Aust. Vet. J.* **53**, 241–244.

13 Mahgoub, E. S. (1976). Medical management of mycetoma. *Bull. W.H.O.* **54**, 303–310.

14 Winslow, D. J. and Steen, F. G. (1964). Considerations in the histologic diagnosis of mycetoma. *Am. J. Clin. Pathol.* **42**, 164–169.

15 Abbott, P. (1956). Mycetoma in the Sudan. *Trans. Roy. Soc. Trop. Med. Hyg.* **50**, 11–30.

16 Winslow, D. J. (1971). Mycetoma In *The Pathologic Anatomy of Mycoses. Human Infection with Fungi, Actinomycetes and Algae.* R. D. Baker, ed. Springer-Verlag, Berlin. pp. 589–613.

17 Bridges, C. H. and Beasley, J. N. (1960). Maduromycotic mycetomas in animals – Brachycladium spiciferum. *J. Am. Vet. Med. Assoc.* **137**, 192–201.

18 MacKinnon, J. E. (1962). Mycetomas as opportunistic would infections. *Lab. Invest.* **11**, 1124–1131.

19 Cameron, H. M., Gatei, D. and Bremner, A. D. (1973). The deep mycoses in Kenya: A histopathological study. 1. Mycetoma. *East Afr. Med. J.* **50**, 382–395.

20 Green, W. O. and Adams, T. E. (1964). Mycetoma in the United States. *Am. J. Clin. Pathol.* **42**, 75–91.

21 Greenblatt, M., Heredia, R., Rubenstein, L. and Alpert, S. (1964). Bacterial pseudomycosis ('botryomycosis'). *Am. J. Clin. Pathol.* **41**, 188–193.

22 Winslow, D. J. (1959). Botryomycosis. *Am. J. Pathol.* **35**, 153–167.

23 Winslow, D. J. and Chamblin, S. A. (1960). Disseminated visceral botryomycosis. Report of a fatal case probably caused by Pseudomonas aeruginosa. *Am. J. Clin. Pathol.* **33**, 43–47.

18 Mycotic keratitis

(Keratomycosis)

Aetiologic agents:

A diversity of microorganisms, including hyaline and dematiaceous filamentous fungi, yeast-like fungi, and actinomycetes. The fungi most frequently implicated are members of the genus *Aspergillus*, most commonly *A. fumigatus*, *A. flavus* and *A. niger;* members of the genus *Candida*, particularly *C. albicans;* and *Fusarium solani*. The actinomycete *Actinomyces israelii* (*bovis*) has also been isolated from corneal ulcers[1].

Definition and background information

Mycotic keratitis is an infection of the cornea by fungi or actinomycetes. Previously a rare disease, it has been observed with increasing frequency in recent years. Both clinical and experimental evidence indicates that the increased incidence of mycotic keratitis is associated with the increased topical use of steroids and antibacterial antibiotics to treat some other inflammatory ocular disease[2]. A long and varied list of fungal agents of mycotic keratitis has been recorded. The organisms involved are not basically pathogenic fungi. Most are airborne or soil saprophytes that have the added capacity, under certain conditions, to invade injured corneal tissue.

The normal cornea is resistant to invasion by fungi. Mycotic infections occur in corneas that have been damaged by mechanical trauma or by some other disease. Often patients with such infections have received topical steroids and antibacterial antibiotics to prevent or control bacterial infections. This combination of factors renders the cornea susceptible to fungal invasion. Thus, mycotic keratitis is essentially an opportunistic fungus disease.

Certain clinical findings strongly suggest a fungal infection of the cornea. The lesions are ulcerative in nature. Their margins are often elevated above the corneal surface, and the lesions characteristically have a fluffy appearance. Radiating lines of infiltrate from the margins of the ulcer are generally observed. Discrete satellite lesions, slightly distant from the main lesion, are also frequently noted. The satellite lesions may coalesce and form a ring around a portion of the main ulcer[3]. Although the clinical picture is distinctive, an accurate diagnosis rests upon the demonstration of fungi within tissue obtained by scraping the bed and edges of the ulcer. Such tissue should be studied by microscopic examination of direct smears, by culture, and if possible by histopathologic procedures with a battery of histologic stains. Usually, it is not possible by direct examination of smears or sections to identify the species of fungus or actinomycete involved in a case of mycotic keratitis. One can only determine whether the agent is a yeast-like fungus, a hyaline or dematiaceous hyphomycete, or an actinomycete. Cultural studies are necessary to identify the aetiologic agent as to species. Cultural examination alone, however, is inadequate for making an accurate diagnosis of mycotic keratitis because the external eye is not sterile[4] and a fungus isolate may merely represent a surface contaminant. It should be emphasised that even when there is microscopic evidence for fungal invasion of tissue, determining whether a given isolate is the cause of the disease may at times be difficult. The correlation of the microscopic morphology of the fungus isolated with that of the fungus observed in tissue must be taken into consideration in interpreting results of cultural studies.

Early and accurate diagnosis and proper management are very important in mycotic keratitis, because fungal infections, if untreated, can lead to corneal perforation, endophthalmitis, and enucleation. Successful management entails removal of infected tissue, withdrawal of corticosteroids, and topical application of antifungal medications[2]. Antifungal drugs reported to be effective for treating mycotic keratitis are amphotericin B, nystatin, and pimaricin[1].

Histopathology (Figures 399–408)

In most instances, mycotic keratitis is confirmed by wet mount examination and culture of corneal scrapings[5]. However, pathologists may be called upon to confirm or refute a diagnosis of mycotic keratitis based solely on the histopathologic examination of excised corneal tissue or corneal scrapings.

Microscopically, H&E-stained sections reveal varying degrees of corneal destruction usually associated with the presence of fungi[2, 3, 6–10]. The central portion of the cornea is usually involved, and peripheral vascularisation or satellite lesions or both may be seen. There may be few, if any, inflammatory cells associated with the presence of fungi, and the absence of an inflammatory response should not preclude a diagnosis of mycotic keratitis. Usually, however, there is a purulent and necrotising inflammatory reaction on the surface of the cornea and at various depths within the underlying stroma. There may be profuse growth of hyphae or yeast-form cells or both within and on the surface of the cornea.

In other cases, only a few actinomycotic or fungal elements may be associated with severe necrotising and purulent reactions. Necrosis and inflammation frequently result in a corneal ulcer that is initially shallow but may continue to develop and eventually may penetrate the anterior chamber of the eye[8, 9]. The progress of tissue destruction and fungal growth may be temporarily blocked, however, by Descemet's membrane, and the accumulation of inflammatory cells and proteinaceous materials may separate this membrane from the corneal stroma. As a result of this separation, Descemet's membrane may be folded, and in some cases a descemetocele is formed. If Descemet's membrane is penetrated, fungal or actinomycete growth may be profuse on the posterior surface of the cornea. Endophthalmitis may also develop with both chambers of the eye filled with exudate and varying numbers of proliferating fungi or actinomycetes.

Because corneal ulcers may be caused by infectious agents other than fungi or actinomycetes, or may result from noninfectious processes[11], it is extremely important to determine whether fungi or actinomycetes are present within the affected tissues. With the exception of most dematiaceous fungi[12–14], those species most frequently implicated as agents of mycotic keratitis are difficult to detect in H&E-stained sections. This is particularly true if fungal or actinomycotic elements are sparse or degenerated. However, with the special stains for fungi and bacteria (actinomycetes), these agents are readily demonstrated within the affected tissues at the base and edge of the ulcer, or in the exudate in the anterior chamber. Although the species of the fungus or actinomycete seen in corneal tissues cannot be determined, tissue invasion by such organisms can be confirmed and certain fungi can sometimes be placed in their proper genus, e.g., species of *Aspergillus* and *Candida*.

In the absence of cultural studies, specific fluorescent antibody tests on corneal scrapings or unstained tissue sections may be valuable for identifying the aetiologic agent as to genus and perhaps species.

References

1 Rippon, J. W. (1974). *Medical Mycology, The Pathogenic Fungi and Pathogenic Actinomycetes*. W. B. Saunders Co., Philadelphia. pp. 475–484.

2 Zimmerman, L. E. (1962). Mycotic keratitis. *Lab. Invest.* **11**, 1151–1160.

3 Kaufman, H. E. and Wood, R. M. (1965). Mycotic keratitis. *Am. J. Ophthalmol.* **59**, 993–1000.

4 Hammereke, J. C. and Ellis, P. O. (1960). Mycotic flora of the conjunctiva. *Am. J. Ophthalmol.* **49**, 1174–1178.

5 Wilson, L. A. and Sexton, R. R. (1968). Laboratory diagnosis in fungal keratitis. *Am. J. Ophthalmol.* **66**, 464–653.

6 Jones, D. B., Sexton, R. R. and Rebell, G. (1969). Mycotic keratitis in South Florida: A review of 39 cases. *Trans. Ophthalmol. Soc. U.K.* **89**, 781–797.

7 Naumann, G., Green, W. R. and Zimmerman, L. E. (1967). Mycotic keratitis. *Am. J. Ophthalmol.* **64**, 668–682.

8 Elliott, I. D., Halde, C. and Shapiro, J. (1977). Keratitis and endophthalmitis caused by Petriellidium boydii. *Am. J. Ophthalmol.* **83**, 16–18.

9 Schwartz, L. K., Loignon, L. M. and Webster, R. G., Jr. (1978). Posttraumatic phycomycosis of the anterior segment. *Arch. Ophthalmol.* **96**, 860–863.

10 Chin, G. N. and Goodman, N. L. (1978). Aspergillus flavus keratitis. *Ann. Ophthalmol.* **10**, 415–418.

11 Conant, N. F., Smith, D. T., Baker, R. D. and Callaway, J. L. (1971). *Manual of Clinical Mycology*, 3rd ed. W. B. Saunders Co., Philadelphia. pp. 541–547.

12 Nityananda, K., Sivasubramaniam, P. and Ajello, L. (1964). A case of mycotic keratitis caused by Curvularia geniculata. *Arch. Ophthalmol.* **71**, 456–458.

13 Wilson, L., Sexton, R. R. and Ahearn, D. (1966). Keratochromomycosis. *Arch. Ophthalmol.* **76**, 811–816.

14 Zapater, R. C., Albesi, E. J. and Garcia, G. H. (1975). Mycotic keratitis by Drechslera spicifera. *Sabouraudia* **13**, 295–298.

19 Nocardiosis

Aetiologic agents:

The principal species are *Nocardia asteroides*, *N. brasiliensis* and *N. caviae*.

Definition and background information

Nocardiosis is a subacute to chronic suppurative or granulomatous disease of humans and lower animals caused by members of the genus *Nocardia*. The species most frequently implicated are *N. asteroides, N. brasiliensis,* and *N. caviae*. Nocardiosis is an exogenous disease, and infections are contracted by exposure to these organisms that live as saprophytes in nature.

By tradition, the *Nocardia* species fall within the province of medical mycology. However, they are bacteria, not fungi, and are classified in the Order Actinomycetales, which includes organisms such as the mycobacteria and *Actinomyces* species. The *Nocardia* species are aerobic organisms that grow well on routine laboratory media which do not contain antibacterial antibiotics. The three species are morphologically similar. They develop slowly on laboratory media, and their colonies are characteristically heaped and folded. They may have a moist, glabrous surface or one covered with a powdery or short downy aerial mycelium. Colonies may be cream to tan or shades of yellow to yellowish orange. When aerial mycelium is conspicuous, the surface is chalky white. Microscopically, both in culture and in clinical materials, the three species appear as branched mycelium which is 1 μm or less in diameter and which fragments into bacillary and coccoid forms. All three species are gram positive and partially acid fast. They may stain unevenly and present a 'beaded' appearance. When they cause systemic and subcutaneous infections, these actinomycetes are usually found free or in loose aggregates in tissue; in mycetomas they occur in the form of granules (see Chapter 17). Because of their close morphological similarities, the nocardiae can be identified as to species only by isolating them in culture and by studying their physiological and biochemical properties[1, 2].

Nocardiosis is extremely variable both clinically and pathologically. The disease may be systemic, usually with a primary pulmonary focus. It may also occur as single or multiple subcutaneous lesions or as a localised form of mycetoma[3].

Systemic nocardiosis is primarily a pulmonary disease characterised by the formation of suppurative lesions in the lungs and other parts of the body. Clinical manifestations of pulmonary infections vary considerably. Some individuals with systemic nocardiosis are relatively asymptomatic; others may have a benign self-limiting bronchopulmonary infection manifested by cough, fever, and pulmonary infiltrates. In more severe cases, the disease appears as a slowly or rapidly progressive pulmonary infection. If untreated, fulminating nocardiosis can be fatal. The more severe forms of pulmonary nocardiosis occur in patients with an underlying disease that reduces their body defenses. The infection may spread from the lungs directly to the pleural cavity. Development of subcutaneous abscesses with sinus tracts that open to the skin surface are characteristic.

Pulmonary infections may disseminate by way of the blood stream and lymphatics to the brain and meninges or other parts of the body, and localised abscesses may develop at the sites of distant spread.

Subcutaneous nocardiosis may be secondary to systemic disease, or may occur as a primary disease resulting from direct inoculation of the organism through the skin. Subcutaneous infections appear as small nodules that heal spontaneously, or they may suppurate and ulcerate. Infections may spread to regional lymph nodes.

All three *Nocardia* species may cause mycetomas. Mycetomas due to nocardiae are discussed and illustrated in Chapter 17.

Nocardiosis has been recorded in a variety of lower animals. Dogs and cattle appear to be the most frequently affected domestic species[4]. Nocardiosis in dogs is similar to that observed in man. Systemic canine infections usually have a pulmonary focus. Common signs are dyspnea, coughing, anorexia, and nasal and ocular discharges. The disease process may remain confined to the lungs or may disseminate to other parts of the body, including the brain. Cutaneous and subcutaneous infections appear to be more common than systemic involvement. Cutaneous and subcutaneous lesions vary in form and severity, but characteristically appear as abscesses with draining sinus tracts.

Bovine nocardiosis may be manifested as mastitis, or there may be pulmonary involvement. Mastitis is the most common form of the disease in cattle. The disease is usually encountered in a single member of a herd. However, it may at times affect many members and cause severe economic losses.

In most cases, infections are confined to the mammary gland. At times, the infection may spread to the supramammary and inguinal lymph nodes. Infections may be acute or chronic and vary from mild to severe, depending upon the host. Systemic and cutaneous *Nocardia* infections have also been diagnosed in nonhuman primates[5], cats[6], and other animal species.

Systemic and subcutaneous forms of nocardiosis occur throughout the world. Mycetomas due to the *Nocardia* species also occur in many parts of the world, but are more common in the tropics and subtropics, regions where individuals commonly walk barefooted. Systemic infections may occur in humans and lower animals after inhalation of the agent. Primary subcutaneous infections and mycetomas occur when the organisms are introduced into the tissues at the time of an injury. In bovine mastitis cases, the organisms enter the gland through the teat canal. Nocardiosis is not transmitted from man to man or from animals to man. Infections are contracted by exposure to sources in nature[4].

Sulfonamides are the drugs of choice for treating nocardiosis. The sulfa drugs can be given alone or in combination with antibacterial antibiotics. To be effective, antimicrobial therapy must be prolonged. Where indicated, surgical therapy is a valuable adjunct, but not a substitute for antimicrobial treatment[3].

Histopathology (Figures 409–419)

In most subjects with nocardiosis, the lungs are the primary site of infection[3, 7, 8], and extension of infection to the pleura may result in empyema. The systemic form of nocardiosis is actually a pyemia that usually results in the formation of small to massive abscesses in many organs and tissues. Secondary lesions can occur in any part of the body but are most frequently seen in the brain, spinal cord, meninges, intestines, and peritoneum[3, 8, 9, 10].

In both the systemic and localised forms of nocardiosis, the tissue response to the *Nocardia spp.* is monotonously similar from specimen to specimen and case to case[4, 8, 11]. Generally, the inflammatory reaction is intensely purulent and, at times, necrotising. One usually sees either multiple confluent abscesses of various sizes or solid sheets of neutrophils and cellular debris that contain slender, gram-positive, branched, filamentous bacteria. In some cases, eosinophils and mononuclear cells may also be present. Although abscesses tend to occur, they may be poorly delimited and may or may not be enclosed by a fibrotic capsule infiltrated with varying numbers and types of inflammatory cells.

In advanced lesions, a chronic inflammatory reaction consisting of macrophages, plasma cells, lymphocytes, and neutrophils may predominate. Mononuclear cells commonly surround an abscess and blend imperceptibly with the purulent material in its centre. Generally, fibrosis tends to be less severe in nocardiosis than in actinomycosis, and when a fibrotic capsule encloses an abscess, it may be narrow and ill-defined. Clusters of epithelioid and multinucleated giant cells may also be seen at the periphery of an abscess, usually embedded within a fibrotic capsule. Although poorly formed granulomas are occasionally present, we have never observed a purely granulomatous response to the aetiologic agents of nocardiosis. Others have had similar experiences[3, 8, 12]. Instead, one may see a microabscess whose purulent centre is enclosed by a granulomatous wall in which histiocytes and multinucleated giant cells of both types are plentiful.

Within abscesses, nocardial filaments are usually abundant. They may be extracellular and intimately surrounded by neutrophils, or intracellular within macrophages. Although organisms are more numerous in the purulent and necrotic areas, they may also be seen in areas of granulomatous inflammation and fibrosing granulation tissue. In the latter sites, organisms are predominantly intracellular.

At times, particularly in immunosuppressed and debilitated patients, focal areas of necrosis develop in the lungs or other organs that are associated with little or no inflammatory reaction. These necrotic areas as well as some abscesses may contain individual filaments, aggregates of tangled filaments and, at times, filaments organised into granules. The granules are generally not associated with Splendore–Hoeppli material as is commonly seen in actinomycosis. (For a description of nocardial granules, see Chapter 17.)

The identification of an organism as a member of the genus *Nocardia* in tissue sections is based on its morphological and staining characteristics[1, 2, 13, 14]. In Gram-stained sections, organisms appear as delicate, branched filaments ranging from 10–30 μm or more in length and 0.5–1.0 μm in width. They frequently appear beaded or granular, especially when the Gram stain is used. Filaments branch at approximately right angles, and when branched and beaded, they are somewhat similar in appearance to Chinese characters. Coccobacillary forms may also be seen and probably result from fragmentation of filaments. When abundant, nocardial filaments are easily demonstrated. At times, however, filaments are sparse, and because of this, they should be diligently searched for under a microscope equipped with a high dry objective. Once located, the organisms should be studied in detail under oil immersion, and characteristic branching should be demonstrated.

In general, the *Nocardia* species react to histological stains as do nonfilamentous bacteria. Individual filaments are very difficult or impossible to see in H&E-stained sections, and they therefore are easily overlooked. Nocardial filaments are also not visible with the GF and PAS stains. Satisfactory results are obtained, however, by using the tissue Gram stains. Of these stains, the Brown and Brenn procedure has given the best results in our laboratory. The nocardiae are also well demonstrated by the GMS procedure, but filaments may be weakly or unevenly stained unless the staining time in the silver nitrate solution is increased from 60 min. to 80–100 min.

The *Nocardia* species are characteristically partially acid-fast in tissue sections stained with the modified Kinyoun or CDC modified Fite–Faraco acid-fast staining procedures. In most of the sections we have examined from subjects with culturally confirmed nocardiosis, some but not all of the filaments have shown strong acid-fast stainability with the latter procedure. A weak decolourising agent such as 0.5–1.0% aqueous sulphuric acid must be used in these procedures instead of acid alcohol, which is the usual decolouriser used for acid-fast staining of the mycobacteria, because nocardial filaments do not as a rule demonstrate acid-fastness when acid alcohol is used. The morphologic and tinctorial features of the *Nocardia* and *Actinomyces* species are reviewed by Robboy and Vickery[13].

If individual filaments of the *Nocardia spp.* are not acid-fast, they cannot be differentiated from those of the *Actinomyces spp.* and members of other actinomycete genera. *Nocardia spp.* in tissues may be organised into granules, as discussed in the chapter on mycetomas. Usually, such granules do not have peripheral eosinophilic clubs[12, 15, 16].

We have seen individual, unbranched filaments of the nocardiae mistaken for *Mycobacterium tuberculosis* because the latter bacterium is also acid-fast and gram-positive. However, the mycobacteria remain acid-fast when an acid alcohol decolouriser is used in the standard acid-fast staining procedures, whereas the nocardiae do not. Also, morphologically, the mycobacteria are shorter bacilli that usually do not appear beaded. (An exception to this would be certain 'atypical' mycobacteria, e.g. *M. intracellulare*, *M. marinum* and *M. ulcerans*, that are sometimes elongated and beaded.)

It should be reemphasised that the inflammatory response to the *Nocardia spp.* is nonspecific and that the causative agents are not visible in H&E-stained tissue sections. Therefore, no clue as to infection with *Nocardia* is given in sections stained by this routine procedure. The diagnosis may be missed unless the pathologist has a high index of suspicion and orders special stains for demonstrating the aetiologic agent. If a battery of special stains is used (Brown and Brenn, Fite–Faraco acid-fast for *Nocardia,* and GMS) a diagnosis of nocardiosis can be made by demonstrating typical gram-positive, partially acid-fast, branched filaments diffusely distributed in lesions. Merely observing unbranched acid-fast bacteria is an insufficient basis for making a diagnosis of nocardiosis. Cultural studies are required for identifying and differentiating the *Nocardia spp.*

References

1 Berd, D. (1973). Laboratory identification of clinically important aerobic actinomycetes. *Appl. Microbiol.* **25**, 665–681.

2 Georg, L. K. (1974). Nocardia species as opportunists and current methods for their identification. In *Opportunistic Pathogens,* pp. 177–201. J. E. Prier and H. Friedman, eds. University Park Press, Baltimore, Md.

3 Causey, W. A. and Lee, R. (1978). Nocardiosis. In *Handbook of Clinical Neurology,* pp. 517–530. P. J. Vinken and G. W. Bruyn, eds. North Holland Publishing Company, Amsterdam.

4 Jungerman, P. F. and Schwartzman, R. M. (1972). *Veterinary Medical Mycology,* pp. 171–183. Lea and Febiger, Philadelphia.

5 McClure, H. M., Chang, J., Kaplan, W. and Brown, J. M. (1976). Pulmonary nocardiosis in an orangutan. *J. Am. Vet. Med. Assoc.* **169**, 943–945.

6 Ajello, L., Walker, W. W., Dungworth, D. L. and Brumfield, G. L. (1961). Isolation of Nocardia brasiliensis from a cat. *J. Am. Vet. Med. Assoc.* **138**, 370–376.

7 Webster, B. H. (1956). Pulmonary nocardiosis. *Am. Rev. Tbc. Pul. Dis.* **73**, 485–500.

8 Pizzolato, P. (1971). Nocardiosis. In *The Pathologic Anatomy of Mycosis. Human Infection with Fungi, Actinomycetes and Algae.* R. D. Baker, ed. Springer-Verlag, Berlin. pp. 1059–1080.

9 Pizzolato, P., Ziskind, J., Derman, H. and Buff, E. E. (1961). Nocardiosis of the brain. Report of three cases. *Am. J. Clin. Pathol.* **36**, 151–156.

10 Frazier, A. R., Rosenow, E. C. III and Roberts, G. D. (1975). Nocardiosis: a review of 25 cases occurring during 24 months. *Mayo Clin. Proc.* **50**, 657–663.

11 Swerczek, T. W., Trautwein, G. and Nielson, S. W. (1968). Canine nocardiosis. *Zentralbe. Vet. Med.* **15**, 971–978.

12 Case Records of the Massachusetts General Hospital. (Pulmonary nodule in a renal-transplant recipient.) Weekly clinicopathological exercises. (1978). *N. Engl. J. Med.* **298(3)**, 154–159.

13 Robboy, S. J. and Vickery, A. L. (1970). Tinctorial and morphologic properties distinguishing actinomycosis and nocardiosis. *N. Engl. J. Med.* **282**, 593–596.

14 Gordon, R. E. and Mihm, J. M. (1962). The type species of the genus Nocardia. *J. Gen. Microbiol.* **27**, 1–10.

15 Peabody, J. W. and Seabury, J. H. (1957). Actinomycosis and nocardiosis. *J. Chronic Dis.* **5**, 374–403.

16 Palmer, D. L., Harvey, R. L. and Wheeler, J. K. (1974). Diagnostic and therapeutic considerations in Nocardia asteroides infection. *Medicine (Baltimore)* **53**, 391–401.

20 Paracoccidioidomycosis

(South American blastomycosis, paracoccidioidal granuloma, Lutz–Splendore–Almeida disease)

Aetiologic agent:

Paracoccidioides brasiliensis

Synonym:

Blastomyces brasiliensis

Definition and background information

Paracoccidioidomycosis is basically a pulmonary mycotic disease of humans that is geographically confined to Latin America. The northern limits of its endemic areas reach Mexico and then extend down through Central America to Argentina. Currently the only South American countries without confirmed autochthonous cases are Chile, Guyana, and Surinam. The nations with the highest incidence and prevalence of the disease are Brazil, Colombia, and Venezuela[1].

Paracoccidioidomycosis is caused by the dimorphic mould, *Paracoccidioides brasiliensis.* Presumably it lives in nature as a free-living saprophyte. Indeed, there are reports of its isolation from soil in Argentina[2] and Venezuela[3]. However, these findings have not been confirmed, nor have they led to the discovery of the ecological niche occupied in nature by *P. brasiliensis.*

In contrast to the other systemic mycoses, cases of paracoccidioidomycosis among lower animals have not been discovered with any degree of certainty[1].

Diagnosis of the various types of paracoccidioidomycosis rests not on their clinical expression but on finding the aetiologic agent's characteristic cells in clinical materials. In tissue, *P. brasiliensis* develops as a yeast with large spherical cells that attain diameters ranging from 10–60 μm. The mother cell of *P. brasiliensis,* unlike that of *Blastomyces dermatitidis,* gives rise to multiple buds that are attached by narrow necks. The buds may become almost as large as the mother cell and then become detached. The freed daughter cells in turn bud, and thus the invading fungus multiplies and spreads by contiguity or lymphatic dissemination.

Along with the yeast cells with large buds, mother cells are formed whose surfaces become studded with numerous small buds that in mid-cross-section appear like a ship's pilot wheel.

Infections that are generally believed to be primarily of pulmonary origin can be divided into three broad categories:

1 Pulmonary
   a. Benign
   b. Progressive
2 Mucocutaneous-Lymphangitic
3 Systemic

1. *Pulmonary paracoccidioidomycosis*

a. Benign: This asymptomatic form of the disease has only recently been described[4]. Discovery was incidental, having been made during autopsies for other reasons. Calcification, with the diagnostic multiple buds of *P. brasiliensis,* was found. However, the predominant tissue form cells were small and single budded and could have been mistaken for the tissue form cells of *Histoplasma capsulatum* var. *capsulatum.* Several sections were needed to discover multiple budded forms. With specific fluorescent antibody conjugates for *P. brasiliensis,* the small form cells of this fungus can readily be identified and can be distinguished from those of other fungi with a yeast-like tissue form[5].

b. Progressive. The symptoms of progressive pulmonary paracoccidioidomycosis are similar to those of respiratory infections in general. In a series of 34 cases[6] the predominant symptoms were cough, expectoration, dyspnea, haemoptysis, weight loss, fever, and lethargy.

Specific diagnosis of paracoccidioidomycosis is often delayed since the symptoms of the progressive form are not pathognomonic. Tuberculosis, cancer, tracheobronchitis, and bronchopneumonia are the diseases most apt to be considered before the true nature of the malady is suspected. Diagnosis can be readily established by microscopic study of sputum preparations. There one would find large, multiple budded yeast cells. Culture of the sputum on such media as blood agar would be expected to be positive in a high percentage of cases. Properly controlled immunodiffusion tests would also be useful in establishing a diagnosis[7,8].

2. *Mucocutaneous-Lymphangitic Paracoccidioidomycosis*

Some clinicians consider the mucocutaneous form of paracoccidioidomycosis to be the result of direct inoculation from an exogenous source[9]. A growing number hold, however, that such a localisation is the result of dissemination from a primary subclinical pulmonary infection[10].

The mucocutaneous lesions generally involve the oral mucosa, the gums, the nasal and anal mucosa, and the conjunctivae. Stomatitis and ulceration are the most striking manifestations of oral infection. The ulcers are granulomatous and slow spreading. The tonsils may eventually be invaded.

The gum and periodontal lesions eventually loosen the teeth and cause them to be shed or require extraction. Oral infections, if severe and not treated in their early stages, may spread to involve the tongue, epiglottis, and uvula.

The regional lymph nodes that drain the affected parts commonly become infected, resulting in lymphadenopathy. The cervical lymph nodes may become strikingly enlarged. The lymph nodes in time rupture and drain, which leads to the development of fistulous tracts. The discharged pus contains numerous fungal cells that are readily detected by direct microscopic examination of wet mounts or stained smears.

3. *Systemic Paracoccidioidomycosis*
Dissemination of a primary infection from the lungs by way of the lymphatics or blood vessels may come to involve any or all of the following organs: liver, spleen, intestines, adrenal glands, bones, and the central nervous system.

Diagnosis of systemic paracoccidioidomycosis is based on either the demonstration of the tissue form elements of *P. brasiliensis* in tissue or its isolation or both. Serological tests would also be of diagnostic value, as would be the use of specific fluorescent antibody conjugates for detecting and identifying the tissue form cells of *P. brasiliensis* in histological sections and smears.

Serological tests are very useful aids to the diagnosis of paracoccidioidomycosis. They are rapid and provide presumptive evidence of infection. Serological determinations also have prognostic value and can be used to follow patients' responses to therapy. The most commonly used serodiagnostic tests for this disease are the complement fixation and immunodiffusion tests.

The drugs of choice in the therapy of paracoccidioidomycosis are the sulfonamides, such as the combination of 2,4-diamino-5 (3,4,5-trimethoxybenzyl)-pyrimidine and sulfamethoxazole, and amphotericin B[11].

P. brasiliensis grows slowly at 25°C or room temperature on Sabouraud dextrose agar or similar media. Early growth is usually glabrous and heaped, but white aerial mycelium eventually covers the colony. Microscopically, the growth will be found to consist of hyaline, septate mycelium that is sterile. Chlamydospores are produced, and cells that resemble conidia may be observed. However, several investigators have reported the production of conidia in some isolates[12, 13].

Because the mycelial growth of this fungus lacks distinctive diagnostic features, suspected isolates should be subcultured onto enriched media, such as blood agar, and grown at 37°C. Under those conditions, isolates of *P. brasiliensis* will be converted to their distinctive yeast-form that is indistinguishable from that produced in tissue.

Histopathology (Figures 420–443)

In tissue sections, cells of *P. brasiliensis* are yeast-like, round to oval, and range from 5–60 μm in diameter. Their refractile cell walls are relatively thin but clearly defined. The cytoplasmic contents stain basophilic or amphophilic with H&E and are often retracted from the rigid cell wall, apparently as a result of shrinkage during fixation or processing. Cells of *P. brasiliensis* are uninucleate and reproduce by both single and multiple budding. The buds are attached to the parent cell by narrow connections, and they often appear to be 'pinched-off' in their formation. Rarely, buds are connected to the parent cell by narrow tube-like structures similar to those of *Loboa loboi*. Bud scars resulting from detachment of blastospores are often seen on the external cell wall of a parent cell. These scars are not evident when stained by H&E. Multiple budding forms of *P. brasiliensis* may be of two types: a) daughter cells or buds which are much smaller than the parent cell, spherical, and all about the same size. When such a budding cell is sectioned near its equatorial plane, it has the distinctive appearance of a ship's steering wheel and is called the 'steering wheel' form. b) daughter cells which are larger than those above and are of unequal sizes and shapes. Large buds up to 10 μm in diameter may occur in the latter type. Since the buds develop from all sides of the parent cell, only one or two attachments can usually be seen in one plane of the section. For this reason, the parent cell appears to have a cluster of unconnected satellite cells around it. Small free fungus cells, 2–5 μm in diameter, that are found scattered in a lesion probably represent detached buds. Chains of three or more budding cells are often seen and may be mistaken for pseudohyphae. Hyphae are rarely formed in tissue.

The histopathologic features of paracoccidioidomycosis are similar to those characteristic of blastomycosis (Chapter 7) and coccidioidomycosis (Chapter 10). Since the inflammatory reaction is not specific for any of these mycoses, a histologic diagnosis cannot be made unless typical forms of the aetiologic agent are seen.

In paracoccidioidomycosis, the lungs are the most common sites of primary infection, and the disease may disseminate to any area of the body, especially the skin, mucous membranes, and viscera[6, 10, 14, 15]. Because *P. brasiliensis* disseminates via the lymphatics and blood stream, regional lymph nodes, and other lymphoid organs such as the tonsils, Peyer's patches, and spleen are commonly involved. Superficial lymph nodes may suppurate and drain through the contiguous skin or mucous membrane. Invasion of tissue by *P. brasiliensis* elicits a mixed purulent and granulomatous inflammatory reaction. Within the same specimen, one area may contain focal or confluent abscesses where neutrophils predominate, while another area may contain epithelioid cell granulomas that are often poorly defined. The granulomas either are solid or contain central areas of caseous necrosis and neutrophils surrounded by variable numbers of foreign body and Langhans' giant cells, macrophages, lymphocytes, plasma cells, and fibroblasts. The amount of peripheral fibrosis varies. Numerous organisms may be found in giant cells, in the centre of abscesses, or scattered throughout the granulomatous tissue.

Necrosis is frequently observed in rapidly progressing lesions where masses of extracellular budding organisms of various sizes and shapes invade tissues. At times, the normal architecture of a small organ such as a lymph node or adrenal gland is totally effaced by rapidly proliferating fungal cells. Large extracellular masses of fungi are usually accompanied by smaller numbers of intracellular organisms within giant and epithelioid cells.

Old fibrogranulomatous and sometimes calcified lesions occur, especially in the lungs[4]. In these old lesions, cells of *P. brasiliensis* may be fragmented, distorted, and poorly or unevenly stained by the special fungus procedures. Typical multiple budding forms are almost never seen. Rather, fungal elements appear as empty shells or rings of various shapes and sizes that may also be calcified. In these instances, the atypical *P. brasiliensis* cells can easily be confused with small empty spherules of *Coccidioides immitis* or with the poorly stained, empty yeast forms of *Blastomyces dermatitidis*.

The mucocutaneous form of paracoccidioidomycosis most often involves the skin and mucous membranes of the nose, mouth, pharynx, gastrointestinal tract, anus, and eye[9, 14]. Microscopically, ulceration and marked pseudoepitheliomatous hyperplasia of the epidermis or mucosa may be seen. Broad rete pegs often penetrate deep into the dermis, and intraepidermal microabscesses are common. (Grossly, these lesions are sometimes mistaken for carcinoma.) In the dermis or submucosa there is granulomatous inflammation with microabscess formation and necrosis. In about 25% of mucocutaneous lesions, the underlying skeletal muscle is also involved[16]. Granulation tissue may be prominent, especially in chronic lesions. Numerous fungi, either free or phagocytised by macrophages or giant cells, are found within the purulent and granulomatous components of the lesion.

In the central nervous system, including the meninges, the tissue reaction to *P. brasiliensis* is predominantly granulomatous[17].

Cells of *P. brasiliensis* are usually visible when stained by H&E, but the details of their morphology are better demonstrated with the special fungus stains, especially GMS. In most cases, diagnostic forms of the fungus are readily found in active lesions. Sometimes, however, organisms may be sparse, or diagnostic forms are not readily detected. In such instances, serial sections may have to be carefully examined before a diagnosis can be made.

Single cells and cells of *P. brasiliensis* with one bud closely resemble other yeasts of similar size, e.g., *B. dermatitidis* and lightly encapsulated *Cryptococcus neoformans*. *P. brasiliensis* and *B. dermatitidis* with single buds can generally be differentiated from each other by the fact that the latter has a characteristic broad basal attachment of the bud to the parent cell. The mucicarmine stain is helpful in differentiating *P. brasiliensis* from *C. neoformans,* especially when prominent capsules do not surround the latter. Occasionally, it may not be possible to differentiate these fungi by morphological and histochemical criteria. In such instances, cultural and immunofluorescence studies are necessary[5].

At times, *B. dermatitidis* may form multiple buds and resemble *P. brasiliensis*. Again, the broad basal attachment of the buds to the parent cell of the former is a useful criterion for differentiating the two.

When a tissue section contains only detached small blastospores of *P. brasiliensis,* these forms may be mistaken for *Histoplasma capsulatum* var. *capsulatum,* especially when they are intracellular. Serial sections must then be examined to demonstrate the diagnostic multiple budding forms of *P. brasiliensis*. If a diagnosis cannot be made by histological examination, cultural and immunofluorescence studies are required[5].

References

1 Ajello, L. (1972). Paracoccidioidomycosis: A historical review. In *Paracoccidioidomycosis,* pp. 3–10. Scientific Publication No. 254. Pan American Health Organization, Washington, D.C.

2 Negroni, P. (1967). Aislamiento del Paracoccidioides brasiliensis de una muestra de tierra del Chaco argentino. *Bol. Acad.* Buenos Aires **45**, 513–516.

3 Albornoz, M. B. (1971). Isolation of Paracoccidioides brasiliensis from rural soil in Venezuela. *Sabouraudia* **9**, 248–253.

4 Angulo-Ortega, A. (1972). Calcifications in paracoccidioidomycosis: are they the morphological manifestations of subclinical infections. In *Paracoccidioidomycosis,* pp. 129–133. Scientific Publication No. 254. Pan American Health Organization, Washington, D.C.

5 Kaplan, W. (1972). Application of immunofluorescence to the diagnosis of paracoccidioidomycosis. In *Paracoccidioidomycosis,* pp. 224–226. Scientific Publication No. 254. Pan American Health Organization, Washington, D.C.

6 Londero, A. T., Ramos, C. D. and Lopes, J. O. S. (1978). Progressive pulmonary paracoccidioidomycosis. A study of 34 cases observed in Rio Grande do Sul (Brazil). *Mycopathologia* **63**, 53–56.

7 Kaufman, L. (1972). Evaluation of serological tests for paracoccidioidomycosis: Preliminary report. In *Paracoccidioidomycosis,* pp. 221–223. Scientific Publication No. 254. Pan American Health Organization, Washington, D.C.

8 Palmer, D. F., Kaufman, L., Kaplan, W. and Cavallaro, J. J. (1977). *Serodiagnosis of mycotic diseases.* Charles C. Thomas, Springfield, Illinois.

9 Sampaio, S. A. P. (1972). Clinical manifestations of paracoccidioidomycosis. In *Paracoccidioidomycosis,* pp. 101–108. Proceedings of the First Pan American Symposium. Scientific Publication No. 254. Pan American Health Organization, Washington, D.C.

10 Yarzabal, L. A. (1972). Pathogenesis of paracoccidioidomycosis in man. In *Paracoccidioidomycosis,* pp. 261–270. Scientific Publication No. 254. Pan American Health Organization, Washington, D.C.

11 Negroni, P. (1972). Prolonged therapy for paracoccidioidomycosis: approaches, complications and risk. In *Paracoccidioidomycosis,* pp. 147–155. Scientific Publication No. 254. Pan American Health Organization, Washington, D.C.

12 Borelli, D. (1955). *Los aleurios de Paracoccidioides brasiliensis.* In *Mem. VI Cong. Venez. Cienc. Med.* **4**, 2241–2253.

13 Restrepo, A. (1970). A reappraisal of the microscopical appearance of the mycelial phase of Paracoccidioides brasiliensis. *Sabouraudia* **8**, 141–144.

14 Kroll, J. J. and Walzer, R. A. (1972). Paracoccidioidomycosis in the United States. *Arch. Dermatol.* **106**, 543–546.

15 Benaim Pinto, H. (1961). La paracoccidioidosis brasiliensis como enfermedad sistemica. *Mycopathologia* **15**, 90–114.

16 Robledo, M. (1972). Myositis in paracoccidioidomycosis. In *Paracoccidioidomycosis,* pp. 168–169. Scientific Publication No. 254. Pan American Health Organization, Washington, D.C.

17 Raphael, A. and Pereira, W. C. (1962). Granuloma blastomicotico cerebral. *Rev. Hosp. Clin. Fac. Med.* Sao Paulo **17**, 430–433.

21 Phaeohyphomycosis

(Phaeosporotrichosis, chromomycosis (in part), phaeomycotic cyst, cerebral dematiomycosis, cerebral chromomycosis, cladosporiosis, cladosporoma, dactylariosis)

Aetiologic agents:

A wide variety of opportunistic dematiaceous fungi, e.g., *Cladosporium bantianum (trichoides), Dactylaria gallopava, Drechslera hawaiiensis, D. rostrata, D. spicifera, Exophiala (Phialophora) jeanselmei, Mycocentrospora acerina, Phialophora parasitica, P. richardsiae, Wangiella dermatitidis.*

Definition and background information

Phaeohyphomycosis is the name given to those subcutaneous and systemic diseases caused by various black moulds that develop in tissue in the form of dark-walled, septate mycelium[1-2]. This name replaces the misleading and inappropriate term 'phaeosporotrichosis'[3], which had been compounded to cover such infections. The term was unacceptable since the clinical expressions of phaeohyphomycosis simply do not resemble those of sporotrichosis and since none of its many aetiologic agents resemble the dimorphic *Sporothrix schenckii* in tissue or in culture.

Phaeohyphomycosis is a cosmopolitan disease. The disease has been reported from most parts of the world. Aside from human cases, infections have also been diagnosed in fish[4], birds[5], cats[6,7] and horses[8].

The clinical forms of phaeohyphomycosis fall into two basic types: subcutaneous and systemic. Infections generally occur in compromised or debilitated hosts. Individuals with such chronic diseases as diabetes and leukemia, and patients on immunosuppressants, steroids, and broad spectrum antibiotics are vulnerable to infection by the opportunistic agents of phaeohyphomycosis.

Subcutaneous Phaeohyphomycosis: In this type of infection abscesses or verrucous lesions may develop on various parts of the body[1,9]. Their growth is generally slow, and the disease tends to become chronic. Abscesses, which break down and discharge serosanguinous fluid, may be mistaken for bacterial infections. The abscesses are frequently tender to touch, fluctuant, and erythematous. Verrucose lesions may resemble the exuberant, cauliflower-like outgrowths of chromoblastomycosis.

Systemic or Disseminated Phaeohyphomycosis: Vital internal organs are invaded by some of the aetiologic agents of phaeohyphomycosis. The route of infection is generally via the respiratory tract. The most commonly encountered agent is *Cladosporium bantianum* (*trichoides*). This fungus is highly neurotropic. In consequence, most infections are confined to the brain, with only rare involvement of the lungs and other parts of the body. Brain lesions, either single or multiple, appear as encapsulated abscesses[10] or generalised inflammatory infiltrations[11]. Symptoms associated with cerebral phaeohyphomycosis include headaches, nausea, vomiting, fever, nuchal pain, and rigidity.

C. bantianum may cause isolated pulmonary infections. In one instance[12] an indurated mass, six centimetres in diameter, developed in the apex of the left lower lobe of a lung. Upon lobectomy the infection was found to be confined to a bronchiectatic cavity that was filled with greyish-white necrotic material.

Diagnosis of both subcutaneous and systemic phaeohyphomycosis rests on the demonstration of dematiaceous, mycelial filaments in wet mounts or in histological sections of biopsied tissue. The hyphae are best visualised with such fungal stains as Gomori's methenamine silver stain or Gridley's stain. They range from 2–6 μm in diameter and vary considerably in length. They may be branched or unbranched. Frequently the mycelial elements are bizarre in shape and size.

Since the aetiologic agents are basically similar in tissue, specific identification can be made only by isolating the organism and identifying it on the basis of gross and microscopic characteristics.

Mycology (Description of selected aetiologic agents):

a. *Cladosporium bantianum* (Synonyms: *Torula bantiana*, *C. trichoides*). Colonies are velvety, olive black, heaped. Dark-walled septate mycelium; erect, septate conidiophores with lateral prolongations at maturity. Single celled, oval conidia (2–5 × 3–11 μm) borne in long, branched chains.

b. *Dactylaria gallopava*. Colonies are velvety and flat, at first grey, but becoming brown to reddish brown on surface. Reverse is characterised by the formation of a soluble, deep purplish-red pigment. Dark-walled, septate hyphae. Simple conidiophores bearing 2-celled dematiaceous conidia at their tips and sides on short denticles. Conidia are hyaline at first but become dark at maturity. Cuneiform uniseptate conidia with thick walls, 15–19 × 2.2–4.4 μm. Grows well at 25° and 37°C but optimum growth attained at 45°C. Growth inhibited on media that contain cycloheximide.

c. *Drechslera hawaiiensis.* Colonies are cottony, dark blackish brown, becoming velvety. Reverse of colony is black. Septate mycelium with dark walls. Dark coloured conidiophores, simple or branched. Growth indeterminate; large conidia borne singly at the tip of the conidiophore through an apical orifice. Because of continuous growth of the conidiophore, new apexes are formed to the side of the previous one, each producing a conidium. Two to seven conidia are formed that are psuedoseptate, dark-walled, cylindrical, and measure 12–37 × 5–11 μm[13].

d. *Exophiala jeanselmei* (Synonyms: *Phialophora jeanselmei* and *P. gougerotii*). In early stages of growth, colonies are yeast-like (pasty) and black, composed of unicellular blastospores, 2–4 μm D. In older colonies, septate, dematiaceous, branched mycelium is formed. Conidiophores are simple extensions of the mycelium or physiologically specialised intercalary portions of the mycelium. Spore-bearing cells are bulbous with a tapered tip having a series of superimposed rings (annelations). Conidia are oval, unicellular, smooth, 1–3 × 1–5 μm, with a strong tendency to aggregate in masses around the conidiophore[14].

e. *Phialophora parasitica.* Colonies are olive black, velvety, becoming funiculose. Reverse is black. Dematiaceous, septate mycelium. Short to elongate, flask-shaped conidiophores with poorly to well developed collarettes. Conidia are smooth, hyaline, cyclindrical to ovoid, 2–4 × 2–8 μm.

f. *Wangiella dermatitidis* (Synonyms: *Hormisicium dermatitidis, Hormodendrum dermatitidis, Phialophora dermatitidis*).

Colonies with an initial yeast-like growth, pasty and black. Mature colonies are mycelial with septate, dematiaceous hyphae. Conidiophores are simple or branched specialised hyphae. Conidiogenous cells are flask-shaped, smooth and light brown, collarettes lacking. Single-celled, smooth, hyaline conidia, subglobose to obovoid, (2–4 × 2.5–6 μm) tend to aggregate in globular masses around the conidiophores[13].

Histopathology (Figures 444–476)

A histopathologic diagnosis of phaeohyphomycosis is made by demonstrating pigmented, septate hyphae that range from 2–6 μm in width and vary considerably in length in tissue sections or smears[2]. The hyphae may be branched or unbranched, are often constricted at their prominent, thick septations, and sometimes contain bizarre thick-walled, vesicular swellings that reach a diameter of 25 μm or more and resemble chlamydospores. The latter structures are occasionally seen either singly or in chains. Cells that appear to be budding may also be noted. Sometimes the innate brown pigmentation of the mycelium may not be readily apparent, but a careful search will almost always reveal at least some dematiaceous hyphae in unstained (cleared and mounted) or H&E-stained tissue sections. The agents of phaeohyphomycosis are best demonstrated with the special fungus stains, but these procedures are usually unnecessary because of the dark pigmentation of these fungi. If the special fungus stains are used, the natural brown colour of the fungal elements is masked and a diagnosis of phaeohyphomycosis cannot be made.

The various agents of subcutaneous or systemic phaeohyphomycosis in tissues are so similar in appearance that they cannot be differentiated solely on the basis of morphology. Culture is always needed for a specific identification of the aetiologic agents.

Exophiala jeanselmei, Phialophora parasitica, and certain other dematiaceous hyphomycetes cause subcutaneous cystic granulomas in humans[1, 3, 14, 15] and animals[16]. These lesions are usually solitary, encapsulated by dense collagenous connective tissue, and almost always confined to the dermis and subcutaneous tissues; the overlying epidermis is rarely affected. Microscopically, the centre of the granuloma is seen to contain a purulent exudate that is often liquefied and cystic. This central material is surrounded by a wide zone of granulation tissue containing numerous giant cells, epithelioid cells, and neutrophils. Eosinophils are also occasionally present. In our experience, dematiaceous hyphae are abundant and are easily demonstrated by H&E in the central necrotic exudate and especially in the peripheral granulomatous zone. The number of hyphal elements present is even more evident when the special fungus stains are used.

Subcutaneous infections due to *Drechslera spicifera* have been recorded in horses[8], cats[7], and a human[17]. In the animal cases, single or multiple nodular lesions that appeared histologically as a mixed granulomatous, purulent, and necrotising process were localised to the dermis and subcutaneous tissues. Focal ulceration and pseudoepitheliomatous hyperplasia of the epidermis were sometimes seen. In the only human case of cutaneous phaeohyphomycosis due to *D. spicifera*[17], the inflammatory response in the dermis was described as histiocytic and lymphocytic.

Dematiaceous fungi also infect internal organs. In cerebral infections caused by *Cladosporium bantianum*, the most commonly encountered agent in systemic phaeohyphomycosis, there is characteristically a mixed purulent and granulomatous inflammatory reaction with abscess formation[6, 10, 18, 19]. Most lesions caused by this fungus are found in the white matter of the frontal lobe of the cerebrum. They are seldom found in the cerebellum and brainstem. The lungs and other organs are only rarely involved[12]. The brain abscesses may be single or multiple and may measure up to 5 cm in diameter; they are composed of a central zone of neutrophils and necrotic debris enveloped by a thick wall of multinucleated giant cells, epithelioid cells, plasma cells, and lymphocytes. The abscesses may or may not be sharply circumscribed, and they usually stimulate varying degrees of peripheral gliosis. Single hyphae and clusters of dematiaceous, septate, moniliform hyphae are found extracellularly in the central purulent exudate and intracellularly within huge giant cells that form the wall of the abscess. In some instances, the necrotic and liquefied centre of an abscess contains few if any fungal elements, whereas the surrounding granulomatous tissue contains numerous dematiaceous hyphae that are easily detected. Granulomatous leptomeningitis due to *C. bantianum*, without involvement of the brain parenchyma, occurs rarely[11].

Mycotic encephalitis due to *Dactylaria gallopava,* another highly neurotropic agent of systemic phaeohyphomycosis, causes fatal infections in young turkeys and chickens[5, 20, 21]. The lesions are found in all regions of the brain and they may be extensive, often involving more than half of the parenchyma. Microscopically, single or multiple irregularly circumscribed areas of suppurative necrosis and granulomatous inflammation are seen. Coagulative necrosis is frequently observed in the centre of the lesions, together with a mixture of heterophils and multinucleated giant cells. This central zone is rimmed by densely packed foreign body and Langhans' giant cells, some of which are huge and contain 100–200 nuclei in a single plane of section. Palisading epithelioid cells may also occasionally rim the central foci of necrosis, and reactive gliosis is prominent at the lesion's periphery. Elongated, weakly dematiaceous hyphal elements (1.2–2.4 μm D) are randomly distributed throughout the lesion. Because the hyphae are so lightly pigmented in H&E-stained sections, careful examination under oil immersion may be necessary to demonstrate their dematiaceous character.

Angioinvasion is uncommon in infections by agents of phaeohyphomycosis. Other than this, the tissue changes caused by *D. gallopava* are somewhat similar to those caused by the *Aspergillus spp.*, and a diagnosis must be based on the morphologic and pigmentation differences between these two fungi. The hyphae of the *Aspergillus spp.* are wider (3–6 μm D), hyaline, show characteristic dichotomous branching, and are often oriented in the same direction. *D. gallopava* hyphae are lightly pigmented, narrower (<4 μm) than those of the *Aspergillus spp.*, branch irregularly, usually are longer, and are randomly oriented throughout the lesion. Although there are distinct differences between these two fungi in tissues, cultural studies should always complement a histopathologic diagnosis.

In histologic sections, phaeohyphomycosis has been confused with eumycotic mycetomas caused by dematiaceous fungi[22]. However, the causative agents of mycetomas form distinct granules as illustrated in Chapter 17. In phaeohyphomycosis, the causative agents do not form granules but appear as scattered individual hyphae and small aggregates of dematiaceous, septate hyphae that may be bordered by and embedded in Splendore–Hoeppli material. These fungal elements are often intracellular, whereas granules of the mycetomas are nearly always extracellular.

The nonmycelial cells of *Wangiella dermatitidis,* an agent of subcutaneous phaeohyphomycosis[14], may have transverse septations. Because of this, some workers have regarded this fungus as an agent of chromoblastomycosis. We do not agree with this interpretation because the *W. dermatitidis* cells have relatively thin walls, are septate in only one plane, and frequently occur in chains. In contrast, the muriform cells that are characteristic of chromoblastomycosis have thick walls, have septations in two planes, and do not form chains.

References

1 Ajello, L., Georg, L. K., Steigbigel, R. T. and Wang, C. J. K. (1974). A case of phaeohyphomycosis caused by a new species of Phialophora. *Mycologia* **66**, 490–498.

2 Ajello, L. (1975). Phaeohyphomycosis: Definition and etiology. In *Mycoses,* pp. 126–133. Scientific Publication No. 304, Pan American Health Organization, Washington, D.C.

3 Mariat, F., Segretain, G., Destombes, P. and Darasse, H. (1967). Kyste souscutanee mycosique (phaeosporotricose) a Phialophora gougerotii (Matruchot 1910) Borelli 1955, observe au Senegal. *Sabouraudia* **5**, 209–219.

4 Ajello, L., McGinnis, M. and Camper, J. (1977). An outbreak of phaeohyphomycosis in rainbow trout caused by Scolecobasidium humicola. *Mycopathologia* **62**, 15–22.

5 Ranck, F. M., Georg, L. K. and Wallace, D. H. (1974). Dactylariosis – a newly recognized fungus disease of chickens. *Avian Dis.* **18**, 4–20.

6 Jang, S. S., Biberstein, E. L., Rinaldi, M. G., Henness, A. M., Boorman, G. A. and Taylor, R. F. (1977). Feline abscess due to Cladosporium trichoides. *Sabouraudia* **15**, 115–123.

7 Muller, G. H., Kaplan, W., Ajello, L. and Padhye, A. A. (1975). Phaeohyphomycosis caused by Drechslera spicifera in a cat. *J. Am. Vet. Med. Assoc.* **166**, 150–154.
8 Kaplan, W., Chandler, F. W., Ajello, L., Gauthier, R., Higgins, R. and Cayouette, P. (1975). Equine phaeohyphomycosis caused by Drechslera spicifera. *Can. Vet. J.* **16**, 205–208.
9 Lie-Kian-Joe, Njo-Injo Tjoei Eng., Kertopati, S. and Emmons, C. W. (1957). A new verrucous mycosis caused by Cercospora apii. *Arch. Dermatol.* **75**, 864–870.
10 Crichlow, D. K., Enrile, F. T. and Memon, M. Y. (1973). Cerebellar abscess due to Cladosporium trichoides (bantianum): Case report. *Am. J. Clin. Pathol.* **60**, 416–421.
11 Bennett, J. E., Bonner, H., Jennings, A. E. and Lopez, R. I. (1973). Chronic meningitis caused by Cladosporium trichoides. *Am. J. Clin. Pathol.* **59**, 398–407.
12 Limsila, T., Stituimankaru, T. and Thasnakorn, P. (1970). Pulmonary cladosporoma. Report of a case. *J. Med. Assoc.* Thailand **53**, 586–590.
13 Fuste, F. J., Ajello, L., Threlkeld, R. and Henry, J. E. (1973). Drechslera hawaiiensis: Causative agent of a fatal fungal meningo-encephalitis. *Sabouraudia* **11**, 59–63.
14 McGinnis, M. (1978). Human pathogenic species of Exophiala, Phialophora and Wangiella. In *The Black and White Yeasts,* pp. 37–59. Scientific Publication No. 356. Pan American Health Organization, Washington, D.C.
15 Ichinose, H. (1971). Subcutaneous abscesses due to brown fungi. In *The Pathologic Anatomy of Mycoses. Human Infection with Fungi, Actinomycetes and Algae*. R. D. Baker, ed. Springer-Verlag, Berlin. pp. 719–730.
16 Haschek, W. M. and Kasali, O. B. (1977). A case of cutaneous feline phaeohyphomycosis caused by Phialophora gougerotii. *Cornell Vet.* **67**, 467–471.
17 Estes, S. A., Merz, W. G. and Maxwell, L. G. (1977). Primary cutaneous phaeohyphomycosis caused by Drechslera spicifera. *Arch. Dermatol.* **113**, 813–815.
18 Binford, C. H., Thompson, R. K., Gorham, M. E. and Emmons, C. W. (1952). Mycotic brain abscess due to Cladosporium trichoides, a new species. *Am. J. Clin. Pathol.* **22**, 535–542.
19 Riley, O., Jr. and Mann, S. H. (1960). Brain abscess caused by Cladosporium trichoides: review of 3 cases and report of fourth case. *Am. J. Clin. Pathol.* **33**, 525–531.
20 Georg, L. K., Bierer, B. W. and Cooke, W. B. (1964). Encephalitis in turkey poults due to a new fungus species. *Sabouraudia* **3**, 239–244.
21 Blalock, H. G., Georg, L. K. and Derieux, W. T. (1973). Encephalitis in turkey poults due to Dactylaria (Diplorhinotrichum) gallopava – a case report and its experimental reproduction. *Avian Dis.* **17**, 197–204.
22 Pritchard, D., Chick, B. F. and Connole, M. D. (1977). Eumycotic mycetoma due to Drechslera rostrata infection in a cow. *Aust. Vet. J.* **53**, 241–244.

22 Protothecosis and infections caused by morphologically similar green algae

Aetiologic agents:

Protothecosis – *Prototheca wickerhamii* and *P. zopfii*
Green algal infections – *Chlorella* species

Definition and background information

Protothecosis is a localised or disseminated disease of man and lower animals caused by members of the genus *Prototheca.* The disease is sporadic and occurs worldwide. Although protothecosis is still uncommon, increasing numbers of cases are being diagnosed, and the disease is being viewed with increased interest.

The *Prototheca* species are achlorophyllous microorganisms with a life cycle morphologically similar to that of species of green algae in the genus *Chlorella.* They produce hyaline cells termed sporangia that, when mature, divide by irregular cleavage to form 2–20 or more endospores. After sporulation is completed, the sporangial wall ruptures and the spores are released. The freed spores enlarge, develop into mature cells, and repeat the reproductive cycle. The cells of the various *Prototheca* species are globose to oval; they range in diameter from 1.3–13.4 μm and in length from 1.3–16.1 μm or more, depending upon the stage of development, the species, the isolate, and the medium used for cultivation[1]. The *Prototheca* species grow rapidly on routine laboratory media, and abundant growth is evident after 48 hours of incubation. Colonies are soft, yeast-like in consistency and white to light tan in colour, depending upon the species and age of the culture. Grossly, they look so much like yeasts that thay may be considered to be such unless examined microscopically. Colonies of one of the species, *P. stagnora,* may be mucoid because of a capsular material that generally surrounds individual cells. With the exception of *P. stagnora,* most isolates of *Prototheca* species grow well at ambient temperature (25–30°) and at 37°C. *P. stagnora* grows well at ambient temperature, but poorly or not at all at 37°C. Although the individual *Prototheca* species differ morphologically, their accurate identification requires sugar and alcohol assimilation tests or immunofluorescence tests[1,2].

Both the phylogeny and taxonomic position of the *Prototheca* species are still in dispute. On the basis of similarities of reproductive morphology, most workers regard these microorganisms as naturally occurring achlorophyllous mutants of green algae, very likely *Chlorella.* Some workers, however, take the position that the *Prototheca* species are fungi, because they are achlorophyllous and heterotrophic. In an attempt to resolve this controversy, several workers have carried out electron microscopic studies to determine whether the *Prototheca* species have chloroplasts. Such studies have shown that cells of *Prototheca* species contain starch granules, some of which are enclosed by a membrane. Such membrane-bound structures are considered by some to be storage plastids, which suggest an algal rather than a fungal nature for the genus, because fungi are not known to produce plastids. True chloroplasts have not been found[3,4].

Three *Prototheca* species are currently recognised: *P. stagnora, P. wickerhamii*, and *P. zopfii. P. wickerhamii* and *P. zopfii* have been incriminated as agents of disease[5].

Protothecosis in man may appear in at least three different clinical forms:

1. cutaneous-subcutaneous infection,
2. olecranon bursitis, and
3. systemic disease[2].

The cutaneous-subcutaneous form is characterised by the development of single or multiple lesions on the skin and underlying tissues, generally on an exposed part of the body. The lesions develop slowly, and generally show no tendency to heal spontaneously. They appear as papulonodular lesions, crusted papules with ulceration, subcutaneous nodules and, rarely, as an extensive granulomatous eruption. The lesions remain localised, and only rarely are regional lymph nodes infected.

Protothecal olecranon bursitis is a distinct clinicopathological entity. The signs and symptoms are those of a chronic, persistent olecranon bursitis, with pain and marked swelling being common complaints. In some patients with this disorder, the disease developed after a nonpenetrating injury to the elbow.

Systemic protothecosis is a rare disorder in man. This form of the disease has been reported in only one patient, a New Zealander. This individual had multiple nodular lesions in the peritoneal cavity and lesions on the forehead and nose. Several workers have attempted to establish a causal relationship between the *Prototheca* species and tropical sprue, without success. As yet, there is no proof that the *Prototheca* species cause this disease.

Protothecosis has been diagnosed in a wide variety of lower animals[2]. Cattle and dogs appear to be the most frequent victims. Protothecal mastitis has been the predominant form of the disease in cattle. These bovine infections have generally been severe and often have involved all four quarters of the udder. In some cases the infection was confined to the mammary gland; in others it had disseminated to the regional lymph nodes. Most of the affected dogs had a severe disseminated form of the disease involving many vital organs. The signs of the disseminated disease varied in kind and severity, depending upon the organs that were affected. Three dogs had intraocular infections, a condition that caused blindness. Only one dog had cutaneous protothecosis.

Protothecosis in other animal species has been reported infrequently. The disseminated form of the disease has been diagnosed in a deer and in a captive fruit bat. A localised infection involving the subcutaneous tissues in the tarsus region has been reported in a cat.

The epidemiology of protothecosis is still poorly understood. The *Prototheca* species occur as saprophytes in the environment. They have been recovered from such diverse sites as slime flux of trees, acidic stream and lake waters, marine waters, collections of stagnant waters, and other habitats in various parts of the world[1]. Protothecosis is generally regarded as an exogenous disease and is not considered to be transmissible from one host to another. However, the means by which infections are acquired, and conditions that can predispose to infection and disease are not known with certainty. Humans and lower animals are very likely often exposed to these organisms in nature. Yet the disease is relatively uncommon. This apparent low prevalence of the disease undoubtedly reflects minimal pathogenicity and suggests that the protothecae are opportunists, requiring an alteration in host resistance before they can act as pathogens.

Treatment of protothecosis, except by surgical excision of the lesions, has generally proved unsuccessful. Various topical medicaments have been used to treat cutaneous and subcutaneous infections in man, but none has given lasting improvement[6]. In the New Zealand case of systemic protothecosis, combined treatment with amphotericin B and transfer factor was effective[7].

In vitro susceptibility studies have shown that the two polyene antimycotics amphotericin B and nystatin are inhibitory to the *Prototheca* species. In one in vitro study a synergistic effect between amphotericin B and tetracycline was observed, suggesting that such combined therapy might be effective.

Unicellular green algae morphologically resembling protothecae have been incriminated in disease processes in mammals[2]. Infections by such algae have been diagnosed in cattle, sheep, and a beaver. The cattle and sheep had been slaughtered in veterinary inspected abattoirs. These animals appeared healthy on antemortem examination, but in each case single or multiple lesions affecting various lymph nodes were noted on postmortem examination, and in some cases other organs were also involved. The lesions were green in colour, except for those in one cow. Four greenish-coloured nodules were present in the dermis of the beaver, which had been trapped in Ontario, Canada. The lesions from each of these animals were studied by light microscopy after being stained with H&E and by special fungal stains. Numerous organisms resembling protothecae were detected in each of the specimens. The organisms appeared to be the same in each of the animals and ranged in size from 5.8–14 μm in diameter, depending upon their developmental stage. Tissue samples from three bovines and two sheep were studied with the transmission electron microscope, which revealed the presence of well-defined chloroplasts in the cytoplasm of the algal cells. A *Chlorella sp.* was isolated from infected tissue from two bovines[4].

Unicellular green algal infections have been recognised in animals in the United States, Australia, and Canada. Such infections have not been recognised, as yet, in man. Green algal infections are very likely exogenous. Source(s) and route(s) of infection, incubation period, host susceptibility, and resistance factors and therapy are not known.

Histopathology (Figures 477–504)

The histopathologic diagnosis of protothecosis is not difficult. *Prototheca* species are generally abundant in affected tissues, can be readily demonstrated with the special fungus stains, have a characteristic morphology, and can be definitively identified as to species in unstained, deparaffinised tissue sections with specific fluorescent antibody tests[5].

The two pathogenic species of *Prototheca, P. wickerhamii* and *P. zopfii,* have similar morphological characteristics in tissue and in culture[8]. The organisms appear hyaline and are either spherical, oval, or polyhedral in shape. Occasionally, collapsed or crescent-shaped forms are observed which usually stain poorly and are presumably dead. *Prototheca* species reproduce by endosporulation, with 2–20 or more daughter cells contained within a mother cell. All developmental stages of the organism can be seen in stained tissue sections. These stages include:

1. small, single undifferentiated forms with a single large nucleus that usually stains basophilic with H&E;
2. intermediate forms showing nuclear and cytoplasmic cleavage; and
3. very large mature forms undergoing endosporulation which corresponds to the configuration of a morula.

Within the latter forms (mother cells), 2–8 or more endospores (daughter cells) can be seen in a single plane of section. When mature, the mother cells wall ruptures and the endospores are released. The freed spores gradually enlarge to repeat the reproductive cycle.

In our opinion, a generic identification of *Prototheca* can usually be made with confidence by examining stained tissue sections. Although the two species of pathogenic protothecae are morphologically similar, differences do exist. Cells of *P. zopfii* measure from 10–25 μm in diameter, while those of *P. wickerhamii* are somewhat smaller, measuring 1.3–11 μm in diameter. The endospores in a mother cell of *P. zopfii* tend to be larger, round to polyhedral, and less compact, while those of *P. wickerhamii* tend to be smaller, round or cuboidal, and very compact. These differences, although subtle, enable an experienced observer to make a presumptive identification of the species. For a definitive identification of the species, we recommend that cultural or immunofluorescence studies be done. In only one instance have we encountered a dual infection with both pathogenic species of *Prototheca.*

The H&E stain is of limited value for studying *Prototheca* cells in detail. In H&E-stained sections, organisms are usually visible but do not stain uniformly. The relatively thick, hyaline, and refractile cell wall stains poorly or not at all. The granular protoplasmic contents of some cells are basophilic, while those of other cells are unstained or stain poorly. Often only the outlines of organisms are observed, and, in the absence of an inflammatory response, the *Prototheca* cells may be overlooked when they are sparse. This is particularly true if the tissue section is understained with haematoxylin. Usually, however, because of their size, distinctive appearance, and tendency to grow in large compact clusters, *Prototheca* cells can be easily detected and a generic identification can usually be made.

The cell wall and internal contents of intact *Prototheca* cells are well delineated with the GF, PAS and GMS stains. These special fungus procedures are superior to the H&E stain for detecting their presence. Often, the protoplasmic contents of *Prototheca* cells are retracted from the rigid cell wall, apparently as a result of fixation, and a clear space of variable width is left between them. For studying internal details of the protothecae, we prefer the GF and PAS stains. With the GMS procedure, the entire organism usually stains intensely and not as selectively as with the GF and PAS procedures.

In the cutaneous-subcutaneous and systemic forms of protothecosis in humans and lower animals, the range of tissue reactions to the invading organisms is very broad[7, 9–14]. In some cases little or no inflammatory reaction may be associated with the presence of protothecae, whereas in others there may be severe inflammation and necrosis. We have no explanation for such variability in host response. Sometimes there is little or no host reaction, and masses of *Prototheca* cells may obliterate the normal architecture of a tissue or organ. In other cases, the inflammatory reaction in protothecosis is mixed and consists of lymphocytes, plasma cells, macrophages, and neutrophils. Organisms can be found singly or in clusters within the inflammatory foci. Necrosis may or may not be present. When seen, necrotic tissue usually surrounds compact clusters of organisms and is in turn surrounded by mixed inflammatory cells or granulomatous tissue. Purely granulomatous lesions may also be seen in association with protothecosis. Here, almost all organisms are within densely packed epithelioid and multinucleated giant cells of both the foreign body and Langhans' types. Such organisms are frequently distorted, fragmented, flattened, and poorly stained, even with the special fungus stains. However, these poorly stained forms are usually mixed with typical, intensely stained ones. Foci of haemorrhage and necrosis may be present within the granulomatous tissue. We have occasionally observed *Prototheca* cells within blood or lymph vessels, especially at the periphery of severe necrotising and granulomatous lesions.

Skin biopsies of humans with the cutaneous-subcutaneous form of protothecosis have usually shown varying degrees of hyperkeratosis, parakeratosis, and acanthosis, with or without intraepidermal abscesses[6, 9, 10, 15]. Pseudoepitheliomatous hyperplasia of the overlying epidermis may be seen, especially if the dermal reaction is of the chronic granulomatous type. Usually, there is a mixed inflammatory reaction in the dermis which consists of lymphocytes, macrophages, and polymorphonuclear leucocytes. Individually discrete organisms or densely packed clusters can be found in either the epidermis, dermis, subcutaneous tissues, or any combination of these sites. In some subjects, abundant organisms were found to be predominantly in the hyperkeratotic layer of the epidermis and within intraepidermal abscesses. In others, the dermis was extensively involved. Spread to regional lymph nodes has also been recorded[2, 7].

An interesting form of protothecosis is that involving the olecranon bursa and contiguous subcutaneous tissues in humans[16]. The more superficial layers of the skin over the bursa are usually not affected. Histologically, lesions in the bursal lining contain a large central zone of caseous necrotic tissue surrounded by a wide layer of palisading epithelioid cells and foreign body and Langhans' giant cells. These cells are in turn surrounded by either dense fibrous tissue or granulation tissue which is infiltrated with mixed inflammatory cells. The caseating centre of the lesion may appear stellate. In lesions of the olecranon bursa, we have never seen large compact masses of *Prototheca* cells as are often found in the cutaneous and systemic forms of the disease. Rather, organisms occur singly or in small clusters within the central caseous material. In our experience, organisms are often found at the interface of the necrotic and intact tissues. They may also be found within epithelioid and giant cells that surround the caseating lesions. The *Prototheca* cells are commonly distorted and stain poorly with H&E. In some cases, we were unable to see organisms in H&E-stained sections, and only after the sections were stained with the GMS, GF, or PAS procedures were the organisms readily apparent.

The *Chlorella* species appear morphologically and tinctorially identical to the protothecae in H&E-stained sections, and it is virtually impossible to differentiate the two if they are stained by this routine procedure[2, 4]. *Chlorella* cells reproduce by endosporulation. They show the same developmental stages as do the protothecae, and range from 5.8–14 μm in diameter. The natural green pigmentation of these unicellular algae is not seen in H&E-stained sections because chlorophylls in the algal cells are apparently removed during fixation and embedding[4]. Organisms are, however, bright green in smears of fresh lesions or when grown in culture[4, 17]. When tissues stained with the special fungus procedures are examined, a striking difference between the *Chlorella* species and the protothecae is immediately evident. This difference is the presence of numerous large irregularly shaped starch granules in the cytoplasm of intact *Chlorella* cells. These granules are uniformly and strongly PAS, GF, and GMS positive, and are PAS-negative after diastase digestion. Under polarised light, the larger granules are birefringent in unstained or H&E-stained sections, but are no longer birefringent after they are stained with the special fungal procedures. We have observed similar cytoplasmic granules in only a few *Prototheca* cells, and when present the granules were smaller and less distinct.

Tissue reactions to invasion by green algae vary from case to case and specimen to specimen[2, 4, 17–19]. The inflammatory spectrum is strikingly similar to that seen in protothecosis. In most cases, the lesions are either granulomatous, necrotising, or a combination of both. *Chlorella* cells are observed within epithelioid and giant cells and also extracellularly. In other specimens, there is only a minimal tissue response.

Because the chlorellae and protothecae cannot be differentiated in H&E-stained sections, a logical approach must be followed when one attempts to diagnose these diseases. In our experience, the triad of

1. green lesions in unfixed tissues;
2. endosporulating spheroidal to elliptical organisms with an average diameter of 9 μm within the lesions; and
3. large, abundant, strongly PAS-, GF-, or GMS-positive granules in the cytoplasm of organisms enables one to make a presumptive diagnosis of a green algal infection. Whenever possible, such organisms should be definitively identified by cultural studies. At present, specific fluorescent antibody tests are available only for the pathogenic protothecae (see Chapter 3).

Endosporulating forms of fungi such as *Coccidioides immitis* and *Rhinosporidium seeberi* may possibly be confused with the endosporulating cells of the protothecae and chlorellae, especially if one has not had an opportunity to study those organisms in tissue sections. Differences in the size of the mother cells along with differences in the number and morphology of endospores make it possible to differentiate these organisms (see Chapters 10 and 24). Similarly, certain tissue components such as Russell bodies and the 'membrane' bound spherical bodies in the phenomenon known as myospherulosis (see Chapters 10 and 24) may possibly be mistaken for protothecae or chlorellae. Such tissue components generally do not stain with the GMS procedure. In those instances when only atypical forms are present or when organisms are sparse, specific immunofluorescence can be a useful diagnostic tool.

References

1 Arnold, P. and Ahearn, D. G. (1972). Systematics of the genus Prototheca with a description of a new species P. filamenta. *Mycologia* **63**, 265–275.

2 Kaplan, W. (1977). Protothecosis and infections caused by morphologically similar green algae. Proc. Fourth International Conf. Mycoses, June, 1977. Scientific Publication No. 356. Pan American Health Organization, Washington, D.C. pp. 218–232.

3 Nadakavukaren, M. J. and McCraken, D. A. (1973). Prototheca: An alga or a fungus? *J. Phycol.* **9**, 113–116.

4 Chandler, F. W., Kaplan, W. and Callaway, C. S. (1978). Differentiation between Prototheca and morphologically similar green algae in tissue. *Arch. Pathol. Lab. Med.* **102**, 353–356.

5 Sudman, M. S. and Kaplan, W. (1973). Identification of the Prototheca species by immunofluorescence. *Appl. Microbiol.* **25**, 981–990.

6 Wolfe, I. D., Sacks, H. G. and Samoradin, C. W. (1976). Cutaneous protothecosis in a patient receiving immunosuppressive therapy. *Arch. Dermatol.* **112**, 829–832.

7 Cox, E. G., Wilson, J. D. and Brown, P. (1974). Protothecosis: a case of disseminated algal infection. *Lancet I* (August 17): 379–382.

8 Sudman, M. S. (1974). Protothecosis. A critical review. *Am. J. Clin. Pathol.* **61**, 10–19.

9 Fetter, B. F., Klintworth, G. K. and Nielsen, H. S., Jr. (1971). Protothecosis – algal infection. In *The Pathologic Anatomy of Mycoses*, pp. 1081–1093. Human Infection with Fungi, Actinomycetes, and Algae. R. D. Baker, ed. Springer-Verlag, Berlin.

10 Tindall, J. P. and Fetter, B. F. (1971). Infections caused by achloric algae (protothecosis). *Arch. Dermatol.* **104**, 490–500.

11 Davies, R. R., Spencer, H. and Wakelin, P. O. (1964). A case of human protothecosis. *Trans. Roy. Soc. Trop. Med. Hyg.* **58**, 448–451.

12 Davies, R. R. and Wilkinson, J. L. (1967). Human protothecosis; Supplementary studies. *Ann. Trop. Med. Parasitol.* **61**, 112–115.

13 Klintworth, G. K., Fetter, B. F. and Nielson, H. S., Jr. (1968). Protothecosis, an algal infection. Report of a case in man. *J. Med. Microbiol.* **1**, 211–216.

14 Kaplan, W., Chandler, F. W., Holzinger, E. A., Plue, R. E. and Dickinson, R. O. (1976). Protothecosis in a cat: First recorded case. *Sabouraudia* **14**, 281–286.

15 Mars, P. W., Rabson, A. R., Rippey, J. J. and Ajello, L. (1971). Cutaneous protothecosis. *Br. J. Dermatol.* **85**, (Supplement 7), 76–84.

16 Nosanchuk, J. S. and Greenberg, R. D. (1973). Protothecosis of the olecranon bursa caused by achloric algae. *Am. J. Clin. Pathol.* **59**, 567–573.

17 Cordy, D. R. (1973). Chlorellosis in a lamb. *Vet. Pathol.* **10**, 171–176.

18 Sileo, L. and Palmer, N. C. (1973). Probable cutaneous protothecosis in a beaver. *J. Wildlife Dis.* **9**, 320–322.

19 Rogers, R. J. (1974). Protothecal lymphadenitis in an ox. *Austral. Vet. J.* **50**, 281–283.

23 Rare infections

The medical mycological literature records occasional infections caused by microorganisms that are generally considered to be saprophytes and that were not known previously to cause disease in animals and humans. In this chapter we will describe such rare infections caused by an actinomycete, an oomycete, and several deuteromycetes.

In certain instances the rarity of opportunistic infections may be more apparent than real. Some of these infections, such as petriellidiosis, undoubtedly remain underdiagnosed mainly because their occurrence is often unsuspected and appropriate mycological studies are not carried out. Other rare infections may not be diagnosed even when their aetiologic agents are isolated by a diagnostic laboratory since these agents are generally instinctively considered to be contaminants and may be discarded. This most often occurs when attending clinicians fail to consider opportunistic actinomycete and fungus infections in their differential diagnosis. Other infections, however, are truly rare since host conditions favouring the latent invasiveness of their aetiologic agents seldom occur.

The diseases under discussion are caused by the microorganisms listed in Table 1. Interestingly enough, we were unable to locate any histological material from a verified case of geotrichosis. Although *Geotrichum candidum* is frequently isolated from clinical materials, to our knowledge, the recent literature contains no instances in which the isolates could be correlated with tissue invasion. A case in point is the canine infection reported by Lincoln and Adcock[1]. Although *G. candidum* was isolated from the dog's lung and bronchial lymph nodes, budding yeast cells were noted in tissue sections without well formed mycelium – findings that make one doubt the aetiologic role of the isolate.

Table 1 Aetiologic agents of rare infections

1 *Fusarium moniliforme*	5 *Pythium sp.*
2 *Paecilomyces lilacinus*	6 *Streptomyces griseus*
3 *Penicillium marneffei*	7 *Trichosporon capitatum*
4 *Petriellidium boydii*	

1 *Fusarium moniliforme* (Figures 505–506)

Perfect state: *Gibberella fujikuroi*

This mould is a well known and important parasite of such crops as corn, rice, sorghum, and sugarcane. It also infects a wide variety of other plants. In plant pathology the diseases that it causes are known as foot rot, hypertrophy, seedling blight, scorch, and stunting. *F. moniliforme* survives in soil and on dead vegetation[2]. This fungus has a cosmopolitan distribution.

In the medical literature *F. moniliforme* has only rarely been incriminated as an agent of human disease. In two instances, it caused mycotic keratitis[3, 4], and in a third it caused a pustular hand lesion that healed spontaneously[5]. A widely disseminated infection in a granulocytopenic patient with malignant lymphoma is the most serious type of infection known to have been caused by *F. moniliforme*[6]. At autopsy, mycelium attributed to this fungus was found in the kidneys, lungs, myocardium, and pancreas of the victim. Arteries in the lungs and pancreas were occluded with mycelium, which produced thrombi and infarcts. The proliferating mycelium had permeated the thrombi and had penetrated the arterial walls and the surrounding parenchyma. Our photomicrographs were made from tissue sections taken at autopsy of this patient. They were supplied by Dr. N. A. Young of the National Institutes of Health, Bethesda, Maryland. Microscopically, the hyphae of *F. moniliforme* were seen to be embedded in foci of parenchymal necrosis that were surrounded by very few mononuclear inflammatory cells. The hyaline, septate hyphae measured 3–7 μm in width. Branching was frequent, with branches generally formed at an angle of approximately 90°. Dichotomous branching as seen in the aspergilli was infrequent. Although the hyphae stained poorly with H&E,

they were readily demonstrated with any of the special fungus stains.

Through the courtesy of Dr. Michael McGinnis of the North Carolina Memorial Hospital, Chapel Hill, we have had the opportunity to study tissue sections from a burn patient infected with *F. oxysporum.* Angioinvasion was also a prominent feature in this case, and, in tissue, the fungus appeared similar to *F. moniliforme*[6]. This propensity for angioinvasion, coupled with the fact that the hyphae of the *Fusarium spp.* are morphologically similar to those of the aspergilli, makes cultural studies necessary for a definitive identification.

In culture, *F. moniliforme* grows rapidly and produces a downy, slightly lavendar colony that becomes violet with age. The reverse of the colony develops a dark violet colour in time. Microconidia are produced in chains and frequently are the only spores present. Hence the isolates may erroneously be considered to be a species of *Acremonium.* However, although rare in some isolates, the curved, multiseptate, hyaline macroconidia typical of the genus *Fusarium* are also produced. For identifying the members of this genus, the monograph by Booth is recommended[2].

Unidentified *Fusarium spp.* have been suspected of being aetiologic agents of mycetomas on several occasions[7], but in only two previous cases were the species identified. One proved to be *F. solani*[8], the other *F. moniliforme*[9] (see Chapter 17).

Several *Fusarium* species, especially *F. solani* and *F. oxysporum,* are frequent causes of mycotic keratitis[10].

2 *Paecilomyces lilacinus* (Figures 507–508)

Synonym: *Penicillium lilacinum*

In describing this species under its previous name, Raper and Thom stated that it was 'among the most abundant of the soil Penicillia'[11].

Our histological material was provided by Dr Elliott Jacobson of the University of Florida, Gainesville. The lung tissue came from three green sea turtles (*Chelonia mydas*) afflicted with a mycotic pneumonia. Histological studies revealed multiple pulmonary cavities whose necrotic walls were heavily infiltrated with branched, septate mycelial elements of *P. lilacinus* that were 2–4 μm wide and strongly GMS-positive. The mycelium projected into and partially filled the lumens of the pulmonary cavities. Within the cavities, and rarely in their walls, conidiophores bearing flask-shaped phialides were seen. Chains of smooth, spherical conidia were either free or attached to the tapered ends of the phialides. Inflammation in the surrounding tissues was minimal and consisted of mononuclear inflammatory cells.

P. lilacinus grows rapidly on Sabouraud dextrose agar, giving rise to a white floccose colony that becomes lilac or vinaceous in time. On slide cultures its mycelium is hyaline, 2–4 μm wide, and septate. Long conidiophores, 400–600 μm, are produced with verticillate branches that bear whorls of several phialides. The phialides are flask-shaped with a tapered neck. The conidia are produced in chains that are 50–75 μm in length. They are ellipsoidal to fusiform, with a smooth to finely roughened surface, and measure 2.5–3.0 × 1.0–2.2 μm. In mass, they have a purplish cast. An infection ascribed to *P. lilacinus* occurred in a Japanese woman with a chronic facial lesion[12]. A sharply delimited dark red plaque developed on her left cheek. It had a pitted surface with semi-hard red papules. The disease was first diagnosed as lupus vulgaris and was so treated. Since there was no therapeutic response, tissue from the plaque was cultured and studied histologically. Infiltrates composed of lymphocytes, epithelioid cells, and a few giant cells were observed in tissue sections. With the PAS stain, fragmented mycelial elements were observed. Culture of biopsied tissue yielded a mould that was identified as *P. lilacinus.*

The most common type of human infection by *P. lilacinum* has been mycotic keratitis[13–15]. In every instance, it occurred as an opportunistic infection after implantation of prosthetic plastic lenses. Epidemiologic investigations traced the source of infection to a solution of fluid that had become contaminated with *P. lilacinus*[14, 15].

Other *Paecilomyces* species found to have caused disease are: *P. fumosoroseus*[16], *P. variotii*[17–21], and *P. viridis*[22].

P. fumosoroseus was incriminated in a fatal pulmonary infection in a captive Aldabra tortoise (*Testudo gigantea elephantina*). The mycelium of this fungus had invaded the bronchi and bronchioles. Masses of septate, branched hyaline mycelium, 3–4 μm D, were present. Various sized granulomas were in the parenchyma. Their outer border was made up of epithelioid and Langhans' giant cells. An amorphous material and inflammatory mononuclear cells filled their centres.

P. variotii has caused endocarditis in two humans[17–18], endophthalmitis in a young man[23], and disseminated infections in a dog[19, 21] and horse[20].

Rodrigues and MacLeod, through a *lapsus memoriae,* attributed the endophthalmitis of their patient[23] and the patient of Uys et al.[17] to *P. viridis* instead of *P. variotii.* We studied the organism isolated by Rodrigues et al. and identified it as *P. variotii.*

A new species of *Paecilomyces, P. viridis,* first described in 1964, caused a systemic fatal infection in four chameleons (*Chameleo lateralis*) imported from Malagasy[22]. At autopsy of the emaciated animals, the liver and spleen were the organs most affected. They were covered with whitish granulations. Histologically the aetiologic agent was in the form of budding yeast cells that were spherical to oval and 2–7 μm in diameter. A few had multiple buds. In areas with few yeast cells, there were pieces of mycelium that were irregularly septate and variable in width.

At room temperature on Sabouraud dextrose agar, *P. viridis* produced a downy green colony. Conidiophores typical of the genus *Paecilomyces* were produced that bore long chains of smooth, subspherical conidia measuring 2.7 × 3.5 μm. *P. viridis* does not grow at 37°C, and it is not pathogenic in mice. However, experimental infections have been produced in cold-blooded animals, such as chameleons and frogs, by intraperitoneal inoculation.

3 *Penicillium marneffei* (Figures 509–513)

Only two isolates of *Penicillium marneffei,* the aetiologic agent of penicilliosis marneffei, are known to exist. The first one was isolated from a captive bamboo rat (*Rhizomys sinensis*) in Vietnam[24]. This rat had been experimentally inoculated with *Rickettsia orientalis* and died 23 days later. At autopsy the animal was found to have an enlarged liver, an enlarged verrucose spleen, viscous ascitic fluid and epiploic nodules. From the rat's organs a mould, identified as *Penicillium* species, was isolated. It proved to be pathogenic to hamsters.

Previous to this, two other captive, uninoculated bamboo rats had died after showing signs of severe illness. At autopsy these animals revealed a slightly hypertrophic spleen, ascites, and epiploic nodules. Fungus cells were found in their macrophages. However, their tissues were not cultured.

In Paris, at the Institut Pasteur, the *Penicillium* isolate was intensely studied and described as a new species[25–26]. In vitro as well as in vivo studies revealed *P. marneffei* to be a dimorphic fungus.

On Sabouraud's dextrose agar, *P. marneffei* grows rapidly. The colony's surface is downy and white. On its reverse a red pigment appears shortly after inoculation and rapidly diffuses throughout the medium. As the conidiophores develop and produce their chains of spores, the surface of the colony assumes a bluish-green hue. The conidiophores produce divaricate branches with four to five metulae which in turn bear groups of bottle-shaped sterigmata. The spore chains are made up of smooth, apiculate spherical to subglobose conidia 2–3 μm D. At 37°C on a variety of media and in animals, the fungus grew as a unicellular yeast. In contrast to most yeasts, the cells multiplied by schizogony rather than by a budding process. The generally elongated mother cell formed one or two septa, at which points the cells separated[27].

The potential pathogenicity of *P. marneffei* was revealed when Segretain accidentally infected his right index finger with a syringe while inoculating rats intravenously with this fungus. A small nodule developed at the puncture site nine days after the laboratory accident. On the lymphatic cord of his biceps, two small nodules also appeared. A few days later his axillary lymph nodes became slightly enlarged. Twelve days after the inoculation the digital nodule was removed and *P. marneffei* was isolated from it. Successful treatment with nystatin was initiated since the fungus has been found to be sensitive to this antibiotic.

The second isolate of *P. marneffei,* which caused the first natural infection in man, was described by Di Salvo et al. in 1973[28]. The patient was a victim of Hodgkin's disease and had received cobalt radiation therapy 4 years previous to his third hospital admission. At that time it was noted that his spleen was enlarged and infarcted. The excised spleen was found to have a necrotic area 9 cm in diameter. The necrotic material was inoculated on tubes of Sabouraud's dextrose agar, and a mould subsequently identified as *P. marneffei* was isolated. Sections of the splenic lesion stained by the GMS and GF procedures revealed small ovoid yeast cells 2.5–4.5 μm D. In addition, elongated forms 3–6 μm long and 1–2 μm wide were present. Both types of cells were found to be septate when carefully examined under the oil immersion lens.

In the tissue form, cells of *P. marneffei* superficially resemble those of *Histoplasma capsulatum* var. *capsulatum*. However, the latter multiply by a budding process and not by schizogony. In tissue, *P. marneffei* cells may also be distinguished from those of *H. capsulatum* by their failure to stain with the specific fluorescent antibody conjugates of *H. capsulatum*[28, 29].

In experimentally infected hamsters, but not in guinea pigs and rabbits, which were found to be resistant to infection, Capponi et al.[24] found an intense macrophagic reticulosis throughout the spleen and lymph nodes with total disappearance of all normal structures. The reticulosis was localised in the liver around the portal spaces but with evidence of invasion of the entire lobule.

4 *Petriellidium boydii* (Figures 514–518)

Synonym: *Allescheria boydii*
Imperfect state: *Scedosporium* (*Monosporium*) *apiospermum*

P. boydii, although primarily an agent of white-grained eumycotic mycetoma, is quite versatile as a pathogen. It also causes pulmonary and disseminated infections that can be called petriellidiosis.

Pulmonary infections with possible subsequent spread to other vital organs are acquired by inhalation of the airborne spores of *P. boydii,* a cosmopolitan soil fungus[30–33].

Cases of systemic petriellidiosis have been recorded in many parts of the world: Canada[34], France[35], Germany[36], India[37], the United States of America[38, 39] and the Union of Soviet Socialist Republics[40].

Literature reports indicate that pulmonary petriellidiosis primarily occurs as a secondary infection in compromised hosts, although primary infections have developed in apparently healthy individuals[41].

The clinical symptoms of pulmonary petriellidiosis include chest pain, cough, chills, fever, and haemoptysis. These signs, of course, are not pathognomonic *per se.* A definitive diagnosis rests on isolation of the aetiologic agent from clinical materials, x-ray findings, and histological evidence of mycotic infection that is compatible with the tissue form of *P. boydii.*

In patients with petriellidiosis, *P. boydii* exists and develops in the form of scattered or compact masses of hyaline, septate mycelial filaments. This is in sharp contrast to the well organised, white granules that this same fungus produces in patients with eumycotic mycetomas (see Chapter 17).

In many instances petriellidiosis has appeared in the form of a fungus ball. That is to say, the invading fungus developed and occupied a pre-existing pulmonary cavity[39, 42]. Such cavities are readily visualised by x-ray. Upon pneumonectomy or pulmonary resection the cavities may be seen to be discrete or interconnected or communicating with bronchi. Dimensions of the cavities range widely. Within the cavity the so-called fungus ball, which may have a brownish colour, is smooth-surfaced and compressed. When sectioned, the mycelial mass frequently is found to be layered and to have an onion-peel appearance. The mycelium is radially arranged, septate and hyaline. Spores occasionally have been found associated with the mycelium[42, 43]. In some cavities, a thick brownish fluid may be present that contains clumps of mycelium. Histopathological study of the wall surrounding the cavity usually reveals a granulomatous reaction with epithelioid cells, lymphocytes, foreign body giant cells, and fibroblasts.

Petriellidiosis of the brain[34, 44, 45], eye[44], paranasal sinuses[46–48], and knee[44] have been described in compromised patients or in patients with traumatic wound infections[42]. With the exception of the sinus infections, the diagnosis rested upon the finding of scattered hyaline, branched, septate hyphae in tissue sections, and upon the isolation of *P. boydii.* In the sinus infections, the fungus appeared as compact masses of hyphae. Conidia were also noted in some cases.

In lower animals, petriellidiosis has been diagnosed as a cause of mycotic abortion in a mare[49] and also in cattle[50]. The mare had produced ten foals and aborted once. There was no history of treatment with antibiotics, and she had not undergone uterine irrigation. Histopathological studies revealed mycotic lesions in the chorion, amnion, and fetal lungs. In the chorion, mycelium had penetrated the deep villi and connective tissue, and it had invaded the necrotic areas in the subepithelial layer. Inflammatory cells of several types abounded. Giant cells were absent. This was also the case in the amnion, where areas of necrosis with karyorrhectic mesenchymal cells were present. The lungs of the fetus had a conspicuous number of whitish nodules, 1–2.5 mm in diameter, which were uniformly distributed throughout the organ. Histologically the nodules were found not to be walled off. Rather, they blended imperceptibly with the surrounding normal tissue. Large numbers of giant cells with peripheral nuclei were present. Mycelial filaments had been engulfed by some of them. The lesions were basically granulomatous without polymorphs. The GF stain revealed abundant septate mycelium. The aetiology of the infection was ascertained by isolation and identification of the fungus. The diagnostic cultural features of *P. boydii* are given in Chapter 17.

In the bovine cases[50], *P. boydii* was isolated from the placentas, and mycelium was demonstrated therein. Histologic examination of the placentas showed 'vascular and perivascular necrosis, suppurative allanto-chorionitis, necrosis of the fetal villi and necrosis of the arcade zone'.

5 *Pythium sp.* (Figures 519–521)

Synonym: *Hyphomyces destruens*

The term pythiosis is proposed as a more appropriate name for an equine disease variously known as bursatie[51], Florida horse leeches[51], granular dermatitis[52], hyphomycosis destruens[51], phycomycotic granuloma[53], and swamp cancer[54].

This change in terminology is based on important studies carried out by Austwick and Copland[54]. Those investigators found that isolates of *Hyphomyces destruens,* considered by many to be a zygomycete[51, 55], produced biflagellate zoospores when grown on bits of rotten corn silage in sterile distilled water. The characteristics of the zoospores and undifferentiated sporangia were such that the organism was considered to be a species of *Pythium.* It is important to note that the members of the genus *Pythium* are properly classified in the Kingdom Protista in the phylum Oomycetes. They are not to be considered members of the Division Zygomycetes in the Kingdom Fungi (see Chapter 1).

Cases of pythiosis have been recorded in tropical and subtropical areas of the world: Australia[53], India[55], Indonesia[55], Japan[52], Papua New Guinea[53] and the United States (in Florida and Texas)[55].

The disease predominantly develops on the fetlocks of horses and other equines and produces extensive areas of granulomatous necrotic tissue[56]. The infection incites intense pruritus. The layman's name 'leeches' is derived from the occurrence of greyish-white masses of mycelium in the necrotic sinus tracts. These mycelial masses have been frequently but mistakenly considered to be the blood sucking annelide worms of the class Hirudinea. The mycelial masses can be readily distinguished from true leeches by studying histological sections. The masses caused by the *Pythium* species will be composed of broad aseptate mycelium; a leech, of course, will not.

Infections apparently begin in sites of traumatic injuries. As the fungus invades the site and proliferates, necrosis occurs and the lesion spreads. Exuberant granulation tissue develops, and frequently the exposed tissue is destroyed by biting and rubbing activities of the host, actions induced by the pruritus that accompanies the infection. The lesions enlarge by subcutaneous extension. However, the bones and tendons are not invaded by the proliferating mycelium. Upon surgical removal of the granulomatous areas, investigators have found firm, yellowish masses of necrotic tissue that measure 1–10 mm in diameter. These may be elongated and tubular in form.

Aside from the fetlocks, the disease may develop in other exposed parts of the body: abdomen, axilla, limbs, mammary glands, nasal septum, and neck[52, 56]. Diagnosis rests on the demonstration of a zygomycetic type of mycelium in tissue observed by direct examination of clinical matter in 10% KOH mounts or in histological sections. The hyphae, which may have an occasional septum, measure 5–6 μm D.

In the past, surgery has been the most effective and widely used procedure for the treatment of pythiosis[55]. It is most efficaceous in early stages of the disease. For animals with advanced cases and loss of function, euthanasia has been required. However, amphotericin B, when used intravenously and locally, has proved to be effective[56]. McMullan et al.[56] recommended as an ideal treatment 'early surgical removal of the lesion followed by daily intravenous and topical administration of amphotericin B, with periodic extirpation of small necrotic tracts as necessary'.

A description of the sterile growth of the aetiologic agent of pythiosis will be found in the publication by Bridges and Emmons[55]. The paper by Austwick and Copland[54] gives a tantalising brief description of zoospore production by this species of *Pythium*.

6 *Streptomyces griseus* (Figures 522–523)

This aerobic actinomycete is well known as the source of two important antibiotics: cycloheximide and streptomycin[57]. It is widespread in nature and it lives in soil as a saprophyte.

Surprisingly, *S. griseus* has been reported to have been the aetiologic agent of a brain infection[58]. It was demonstrated to have caused a brain abscess in a woman who had been hospitalised in a stuporous state. There, a provisional diagnosis of orbital cellulitis and frontal-lobe abscess was made. During exploratory surgery, thick pus was withdrawn from the abscess that was located in the right lobe of the cerebellum. Microscopic examination of the pus revealed fragments of beaded narrow mycelium. An aerobic actinomycete was isolated and identified as a member of the *S. griseus* complex with the specific name *S. coelicolor.* Under treatment with penicillin and streptomycin the patient steadily improved, and at the time of discharge her brain abscess had shrunk to the size of a pea.

Diagnosis of infections caused by actinomycetes rests on demonstration of delicate ($\leq 1\ \mu$m D), aseptate, hyaline mycelium in clinical materials and on the isolation and identification of these filamentous bacteria by using appropriate biochemical tests as described in Bergey's manual[59].

We recently studied and photographed lung tissue from a human case confirmed by culture and found myriads of gram-positive, branched, and often beaded *S. griseus* filaments embedded in a focus of parenchymal necrosis. The necrotic tissue contained few if any inflammatory cells and was surrounded by a thin, incomplete fibrotic capsule. Numerous *S. griseus* filaments were haphazardly arranged and formed a loose aggregate. Granules as seen in actinomycosis (Chapter 4) were not observed.

7 *Trichosporon capitatum* (Figures 524–525)

This filamentous yeast exists in nature as a saprophyte. It has been isolated from a sewage trickling filter[60] and wood pulp[61]. *T. capitatum* is also commonly encountered in clinical materials but usually without any evidence of tissue invasion[62, 63].

However, a fatal, systemic infection has been described in an immunosuppressed host[64]. The patient was being treated for idiopathic aplastic anaemia by bone marrow transplantation. In the course of his treatment, he received facilitation therapy with cyclophosphamide along with methotrexate as a prophylactic. The patient's condition did not improve since the bone marrow graft was rejected. He returned to the hospital because of recurrent fatigue, generalised malaise, fever, and mandibular joint swelling. After treatment with antibiotics and a second bone marrow transplant, the patient died. *T. capitatum* was isolated from blood cultures taken before his death. At autopsy, fungal emboli were found to have occluded his blood vessels in virtually all organs, including the heart and kidneys. Histologically, the emboli contained many hyaline, branched septate hyphae and budding yeast cells. *T. capitatum* was isolated from several of the organs. Our photomicrographs were taken of tissue sections that were generously given to us by Dr. Drew J. Winston of the University of California at Los Angeles. In our experience, cultural studies would be needed to accurately identify this fungus.

Spontaneous animal infections by *T. capitatum* have been reported in cows[65, 66]. In these studies, *T. capitatum* was isolated from the afterbirth of a fetus or from fetal gastric contents.

Among the other species of *Trichosporon, T. beigelii* (*T. cutaneum*) is the well known agent of white piedra. This species has also been implicated as the cause of a brain abscess in a cancer victim[67]. Diagnosis rested on isolation of *T. beigelii* from the pus obtained from the abscess at autopsy, and demonstration of fungal elements in brain tissue.

A fatal disseminated infection was diagnosed in a 12-year-old boy with leukemia in Texas[68]. *T. beigelii* was isolated from his blood cultures, urine, tracheal aspirate, throat, and stools. At necropsy, study of tissue sections revealed the fungus in the bone marrow, kidneys, liver, lungs, and other organs.

Members of the genus *Trichosporon* are characterised morphologically by the development of yeast-like colonies that are composed of mycelium and pseudomycelium that produce blastospores and arthrospores. Physiologically they do not ferment sugars, but they assimilate carbon compounds.

T. capitatum and *T. beigelii* are distinguished from each other and other *Trichosporon sp.* on the basis of their individualistic assimilation patterns[61].

References

1 Lincoln, S. D. and Adcock, J. L. (1968). Disseminated geotrichosis in a dog. *Pathol. Vet.* **5**, 282–289.

2 Booth, C. (1971). *The Genus Fusarium.* Commonwealth Mycological Institute, Kew, Surrey, England.

3 Anderson, B., Roberts, S. S., Jr., Gonzalez, C. and Chick, E. W. (1959). Mycotic ulcerative keratitis. *Arch. Ophthalmol.* **62**, 169–179.

4 Kidd, G. H. and Wolf, F. T. (1973). Dimorphism in a pathogenic Fusarium. *Mycologia* **65**, 1371–1375.

5 Collins, M. S. and Rinaldi, M. G. (1977). Cutaneous infection in man caused by Fusarium moniliforme. *Sabouraudia* **15**, 151–160.

6 Young, N. A., Kwon-Chung, K. J., Kubota, T. T., Jennings, A. E. and Fisher, R. I. (1978). Disseminated infection by Fusarium moniliforme during treatment for malignant lymphoma. *J. Clin. Microbiol.* **7**, 589–594.

7 Destombes, P., Mariat, F., Rosati, L. and Segretain, G. (1977). Les mycetomes en Somalie-conclusions d'une enquete menée de 1959 à 1964. *Acta Tropica* **34**, 355–373.

8 Peloux, Y. and Segretain, G. (1966). Mycetome à Fusarium. *Bull. Soc. Fram. Mycol. Med.* **11**, 31–32.

9 Alberici, F., Morganti, L., Ajello, L. and Chandler, F. (1979). Fusarium moniliforme. A new mycetoma agent. *Current Microbiol.* (in press).

10 Zapater, R. C., Brunzini, M. A., Albesi, E. J. and Silicaro Arturi, C. A. (1976). El genero Fusarium como agente etiologico de micosis oculares. *Archivos Oftalmologia* (Buenos Aires) **51**, 279–286.

11 Raper, K. B. and Thom, C. (1949). *A Manual of the Penicillia.* Wiiliams & Wilkins Co., Baltimore, Maryland.

12 Takayasu, S., Akagi, M. and Shimizu, Y. (1977). Cutaneous mycosis caused by Paecilomyces lilacinus. *Arch. Dermatol.* **113**, 1687–1690.

13 Webster, R. G., Martin, W. J., Rhodes, T. H., Boni, B., Midura, T. and Skinner, M. D. (1975). Eye infections after plastic implantation. *Morb. Mort. Weekly Report* **24**, 437–438.

14 Mosier, M. A., Lusk, B., Petit, T. H., Howard, D. H. and Rhodes, J. (1977). Fungal endophthalmitis following intraocular lens implantation. *Am. J. Ophthalmol.* **83**, 1–8.

15 O'Day, D. M. (1977). Fungal endophthalmitis caused by Paecilomyces lilacinus after intraocular lens implantation. *Am. J. Ophthalmol.* **83**, 130–131.

16 Georg, L. K., Williamson, W. M., Tilden, E. B. and Getty, R. E. (1962). Mycotic pulmonary disease of captive giant tortoises due to Beauvaria bassiana and Paecilomyces fumoso-roseus. *Sabouraudia* **2**, 80–86.

17 Uys, C. J., Don, P. A., Schrire, V. and Barnard, C. N. (1963). Endocarditis following cardiac surgery due to the fungus Paecilomyces. *S. Afr. Med. J.* **37**, 1276–1280.

18 Silver, M. D., Tuffnell, P. G. and Bigelow, W. G. (1971). Endocarditis caused by Paecilomyces varioti affecting an aortic valve allograft. *J. Thoracic and Cardiovasc. Surg.* **61**, 278–281.

19 Patnaik, A. K., Liu, S. K., Wilkins, R. J., Johnson, G. F. and Seitz, P. E. (1972). Paecilomycosis in a dog. *J. Am. Vet. Med. Assoc.* **161**, 806–813.
20 Redaelli, G., Guallini, L. and Mandelli, G. (1968). Osservazioni sull' azione patogena sperimentale di 'Paecilomyces varioti Bainier 1907'. *Arch. Vet. Ital.* **19**, 185–197.
21 Jang, S. S., Biberstein, E. L., Slauson, D. O. and Suter, P. F. (1971). Paecilomyces in a dog. *J. Am. Vet. Med. Assoc.* **159**, 1775–1779.
22 Segretain, G., Fromentin, H., Destombes, P., Brygoo, E. R. and Dodin, A. (1964). Paecilomyces viridis n. sp. champignon dimorphique, agent d'une mycose generalisée de Chameleo lateralis Gray. Note. *C. R. Acad. Sc.* (Paris) **259**, 258–261.
23 Rodrigues, M. M. and MacLeod, D. (1975). Exogenous fungal endophthalmitis caused by Paecilomyces. *Am. J. Ophthalmol.* **79**, 687–690.
24 Capponi, M., Sureau, P. and Segretain, G. (1956). Penicillose de Rhizomys sinensis. *Bull. Soc. Pathol. Exot.* **49**, 418–421.
25 Segretain, G. (1959). Penicillium marneffei n. sp., agent d'une mycose du systeme reticuloendothelial. *Mycopathol. Mycol. Appl.* **11**, 327–353.
26 Segretain, G. (1959). Description d'une nouvelle espece de Penicillium: Penicillium marneffei n. sp. *Bull. Soc. Mycol. Fr.* **75**, 412–416.
27 Garrison, R. G. and Boyd, K. S. (1973). Dimorphism of Penicillium marneffei as observed by electron microscopy. *Can. J. Microbiol.* **19**, 1305–1309.
28 DiSalvo, A. F., Fickling, A. M. and Ajello, L. (1973). Infection caused by Penicillium marneffei. *Am. J. Clin. Pathol.* **60**, 259–263.
29 Kaufman, L. and Kaplan, W. (1961). Preparation of a fluorescent antibody specific for the yeast phase of Histoplasma capsulatum. *J. Bacteriol.* **82**, 729–735.
30 Ajello, L. (1952). The isolation of Allescheria boydii Shear, an etiologic agent of mycetomas, from soil. *Am. J. Trop. Med. Hyg.* **1**, 227–238.
31 Bell, R. G. (1976). The development in beef cattle manure of Petriellidium boydii (Shear) Malloch, a potential pathogen for man and cattle. *Can. J. Microbiol.* **22**, 552–556.
32 Gugnani, H. C. and Shrivastav, J. B. (1972). Occurrence of pathogenic fungi in soil in India. *Indian J. Med. Res.* **60**, 40–47.
33 Mackinnon, J. E., Conti-Diaz, I. A., Gezuele, E. and Civilia, E. (1971). Datos sobre ecologia de Allescheria boydii Shear. *Rev. Uruguaya Pat. Clin. y Microbiol.* **9**, 37–43.
34 Rosen, F., Deck, J. H. N. and Rewcastle, N. B. (1965). Allescheria boydii – unique systemic dissemination to thyroid and brain. *Can. Med. Assoc. J.* **93**, 1125–1127.
35 Oury, M., Hocquet, P., Simard, C., Tuchais, E. and Cocaud, J. (1968). Allescheriase pulmonaire (Mycetome à Allescheria boydii). *J. Fr. Med. Chir. Thorac.* **22**, 425–437.
36 Stoeckel, H. and Ermer, C. (1960). Ein Fall von Monosporium-Mycetoma de Lunge. *Beitrag Klin. Tuberk.* **122**, 30–38.
37 Misra, S. P., Shende, G. Y., Yerwadekar, S. N., Padhye, A. A. and Thirumalachar, M. J. (1966). Allescheria boydii and Emmononsia ciferrina, isolated from patients with chronic pulmonary infections. *Hindustan Antibiot. Bull.* **9**, 99–103.
38 Rippon, J. W. and Carmichael, J. W. (1976). Petriellidiosis (Allescheriosis): Four unusual cases and review of literature. *Mycopathologia* **58**, 117–124.
39 Jung, J. Y., Salas, R., Almond, C. H., Saab, S. and Reyna, R. (1977). The role of surgery in the management of pulmonary monosporosis. *J. Thorac. Cardiovasc. Surg.* **73**, 139–144.
40 Ariewitsch, A. M., Stepaniszewa, S. G. and Tiufilina, O. W. (1969). Ein Fall des durch Monosporium apiospermum Hervorgerufenen Lungenmyzetoma. *Mycopathol. Mycol. Appl.* **37**, 171–178.
41 Deloach, E. D., Di Benedetto, R. J., Hitch, W. S. and Russell, P. (1979). Pulmonary infection with Petriellidium boydii. *S. Med. J.* **72**, 479–481.
42 Bakerspigel, A., Wood, T. and Burke, S. (1977). Pulmonary allescheriasis. *Am. J. Clin. Pathol.* **68**, 299–303.
43 McCarthy, D. S., Longbottom, J. L., Riddell, R. W. and Batten, J. C. (1969). Pulmonary mycetoma due to Allescheria boydii. *Am. Rev. Resp. Dis.* **100**, 213–216.
44 Lutwick, L. I., Galgiani, J. N., Johnson, R. H. and Stevens, D. A. (1976). Visceral fungal infections due to Petriellidium boydii. *Am. J. Med.* **61**, 632–640.
45 Winston, D. J., Jordan, M. C. and Rhodes, J. (1977). Allescheria boydii infections in the immunosuppressed host. *Am. J. Med.* **63**, 830–835.
46 Gluckman, J. J., Ries, K. and Arbutyn, E. (1977). Allescheria (Petriellidium) boydii sinusitis in a compromised host. *J. Clin. Microbiol.* **5**, 481–484.
47 Hecht, R. and Montgomerie, J. Z. (1978). Maxillary sinus infection with Allescheria boydii (Petriellidium boydii). *Johns Hopkins Med. Bull.* **142**, 107–109.
48 Mader, J. T. and Heath, P. W. (1978). Petriellidium boydii (Allescheria boydii) sphenoidal sinusitis. *J. Am. Med. Assoc.* **239**, 2368–2369.
49 Mahaffey, L. W. and Rossdale, P. D. (1965). An abortion due to Allescheria boydii and general observations concerning mycotic abortions of mares. *Vet. Rec.* **77**, 541–545.
50 Knudtson, W. U., Wohlgemuth, K., Kirkbride, C. A., Robl, M. G., Vorhies, M. W. and McAdaragh, J. P. (1974). Mycologic, serologic and histologic findings in bovine abortion associated with Allescheria boydii. *Sabouraudia* **12**, 81–86.
51 Emmons, C. W., Binford, C. H., Utz, J. P. and Kwon-Chung, K. J. (1977). *Medical Mycology*. Lea & Febiger, Philadelphia.
52 Amemiya, J. and Nishiyama, S. (1966, 1968, 1969). On the granular dermatitis in horses which contains a kind of true fungus in the foci. Parts 1–3. *Bull. Fac. Agric.* Kagoshima Univ. No. **17**, 215–224 (1966), No. **18**, 185–191 (1968), No. **19**, 31–50 (1969).
53 Johnston, K. G. and Henderson, A. W. K. (1974). Phycomycotic granuloma in horses in the Northern Territory. *Austral. Vet. J.* **50**, 105–107.
54 Austwick, P. K. C. and Copland, J. W. (1974). Swamp cancer. *Nature* **250**, 84.
55 Bridges, C. H. and Emmons, C. W. (1961). A phycomycosis of horses caused by Hyphomyces destruens. *J. Am. Vet. Med. Assoc.* **138**, 579–589.
56 McMullan, W. C., Joyce, J. R., Hanselka, D. V. and Heitmann, J. M. (1977). Amphotericin B for the treatment of localised subcutaneous phycomycosis in the horse. *J. Am. Vet. Med. Assoc.* **170**, 1293–1298.
57 Waksman, S. A. (1950). *The Actinomycetes.* Chronica Botanica Co., Waltham, Mass.
58 Clarke, P. R. R., Warnock, G. B. R., Blowers, R. and Wilkinson, M. (1964). Brain abscess due to Streptomyces griseus. *J. Neurosurg. Psychiatr.* **27**, 553–555.
59 Buchanan, R. E. and Gibbons, N. E. (1974). *Bergey's Manual of Determinative Bacteriology,* 8th ed. Williams & Wilkins Co., Baltimore.
60 Cooke, W. B., Phaff, H. J., Miller, M. W., Shifrine, M. and Knapp, E. P. (1960). Yeasts in polluted water and sewage. *Mycologia* **52**, 210–230.
61 Lodder, J. (1970). *The Yeasts.* North-Holland Publishing Co., Amsterdam.
62 Rose, A. H. and Harrison, J. S. (1969). *The Yeasts.* Academic Press, London.
63 Gemeinhardt, H. (1965). Lungenpathogenität von

Trichosporon capitatum beim Menschen. *Zentralbe. Bakteriol.* **196**, 121–133.
64 Winston, D. J., Balsley, G. E., Rhodes, J. and Linne, S. R. (1977). Disseminated Trichosporon capitatum infection in an immunosuppressed host. *Arch. Intern. Med.* **137**, 1192–1195.
65 Hellmann, E. and Raethel, S. (1964). Trichosporon capitatum als Ursache eines Abortes beim Rind. *Berl. Munch. Tierarztl Wochenschr.* **77**, 380–381.
66 Hajsig, M. and Topolko, S. (1967). Yeasts and yeast-like fungi in the genital organs of cows and heifers. *Vet. Arh.* **37**, 193–196.
67 Watson, K. C. and Kallichurum, S. (1970). Brain abscess due to Trichosporon cutaneum. *J. Med. Microbiol.* **3**, 191–193.
68 Rivera, R. and Cangir, A. (1975). Trichosporon sepsis and leukemia. *Cancer* **36**, 1106–1110.

24 Rhinosporidiosis

Aetiologic agent:

Rhinosporidium seeberi

Common synonyms:

Coccidium seeberi, Rhinosporidium kinealyi, R. equi, R. ayyari

Definition and background information

Rhinosporidiosis is a chronic, granulomatous disease of man and lower animals. It is characterised by the development of polypoid lesions on the mucosa of the nose, eyes and, occasionally, other body sites. The disease occurs worldwide but appears to be most common in India and Sri Lanka. *Rhinosporidium seeberi* has never been cultured and is known only in the form seen in infected tissue. There it develops as spherical sporangia that range from 6–300 μm or more in diameter, depending upon the stage in its growth cycle. As the sporangia mature, they develop thick refractile walls. Their nuclei divide and the cytoplasm undergoes progressive cleavage, forming numerous uninucleate endospores. The individual spores appear lobulated and are 6–7 μm in diameter. When the sporangium matures, its spores are released through a break in the cell wall. The free spores gradually enlarge to become mature sporangia[1].

In man, rhinosporidiosis is characterised by the development of polyps on the mucosa of the nose, eyes, larynx, trachea, bronchi, and occasionally on the ears, genitals, and rectum. Clinically, nasal lesions are often confused with allergic polyps, but the pathologist should have no difficulty in differentiating the two. The polyps caused by *R. seeberi* are soft, red, friable and lobed, and they bleed readily when traumatised. They may arise directly from the mucosa or be borne on short pedicles. Multiple minute white foci may be seen on their surfaces and represent the larger spherules filled with sporangiospores. The polyps are not painful but may obstruct breathing and interfere with speech if present in the nose or larynx[2]. Dissemination to other body parts is extremely rare. The disease is seldom fatal.

Rhinosporidiosis has been diagnosed in cattle, horses, mules, and dogs[3], and in a goose and two ducks[4]. In most of the affected animals the disease occurred as a chronic polypoid rhinitis. In most cases the growths were of sufficient size to interfere with breathing.

The source of infection is not known. However, the disease in man in India and Sri Lanka has been associated with swimming and working in stagnant water, which suggests that water is a natural habitat of *R. seeberi*. The disease is not contagious, and the treatment of choice is surgical excision.

Histopathology (Figures 526–537)

In humans and animals, *R. seeberi* typically incites a chronic inflammatory reaction in the submucosa or dermis where lymphocytes, plasma cells, highly vascular granulation tissue, and varying numbers of epithelioid cells and neutrophils predominate[5–8]. Eosinophils are extremely rare. The number of neutrophils depends on the reproductive stage in contact with host tissue, i.e., recently released sporangiospores may stimulate a pronounced neutrophilic response with variable necrosis, whereas developing, mature, and empty sporangia are associated with a chronic inflammatory response. In some cases, recently released spores may stimulate a granulomatous reaction with few, if any, neutrophils. Multinucleated giant cells of both types may be mixed with other inflammatory cells. They usually surround empty sporangial shells and mature sporangia containing spores. It is not uncommon to find epithelioid and giant cells within empty sporangia, having entered through their ruptured walls. Empty, partially collapsed sporangia are often semilunar in shape, and their walls may be fragmented.

The chronic inflammatory reaction to *R. seeberi* may persist for many years and usually causes the formation of sessile or pedunculated polyps that are friable and of varying shapes and sizes[7, 9, 10]. Generalised rhinosporidiosis due to haematogenous and lymphatic dissemination is very rare. In two reported cases[11, 12] multinucleated giant cells and lymphocytes surrounded sporangia and spores, a reaction similar to those described above.

Because *R. seeberi* cannot as yet be cultured, a diagnosis is made solely by demonstrating the organism in clinical material by direct microscopy. Histologic specimens are of particular value. In tissue, many sporangia, 6–300 μm in diameter, in various stages of development are usually embedded in the inflamed stroma of a nasal or other mucosal polyp. The overlying mucosa may be hyperplastic and inflamed and may also contain sporangia. The various forms of sporangia observed in tissue sections include:

1. young 'trophic' forms, 10–100 μm in diameter, with a single, central, basophilic karyosome (nucleus) and amorphous, lacy cytoplasmic contents,
2. mature forms, 100–300 μm in diameter, which contain sporangiospores that usually develop on one side within the sporangium, fill the centre as they mature, and escape through a break in the sporangial wall, and
3. empty, collapsed forms usually contiguous to free sporangiospores.

The largest sporangia usually lie just beneath the epithelial surface. They have walls that may be up to 5 μm thick, and they contain innumerable spores. Ruptured sporangia are often seen with sporangiospores lying free on the epithelial surface or in the underlying stroma. The drag of the microtome knife during sectioning may be responsible for the large number of ruptured sporangia observed in some tissue sections.

R. seeberi can be easily identified in H&E-stained sections, and the pathologist should be able to make a diagnosis without the aid of special fungus stains. The larger sporangia are visible even to the naked eye and appear as holes when a tissue section is held up to the light before microscopic examination. Special stains are useful for delineating entire sporangiospores and the hyaline, often laminated (chitinous) walls of mature sporangia, both of which stain uniformly with the GMS, GF, and PAS procedures[1]. In our experience, the last two procedures will not uniformly stain the smaller, developing 'trophic' forms in tissue sections. For this reason, the GMS or GMS-H&E procedures are preferred. It should also be pointed out that the often convoluted and fragmented walls of old, empty sporangia may only be partially stained by the special fungus procedures. Although Mayer's mucicarmine procedure stains *Cryptococcus neoformans* and may also stain the walls of sporangiospores and the inner walls of the sporangia of *R. seeberi*[1], there should be no difficulty in distinguishing the two fungi because each of them is morphologically distinct.

The sporangia of *R. seeberi* may possibly be confused with spherules of *Coccidioides immitis*. However, the mature sporangia of *R. seeberi* are much larger than mature *C. immitis* spherules. The latter are seldom more than 80–200 μm in diameter. In addition, the sporangiospores of *R. seeberi* are stained uniformly with the special fungus stains. They usually contain 10 or more globular eosinophilic bodies. Also, they are flattened and smaller at the periphery. Sporangiospores usually are situated on one side of the sporangium, where they initially develop before attaining a spherical shape and filling the centre. Mature spores may also orient on the opposite side of developing sporangia. The endospores of *C. immitis* are round regardless of their location within the spherule. They lack internal globular bodies, and only their walls stain with the special fungus procedures. On occasion, small, empty, degenerated sporangia of *R. seeberi* may be mistaken for empty spherules of *C. immitis* or for large, empty cells of *Blastomyces dermatitidis*. Here, one must search for the typical reproductive forms of *R. seeberi*. If typical sporangia are not found, specific immunofluorescence tests for *B. dermatitidis, C. immitis,* and *C. neoformans* can be useful in making a differential diagnosis. Examination of serial sections may be necessary. Large, empty sporangia of *R. seeberi* may be confused with the adiaspores of *Chrysosporium parvum* var. *crescens,* and, again, one should search for characteristic sporangia containing spores of *R. seeberi*. In addition, the walls of the adiaspores of the *crescens* variety of *Chrysosporium parvum* are trilaminar and much thicker than the sporangial wall of *R. seeberi*[13]. The membrane-enclosed spherical bodies seen in the phenomenon known as myospherulosis[14] may be mistaken for the mature sporangia of *R. seeberi*. Intramembranous round bodies in myospherulosis generally do not stain with the GMS procedure, but are positive with the various stains for haemoglobin[14].

References

1 Bader, G. and Gruber, H. L. E. (1970). Histochemical studies of Rhinosporidium seeberi. *Virchows Arch.* [*Pathol. Anat.*] **350**, 76–86.

2 Karunaratne, W. A. E. (1964). *Rhinosporidiosis in man.* Athlone Press, University of London, London.

3 Stuart, B. P. and O'Malley, N. (1975). Rhinosporidiosis in a dog. *J. Am. Vet. Med. Assoc.* **167**, 941–942.

4 Davidson, W. R. and Nettles, V. P. (1977). Rhinosporidiosis in a wood duck. *J. Am. Vet. Med. Assoc.* **171**, 989–990.

5 Weller, C. V. and Riker, A. D. (1930). Rhinosporidium seeberi. *Am. J. Pathol.* **6**, 721–732.

6 Karunaratne, W. A. E. (1936). Pathology of rhinosporidiosis. *J. Pathol. Bacteriol.* **42**, 193–202.

7 Satyanarayana, C. (1960). Rhinosporidiosis with a record of 255 cases. *Acta Otolaryngol.* (Stockh.) **51**, 348.

8 Cameron, H. M., Gatei, D. and Bremner, A. D. (1973). The deep mycoses in Kenya: a histopathological study. 4. Rhinosporidiosis. *East Afr. Med. J.* **50**, 413–416.

9 David, S. S. (1974). Nasal rhinosporidiosis. *J. Indian Med. Assoc.* **62**, 301–306.

10 Pillai, O. S. (1974). Rhinosporidiosis of the larynx. *J. Laryngol. Otol.* **88**, 277–280.

11 Rajam, R. V., Viswanathan, G. S., Rao, A. R., Rangiah, P. N. and Anguli, V. S. (1955). Rhinosporidiosis: a study with report of a fatal case of systemic dissemination. *Indian J. Surg.* **17**, 269–298.
12 Agrawal, S., Sharma, K. D. and Shrivastava, J. B. (1959). Generalised rhinosporidiosis with visceral involvement: report of a case. *Arch. Dermatol.* (Chicago) **80**, 22–26.
13 Watts, J. C., Callaway, C. S., Chandler, F. W. and Kaplan, W. (1975). Human pulmonary adiaspiromycosis. *Arch. Pathol.* **99**, 11–15.
14 Rosai, J. (1978). The nature of myospherulosis of the upper respiratory tract. *Am. J. Clin. Pathol.* **69**, 475–481.

25 Sporotrichosis

Aetiologic agent:

Sporothrix schenckii

Synonym:

Sporotrichum schenckii

Definition and background information

Sporotrichosis is a subacute or chronic disease of humans and lower animals caused by the fungus *Sporothrix schenckii*. The disease is worldwide in distribution. Sporotrichosis is usually limited to the skin and subcutaneous tissues. In rare cases the infection may disseminate to the bones and internal organs. Occasionally, sporotrichosis may be primarily a systemic disease having a pulmonary inception.

Sporothrix schenckii is dimorphic[1]. When it grows at room temperature, it develops in a mycelial form. When it grows at 37°C in vitro or in tissues of a living host, it develops in a yeast-form. Mycelial-form cultures usually grow rapidly and characteristically have a wrinkled or folded membranous surface which at first is whitish in colour but in time becomes brownish or, in some isolates, black. In some isolates, fine, greyish, velvety aerial mycelium may form at the outer borders. Microscopic examination reveals relatively fine, branched, septate, hyaline mycelium and numerous conidia. Conidia measuring $2 \times 3\ \mu m$ to $3 \times 6\ \mu m$ are produced in abundance on delicate sterigmata along the hyphae and terminally on conidiophores.

Yeast-form colonies are moist, creamy, and whitish in colour. Microscopic examination reveals single and budding yeast-like cells that vary in size and form. These cells may be round, oval, or cigar-shaped. Round or oval forms are generally 2–6 μm or more in diameter; cigar-shaped cells attain a size of 2×3 to $3 \times 10\ \mu m$. Single and budding cells identical in appearance to those observed in yeast-form cultures occur in infected tissues and are observed in exudates. In most cases, very few of these yeast-like cells are found in clinical materials from lesions in man.

Recently a new variety of *S. schenckii* was described and named *S. schenckii* var. *luriei*[2]. It was isolated from a fixed type of sporotrichosis characterised by development of a tumour on the left frontal region of a South African native. Bony erosion had occured, creating a connection with the skull cavity. In culture, *S. schenckii* var. *luriei* is indistinguishable from the typical form of *S. schenckii*. However, in tissue, it forms not only small budding yeast cells, but also large spheroidal, thick-walled cells. The huge cells are 16–18 μm in diameter and divide by partitioning or by a budding process or both.

S. schenckii exists in nature as a saprophyte[3]. It is found in soil, on plants, and on various plant materials. Infections are usually contracted by the accidental inoculation of the fungus into the skin or subcutaneous tissue. Pulmonary infections, however, may result from the inhalation of the fungus.

The most common form of sporotrichosis in man is a linear series of chronic subcutaneous nodules[4]. The initial lesion usually occurs on an exposed part of the body, commonly on the hand, arm, or neck and occasionally on the foot or leg, from which site the infection spreads along the path of lymphatic drainage of the area. The lymphatic vessels become corded, and a series of secondary nodules is formed. Eventually the nodules break down, ulcerate, and discharge pus. Single lesions of the skin and underlying tissues are not uncommon. Occasionally, individual or coalesced subcutaneous nodules are formed in many parts of the body. Infections of the bones, joints, lungs and other internal organs are also occasionally observed[5].

Sporotrichosis has been recognised in a diversity of lower animals[6]. In horses, mules and donkeys, the disease is generally limited to the skin, subcutaneous tissues, and lymphatics. Characteristically, in these solipeds, the disease appears as a series of subcutaneous nodules that develop along the course of the lymphatics that drain the area of a primary lesion. The nodules eventually break down, ulcerate, and discharge pus. In addition to this classical, lymphangitic form, a subcutaneous form in which nodules develop without involvement of the lymphatics has also been described in horses. In dogs, both cutaneous and disseminated forms of the disease as well as the classical lymphangitic form have been described. The disease is too infrequent in other animal species to permit its characterisation.

Sporotrichosis is not transmitted from host to host. However, one may become infected by accidental inoculation or contamination of the broken skin with lesion exudates or other infectious material.

Serological tests can be used to advantage for the diagnosis of sporotrichosis. A wide variety of serodiagnostic tests have been developed for this mycosis. The tube agglutination and the latex agglutination tests, considered by many workers to be the most reliable and specific tests for sporotrichosis, are of particular value for the diagnosis of extracutaneous or systemic infections.

Saturated potassium iodide administered orally is the treatment of choice for cutaneous and subcutaneous forms of the disease[7]. Amphotericin B administered intravenously has been used successfully to treat extracutaneous sporotrichosis[8].

Histopathology (Figures 538–559)

S. schenckii usually incites a mixed purulent and granulomatous inflammatory reaction that is often accompanied by fibrosis[9–11]. This mixed inflammatory response is typical of all forms of the disease, but it is not specific and may be indistinguishable from those lesions seen in certain other mycoses, and in certain bacterial diseases such as tuberculosis, anthrax, glanders, syphilis, and tularemia.

On clinical examination, primary skin lesions of sporotrichosis may be mistaken for a neoplasm and surgically excised[9, 12–15]. Microscopically, these lesions are characterised by hyperkeratosis, parakeratosis, and varying degrees of pseudoepitheliomatous hyperplasia and ulceration of the epidermis. Intraepidermal microabscesses may occur. In the dermis and at times the subcutaneous tissues, *S. schenckii* causes either a nodular (often referred to as sporotrichotic nodules) or diffuse granulomatous reaction, or a combination of both. Typical solid granulomas may be present, but granulomas with central microabscesses are most common. In addition to intact polymorphonuclear leucocytes, such granulomas may contain cellular debris, caseous material, and yeast-form cells of *S. schenckii.* When present in solid granulomas, organisms are usually within giant cells. If the dermal reaction is diffuse, one frequently sees small clusters of epithelioid and multinucleated giant cells among variable numbers of lymphocytes, plasma cells, polymorphonuclear leucocytes and fibroblasts. Here, the fungus may be intracellular or extracellular. In chronic skin lesions (>6 months duration) there is variable fibrosis, the inflammatory response may be less severe, and yeast form cells may be very scarse and distorted[16].

A mixed inflammatory response, as described above, and the demonstration of one or more yeast cells either free or surrounded by Splendore–Hoeppli material (the asteroid body) and morphologically compatible with *S. schenckii* is highly suggestive of sporotrichosis and enables a presumptive diagnosis to be made. The asteroid body consists of a single or budding yeast cell(s) intimately surrounded by a stellate, radial corona that is brightly eosinophilic with H&E and may be up to 100 μm in diameter. At times the centrally located yeast cell will not be visible. Splendore–Hoeppli material is thought to be glycoprotein primarily of host origin resulting from a localised antigen-antibody reaction on the surface of the yeast in the hypersensitised host[17]. Similar material is deposited around the yeast cells of *S. schenckii* in vitro when they are suspended in specific antiserum[18].

We can recall only a few times when the asteroid body in tissue sections was not surrounded by purulent or necrotic material, usually in the centre of a granuloma. Others have also reported this. In one study[15], asteroid bodies were detected in 36 of 39 cases of sporotrichosis, and they were always found in purulent centres of granulomas or in intraepidermal abscesses. In a few cases, we have also observed asteroid bodies within huge, multinucleated giant cells at the periphery of an abscess. Several authors have also reported that asteroids were more common in the cutaneous form of sporotrichosis than in the lymphangitic and disseminated forms[5, 17].

Although the Splendore–Hoeppli reaction may be associated with *S. schenckii* in tissues, it is not pathognomonic for sporotrichosis. Splendore–Hoeppli material may be seen surrounding colonies of bacteria, parasite ova[19], foreign objects such as suture material[20], and other species of fungi, particularly *Coccidioides immitis, Aspergillus spp., Candida spp.,* and certain of the species that cause mycetomas. It is imperative that the pathologist realise this fact because we have seen diagnoses of sporotrichosis based solely on the presence of asteroid bodies. It should be emphasised that in many cases of sporotrichosis, asteroid formation does not occur. Therefore, the absence of asteroids in an H&E-stained tissue section does not rule out the possibility of sporotrichosis.

We have seen several cases of pulmonary sporotrichosis that were presumed to be primary[21]. In these, the pneumonia consisted of focal granulomas with large caseous centres which in turn were surrounded by concentric zones of epithelioid cells mixed with giant cells and proliferating fibroblasts. Organisms were usually found within the caseous material or within giant and epithelioid cells at the periphery. We have also seen chronic lung lesions that in H&E-stained sections were indistinguishable from the old fibrocaseous nodules caused by infection with *Histoplasma capsulatum* var. *capsulatum* or *Coccidioides immitis*. In these instances, fluorescent antibody procedures may be required for a diagnosis.

Lesions in the rare disseminated form of sporotrichosis are similar to those of the primary cutaneous and lymphangitic forms, but usually contain more yeast cells[5, 9, 22–25]. In disseminated lesions, large giant cells may contain many *S. schenckii* organisms.

The morphology of the cells of *S. schenckii* var. *luriei* in tissues is distinctly different from the typical form of this species[2]. Mosf cells of the *luriei* variety are much larger (15–20 μm or more in D), have thick walls, and divide by septation (fission) and also by budding. A mixture of large and typical forms is usually present in experimentally induced lesions in animals[2]. To our knowledge, only one human infection due to the *luriei* variety has been reported[2]. In that case (see background information), the histopathology was similar to that described for the typical form of *S. schenckii*. Typical sporotrichotic granulomas were present and consisted of central microabscesses composed of polymorphonuclear leucocytes surrounded by epithelioid and foreign body type giant cells. The giant cells were often huge, measuring up to 130 μm and containing 50–60 nuclei in a single plane of section. Fungus cells, some of which were coated by stellate, eosinophilic Splendore–Hoeppli material, were present within the granulation tissue, predominantly in the centres of sporotrichotic granulomas. An asteroid was occasionally seen within large, bizarre foreign body giant cells.

In primary lesions caused by the typical form of *S. schenckii*, free yeast-form cells are almost never found in tissue sections stained with H&E. The yeast-form cells of *S. schenckii* stand out clearly with the special fungus stains, but because of their scarcity, serial sections may be needed to demonstrate a single yeast cell either free or surrounded by Splendore–Hoeppli material. Tissue Gram stains are not of much value since the few organisms present are difficult to differentiate from other tissue elements. Because organisms are usually found in microabscesses, the GMS procedure with H&E counterstain is extremely helpful in making the fungus visible while still allowing one to visualise the background tissue response. When present, the asteroid body stains deeply eosinophilic with H&E, but the GMS procedure does not selectively stain Splendore–Hoeppli material. If GMS-H&E stained serial sections of primary cutaneous lesions are thoroughly searched, yeast forms of *S. schenckii* that stain dark-brown to black can be demonstrated in most cases. However, in some instances organisms are never found, despite a positive culture.

In tissue sections, *S. schenckii* appears as round, oval, or elongated ('cigar' shaped) single or budding cells that are usually 2–6 μm or more in diameter. In some instances, multiple budding is seen. Although considered by some to be the classic form of the organism in tissue, cigar-shaped forms are, in our experience, not regularly found. Large round yeast form cells up to 10 μm in diameter and branching hyphae of *S. schenckii* may occasionally be found in solid lesions, particularly in disseminated cases or experimental lesions in animals[9, 11, 21, 26, 27].

Occasionally, the large yeast-form cells of *S. schenckii* show only peripheral staining and appear as empty rings. These forms must be differentiated from small empty spherules of *Coccidioides immitis* or large empty yeast form cells of *Blastomyces dermatitidis*. Moreover, smaller intracellular *S. schenckii* cells, when abundant, may resemble those of *Histoplasma capsulatum* var. *capsulatum*. In those instances, specific immunofluorescence procedures are invaluable for confirming a diagnosis[28] (see Chapter 3). On two occasions, we have seen Russell bodies mistaken for *S. schenckii*, but the former are GMS negative.

References

1 Mariat, F., Lavalle, P. and Destombes, P. (1962). Recherches sur la sporotrichose. Etude mycologique et pouvoir pathogene de souches Mexicaines de Sporotrichum schenckii. *Sabouraudia* **2**, 60–79.
2 Ajello, L. and Kaplan, W. (1969). A new variant of Sporothrix schenckii. *Mykosen* **12**, 633–644.
3 Mackinnon, J. E., Conti-Diaz, I. A., Gezuele, E., Civila, E. and da Luz, S. (1969). Isolation of Sporothrix schenckii from nature and considerations on its pathogenicity and ecology. *Sabouraudia* **7**, 38–45.
4 *Sporotrichosis infection on mines of the Witwatersrand.* A symposium. Proceedings Transvaal Mine Medical Officer's Association. Transvaal Chamber of Mines, Johannesburg, 1947.
5 Lynch, P. J., Voorhees, J. J. and Harrell, E. R. (1970). Systemic sporotrichosis. *Ann. Intern. Med.* **73**, 23–30.
6 Jungerman, P. F. and Schwartzman, R. M. (1972). *Sporotrichosis*, pp. 31–39. Veterinary Medical Mycology. Lea & Febiger, Philadelphia.
7 Orr, E. R. and Riley, H. D. (1971). Sporotrichosis in childhood: Report of ten cases. *J. Pediatr.* **78**, 951–957.
8 Parker, J. D., Sarosi, G. A. and Tosh, F. E. (1970). Treatment of extracutaneous sporotrichosis. *Arch. Int. Med.* **125**, 858–863.
9 Lurie, H. I. (1963). Histopathology of sporotrichosis. *Arch. Pathol.* **75**, 92–109.
10 Davis, H. H. and Worthington, E. W. (1964). Equine sporotrichosis. *J. Am. Vet. Med. Assoc.* **145**, 692–693.
11 Scott, D. W., Bentinck-Smith, J. and Hagerty, G. F. (1974). Sporotrichosis in three dogs. *Cornell Vet.* **64**, 416–426.
12 Fetter, B. F. and Durham, N. C. (1961). Human cutaneous sporotrichosis. *Arch. Pathol.* **71**, 416–419.

13 Fetter, B. F. and Tindall, J. P. (1964). Cutaneous sporotrichosis. *Arch. Pathol.* **78**, 613–617.

14 Khan, K. P. (1975). Sporotrichosis. A histological study of four cutaneous cases. *Indian J. Dermatol.* **21**, 8–11.

15 Bullpitt, P. and Weedon, D. (1978). Sporotrichosis: a review of 39 cases. *Pathol.* **10**, 249–256.

16 Carr, R. D., Storkan, M. A., Wilson, J. W. and Swatek, F. E. (1964). Extensive verrucous sporotrichosis of long duration. *Arch. Dermatol.* **89**, 124–130.

17 Lurie, H. I. (1963). Histopathology of sporotrichosis: notes on the nature of the asteroid body. *Arch. Pathol.* **75**, 421–437.

18 Lurie, H. I. and Still, W. J. S. (1969). The 'capsule' of Sporotrichum schenckii and the evolution of the asteroid body. A light and electron microscopic study. *Sabouraudia* **7**, 64–70.

19 Von Lichtenberg, F., Smith, J. H. and Cheever, A. W. (1966). The Hoeppli phenomenon in schistosomiasis: Comparative pathology and immunopathology. *Am. J. Trop. Med. Hyg.* **15**, 886–895.

20 Liber, A. F. and Choi, H. S. (1973). Splendore–Hoeppli phenomenon about silk sutures in tissue. *Arch. Pathol.* **95**, 217–220.

21 Berson, S. D. and Brandt, F. A. (1977). Primary pulmonary sporotrichosis with unusual fungal morphology. *Thorax* **32**, 505–508.

22 Shoemaker, E. H., Bennett, H. D., Fields, W. S., Whitcomb, F. C. and Halpert, B. (1957). Leptomeningitis due to Sporotrichum schenckii. *Arch. Pathol.* **64**, 222–227.

23 Marrocco, G. R., Tihen, W. S., Goodnough, C. P. and Johnson, R. J. (1975). Granulomatous synovitis and osteitis caused by Sporothrix schenckii. *Am. J. Clin. Pathol.* **64**, 345–350.

24 Font, R. L. and Jokobiec, F. A. (1976). Granulomatous necrotizing retinochoroiditis caused by Sporotrichum schenckii. Report of a case including immunofluorescence and electron microscopical studies. *Arch. Ophthalmol.* **94**, 1513–1519.

25 Lurie, H. I. (1963). Five unusual cases of sporotrichosis from South Africa, showing lesions in muscles, bones, and viscera. *Brit. J. Surg.* **50**, 585–591.

26 Maberry, J. D., Mullins, J. F. and Stone, O. J. (1966). Sporotrichosis with demonstration of hyphae in human tissue. *Arch. Dermatol.* **93**, 65–67.

27 Barbee, W. C., Ewert, A. and Davidson, E. M. (1977). Animal model of human disease: sporotrichosis in the domestic cat. *Am. J. Pathol.* **86**, 281–284.

28 Kaplan, W. and Gonzalez-Ochoa, A. (1963). Application of the fluorescent antibody technique to the rapid diagnosis of sporotrichosis. *J. Lab. Clin. Med.* **62**, 835–841.

26 Superficial and cutaneous mycoses

Fungus diseases that affect the epidermal tissues can be divided into two groups: the superficial mycoses and the cutaneous mycoses. The superficial mycoses are disorders involving the outermost layer of the skin and hair. The diseases included in this group are tinea nigra, tinea versicolour, white piedra, and black piedra. These diseases are primarily of cosmetic importance, but severe infections can cause discomfort. Cutaneous mycoses are those disorders that involve the skin and its appendages to a greater degree than do the diseases classified as superficial mycoses. The lesions produced vary in extent and severity, and the signs and symptoms range from mild to severe. Dermatophytosis is the most important cutaneous mycosis.

The lesions caused by the agents of the superficial and cutaneous mycoses are usually confined to the skin and its appendages. These fungi are readily demonstrated by direct examination of skin scrapings or hairs in KOH preparations, and they can be definitively identified by cultural studies. Generally, when the skin is involved, dermatophytes grow within or upon the stratum corneum and may invade hair follicles. They seldom invade the deeper skin layers, and only rarely are pathologists asked to diagnose such superficial infections. Usually they are consulted only when the lesions are atypical and when the clinician suspects a disease other than a superficial or cutaneous mycosis. Pathologists may also encounter these infections when they coexist with another disease for which a histopathological evaluation is requested. Thus, one needs to be familiar with the appearance of the agents of the superficial and cutaneous mycoses in tissues so that the microscopic findings can be interpreted properly. In this chapter, we cover dermatophytosis, tinea nigra, and tinea versicolour because these mycoses affect the skin and may therefore be encountered when skin biopsies are examined. The mycoses that exclusively involve the hair, such as white and black piedra, are not discussed because histopathological techniques are not used for their diagnosis.

A Dermatophytoses

(Ringworm, tinea, dermatomycosis)

Aetiologic agents:

Pathogenic members of the genera *Epidermophyton, Microsporum,* and *Trichophyton* (Table 1) (Perfect states: *Microsporum* = *Nannizzia, Trichophyton* = *Arthroderma, Epidermophyton* = not known) (Table 2)

Definition and background information

Dermatophytosis is a clinical entity caused by members of a group of taxonomically related fungi known as dermatophytes. The dermatophytes parasitise the skin, hair, and nails of man and lower animals and only rarely infect deeper tissues. The diseases that they produce are also known as tineas or ringworm. These disorders include: 1) tinea pedis (ringworm of the feet); 2) tinea corporis (ringworm of the body); 3) tinea capitis (ringworm of the scalp); 4) tinea cruris (ringworm of the groin); and 5) tinea unguium (ringworm of the nail).

Table 1 Recognised dermatophyte species*

Epidermophyton	*Trichophyton*
E. floccosum	*T. concentricum*
Microsporum	*T. equinum*
M. audouinii	*T. gourvilii*
M. canis	*T. megninii*
M. cookei	*T. mentagrophytes*
M. distortum	*T. rubrum*
M. equinum	*T. schoenleinii*
M. ferrugineum	*T. simii*
M. fulvum	*T. tonsurans*
M. gallinae	*T. verrucosum*
M. gypseum	*T. violaceum*
M. nanum	*T. yaoundei*
M. persicolor	
M. praecox	
M. racemosum	
M. vanbreuseghemii	

*The non-pathogenic species in these three genera are omitted from this table.

Table 2 Dermatophytes with perfect states*

Imperfect States	Perfect States
Microsporum canis	*Nannizzia otae*
M. cookei	*N. cajetani*
M. fulvum	*N. fulva*
M. gypseum complex	*N. gypsea*
	N. incurvata
M. nanum	*N. obtusa*
M. persicolor	*N. persicolor*
M. racemosum	*N. racemosum*
M. vanbreuseghemii	*N. grubyia*
Trichophyton mentagrophytes complex	*Arthroderma benhamiae*
	A. vanbreuseghemii
T. simii	*A. simii*

*The non-pathogenic species of *Microsporum* and *Trichophyton* with perfect states are omitted from this table.

Twenty-seven different species of dermatophytes are currently recognised (Table 1). Most of them produce two types of asexual spores in vitro: small unicellular microconidia and large septate macroconidia. The macroconidia of each genus and species vary in size, shape, and character of their walls and in the manner in which they are borne on the mycelium. The microconidia are oval or pear-shaped, single-celled spores that are borne along the sides of the mycelium or terminally in grape-like clusters. The species and genera of dermatophytes cannot be identified on the basis of their microconidial characteristics, but variations in their size, form, and arrangement aid in the identification of the fungi. On the basis of the conidia, particularly the macroconidia, dermatophytes are classified in three genera: *Microsporum*, *Trichophyton*, and *Epidermophyton*[1]. Members of the genus *Microsporum* produce numerous macroconidia whose surfaces are rough. With some exceptions, the macroconidia are produced in abundance and their walls are thick. Members of this genus also produce microconidia. *Trichophyton* species produce macroconidia with smooth walls. The walls may be thick or thin. These spores are borne singly. *Trichophyton* species also produce microconidia. Members of the genus *Epidermophyton* produce abundant smooth-walled macroconidia borne in groups of 2–3; microconidia are not produced. Identification of most dermatophytes as to species is based upon their gross and microscopic morphology[2]. Morphological criteria, however, are not adequate for the identification of some dermatophyte species. Physiological studies, such as tests for nutritional requirements[3] and tests for ability to perforate hair in vitro[4], are useful in identifying these dermatophytes. Studies of mating reactions with tester strains of known cultures may also be helpful in identifying atypical isolates of some dermatophyte species[5].

Dermatophytes do not form conidia in tissues of an infected host. In vivo they occur as hyaline, septate hyphae that may break up into chains of arthrospores. When hair is infected, the pattern of invasion varies with the dermatophyte species. There are three general patterns of hair attack: the ectothrix, endothrix, and favic types. Mycelium can be found within the hair in all three types. In the ectothrix type of invasion, arthrospores are formed on the outside of the hair; in the endothrix type, arthrospores are formed inside the hair; in the favic type, the infected hair contains hyphae, empty spaces, and only a few arthrospores[6].

In dermatophytosis of the glabrous skin, lesions vary in form. They may be circular or ring shaped and discrete, or they may be diffuse, covering extensive areas. The tissue reaction also varies from erythema and scaliness to heavily crusted, suppurative or, rarely, granulomatous lesions. The lesions may be asymptomatic, pruritic, or painful. In tinea capitis, scattered loss of hair may be the only sign of infection or there may be discrete, usually circular patches with loss of hair and scaling, vesiculation, and suppuration. In some cases large raised suppurative lesions known as kerions occur. In tinea unguium, nails are thickened, discoloured, and deformed. Usually the tissue around the nail is not inflamed and there is no pain.

Dermatophytosis has been recorded in many different lower animal species, including domestic and wild mammals, and also birds. As in man, the host response and the appearance of the lesions vary considerably. In typical cases, lesions appear as circular, scaly, erythematous patches of alopecia that may or may not be covered with crusts. Sometimes only minimal lesions are observed, with only a few broken or missing hairs being the only sign of infection. Lesions, however, may be vesicular or suppurative[7].

Dermatophytosis is a common disease of worldwide distribution in human and lower animal populations. However, the individual dermatophyte species vary in their geographic distribution. Some are cosmopolites; others have a limited distribution. On the basis of their host preference and natural habitat, the dermatophytes may be divided into three groups: anthropophilic, zoophilic and geophilic. Anthropophilic dermatophytes are primarily adapted for parasitism of humans and rarely, if ever, infect lower animals. Infections by these agents are spread from host to host by direct contact or indirectly by exposure to contaminated fomites. Zoophilic dermatophytes are basically lower animal pathogens; however, they are infectious for humans also. Again, transmission may result from direct contact or indirectly by exposure to contaminated fomites. In contrast to the other two types, the geophilic dermatophytes live in soil as saprophytes but have the added capacity under certain conditions to infect humans and lower animals and to cause ringworm[8].

Topical antifungal and keratolytic agents are often effective for treatment of dermatophyte infections of the glabrous skin. Griseofulvin administered orally may be used from the outset or may be prescribed later on if the disease is resistant to topical therapy. In the treatment of dermatophyte infections of the nails and hairy skin, oral griseofulvin therapy is generally required[9].

Histopathology (Figures 560–576)

Microscopically, epidermal changes usually consist of hyperkeratosis and varying degrees of acanthosis. Spongiosis, intracellular edema, and vesicle formation are also occasionally seen. These changes may or may not be accompanied by an inflammatory infiltrate of varying severity in the dermis. When present, inflammation is usually mild and predominantly mononuclear. In H&E-stained sections, dermatophytes may be visible as hyphae, chains of arthrospores, or disassociated chains of arthrospores within the stratum corneum, hair follicles, and hairs[10–12]. However, these fungi are best demonstrated with the special fungus stains. When the hairs are infected, histopathologic examination may reveal the pattern of hair invasion (ectothrix, endothrix, and favic types).

On rare occasions, dermatophytes infect the deeper nonkeratinised layers of the skin where they may produce an acute purulent reaction with abscess formation or a granulomatous reaction that is usually of the nodular type. Pseudoepitheliomatous hyperplasia of the overlying epidermis may be seen. In some of these deep-seated lesions, fungi appear as individual hyphae* or as groups of hyphae. Some investigators have interpreted the fungal aggregates as granules and have called the infections mycetomas[13–15]. We have had the opportunity to study sections from two such cases, one caused by *Microsporum canis* and the other by a *Trichophyton* species. In both cases, a nodular granulomatous inflammatory reaction was present in the dermis which contained individual hyphae surrounded by a thick radiating coat of Splendore–Hoeppli material. In addition, aggregates of hyphae were embedded in and surrounded by this same material. Fungal aggregates were intimately surrounded by giant cells, palisading epithelioid cells and sometimes polymorphonuclear leucocytes. Draining sinuses lined by epithelioid and multinucleated giant cells were seen in one case. Rupture of hair follicles was clearly evident, and fungal elements from within the follicles could be seen invading the dermis through defects in the follicle walls. In these cases, we do not believe that the fungal aggregates represent mycetomal granules and that the dermatophyte infections can be properly termed mycetomas. This opinion is based on the fact that the hyphae in the aggregates were not organised into granules and that the eosinophilic Splendore–Hoeppli-like material was unlike cement substance, notwithstanding the fact that true granules of some mycetoma agents do not contain a cement matrix. We believe that such aggregates merely represent the clustering of individual hyphae, each surrounded by abundant Splendore–Hoeppli material. We prefer to call such aggregates 'pseudogranules'. The microscopic appearance of the 'pseudogranules' was strikingly similar in both cases, irrespective of the aetiologic agent.

*The term Majocchi's dermatophytic granuloma is applied to certain cases in which individual dermatophyte hyphae are found in granulomatous lesions of the dermis.

B Tinea nigra

(Keratomycosis nigricans palmaris, pityriasis nigra, cladosporiosis epidermica, microsporosis nigra)

Aetiologic agents:

Exophiala werneckii
Stenella araguata

Synonym:

Cladosporium werneckii (Perfect state – not known)
Cladosporium castellanii (Perfect state – not known)

Definition and background information

Tinea nigra is a superficial mycotic infection of the dermis, characterised by the formation of brownish or black macules usually on the palm of the hand. The lesions are flat, not scaly or inflammatory, and pigmentation is most intense at their border. The disease is usually asymptomatic[16, 17].

Tinea nigra occurs most commonly in tropical and subtropical regions. Occasional cases are encountered in temperate areas. There is evidence to indicate that the infections are contracted by traumatic inoculation of the causative agent into the skin from sources in the environment.

Tinea nigra is a benign disease of cosmetic importance. However, it warrants greater awareness, because it may be mistaken for a rapidly growing nevus[18]. On several occasions, confusion of tinea nigra with nevi has resulted in surgical excision or biopsy of the lesion. Greater awareness of this disease and its accurate diagnosis is important from the standpoint of avoiding unnecessary surgery.

Tinea nigra has not been reported in lower animals.

Exophiala werneckii, one of the aetiologic agents, grows well on routine laboratory media. Young colonies are moist, shiny, and black or greenish black. As colonies mature, they become drier and develop greyish black aerial mycelium on their surface. Microscopically the black, moist growth is composed of oval, dematiaceous, budding yeast-like cells that have a septum. These cells are produced laterally from dark hyphal elements. Older colonies with aerial mycelium have clusters or short chains of conidia borne on the ends of simple conidiophores. Mycelium and conidia are dark, and conidia are usually uniseptate[19].

In the epidermis, *E. werneckii* appears in the form of dematiaceous, branched septate hyphae 1.5–3.0 μm in diameter. Elongated budding cells 1.5–5.0 μm in diameter may also be present.

The disease usually responds to local therapy with keratolytic agents.

Stenella araguata[20] forms slow growing velvety olive grey to olive green colonies with a grey to black reverse. The colony's dematiaceous mycelium gives rise to simple or branched conidiophores that may be as long as 65 μm. They give rise to cylindrical to obclavate, pale to olive brown chains of 0–4 septate, rough walled conidia. Uniseptate conidia predominate, which range from 7.0–21.2 × 2.2–4.8 μm.

Histopathology (Figures 577–578)

The pathologic changes that occur in tinea nigra and tinea versicolor (part C) are not as profound and destructive as those that characterise the diseases classified as the cutaneous mycoses[10, 11]. Microscopically, there is mild to moderate hyperkeratosis of the epidermis in tinea nigra, often with linear separation of the keratin layer. Short, septate hyphae and elongated budding cells are usually confined to the outer portion of the stratum corneum. The fungal elements are naturally pigmented and appear light brown in H&E-stained skin sections. One may overlook their dematiaceous nature unless sections are examined under reduced light. There is little or no inflammatory reaction in the dermis. When present, it usually consists of small collections of mononuclear cells.

C Tinea versicolor

(Pityriasis versicolor, tinea flava, dermatomycosis furfuracea, 'liver spots')

Aetiologic agent:

Malassezia furfur

Synonyms:

Pityrosporum furfur, P. orbiculare, P. ovale (Perfect state – not known)

Definition and background information

Tinea versicolor is a fungus disease of the skin characterised by the development of flat or slightly raised scaly spots that gradually enlarge and coalesce. In light-skinned individuals the lesions are brownish, unless the skin is tanned, in which case they are found to be lighter in colour than the surrounding skin. In dark-skinned individuals the lesions are lighter in colour than the surrounding areas. In rare cases, hair follicles are involved and lesions are small, raised, and vesicular.

The infection is most common on the upper chest, back, arms and neck. The disease is generally chronic, and lesions may persist, spread, or reappear for years. Infections are usually asymptomatic, but in severe cases there may be itching. The disease is primarily of cosmetic importance[21].

Tinea versicolor is a common disease of worldwide distribution. It is, however, most prevalent in tropical and subtropical regions. The aetiologic agent has not been found to exist in nature as a saprophyte, and it is thought that the infection spreads from person to person directly or indirectly by exposure to infected desquamated epidermal scales.

Tinea versicolor has not been recorded in animals.

Cultural examinations are not routinely carried out for the diagnosis of tinea versicolor, because they are not necessary. The diagnosis is made microscopically by observing the aetiologic agent in epidermal scales. In such materials, *M. furfur* appears as short somewhat curved and bent hyphal elements, 2.5–4.0 μm in diameter, associated with clusters of oval or round thick-walled cells, 3.0–8.0 μm in diameter. These round or oval cells are considered to be phialospores[22]. They are pushed out from the end of a hypha through a collarette. Secondary buds are also produced in the same manner.

M. furfur can be cultivated on routine mycological media that have been overlaid with 1–2 ml of sterile olive oil[23]. Colonies are cream to tan in colour and are yeast-like. In culture, budding yeast-like cells predominate. Under certain conditions hyphae are also formed. The fungus has a nutritional requirement for lipids.

Treatment generally consists of the topical application of aqueous solutions of 20% sodium hyposulfite or 2.5% selenium sulfide suspension in a detergent vehicle[21].

Histopathology (Figures 579–580)

The histopathology of tinea versicolor is similar to that of tinea nigra. There is mild to moderate hyperkeratosis of the epidermis that may be associated with a minimal mononuclear cell infiltrate in the dermis. Elements of *M. furfur* appear as short, somewhat curved and bent hyphal elements associated with clusters of round or oval thick-walled cells, some of which are seen to be budding. These forms are usually found in the middle and deep portions of the stratum corneum. Fungal elements may be visible in H&E-stained sections, but are best demonstrated with the Giemsa and special fungus stains[10, 11].

References

1 Ajello, L. (1977). Taxonomy of the dermatophytes: A review of their imperfect and perfect states. In *Recent Advances in Medical and Veterinary Mycology,* pp. 289–297. K. Iwata, ed. University of Tokyo Press, Tokyo.

2 Rebell, G. and Taplin, D. (1970). *Dermatophytes.* Their Recognition and Identification. University of Miami Press, Coral Gables, Florida.

3 Georg, L. K. and Camp, L. B. (1957). Routine nutritional tests for the identification of dermatophytes. *J. Bacteriol.* **74**, 113–121.

4 Ajello, L. and Georg, L. K. (1957). In vitro hair cultures for differentiating between atypical isolates of Trichophyton mentagrophytes and Trichophyton rubrum. *Mycopathol. Mycol. Appl.* **8**, 3–17.

5 Padhye, A. A. (1975). Mating reactions for the identification of dermatophytes and other pathogenic fungi, pp. 111–117. Proc. Third International Conference on the Mycoses. Scientific Publication No. 304. Pan American Health Organization, Washington, D.C.

6 Ajello, L., Georg, L. K., Kaplan, W. and Kaufman, L. (1963). *Laboratory Manual for Medical Mycology.* Public Health Service Publication No. 994. Government Printing Office, Washington, D.C.

7 Georg, L. K. (1960). *Animal Ringworm in Public Health.* Public Health Service Publication No. 727. Government Printing Office, Washington, D.C.

8 Ajello, L. (1962). Present day concepts of the dermatophytes. *Mycopathol. Mycol. Appl.* **17**, 315–324.

9 Hildick-Smith, G., Blank, H. and Sarkany, I. (1964). *Fungus Diseases and Their Treatment.* Little, Brown & Co., Boston, Mass.

10 Graham, J. H. and Barroso-Tobila, C. (1971). Dermal pathology of superficial fungus infections. In *The Pathologic Anatomy of Mycoses,* pp. 211–382. Human Infection with Fungi, Actinomycetes and Algae. R. D. Baker, ed. Springer-Verlag, Berlin.

11 Graham, J. H. (1972). Superficial fungus infections. In *Dermal Pathology.* J. H. Graham, W. C. Johnson and E. G. Helwig, eds. Harper and Row, Hagerstown.

12 Connole, M. D. (1963). A review of dermatomycoses of animals in Australia. *Austral. Vet. J.* **39**, 130–134.

13 Camain, R., Baylet, R., Nonhouahi, Y. and Faye, I. (1971). Note sur les mycetomes de la nuque et du cuir chevelu de l'Africain. *Bull. Soc. Pathol. Exot.* **64**, 447–454.

14 Baylet, R., Camain, R., Juminer, B. and Faye, I. (1973). Microsporum ferrugineum Ota, 1921, agent de mycetomes du cuir chevelu en afrique noire. *Pathol. Biol.* **21**, 5–12.

15 Frey, D. and Lewis, M. B. (1976). Mycetoma of the scalp in an aboriginal child. *Australas. J. Dermatol.* **17**, 7–9.

16 Pillsbury, D. M., Shelley, W. B. and Kligman, A. M. (1956). *Dermatology,* p. 582. W. B. Saunders Co., Philadelphia.

17 Pardo-Costello, V. (1938). Keratomycosis nigricans palmaris. *Rev. Argent. de Dermatosif.* **22**, 255–264.

18 Smith, J. G., Sams, W. M. and Roth, F. J. (1958). Tinea nigra palmaris. A disorder easily confused with junction nevus of the palm. *J. Am. Med. Assoc.* **167**, 312–314.

19 McGinnis, M. R. (1978). *Human pathogenic species of Exophiala, Phialophora, and Wangiella,* pp. 37–59. Proc. Fourth International Conference on the Mycoses. Scientific Publication No. 356, Pan American Health Organization, Washington, D.C.

20 McGinnis, M. R. and Padhye, A. A. (1978). Cladosporium castellanii is a synonym of Stenella araguata. *Mycotaxon* **7**, 415–418.

21 Conant, N. F., Smith, D. T., Baker, R. D. and Callaway, J. L. (1971). *Manual of Clinical Mycology*, pp. 644–651. W. B. Saunders Co., Philadelphia.

22 Vanbreuseghem, R. (1954). Morphologie parasitaire de l'agent du Pityriasis versicolor: Malassezia furfur. *Ann. Soc. Belg. Med. Trop.* **35**, 251–254.

23 Gordon, M. A. (1951). The lipophilic mycoflora of the skin. I. In vitro culture of Pityrosporum orbiculare n. sp. *Mycologia* **43**, 524–535.

27 Zygomycosis

(Phycomycosis, mucormycosis, entomophthoromycosis, hyphomycosis, subcutaneous phycomycosis, rhinophycomycosis, phycomycosis entomophthorae, basidiobolomycosis, oomycosis, rhino-entomophthoromycosis)

Aetiologic agents:

Eleven species of zygomycetes, classified in eight genera, are well authenticated causative agents of human zygomycosis[1–6]:

Absidia corymbifera	*Mucor ramosissimus*
*Basidiobolus haptosporus**	*Rhizopus microsporus*
Conidiobolus coronatus	*R. oryzae*
C. incongruus	*R. rhizopodiformis*
Cunninghamella bertholletiae	*Saksenaea vasiformis*
Rhizomucor pusillus	

Definition and background information

Zygomycosis is a polymorphic disease of multiple aetiology. Its clinical forms develop as cutaneous, subcutaneous, systemic, and rhinocerebral infections. As noted in the list of synonyms for zygomycosis, infections caused by the various zygomycetes have, in the course of time, been given a wide variety of names. As stated in previous publications, the general term zygomycosis was adopted to replace the various names since fundamental changes in the classification of fungi have made the term 'phycomycosis' obsolete[1,2]. Other names based on the orders and genera of the zygomycetes involved are considered superfluous and confusing to use. The umbrella term zygomycosis adequately and clearly covers all zygomycete infections regardless of the classification of the aetiologic agents. When necessary, specific types of infections can be designated by coupling the term zygomycosis with an appropriate descriptive adjective, e.g. cutaneous zygomycosis, subcutaneous zygomycosis, etc.

Regardless of the clinical expression of zygomycosis, the unifying diagnostic hallmark of the disease is the form assumed by the aetiologic agents in tissue. The invasive form is mycelial in nature. This mycelium is infrequently septate and is significantly broader than that of any other of the fungi with a filamentous tissue form (*Aspergillus sp.*; *Candida sp.*, the agents of phaeohyphomycosis). The hyaline mycelium ranges from 6–25 μm in diameter, although on occasion, narrow hyphae that are 3–4 μm in width may be present. Branched filaments are not uncommon, and frequently the mycelium may be distorted and assume bizarre forms. On rare occasions, sporangiophores with or without rhizoids and sporangia may develop in certain tissues such as the nasal turbinates or ethmoid sinuses[3,7].

Cutaneous zygomycosis

Primary infections of this type of zygomycosis have been rare. When cultured, the aetiologic agents involved were identified as *Mucor ramosissimus*[8,9] and *Rhizopus rhizopodiformis*[10–12].

The one known *M. ramosissimus* infection in a patient with no predisposing conditions involved the face and neck as well as the nasal septum. This chronic infection of 24 years duration began with the development of a flat, erythematous lesion on the left cheek that had undefined boundaries and a soft consistency. The infection spread centrifugally and formed a 'papular, congestive, infiltrated plaque' that was painless[8]. As the disease progressed, the infection came to involve the cutaneous area of both lips, the nasal septum, and chin. After 24 years of development of the disease without a diagnosis, the skin was drawn and shiny, with a waxy-whitish hue. Irregularly distributed, firm papules of 2–3 mm D were present. The diagnosis of zygomycosis was based on histological study of biopsied tissue that revealed the presence of aseptate, broad, hyaline mycelial filaments, and on the isolation and identification of the aetiologic agent[9].

Hospital-acquired infections have been attributed to *R. rhizopodiformis* in Argentina[11], Louisiana[10],

*There is a growing consensus that all of the human isolates should be referred to as *Basidiobolus ranarum*[50].

New York[12], Minnesota, and elsewhere[13]. These nosocomial infections developed on the skin of patients with various primary medical problems. From the epidemiological point of view, the most interesting cases[12, 13] were those involving infections which began in gauze-dressed wounds covered with a specific brand of tape. *R. rhizopodiformis* was isolated from fresh packs of the tape that were to be used on the patients[13]. The infections manifested themselves by the development of erythematous, papular lesions. The infected tissue often became necrotic, and the lesions spread progressively. Biopsied tissue revealed the presence of coenocytic, broad, branched, hyaline hyphae. Cultures were grown successfully, and the aetiologic agents were identified as *R. rhizopodiformis*.

Subcutaneous zygomycosis

Two types of infection fall in this category:

1 subcutaneous infections not restricted to any particular area of the body. Almost invariably, these have been caused by *Basidiobolus haptosporus;*

2 subcutaneous infections confined to the nasal mucosa and adjacent tissues. The single causative agent in these infections has been *Conidiobolus coronatus*.

Almost all of the *B. haptosporus* infections have occurred in Africa and Asia[14]. The case attributed to the United States by Coremans–Pelseneer[14] was actually caused by *Absidia corymbifera*[15]. The one New World subcutaneous case of *B. haptosporus* infection was diagnosed in a Brazilian child who had developed an infection in her left thigh[16].

An invasive infection of the palate and maxillary sinus was attributed to *B. haptosporus* in a Missouri, USA, patient[17].

Clinically, *B. haptosporus* infections involve the trunk and limbs. In the earliest stage, such an infection begins as a painless nodule that develops slowly. Within a few months a large, firm mass, sharply delimited from the surrounding tissues has formed. The skin covering the tumefaction may remain normal in appearance or become scaly and discoloured. In some cases, superficial ulcers may develop. Their occurrence is dependent on the size of the subcutaneous mass and the duration of the infection. Multiple lesions are rare. Spontaneous regression may occur. In persistent cases, treatment with iodides has been highly effective.

Culturally confirmed cases of *Conidiobolus coronatus* infection have been reported with the highest frequency in Africa, particularly Nigeria[18]. Outside of Africa, cases have been diagnosed only in the Caribbean area[19, 20] and South America[21, 22]. *C. coronatus* infections are chronic, with a history of nasal obstruction and gradual but progressive swelling of the nose, cheeks, and upper lip. Extremes in this form of tumefaction are dramatically illustrated in a case from the Cameroon[23].

Diagnosis of most of the described cases of *C. coronatus* infection was based on the presence of infrequently septate, broad, mycelial filaments in tissue and by the cultural identification of *C. coronatus*. In some cases, diagnosis has been tenuously based on clinical developments and, in particular, on the occurrence of a Splendore–Hoeppli reaction around mycelial filaments[24, 25]. Since this host tissue reaction is not limited to *C. coronatus* infections, such diagnoses must be viewed with skepticism. Histologically, the mycelium of the agents of zygomycosis cannot be distinguished one from the other.

C. coronatus infections have been treated most successfully with oral potassium iodide. Resistant cases have responded to amphotericin B. In extreme cases, drug therapy has been combined with surgical intervention[19, 23].

Systemic zygomycosis

Systemic infections with or without a primary pulmonary focus have been reported with relatively high frequency[26]. However, in only a few of these cases were the aetiologic agents isolated and identified. The documented species have been *Absidia corymbifera*[27], *Conidiobolus incongruus*[4, 28, 29], *Cunninghamella bertholletiae* (*elegans*)[5], *Rhizomucor pusillus*[30], *Rhizopus microsporus*[31], *R. oryzae*[32–35] and *Saksenaea vasiformis*[2].

The clinical signs of pulmonary zygomycosis are not pathognomonic. They closely resemble those elicited by bacterial and viral pathogens. Pain may develop, and frequently bloody sputum is raised. Densities indicative of pneumonia and infarction may be observed by x-ray. Pulmonary infections are progressive, and unless controlled, they spread to involve other vital organs such as the spleen, heart, and stomach[26]. Solitary, localised pulmonary infections caused by unspecified zygomycetes have been recorded[36]. Lobectomy has been successfully used in treating such cases.

A severe cranial infection due to *Saksenaea vasiformis* was initiated by the contamination of head wounds suffered in an automobile accident. The fungus invaded the orbital tissues and the brain. Smears of seropurulent drainage fluid and histological sections of orbital and brain tissues revealed the presence of broad, aseptate hyphae. The aetiologic agent was isolated from excised tissue[2].

Some of the human pathogenic species (*A. corymbifera, C. coronatus, R. pusillus, R. oryzae, R. microsporus, R. rhizopodiformis*) are capable of causing a variety of diseases and complications in lower animals, including abortion in cattle. Several other zygomycetes, not as yet implicated in human diseases, have also been found to cause diseases in lower animals (*Mortierella alpina, M. polycephala, M. wolfii, M. zychae, Mucor dispersus, M. hiemalis, M. racemosus* and *Syncephalastrum racemonus*[37].

Rhinocerebral zygomycosis

This is a disease almost invariably associated with acute diabetes. It is undoubtedly the most fulminating of all of the mycotic diseases. Death ensues in a matter of a few days after the infection has begun if it remains unrecognised and untreated. All verified cases have been due to the

---

Synonyms of the Pathogenic Zygomycetes

Absidia corymbifera
Synonyms:
= *A. cornealis* = *L. italiana*
= *A. italiana* = *L. italica*
= *A. lichtheimii* = *L. ramosa*
= *A. ramosa* = *Mucor cornealis*
= *Lichthemia cornealis* = *M. corymbifera*
= *L. corymbifera* = *M. lichtheimii*

Conidiobolus coronatus
Synonyms:
= *Delacroixia coronata* = *Entomophthora coronatus*

Cunninghamella bertholletiae
Synonyms:
= *Actinocephalum japonicum* = *C. elegans*
= *C. blakesleeana*

Rhizomucor pusillus
Synonym:
= *M. miehei*

Rhizopus microsporus
Synonyms:
= *Mucor speciosus* = *R. minimus*
= *R. equinus* = *R. speciosus*

Rhizopus oryzae[39, 43]
Synonyms:
= *Mucor arrhizus* = *R. formosaensis*
= *M. cambodja* = *R. hangchow*
= *M. norvegicus* = *R. japonicus*
= *Rhizopus achlamydosporus* = *R. kasanensis*
= *R. arrhizus* = *R. maydis*
= *R. boreas* = *R. nodosus*
= *R. bovinus* = *R. ramosus*
= *R. cambodja* = *R. tritici*
= *R. chiuniany* = *R. trubinii*
= *R. chunkuvensis* = *R. usamii*
= *R. delemar*

Rhizopus rhizopodiformis
Synonyms:
= *R. chinensis* = *R. cohnii*

Basidiobolus haptosporus has been variously misidentified as *B. meristosporus* and *B. ranarum*.

Rhizopus stolonifer (*R. nigricans*), although cited as an agent of zygomycosis by some investigators, is believed either to have been misidentified or to have only played the role of a contaminant[2].

single species, *Rhizopus oryzae.** The victims of this widely distributed fungus are almost invariably uncontrolled diabetics in the acidotic state. The infection has occurred in infants and in persons up to 75 years of age[26]. The primary sites of infection are the nasal turbinates and paranasal sinuses. However, a primary infection of the oral mucosa in a diabetic after tooth extraction has been documented[38]. Spread from the primary sites occurs by direct extension.

The symptoms that quickly develop involve the nose, eyes, and brain. Nasal discharges of black and blood-tinged mucus are seen, and necrotic tissue is observed in the nasal septum and turbinates. The patients usually complain of severe frontal headaches, chills, and fever. Orbital swelling generally is an ominous development since it portends invasion of the brain and the meninges. The cardinal signs in rhinocerebral zygomycosis in diabetics with acidosis are the rapid development of sinusitis, inflammation of the orbital tissues, generally unilateral, with the development of ophthalmoplegia, proptosis, and signs of meningo-encephalitis.

Prompt control of the acidotic state may lead to spontaneous remission of the disease in some cases. However, amphotericin B is recommended for the control of this highly fatal form of zygomycosis.

Serological tests to aid in diagnosing zygomycosis and in monitoring the course of the disease have been developed and evaluated[40]. The immunodiffusion tests with appropriate antigens promise to be highly useful for these purposes.

Zygomycosis is not a contagious disease. It does not spread from person to person or from animals to man. All of the zygomycetes known to cause human and animal disease occur in nature as saprophytes and as agents of decay. They are frequently isolated from the soil and air.

The zygomycetes present identification problems because keys to the several orders, families, genera, and species are not readily available or have not been recently revised to include newer taxonomic concepts. The reader should consult references[41–43] for taxonomic assistance.

To help the reader to properly understand and interpret the literature, the synonyms of the pathogenic zygomycetes are presented in tabular form (page 124).

Histopathology (Figures 581–604)

Fungi in the Order Mucorales usually elicit a pyogenic inflammatory reaction characterised by abscess formation and suppurative necrosis[15, 26, 31, 44, 45]. In most cases of zygomycosis caused by these fungi, a narrow zone of polymorphonuclear leucocytes surrounds broad hyphae embedded in necrotic tissue. Heavily infected tissues may reveal extensive necrosis with diffuse infiltration of polymorphonuclear leucocytes. In the less common chronic infections, a purely granulomatous or mixed purulent and granulomatous inflammatory reaction with or without the formation of granulation tissue is seen.

Because of the great propensity for the zygomycetes to invade blood vessels, necrosis of vessel walls and mycotic thrombi are frequently seen in any infected tissue[15, 26, 44]. Thrombosis often leads to infarction and haematogenous or lymphatic dissemination. Large vessel thrombosis is common and may even involve the carotid arteries. In areas of ischemic necrosis, inflammation is sometimes minimal, despite the presence of numerous typical hyphae.

Zygomycetes are frequently found in ulcers of the gastrointestinal tract of humans and animals, more so than any of the other filamentous fungi[15, 26, 46, 47]. Typical hyphae can be seen invading the necrotic margins of ulcers and extending, at times, through the muscular layers of the gut wall. Angioinvasion is almost always seen in the depths of and at the periphery of these ulcers. Here, numerous broad hyphae are found in and around blood vessels, infiltrating their walls and producing thrombi in their lumens.

In tissue, hyphae of the zygomycetes are characteristically broad, infrequently septate, and thin-walled; they have nonparallel sides and range in width from 3–25 μm (avg. 12 μm) and in length up to 200 μm. They often appear empty, have focal bulbous dilatations and show non-dichotomous, irregular branching that may sometimes be at right angles. Folded, twisted, and compressed hyphae may also be seen, and compression folds that stain deeper than the adjacent hyphal segments have been mistaken for septations. Transected hyphae may mimic large empty yeast cells or empty spherules of *Coccidioides immitis.* Sporangia are rarely seen in tissue[3, 7].

In contrast to most filamentous fungi, the zygomycetes are best observed in tissue sections stained by H&E. With this stain, the hyphae are usually basophilic or amphophilic and are easily detected when a tissue section is scanned under the low power objective. The special fungus stains (GMS, GF, PAS) are useful, but generally do not colour the zygomycetes as deeply as they do other fungi. In rare instances when zygomycete hyphae are not stained by H&E, special fungus stains should be tried, especially GMS. When GMS is used, however, it may be necessary to prolong the staining time in the silver nitrate solution. Some-

*The opinion expressed by Scholer and Miller[39] that *R. arrhizus* is a synonym of *R. oryzae* is accepted.

times the combination of GMS and H&E intensifies the staining of zygomycete hyphae.

At times, it may be difficult to distinguish zygomycetes from aspergilli in tissue sections, especially when the former contain septations and are narrower than usual. (Merely observing septations does not rule out the possibility of a zygomycete, because these fungi are not completely aseptate.) In general, however, hyphae of the aspergilli have characteristic dichotomous branching, parallel walls, and numerous septa. They are also narrower and stain deeper with the special fungus stains than do the zygomycetes.

The characteristic affinity of the zygomycetes for haematoxylin, together with their broad, infrequently septate and irregularly branched hyphae, usually enables the microscopist to identify these fungi. However, a zygomycete cannot be identified as to genus and species because all members in this group are morphologically similar in tissue; cultural studies are always necessary for a differential identification.

When subcutaneous zygomycosis is caused by *B. haptosporus*, a zygomycete belonging to the Order Entomophthorales, the buttocks, thighs, trunk and perineum are the sites most commonly involved[10, 29, 45, 48]. Although at first localised, in later stages the disease may spread laterally and penetrate deep into underlying tissues including the muscles and thoracic, abdominal, and pelvic viscera. However, in contrast to the clinical manifestations caused by members of the Order Mucorales, metastatic lesions seldom occur and there is less tendency to invade blood vessels. Microscopically, the deep dermis and subcutaneous tissues are obliterated by granulation tissue containing foreign body giant cells and numerous eosinophils. Generally, very few fungal elements are found, and they usually appear as short, poorly stained hyphal fragments with extremely thin walls. The fragments are characteristically bordered by an irregular, brightly eosinophilic zone of granular or club-like Splendore–Hoeppli material and are embedded in necrotic eosinophilic microabscesses. Foreign body giant cells and palisading epithelioid cells may surround these abscesses, and these phagocytes sometimes contain hyphal fragments. When intracellular, some hyphae still retain their conspicuous eosinophilic border. Degranulating eosinophils are sometimes evident, and, in one case, we have observed Charcot–Leyden crystals within and contiguous to eosinophilic abscesses.

Hyphae of *B. haptosporus* range from 6–25 μm in diameter (avg. 12 μm), and they either appear empty or contain faintly basophilic, flocculent cytoplasmic material. Irregular branching and septations are sometimes seen, and in our experience, the latter are more frequently observed in hyphae of the agents of subcutaneous zygomycosis than in those of the Mucorales. In a few lesions, however, branching or septations may not be evident. The hyphae are irregular in width and stain poorly with H&E as well as with the special fungus stains. Of the histologic stains, we prefer H&E simply because the Splendore–Hoeppli material that intimately and selectively surrounds most of the poorly stained hyphae is coloured brightly eosinophilic, thus outlining fungal elements and making them evident even on low power examination.

C. coronatus, another zygomycete belonging to the Order Entomophthorales and the aetiologic agent of nasofacial zygomycosis, causes lesions that are histologically similar to those produced by *B. haptosporus*[10, 19, 48, 49]. Although these two zygomycetes belong to different genera, they are morphologically and tinctorially identical in tissue. However, for unknown reasons, infections by *C. coronatus* are limited to the nasal mucosa, nasal sinuses, and subcutaneous tissues of the nose and face.

References

1 Ajello, L. (1977). Medically important infectious fungi. *Contrib. Microbiol. Immunol.* **3**, 7–19 (Karger, Basel, Pub.).

2 Ajello, L., Dean, D. F. and Irwin, R. S. (1976). The zygomycete Saksenaea vasiformis as a pathogen of humans with a critical review of the etiology of zygomycosis. *Mycologia* **68**, 52–62.

3 Bauer, H., Ajello, L., Adams, E. and Useda Hernandez, D. (1955). Cerebral mucormycosis: pathogenesis of the disease. *Am. J. Med.* **18**, 822–831.

4 King, D. S. and Jung, S. C. (1976). Identity of the etiological agent of the first deep entomophthoraceous infection of man in the United States. *Mycologia* **68**, 181–183.

5 Kwon-Chung, K. J., Young, R. C. and Orlando, M. (1975). Pulmonary mucormycosis caused by Cunninghamella elegans in a patient with chronic myelogenous leukemia. *Am. J. Clin. Pathol.* **64**, 544–548.

6 Weitzman, I. and Crist, M. Y. (1979). Studies with clinical isolates of Cunninghamella. I. Mating behavior. *Mycologia* **71**, 1024–1033.

7 LaTouche, C. J., Sutherland, T. W. and Telleng, M. (1964). Histopathological and mycological features of a case of rhinocerebral mucormycosis (phycomycosis) in Britain. *Sabouraudia* **3**, 148–150.

8 Vignale, R., Mackinuon, J. E., Casella de Vilaboa, E. and Burgoa, F. (1964). Chronic, destructive, mucocutaneous phycomycosis. *Sabouraudia* **3**, 143–147.

9 Hesseltine, C. W. and Ellis, J. J. (1964). An interesting species of Mucor, M. ramosissimus. *Sabouraudia* **3**, 151–154.

10 Baker, R. D., Seabury, J. H. and Schneidau, J. D. (1962). Subcutaneous and cutaneous mucormycosis and subcutaneous phycomycosis. *Lab. Invest.* **11**, 1091–1102.

11 Negroni, R. and Paladino, A. M. (1973). Phycomycosis cutanea por Rhizopus cohnii. *Arch. Argent. Dermatol.* **28**, 27–34.

12 Gartenberg, G., Bottone, E. J., Keusch, G. T. and Weitzman, I. (1978). Hospital acquired mucormycosis (Rhizopus rhizopodiformis) of skin and subcutaneous tissue: Epidemiology, mycology and treatment. *N. Engl. J. Med.* **299**, 1115–1118.

13 Anonymous. (1978). Follow-up on Rhizopus infections associated with Elastoplast bandages – United States. *Morb. Mort. Weekly Report* **27**, 243–244.

14 Coremans-Pelseneer, J. (1972). Epidemiologie de la basidiobolomycose. *Ann. Soc. Belge. Med. Trop.* **52**, 315–328.

15 Straatsma, B. R., Zimmerman, L. E. and Gass, J. D. M. (1962). Phycomycosis. A clinicopathologic study of fifty-one cases. *Lab. Invest.* **11**, 963–985.

16 Bittencourt, A. L., Melo, C. R., Jalil, O. A. M. and Andrade, Z. A. (1977). Basidiobolomicose. Apresentação de um caso. *Rev. Inst. Med. Trop.* Sao Paulo **19**, 208–212.

17 Dworzack, D. L., Pollock, A. S., Hodges, G. R., Barnes, W. G., Ajello, L. and Padhye, A. (1978). Zygomycosis of the maxillary sinus and palate caused by Basidiobolus haptosporus. *Arch. Intern. Med.* **138**, 1274–1276.

18 Fromentin, H. and Ravisso, P. (1977). Les entomophthoromycoses tropicales. *Acta Trop.* **34**, 375–394.

19 Herstoff, J. K., Bogaars, H. and McDonald, C. J. (1978). Rhinophycomycosis entomophthorae. *Arch. Dermatol.* **114**, 1674–1678.

20 Bras, G., Gordon, C. C., Emmons, C. W., Prendegast, K. M. and Sugar, M. (1965). A case of phycomycosis observed in Jamaica; infection with Entomophthora coronata. *Am. J. Trop. Med. Hyg.* **14**, 141–145.

21 Andrade, Z. A., Paula, L. A., Sherlock, I. A. and Cheever, A. W. (1967). Nasal granuloma caused by Entomophthora coronata. *Am. J. Trop. Med. Hyg.* **16**, 31–33.

22 Restrepo, M. A., Greer, D. L., Robledo, V. M., Diaz, G. C., Lopez, M. R. and Bravo, R. C. (1967). Subcutaneous phycomycosis: Report of the first case observed in Colombia, South America. *Am. J. Trop. Med. Hyg.* **16**, 34–39.

23 Misson, R., Guenard, C., Bobin, P., Millet, P., Arnoux, D., Grateau, P., Pons, J. and Antoine, H. (1973). Rhino-bucco-phycomycose. *Ann. Dermatol. Syphiligt.* (Paris) **100**, 409–416.

24 Silva, J. F. da, Silva, W. M. da, Dantas, J. C., Assunção, A. C. R. de y S. Teive Oliveira, M. M. da (1975). Rinoentomoftorose – Registro de um caso. *Rev. Pat. Trop.* **4**, 101–106.

25 Williams, A. O., Lichtenberg, F. von, Smith, J. H. and Martinson, F. D. (1969). Ultrastructure of phycomycosis due to Entomophthora, Basidiobolus and associated 'Splendore–Hoeppli' phenomenon. *Arch. Pathol.* **87**, 459–468.

26 Baker, R. D. (1971). Mucormycosis. In *The Pathologic Anatomy of Mycoses,* pp. 832–918. R. D. Baker, ed. Springer-Verlag, Berlin.

27 Darja, M. and Dary, M. I. (1963). Pulmonary mucormycosis with cultural identification. *Can. Med. Assoc. J.* **89**, 1235–1238.

28 Eckert, H. L., Khoury, G. H., Pore, R. S., Gilbert, E. F. and Gaskell, J. R. (1972). Deep entomophthora phycomycotic infection reported for the first time in the United States. *Chest* **61**, 392–394.

29 Gilbert, E. F., Khoury, G. H. and Pore, R. S. (1970). Histopathological identification of Entomophthora phycomycosis. *Arch. Pathol.* **90**, 583–587.

30 Erdos, M. S., Butt, K. and Weinstein, L. (1972). Mucormycotic endocarditis of the pulmonary valve. *J. Am. Med. Assoc.* **222**, 951–953.

31 Neame, P. and Rayner, D. (1960). Mucormycosis. A report on twenty-two cases. *Arch. Pathol.* **70**, 261–268.

32 McCall, W. and Strobos, R. R. J. (1957). Survival of a patient with central nervous system mucormycosis. *Neurology* **7**, 290–292.

33 Battock, D. J., Grausz, H., Bobrowsky, M. and Littman, M. L. (1968). Alternate-day amphotericin B therapy in the treatment of rhinocerebral phycomycoses (mucormycosis). *Ann. Intern. Med.* **68**, 122–127.

34 Gloor, F., Loffler, A. and Scholer, H. J. (1961). Mucormykosen. *Pathol. Microbiol.* **24**, 1043–1064.

35 McBride, R. A., Corson, J. M. and Dammin, G. J. (1960). Mucormycosis. *Am. J. Med.* **28**, 832–846.

36 Gale, A. M. and Kletisch, W. P. (1972). Solitary pulmonary nodule due to phycomycosis (mucormycosis). *Chest* **62**, 752–755.

37 Ainsworth, G. C. and Austwick, P. K. C. (1973). *Fungal Diseases of Animals,* 2nd ed. Commonwealth Agricultural Bureaux, Farnham Royal, Slough, England.

38 Limongelli, W. A., Clark, M. S., Saglimbene, R., Baden, E., Washington, J. A. and Williams, A. C. (1975). Successful treatment of mucocutaneous mucormycosis after dental extractions in a patient with uncontrolled diabetes. *J. Oral Surg.* **33**, 705–712.

39 Scholer, H. J. and Miller, E. (1971). *Taxonomy of the pathogenic species of Rhizopus.* 7th annual meeting Br. Soc. Mycopathology. Edinburgh, April 5–7.

40 Jones, K. W. and Kaufman, L. (1978). Development and evaluation of an immunodiffusion test for diagnosis of systemic zygomycosis (Mucormycosis): Preliminary report. *J. Clin. Microbiol.* **7**, 97–103.

41 Hesseltine, C. W. and Ellis, J. J. (1973). *Mucorales.* The Fungi, vol. IVB. G. C. Ainsworth, F. K. Sparrow and A. S. Sussman, eds. Academic Press, New York.

42 Hamlin, R. T. (1973). *Keys to the families and species of the Mucorales.* Strauss & Cramer, Leuterhousen, Germany.

43 Zycha, H. and Siepmann, R. (1969). *Mucorales.* J. Cramer, Lehre, Germany.

44 Gregory, J. E., Golden, A. and Haymaker, W. (1953). Mucormycosis of the central nervous system. *Bull. Johns Hopkins Hosp.* **73**, 405–419.

45 Cameron, H. M., Gatei, D. and Bremner, A. D. (1973). The deep mycoses in Kenya: a histopathological study. 2. Phycomycosis. *East Afr. Med. J.* **50**, 396–405.

46 Davis, C. L., Anderson, W. A. and McCrory, B. R. (1955). Mucormycosis in food producing animals. *J. Am. Vet. Med. Assoc.* **126**, 261–267.

47 Gisler, D. B. and Pitcock, J. A. (1962). Intestinal mucormycosis in the monkey (Macaca mulatta). *Am. J. Vet. Res.* **23**, 365–366.

48 Williams, A. O. (1969). Pathology of phycomycosis due to Entomophthora and Basidiobolus species. *Arch. Pathol.* **87**, 13–20.

49 Martinson, F. D. and Clark, B. M. (1967). Rhinophycomycosis entomophthorae in Nigeria. *Am. J. Trop. Med. Hyg.* **16**, 40–47.

50 Hutchison, J. A., King, D. S. and Nickerson, M. A. (1972). Studies on temperature requirements, odor production and zygospore wall undulation of the genus Basidiobolus. *Mycologia* **64**, 467–474.

Pictorial section

The magnifications given for the illustrations relate to the original 35 mm transparencies

3 Immunofluorescence diagnosis

Text pages: 23–25

1

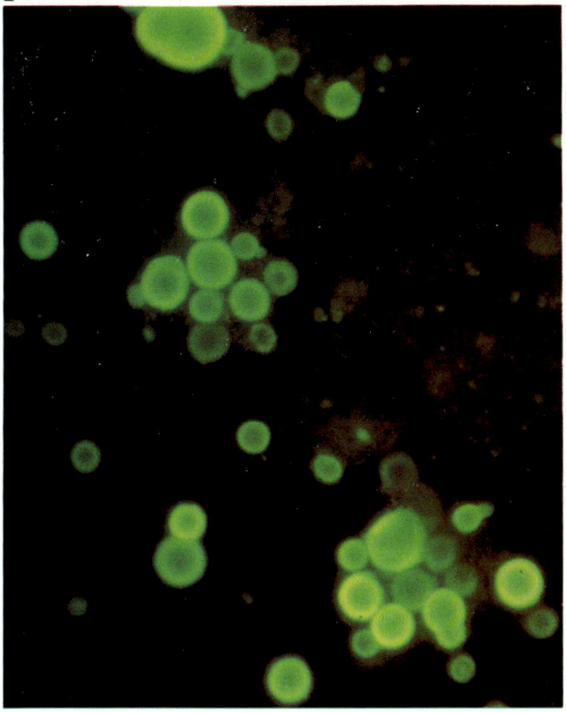

1 **Cryptococcus neoformans** cells in a smear of the sediment from a centrifuged urine sample stained by fluorescein-labelled antiglobulin specific for this fungus. (×240)

2

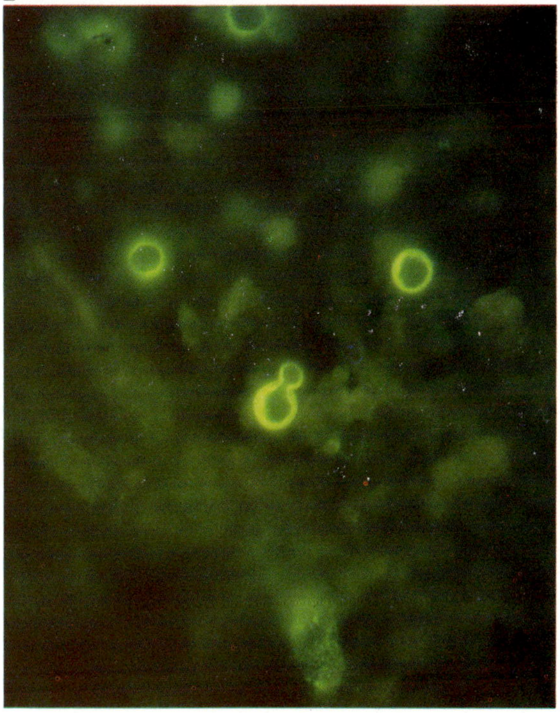

2 **Blastomyces dermatitidis** tissue-form cells in section of lung stained by specific fluorescein-labelled antiglobulins. One cell is budding. (×160)

3

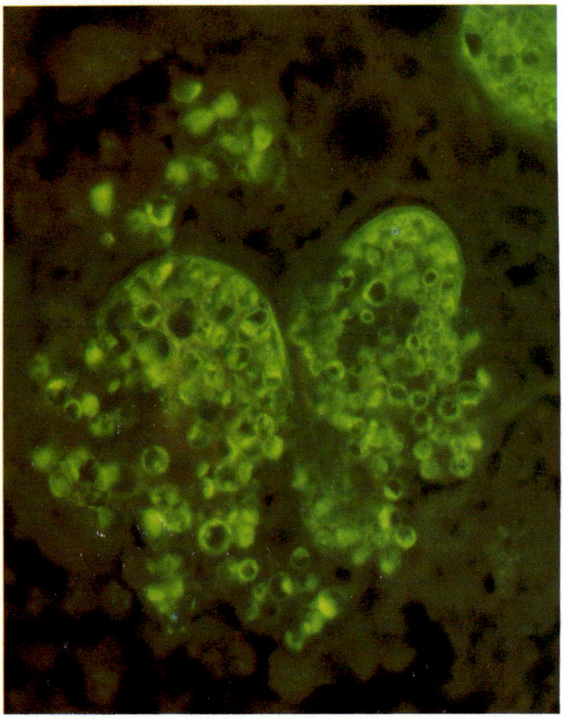

3 Coccidioides immitis in section of formalin-fixed human lung. Two spherules in the centre of the photomicrograph have ruptured and their brightly fluorescing endospores are in the process of being liberated (compare with **192** and **193**). (×240)

4

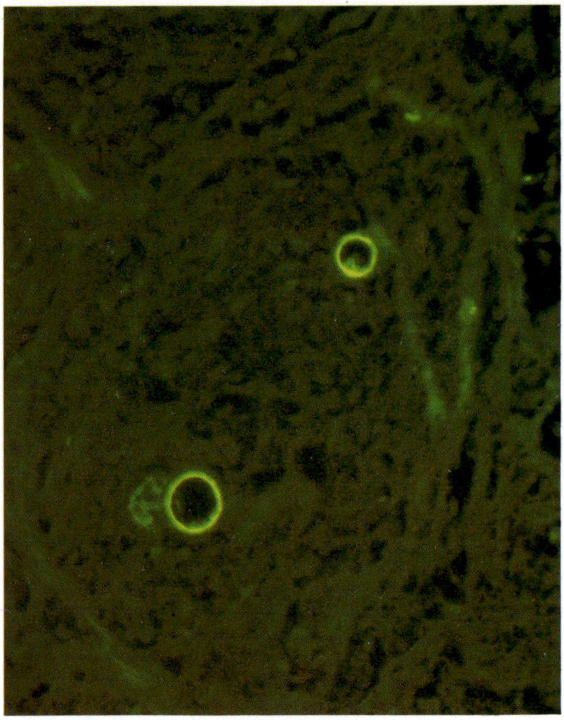

4 Coccidioides immitis in epithelioid cell granuloma of human lung. Two brightly fluorescing, empty spherules stand out in sharp contrast to the surrounding tissue. Such empty spherules are not diagnostic for *C. immitis* and they may be morphologically confused with other fungi. However, as shown here, they can be definitively identified by immunofluorescence. (×240)

5

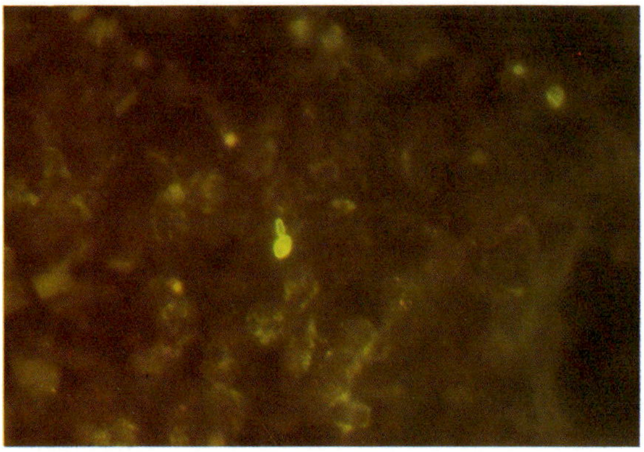

5 Sporothrix schenckii A single budding cell is seen within a dermal microabscess in a human. The skin section was stained by the specific FA procedure. (×384)

6

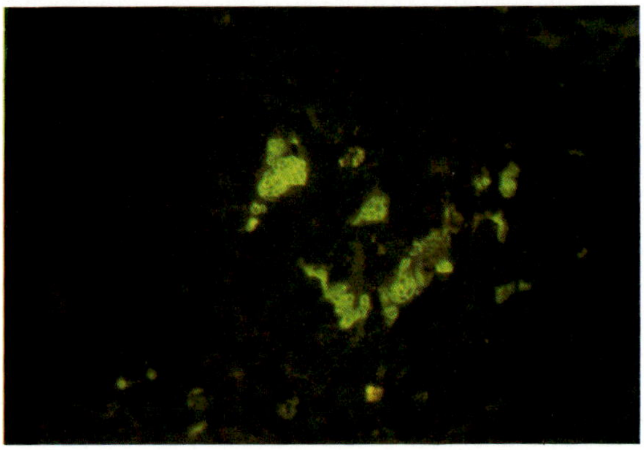

6 Histoplasma capsulatum var. capsulatum Aggregates of yeast cells within macrophages in a section of lymph node from a patient with acute histoplasmosis. The cells were stained by fluorescein-labelled antiglobulins to this fungus that had been adsorbed with cells of *Candida albicans*. (×560)

7

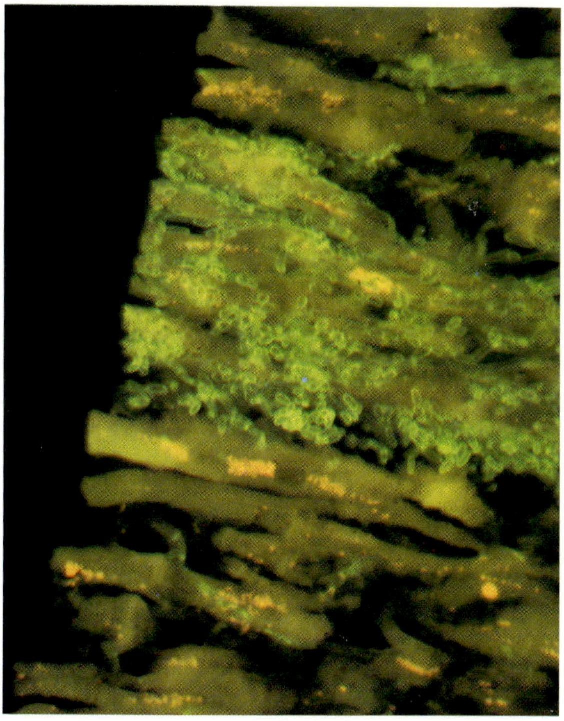

7 Candida spp. Numerous fungal cells in myocardium of a patient who died from a haematological malignancy. Fluorescein-labelled antiglobulins specific for the *Candida* species were used for staining. Note the absence of an inflammatory response. (×450)

8

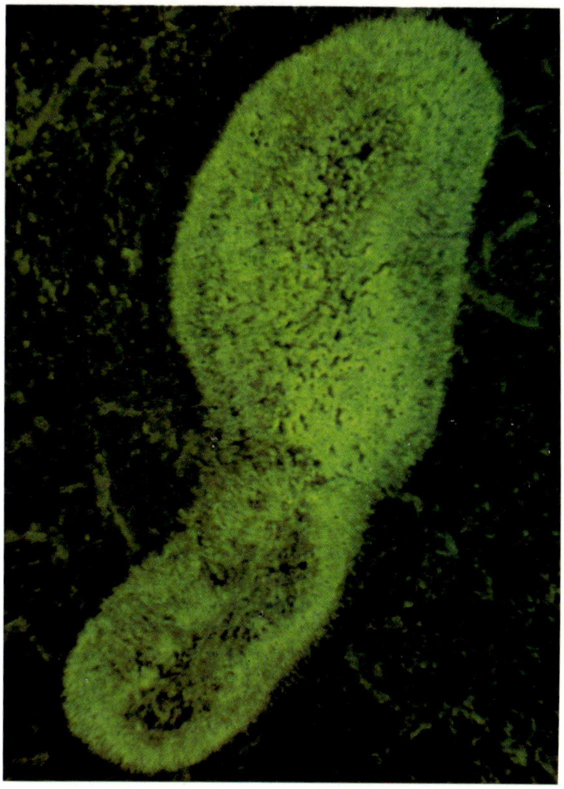

8 Petriellidium (Allescheria) boydii granule in a human lung section stained by specific fluorescein-labelled antiglobulins. (×160)

9

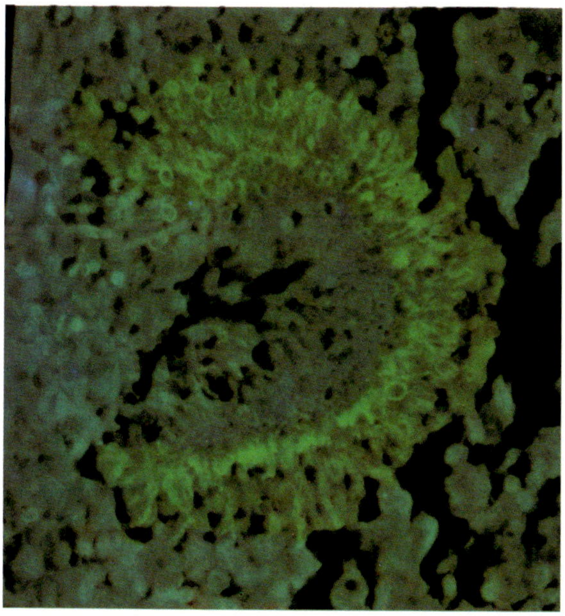

9 Petriellidium boydii Another granule in a section of human lung stained by fluorescein-labelled antiglobulins. (×320)

10

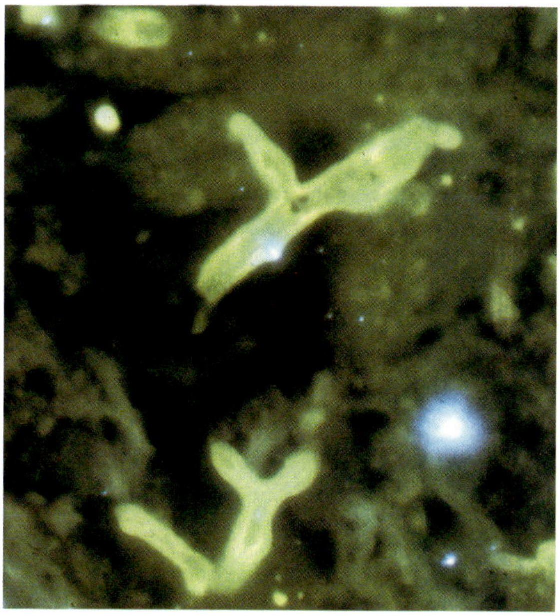

10 Rhizopus oryzae Aseptate hyphae in brain section stained by fluorescein-labelled antiglobulins. (×450)

11

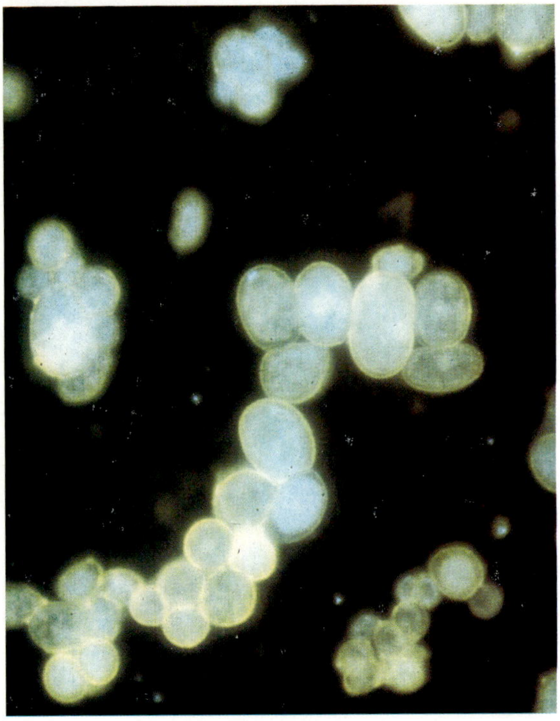

11 Prototheca zopfii cells stained by specific fluorescein-labelled antiglobulins. (×570)

12

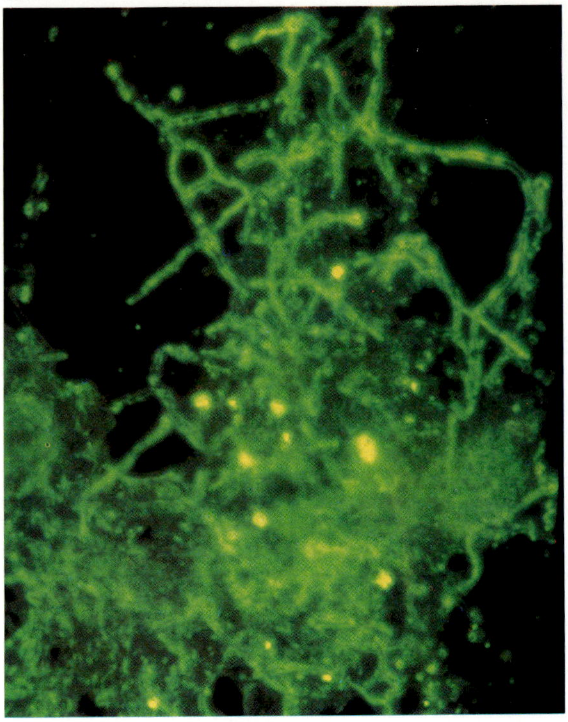

12 Arachnia propionica An aggregate of filaments in a smear of human lung tissue stained by fluorescein-labelled antiglobulins specific for this actinomycete. (×1300)

4 Actinomycosis

Text pages: 26–29

13

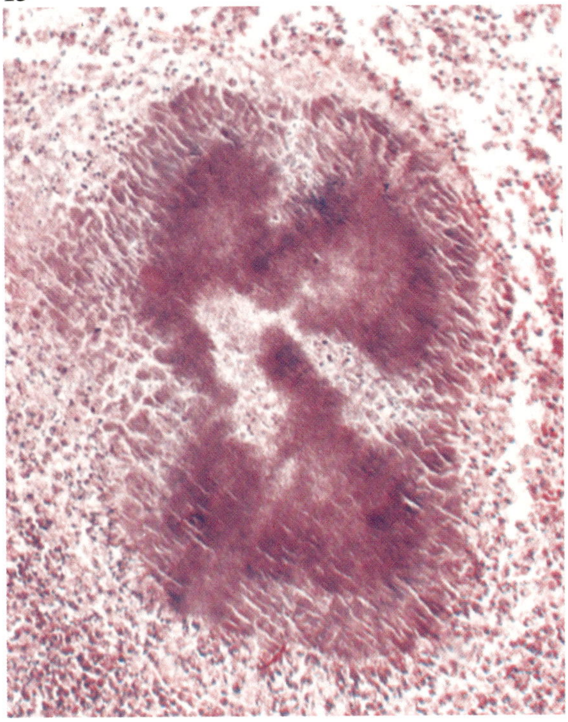

13 Actinomycosis of human liver. An *Actinomyces israelii* granule in an abscess is well stained, but its individual filaments are not visible when stained by H&E. Peripheral clubs are present but not prominent in this case. (H&E, ×50)

14

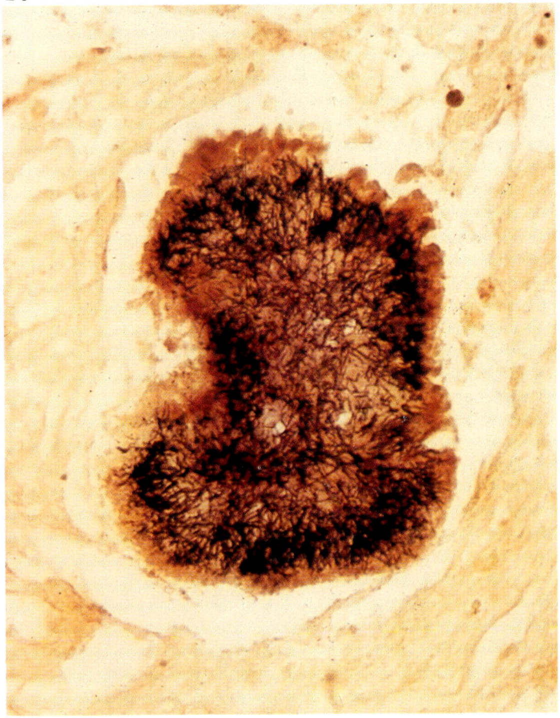

14 Actinomyces israelii Replicate section of granule in 13. Gram-positive filaments are clearly visible within the matrix of the granule. The GMS, Giemsa or tissue Gram stains are required to demonstrate the actinomycetes. (B&B, ×50)

15

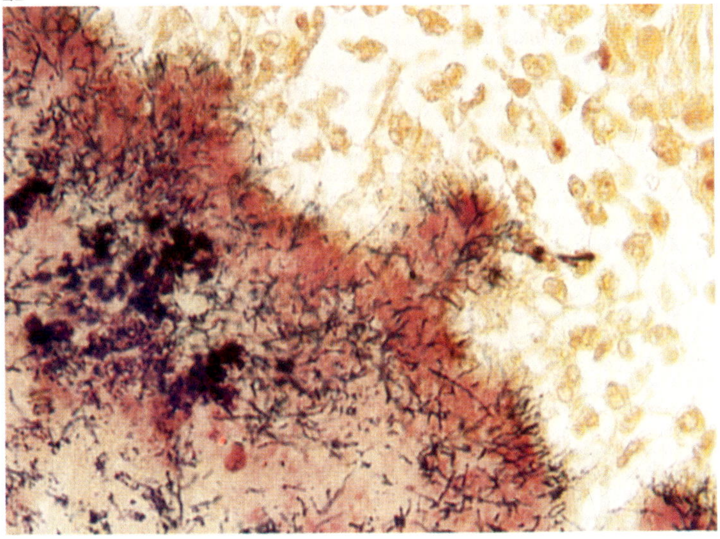

15 Actinomyces israelii granule in human liver. Branching filaments (≤1 μm D) and coccoid elements within the granule are well-stained by the Brown and Brenn procedure, a tissue Gram stain. (B&B, ×500)

16

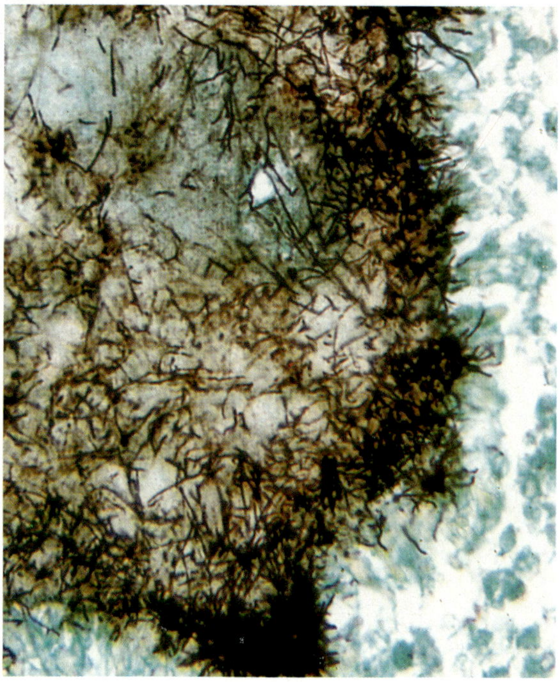

17

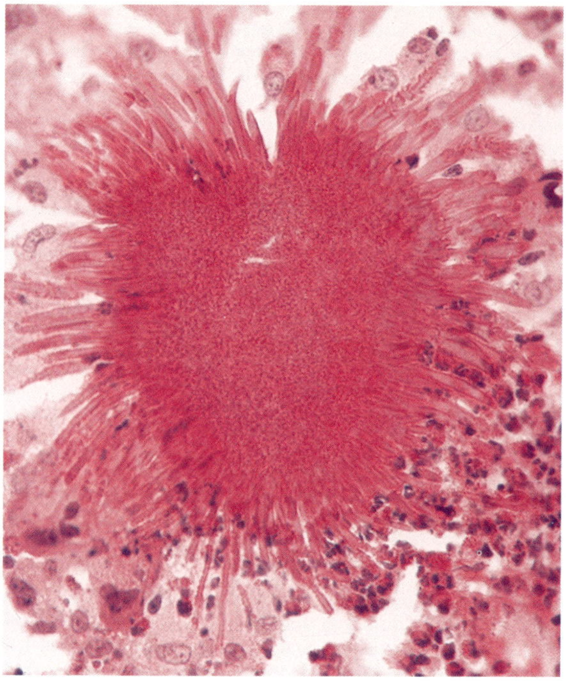

16 Actinomyces israelii Replicate section of granule in **15** but stained by GMS. Note that the delicate filaments and coccoid elements are well delineated by this special fungus stain. Actinomycetes do not stain with the GF, PAS and H&E procedures. (GMS, ×500)

17 Actinomyces israelii Experimental infection in rabbit lung. Granule with prominent peripheral clubs of deeply eosinophilic Splendore–Hoeppli material is surrounded by polymorphonuclear leucocytes. (H&E, ×200)

18

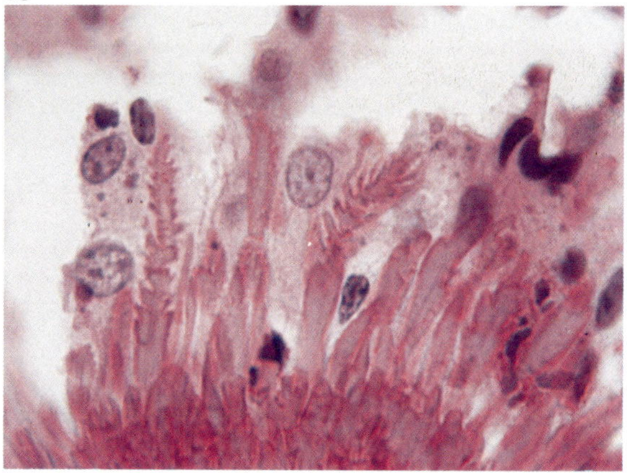

18 Actinomyces israelii Experimental infection in a rabbit. Detailed view of peripheral clubs (Splendore–Hoeppli phenomenon) with serrated borders. Filaments are not visible. (H&E, ×500)

19

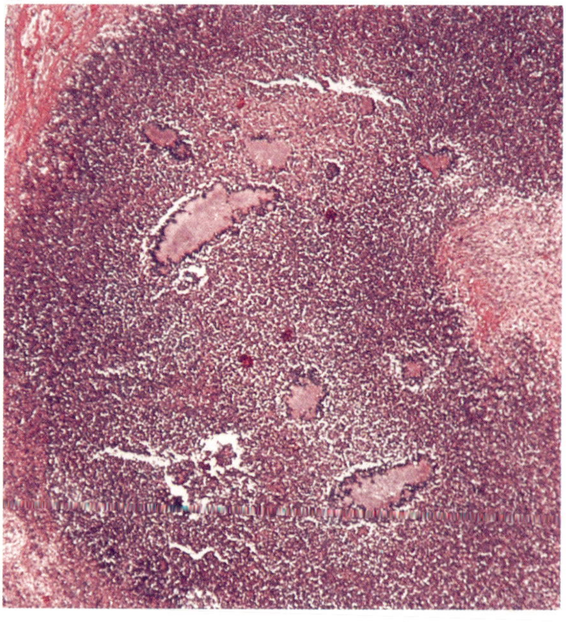

19 Actinomyces naeslundii Tissue from experimentally infected mouse. Note the numerous granules embedded in a large abscess. (H&E, ×20)

20

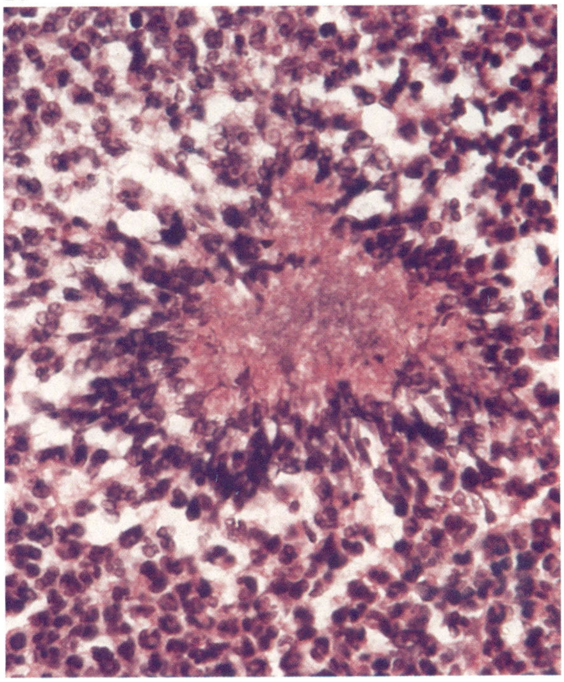

20 Actinomyces naeslundii Higher magnification of **19** showing a single granule intimately surrounded by neutrophils. Filaments within the granule are not visible. In this case, peripheral clubs are not present. (H&E, ×200)

21

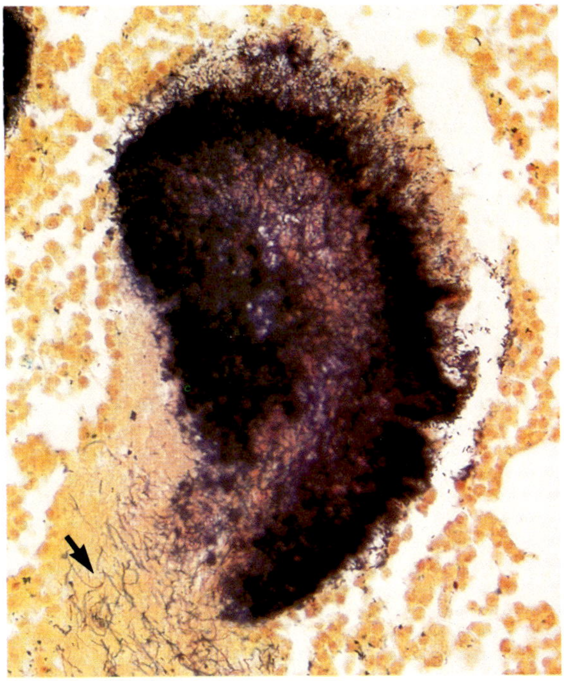

21 Actinomyces viscosus in a dog with pulmonary actinomycosis. Note granule composed of tangled masses of gram-positive filaments. Also observe the numerous individual filaments of this actinomycete in purulent exudate outside of the granule (arrow). (B&B, ×100)

22

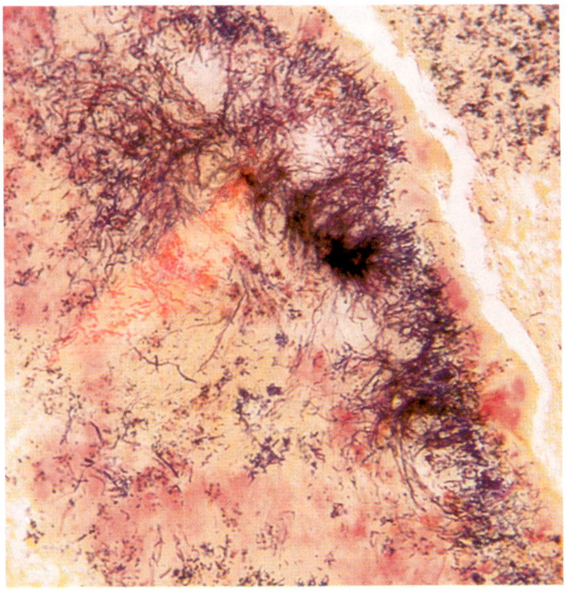

22 Actinomyces viscosus in lung of another dog. Note the aggregates of delicate, gram-positive filaments, scattered rods and coccoid forms. (B&B, ×200)

23

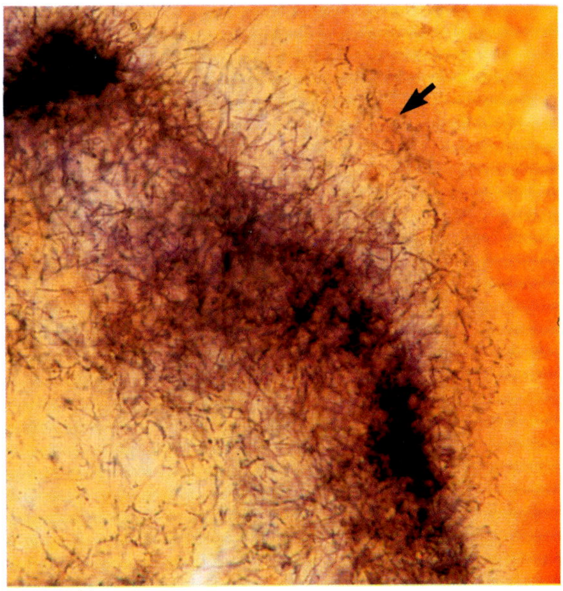

23 Actinomyces viscosus granule in dog lung. Note the tangled mass of gram-positive filaments in the granule. Mycelial filaments are also seen in the reddish (gram-negative) Splendore–Hoeppli material at the periphery of the granule (arrow). (B&B, ×500)

24

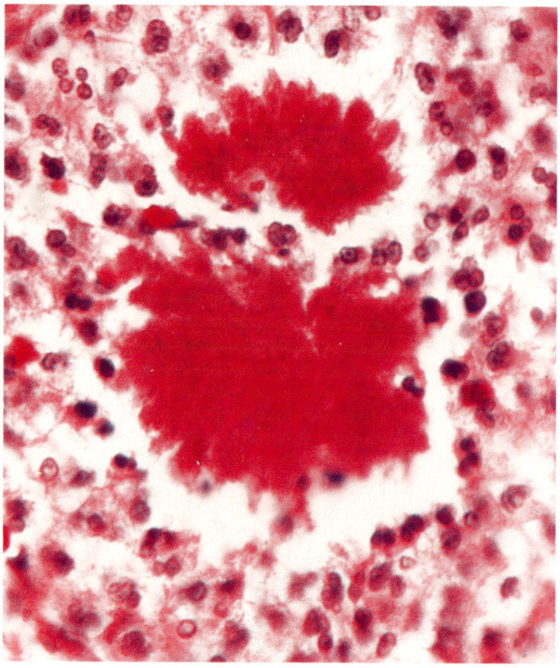

25

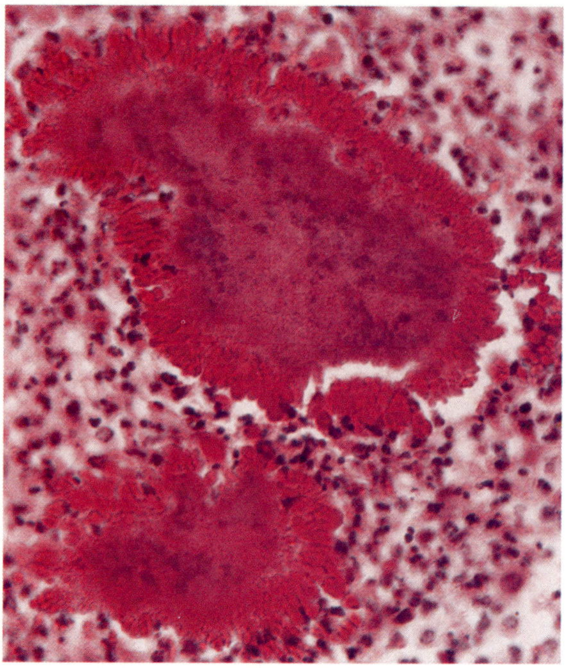

24 Actinomyces odontolyticus as the aetiologic agent of actinomycosis of human appendix. The granule, with its eosinophilic peripheral clubs, is well stained by H&E, but the filaments within the matrix of the granule are not visible. (H&E, ×400)

25 Actinomyces bovis as the aetiologic agent of bovine actinomycosis. The basophilic granules are bordered by prominent eosinophilic clubs. These granules appear identical to those produced by *Actinomyces israelii* and by other *Actinomyces spp.* (H&E, ×200)

26

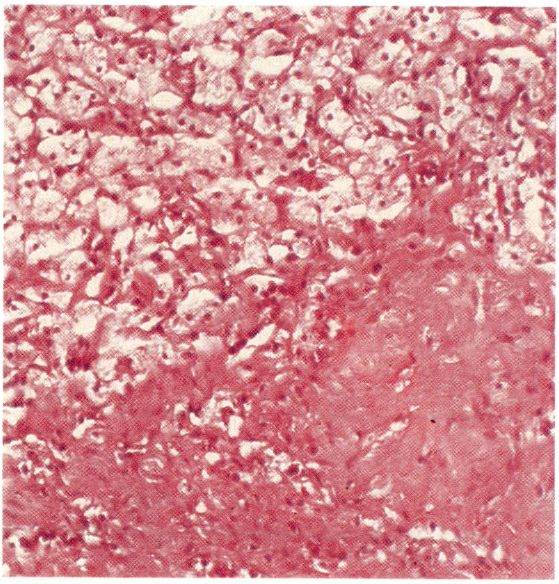

27

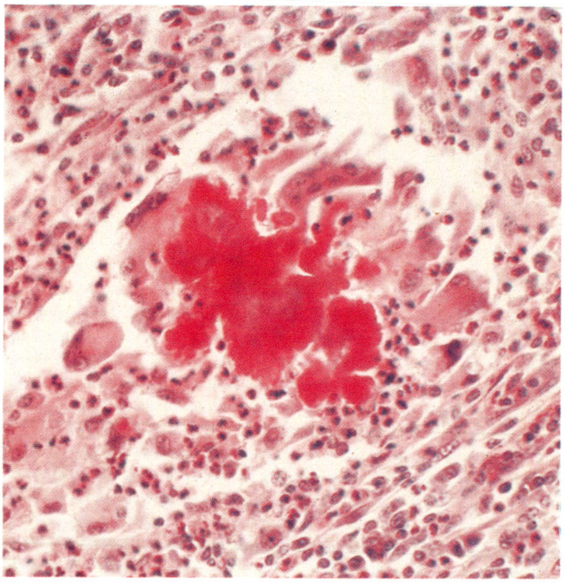

26 Wall of an actinomycotic abscess The innermost portion shown at the top of the photomicrograph is composed of a wide zone of foamy macrophages (lipophages) that is surrounded by a thick fibrotic capsule. Such foamy macrophages are often seen in walls of abscesses caused by actinomycetes as well as certain non-filamentous bacterial species. (H&E, ×100)

27 Actinomyces bovis causing infection of bovine lymph node. Small granules with abundant Splendore–Hoeppli material are surrounded by a mixed granulomatous and purulent inflammatory reaction. (H&E, ×100)

28

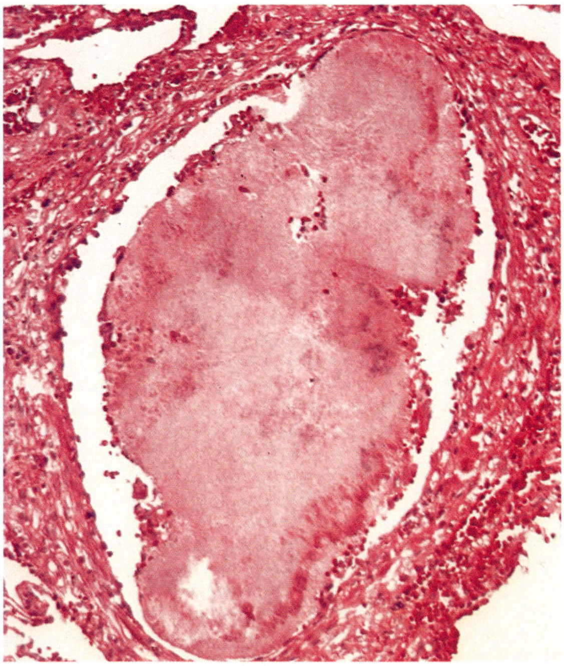

28 Arachnia propionica granule surrounded by fibrinopurulent exudate in human lung. Peripheral clubs are not prominent. (H&E, ×50)

29

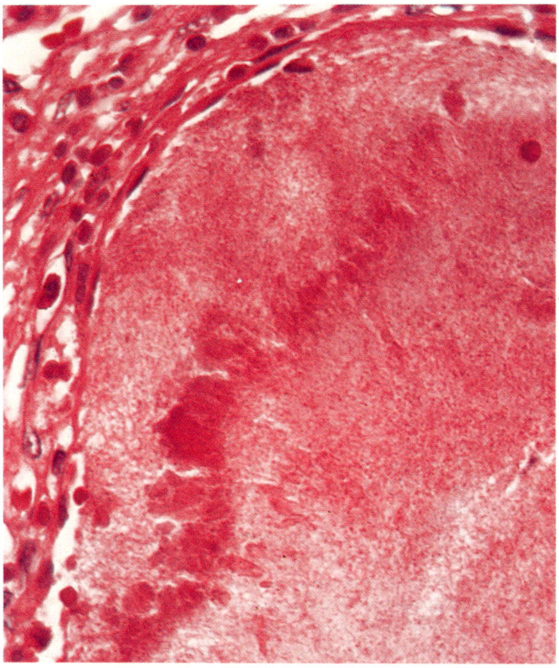

29 Arachnia propionica Higher magnification of the granule in **28**. Note the linear zone of eosinophilic Splendore–Hoeppli material within the granule. Filaments are not visible. (H&E, ×200)

30

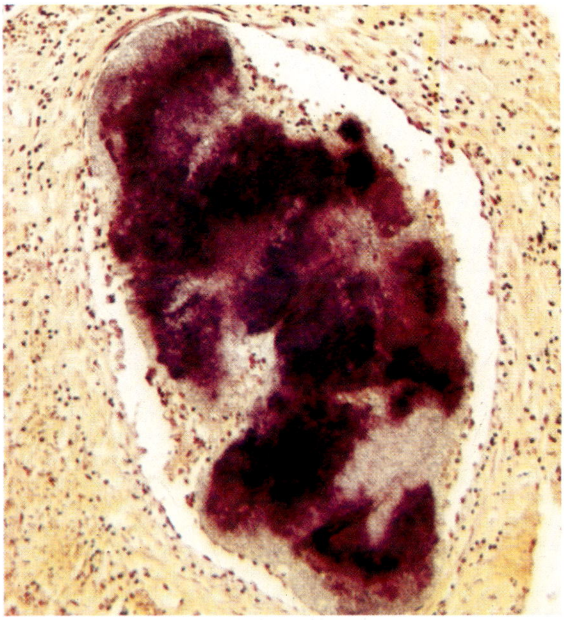

30 Arachnia propionica Replicate section of the granule in **28**, but stained by a tissue Gram procedure. At this magnification, the masses of the deep purple gram-positive filaments are visible but the individual filaments cannot be discerned. (B&B, ×50)

31

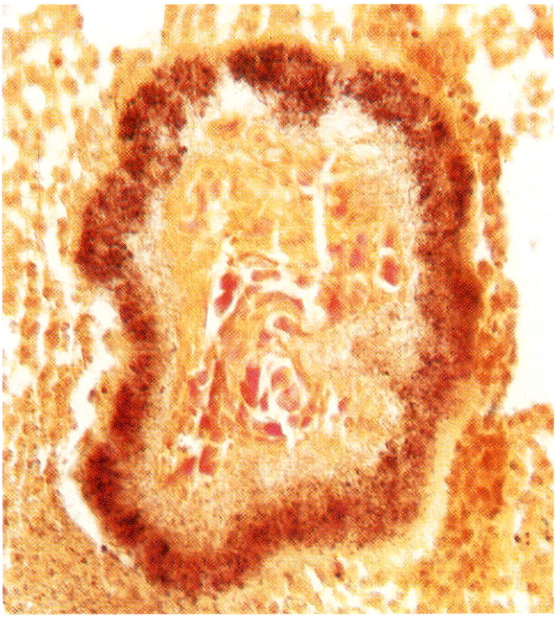

31 Arachnia propionica as the aetiologic agent of actinomycosis of human lung. Note the peripheral arrangement of gram-positive filaments within the matrix of the granule. This orderly arrangement of filaments is sometimes seen in actinomycete granules. (B&B, ×100)

5 Adiaspiromycosis

Text pages: 30–33

32

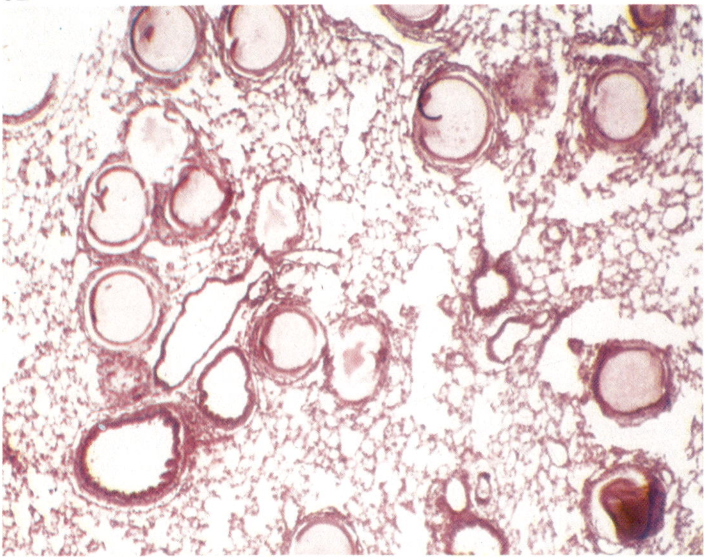

32 Chrysosporium parvum var. **crescens** causing pulmonary adiaspiromycosis in a *Peromyscus sp.* Numerous adiaspores, all in the same stage of development, are surrounded by a minimal inflammatory response. (H&E, ×20)

33

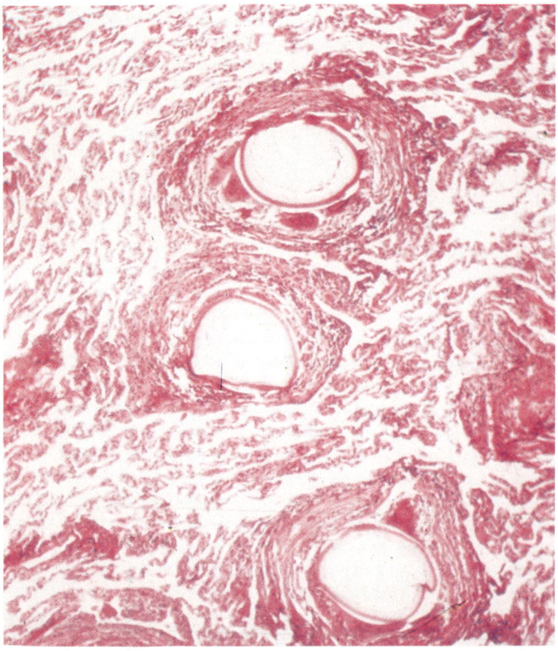

33 Chrysosporium parvum var. **crescens** causing pulmonary adiaspiromycosis in a Guatemalan. In this patient, the adiaspores are surrounded by a fibrogranulomatous reaction. (H&E, ×20)

34

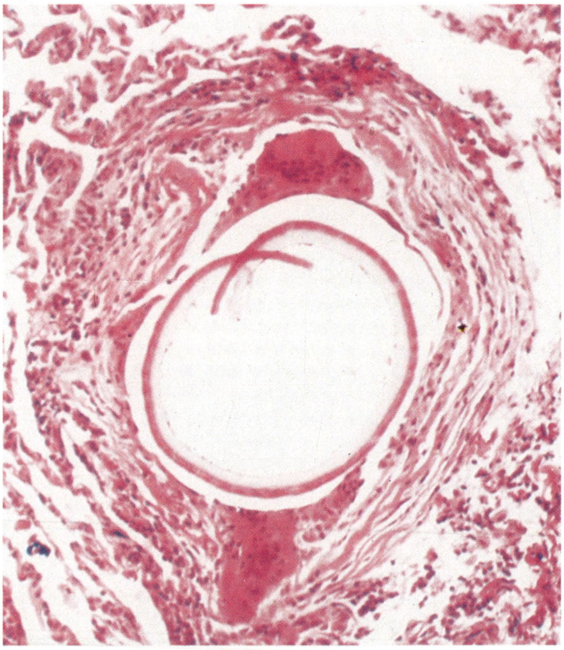

34 Chrysosporium parvum var. **crescens** Another area in **33** that shows an adiaspore enveloped by huge giant cells and concentric rings of fibrous connective tissue infiltrated by mononuclear inflammatory cells. The breakage of the adiaspore wall was apparently due to the microtome knife. (H&E, ×50)

35

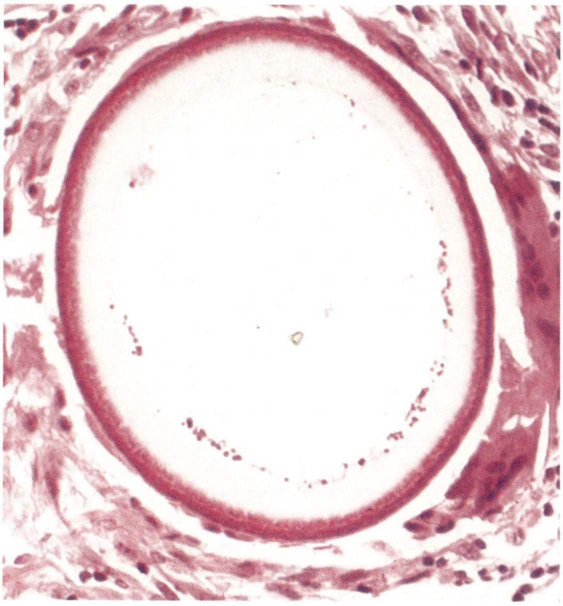

36

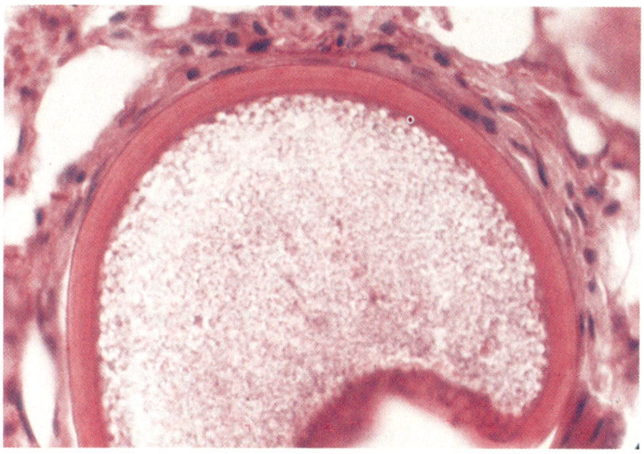

36 Chrysosporium parvum var. **crescens** adiaspore in human lung. Note the internal globular contents of this spore. (H&E, ×200)

35 Chrysosporium parvum var. **crescens** Higher magnification of **33** showing the surrounding inflammatory reaction in greater detail. Note that the centre of the adiaspore is empty. (H&E, ×100)

37

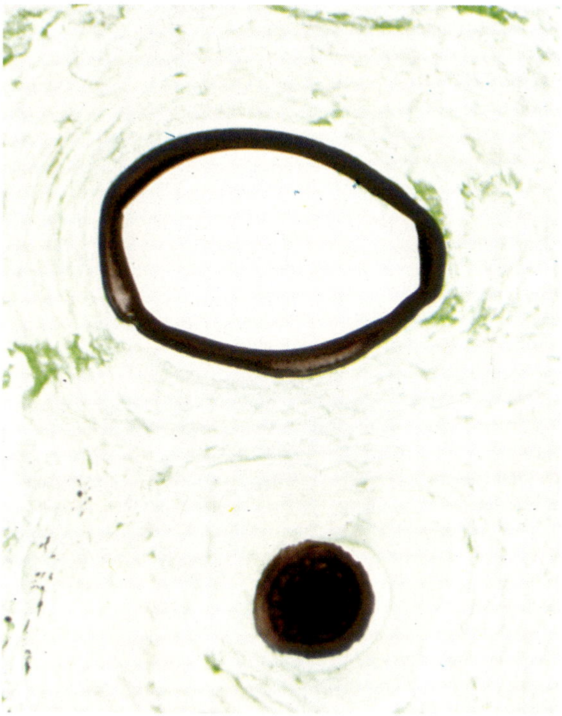

37 Chrysosporium parvum var. **crescens** Replicate section of **33** containing two adiaspores. The larger one was sectioned near its equatorial plane whereas the smaller one that appears solid was sectioned tangentially. (GMS, ×50)

38

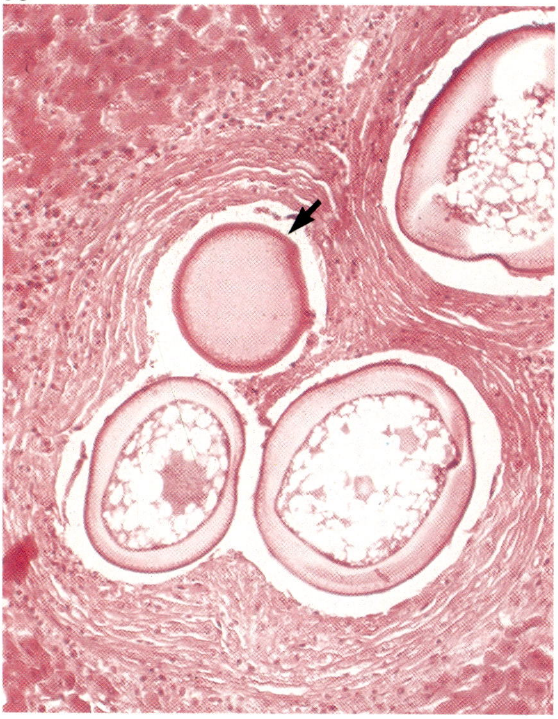

38 Chrysosporium parvum var. **crescens** Liver of monkey infected experimentally. Note fibrogranuloma containing four adiaspores. One spore is sectioned tangentially (arrow). (H&E, ×50)

39

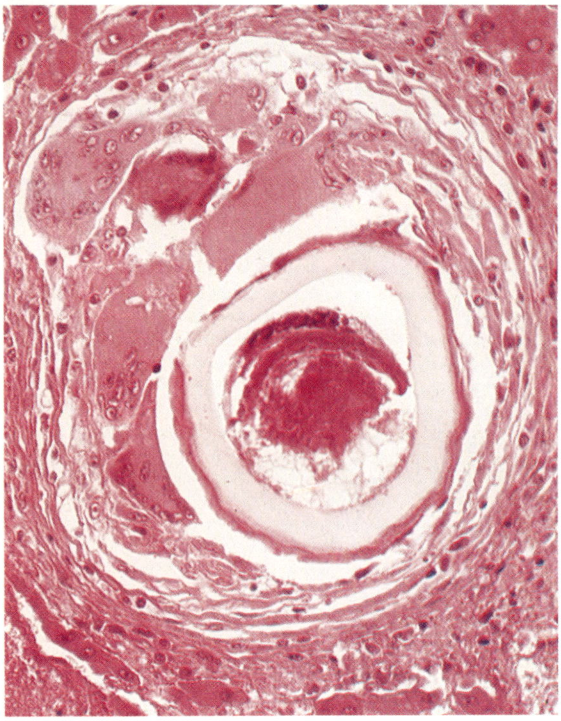

40

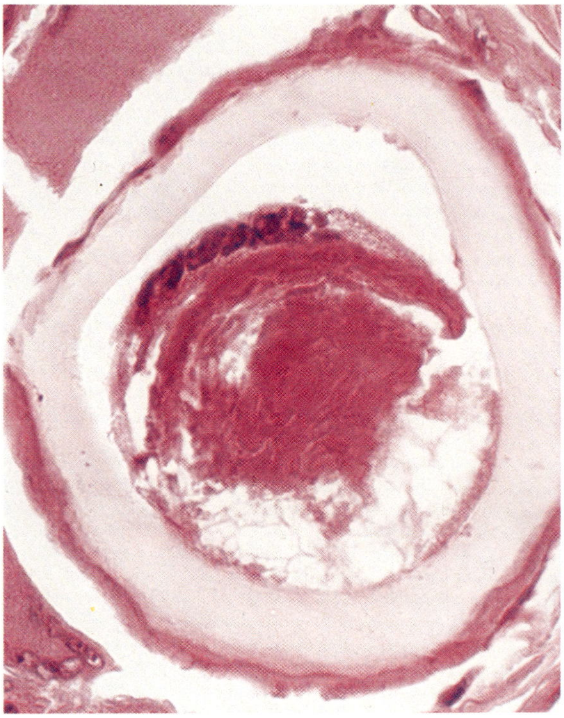

39 Chrysosporium parvum var. **crescens** Another area in **38** that shows a single degenerating adiaspore containing a large Langhans' giant cell. Giant cells and thin concentric rings of fibrous connective tissue surround the adiaspore. (H&E, ×100)

40 Chrysosporium parvum var. **crescens** Higher magnification of **39** showing details of a degenerating adiaspore containing a giant cell. With this routine stain, two distinct zones can be seen in the adiaspore wall. (H&E, ×200)

41

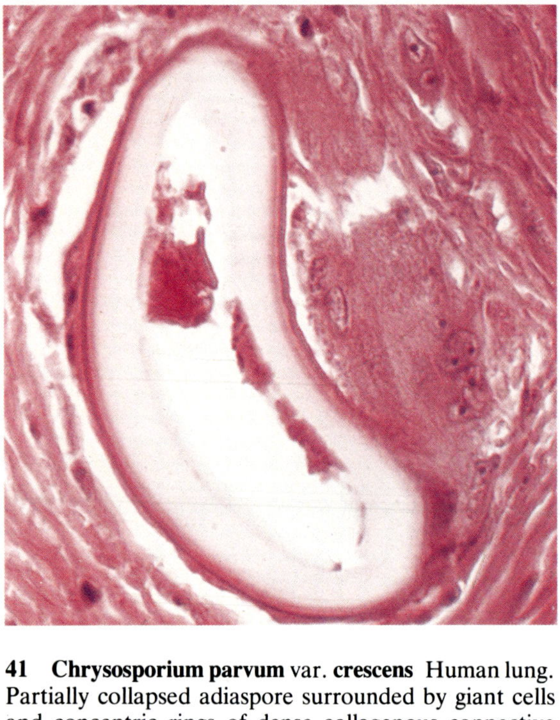

42

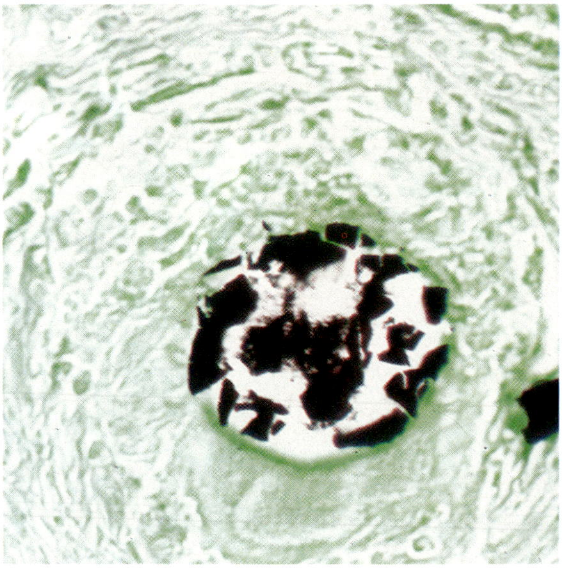

41 Chrysosporium parvum var. **crescens** Human lung. Partially collapsed adiaspore surrounded by giant cells and concentric rings of dense collagenous connective tissue. (H&E, ×200)

42 Chrysosporium parvum var. **crescens** causing human pulmonary adiaspiromycosis. A single fragmented and degenerated adiaspore is sectioned tangentially. (GMS, ×100)

43

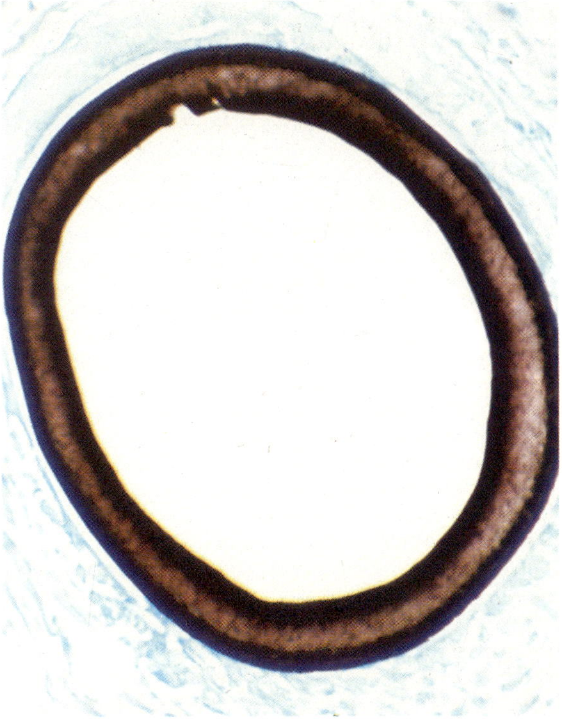

43 Chrysosporium parvum var. **crescens** Another field in **42** that shows an intact but empty adiaspore. The entire wall of the adiaspore is GMS positive, but there are zonal differences in staining intensity, and three distinct zones are discernible. (GMS, ×100)

44

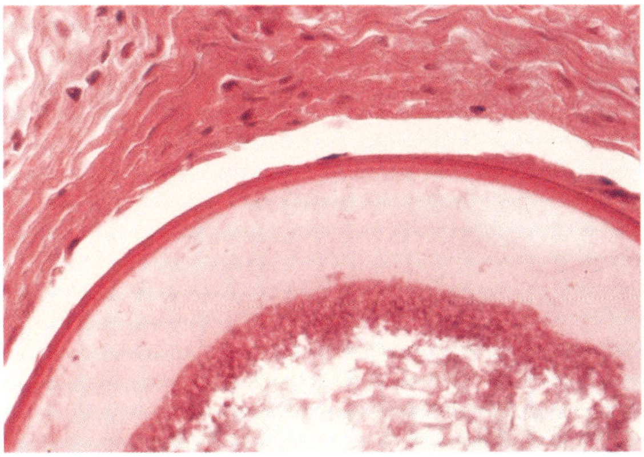

44 Chrysosporium parvum var. **crescens** Another field in **41** showing details of an adiaspore. When stained by H&E, two zones are visible in the thick wall. There are many minute nuclei in the peripheral portion of the cytoplasm adjacent to the wall. (H&E, ×500)

45

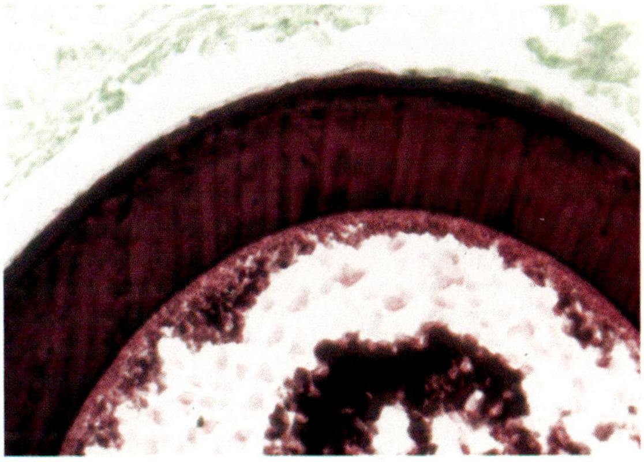

45 Chrysosporium parvum var. **crescens** Replicate section of the adiaspore in **44** but stained by GMS. Note the trilaminar mural substructure. The linear cross-pattern of the thick chitinous wall was apparently caused by the microtome knife. The internal contents of the spore are also stained. (GMS, ×500)

46

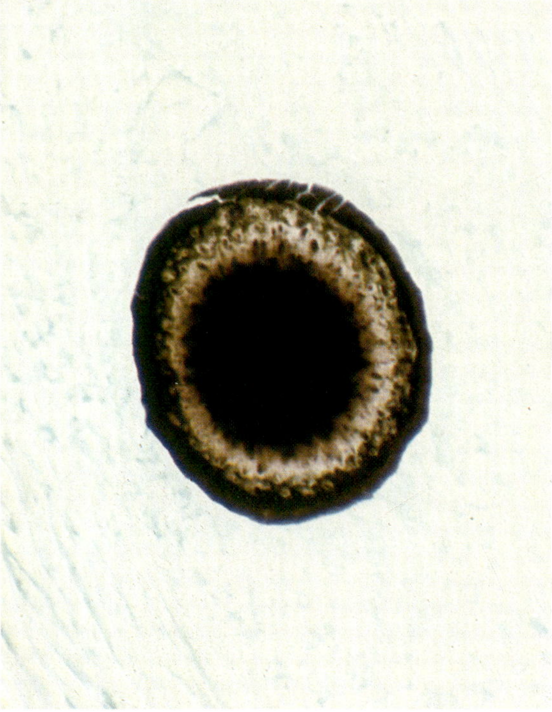

47

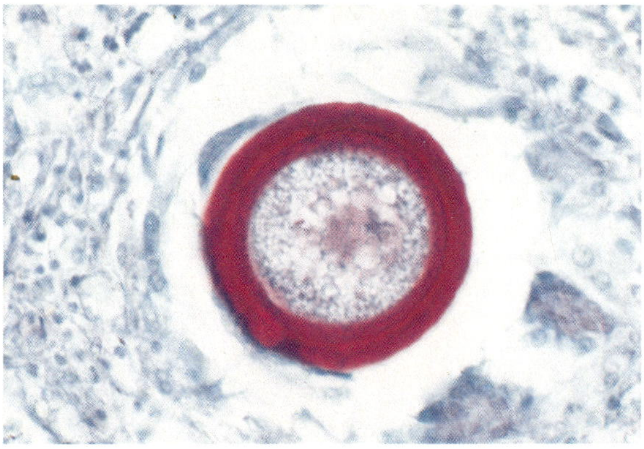

46 Chrysosporium parvum var. **crescens** Tangential section of an adiaspore. The fenestrated layer lining the inner aspect of the middle zone in the spore wall contains cribriform perforations. (GMS, ×100)

47 Chrysosporium parvum var. **crescens** Young adiaspore in human lung. The spore wall is well stained and the internal contents are unstained but discernible. (PAS, ×200)

48

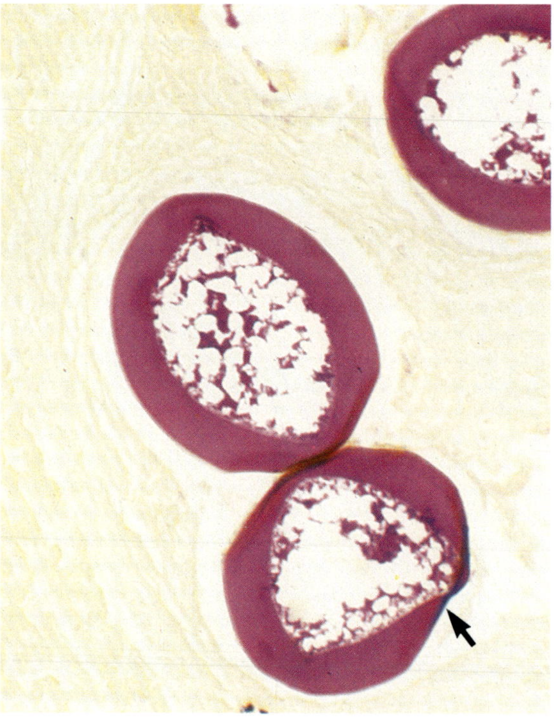

49

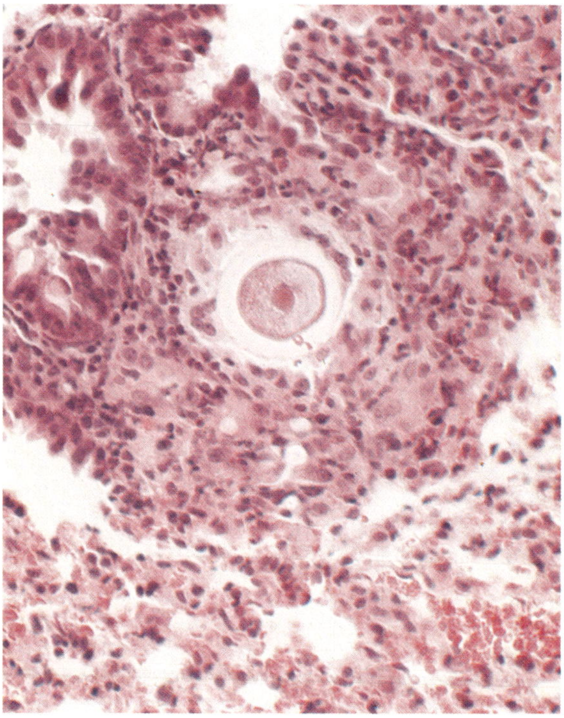

48 Chrysosporium parvum var. **crescens** Tissue containing adiaspores. Note that the spore walls and internal contents are well stained. The wall of one adiaspore is partially folded (arrow), a commonly observed phenomenon. (GF, ×50)

49 Chrysosporium parvum var. **parvum** causing pulmonary adiaspiromycosis in a rodent. A single peribronchiolar adiaspore ca. 25 μm in diameter is present in the centre of a small granuloma. (H&E, ×100)

50

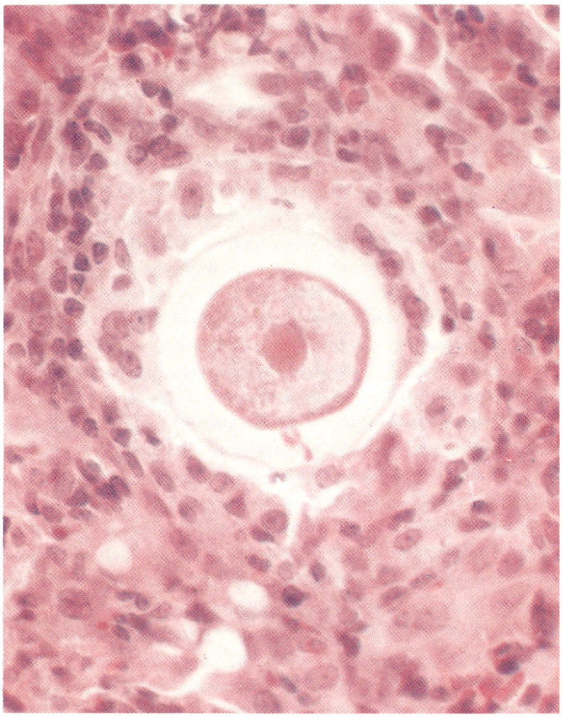

51

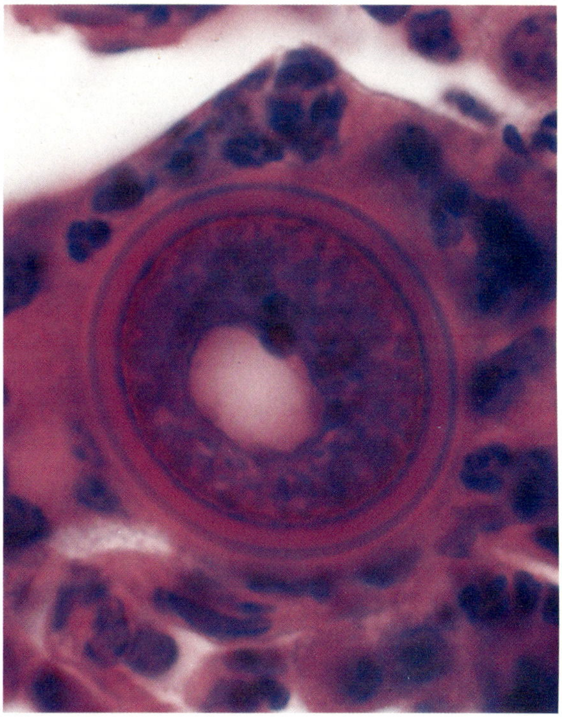

50 Chrysosporium parvum var. **parvum** Higher magnification of **49** showing an adiaspore in the centre of a granuloma. The spore contains a single nucleus and its wall is poorly stained. (H&E, ×200)

51 Chrysosporium parvum var. **parvum** Details of a single adiaspore in rodent lung. The thick wall and cytoplasmic contents are well stained. Note the single nucleus. (PAS, ×500)

6 Aspergillosis

Text pages: 34–38

52

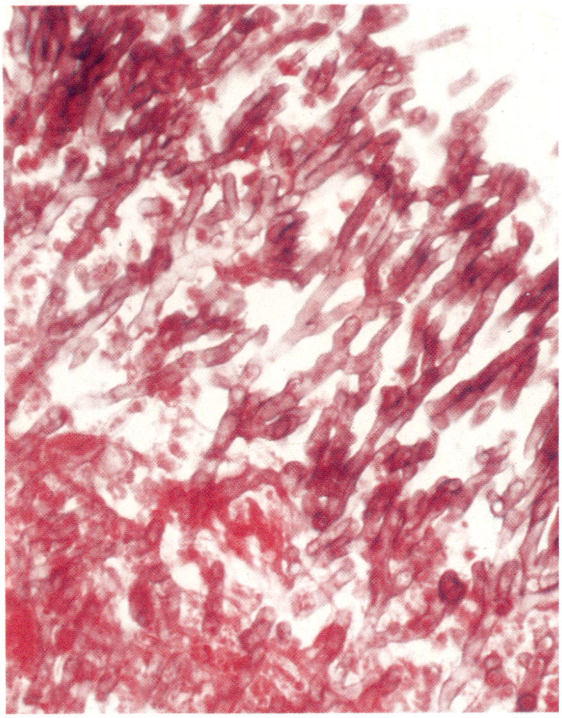

53

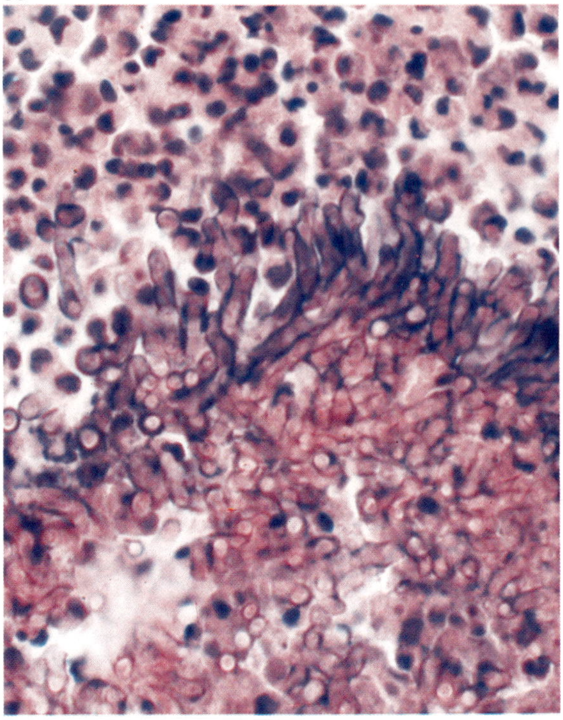

52 Invasive aspergillosis of the human lung. Branched septate hyphae (ca. 4–5 μm wide) are variably stained. (H&E, ×200)

53 Aspergillosis of bovine lung. An aggregate of *Aspergillus sp*. hyphae is surrounded by polymorphonuclear leucocytes. The hyphae at the periphery are basophilic whereas those in the centre of the aggregate stain poorly. (H&E, ×200)

54

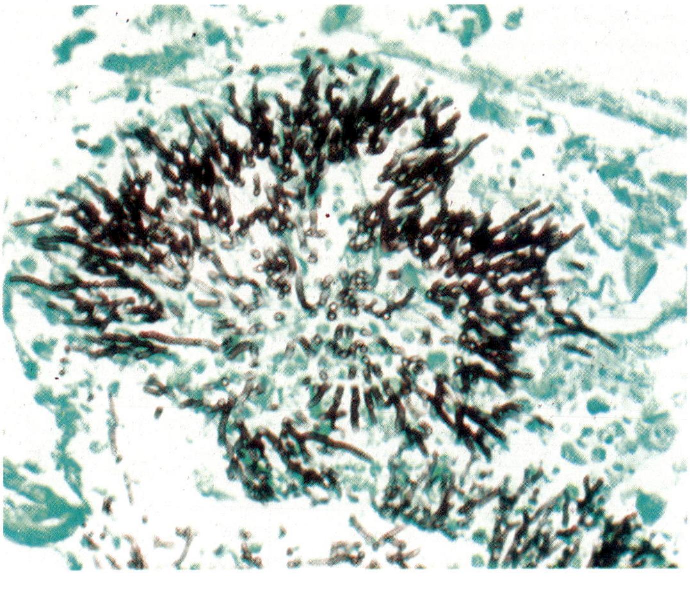

54 Aspergillus fumigatus causing invasive aspergillosis of human lung. Note the characteristic radial or 'sunburst'-like arrangement of the mycelium. (GMS, ×100)

55

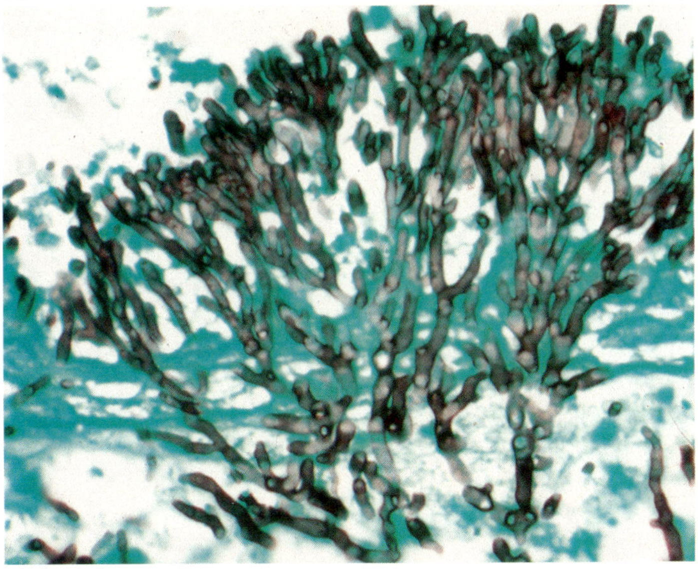

55 Aspergillus fumigatus Higher magnification of **54** to show the characteristic dichotomous branching of *Aspergillus* hyphae. (GMS, ×200)

56

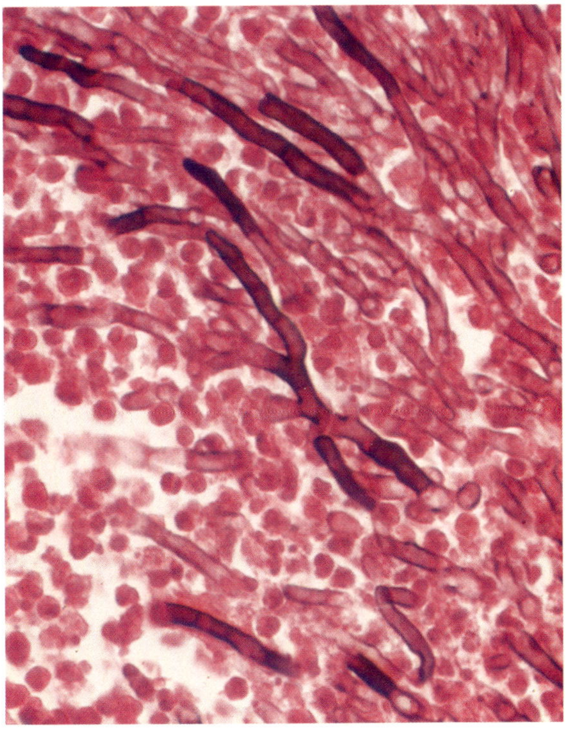

57

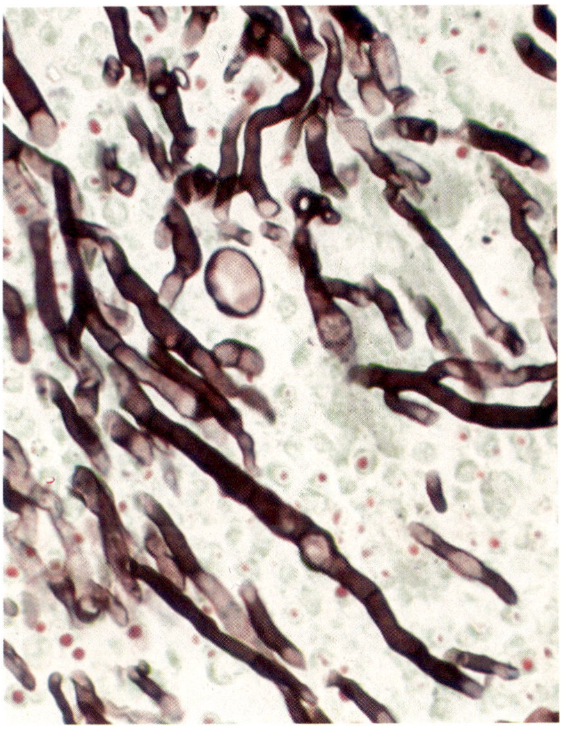

56 Acute aspergillus infection of human lung. Although the hyphae are variably stained by GMS, they stand out in sharp contrast to the recognisable purulent exudate. (GMS–H&E, ×200)

57 Aspergillus infection of bovine lung. The hyphae that contain vesicular swellings are well stained. (GMS, ×200)

58

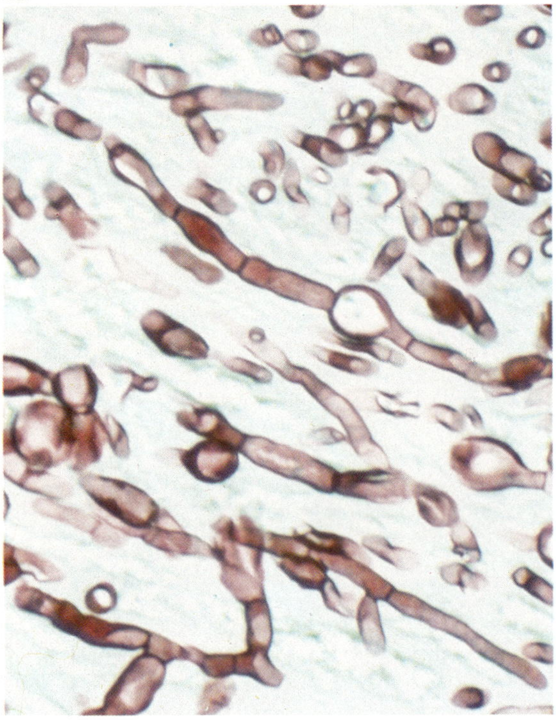

59

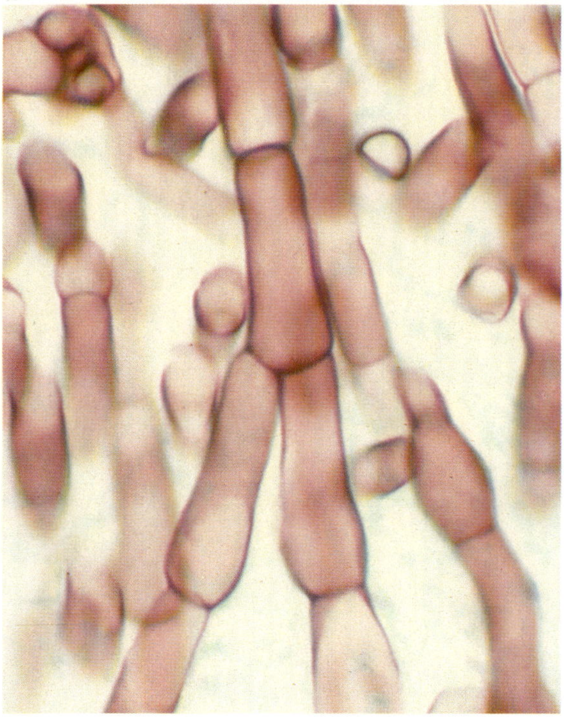

58 Aspergillus sp. causing vegetative valvular endocarditis of human mitral valve. Well stained hyphae that contain vesicular swellings are also seen in this lesion. (GMS, ×200)

59 Aspergillus sp. Another field in **58** to show in detail the septations and dichotomous branching of the *Aspergillus* hyphae. (GMS, ×500)

60

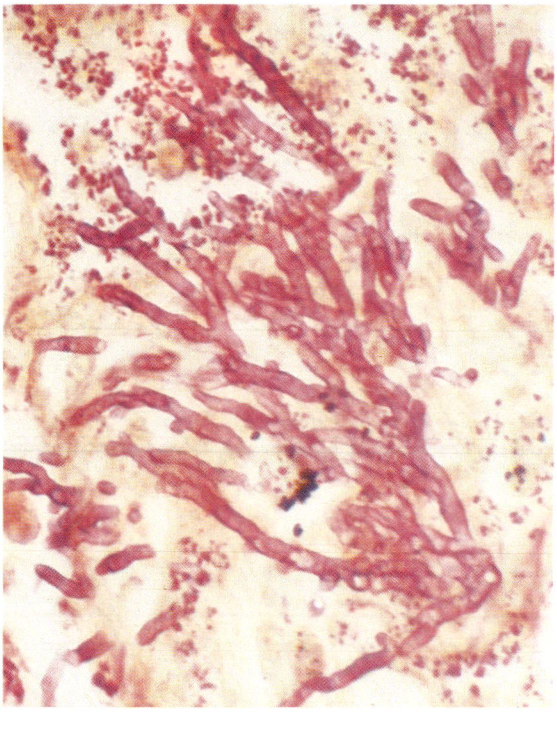

60 Invasive pulmonary aspergillosis in a human who died of Legionnaires' disease. Note that the hyphae are well delineated by the tissue Gram stain, a procedure not routinely used for demonstrating fungi. Some hyphae show characteristic dichotomous branching. (Brown–Hopps, ×100)

61

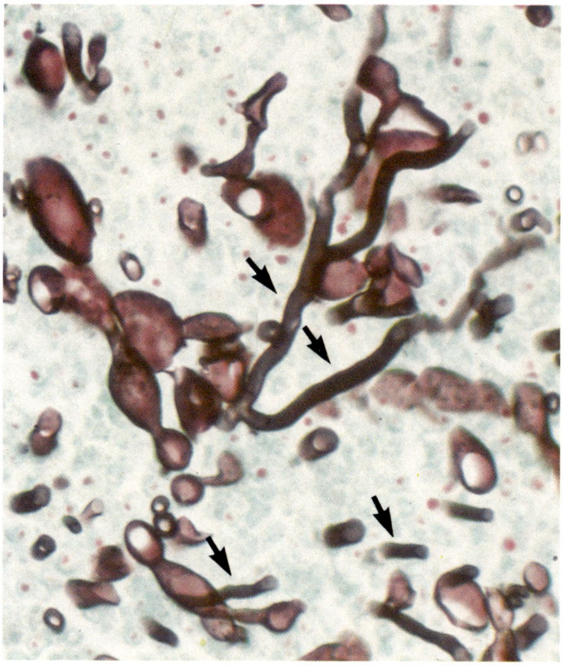

62

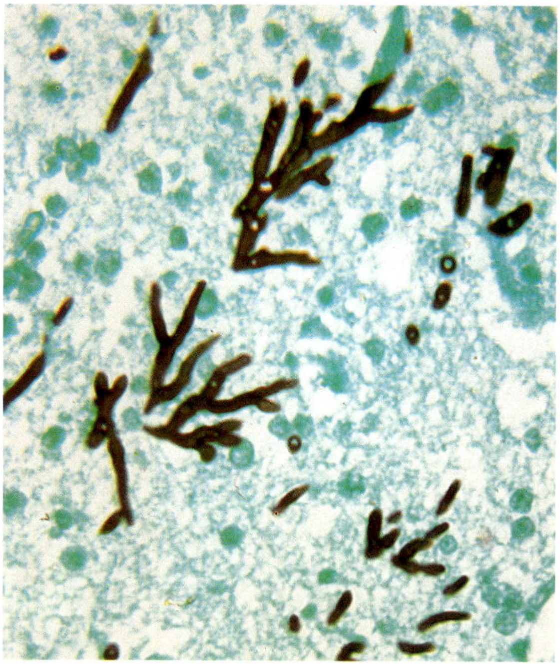

61 Aspergillus sp. (arrows) and a zygomycete causing dual infection in a bovine lung. The *Aspergillus* hyphae are narrow, septate, of uniform width and deeply stained by GMS. In contrast, the zygomycete hyphae are wider, infrequently septate, of varying width and less intensely stained. (GMS, ×200)

62 Aspergillus sp. causing mycotic encephalitis. Note the short hyphae that stain intensely by GMS and show dichotomous branching; in general, the branches are oriented in the same direction. (GMS, ×100)

63

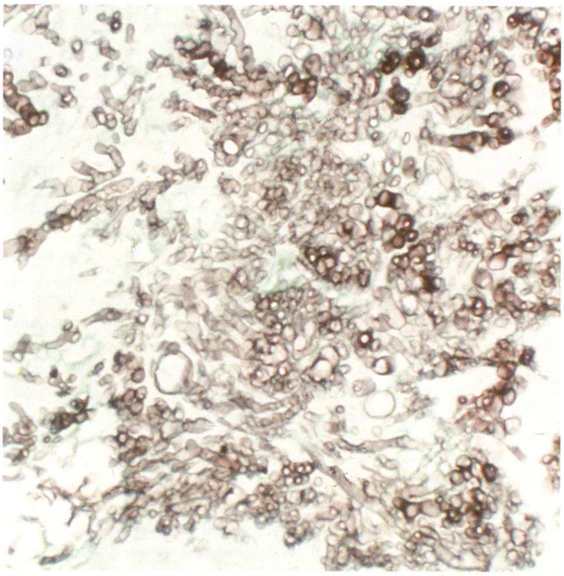

64

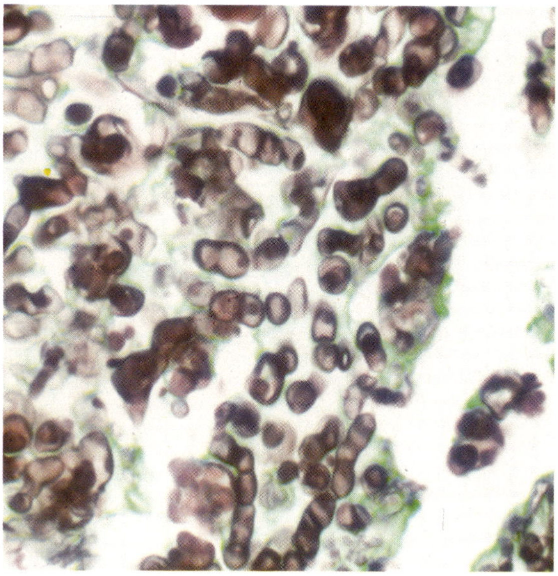

63 Aspergillus sp. causing chronic granulomatous lymphadenitis. Distorted, aberrant and bulbous hyphae are mixed with typical forms. (GMS, ×100)

64 Aspergillus sp. Higher magnification of the lymph node lesion in **63** showing masses of closely septate, aberrant hyphae. Aberrant forms are often found in chronic lesions. (GMS, ×200)

65

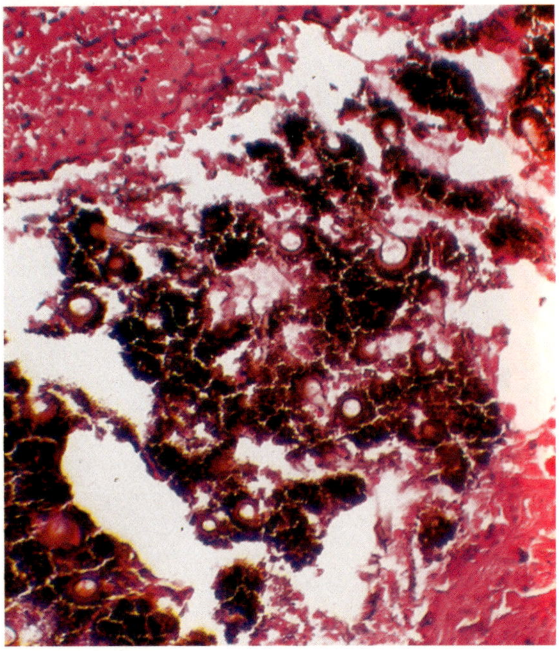

66

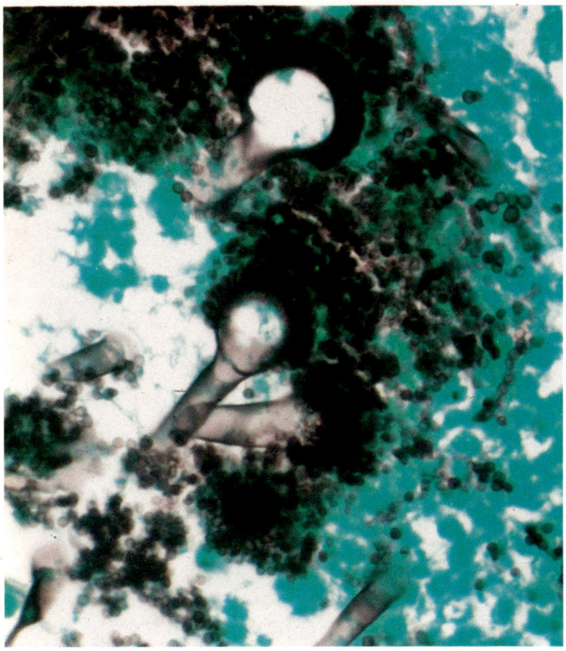

65 Aspergilli in bronchiectatic cavity of lung from a human who died of Legionnaires' disease. Note the large number of conidial heads resulting from exposure of the fungus to air. (GMS–H&E, ×50)

66 Aspergilli Higher magnification of replicate section of **65**. Observe that the conidiophore vesicles are flask-shaped and fertile on their upper half – features characteristic of the *Aspergillus fumigatus* group. (GMS, ×200)

67

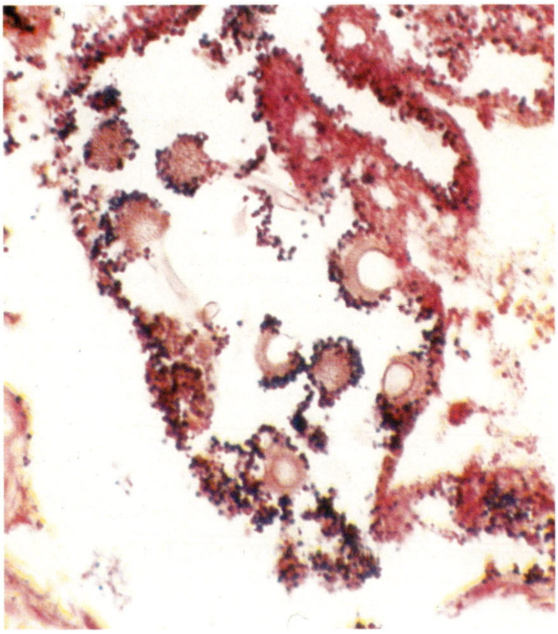

68

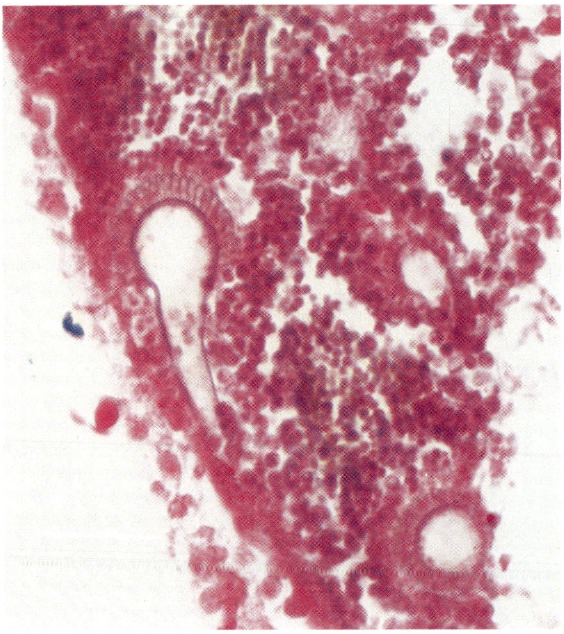

67 Aspergilli Replicate section of **65** but stained by a tissue Gram procedure. The conidia are strongly gram-positive and readily discerned. (Brown–Hopps, ×100)

68 Aspergilli Replicate section of **65**. Note the flask-shaped vesicles bearing crowded sterigmata in a single series on their upper half – diagnostic features of the *Aspergillus fumigatus* group. Chains of conidia are seen among the inflammatory cell debris. (H&E, ×200)

69

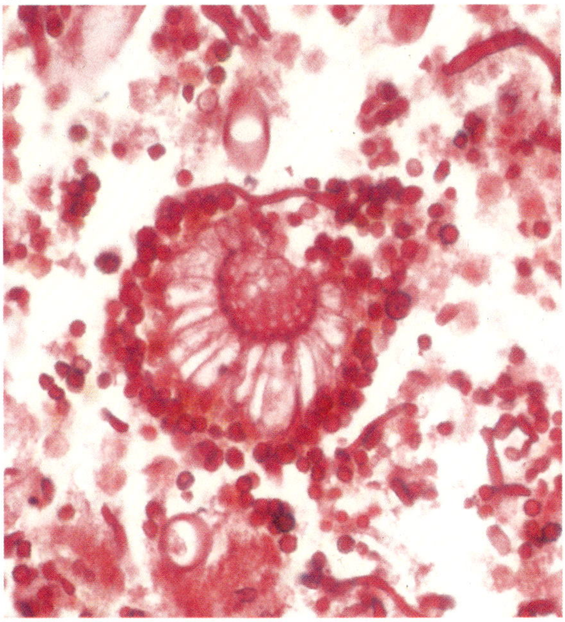

70

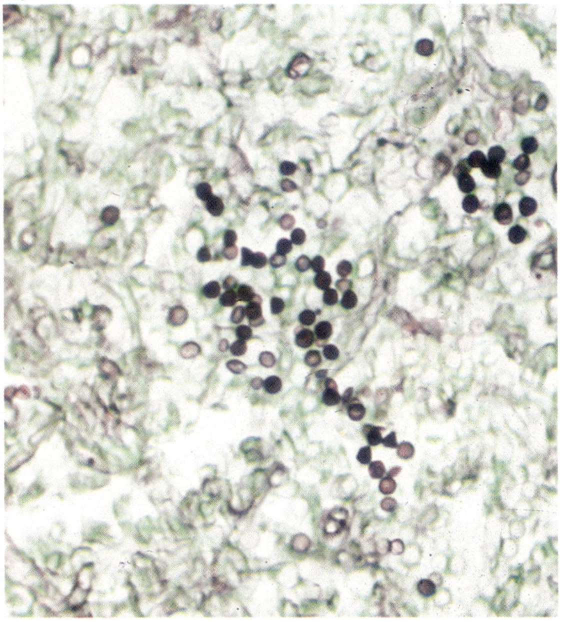

69 Aspergillus niger in human lung cavity. A conidial head, conidia, and hyphae are seen. Observe that the conidiophore's vesicle is globose and that its entire surface is covered by sterigmata. Conidia are found on the ends of the sterigmata and are also free, mixed with inflammatory cells and hyphae. (H&E, ×200)

70 Aspergillus fumigatus fungus ball in a human pulmonary cavity. Numerous well stained conidia mixed with poorly stained hyphae are present. In this section, conidial heads could not be detected. (GMS, ×200)

71

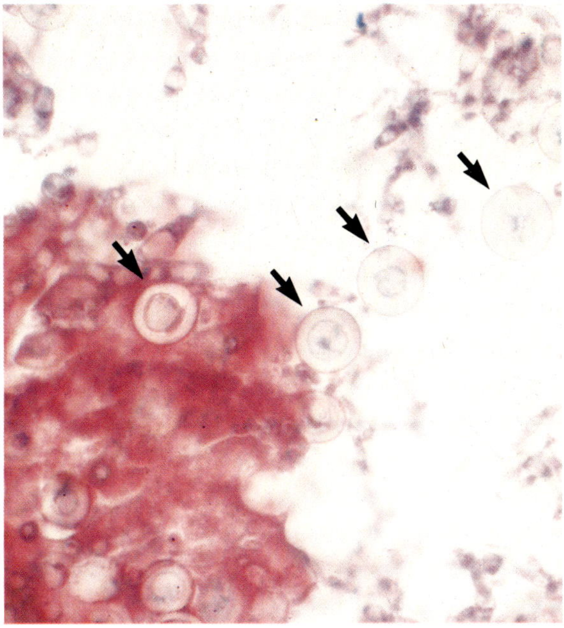

72

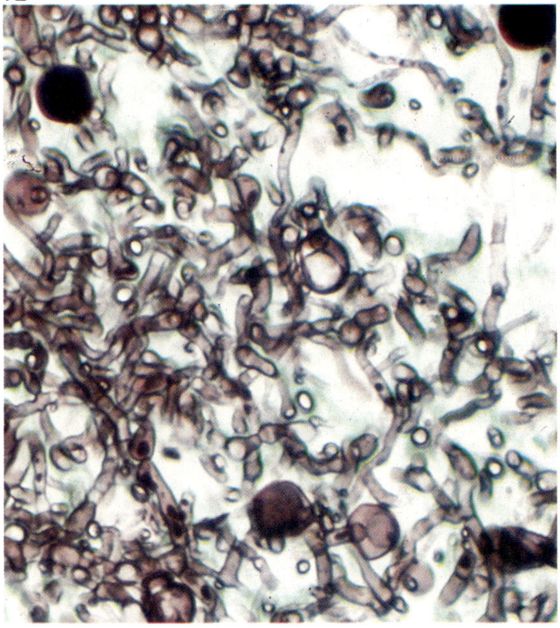

71 Aspergillus nidulans in a pulmonary cavity of a captive rhinoceros. The large, relatively thick-walled Hülle cells (arrows) that are produced by this fungus are mixed with cellular debris and hyphae. (H&E, ×200)

72 Aspergillus nidulans Replicate section of **71**. Note that the Hülle cells are uniformly stained, thus obscuring their internal details. Hyphae are also well stained. (GMS, ×200)

73

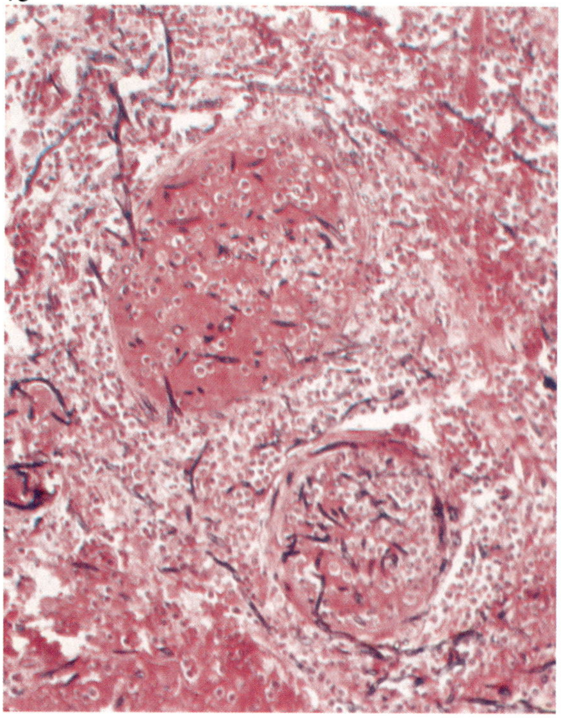

74

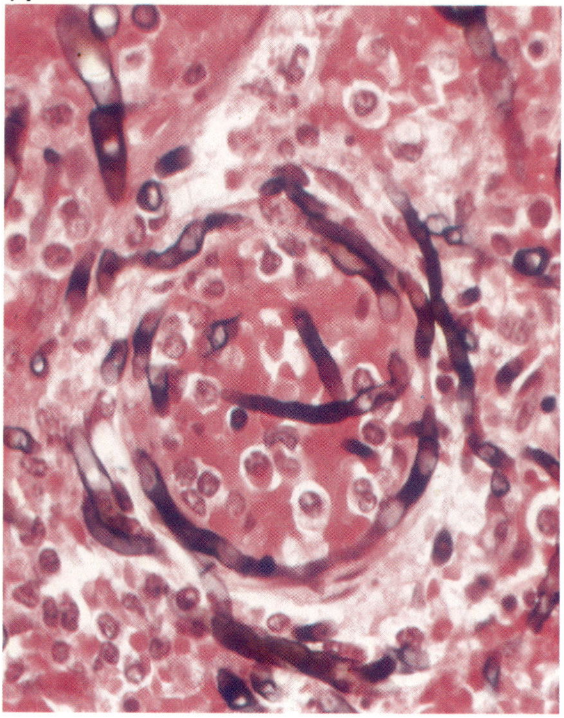

73 Aspergillus sp. causing mycotic angiitis in the submucosa of a human colon. Note that the blood vessel walls are penetrated by many hyphae and that the lumens of the vessels are thrombosed. Hyphae have also invaded tissues outside of blood vessels. (GMS–H&E, ×50)

74 Aspergillus sp. Higher magnification of **73**. Note that the combined GMS–H&E stain clearly demonstrates the fungus, its pattern of invasion, and the host response. Hyphae have invaded the blood vessel wall and have filled its lumen, causing thrombosis. (GMS–H&E, ×200)

75

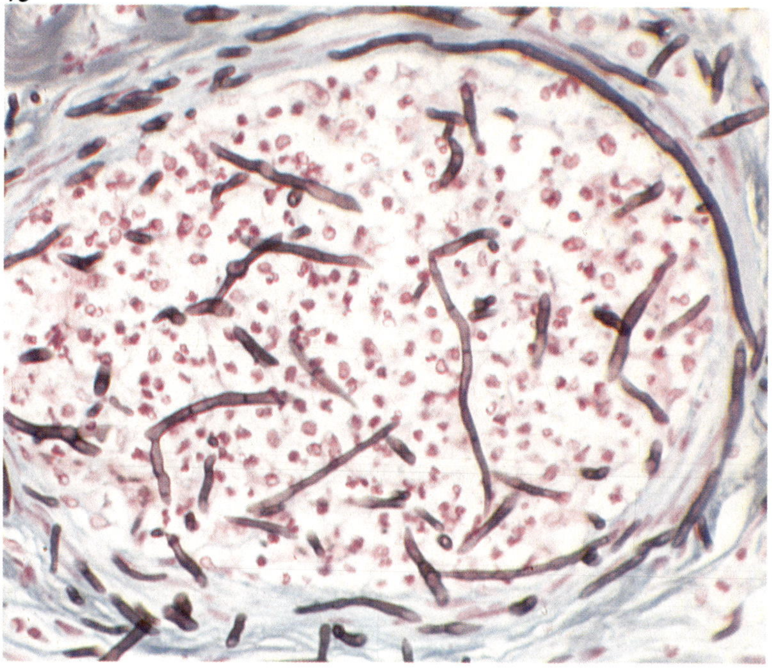

75 Fusarium sp. Angio-invasion in the subcutaneous tissues of a human. Branched, septate hyphae have penetrated the blood vessel wall and are present in its lumen. The propensity of *Fusarium spp.* to invade blood vessels, and their morphological resemblance to *Aspergillus spp.*, make the histological differentiation of these fungi difficult. (GMS, ×100)

76

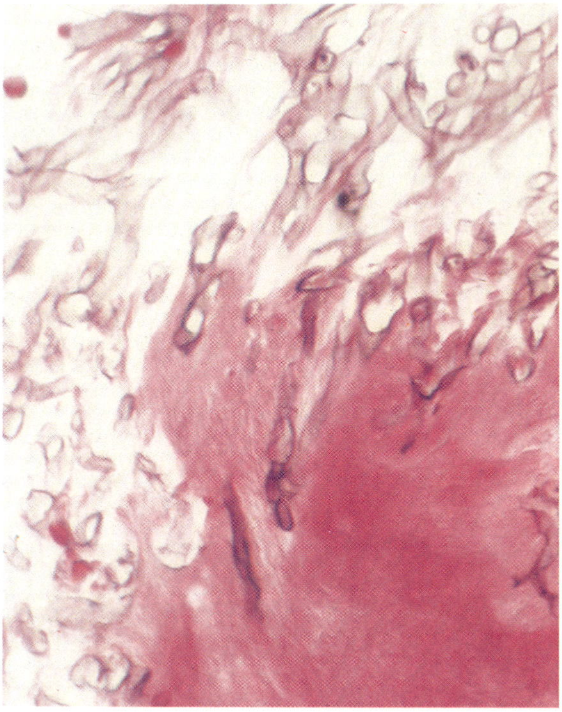

77

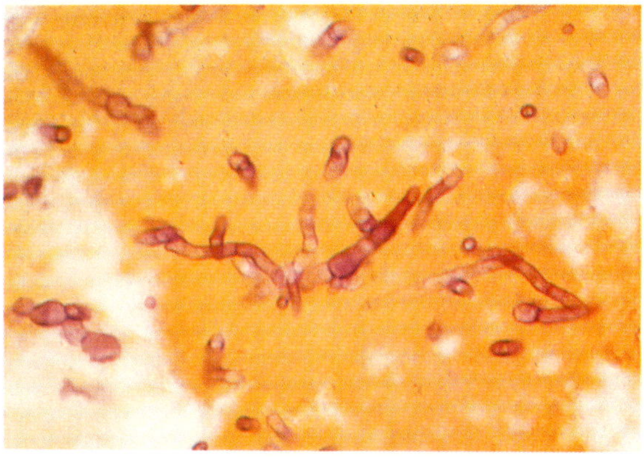

76 Aspergillosis of human bone. Note invasion of the marrow space and erosion of trabecular bone by proliferating hyphae. (GMS–H&E, ×200)

77 Aspergillus infection of bovine lung. In this case, the hyphae are well stained by GF, and the details of branching and septation are evident. (GF, ×200)

78

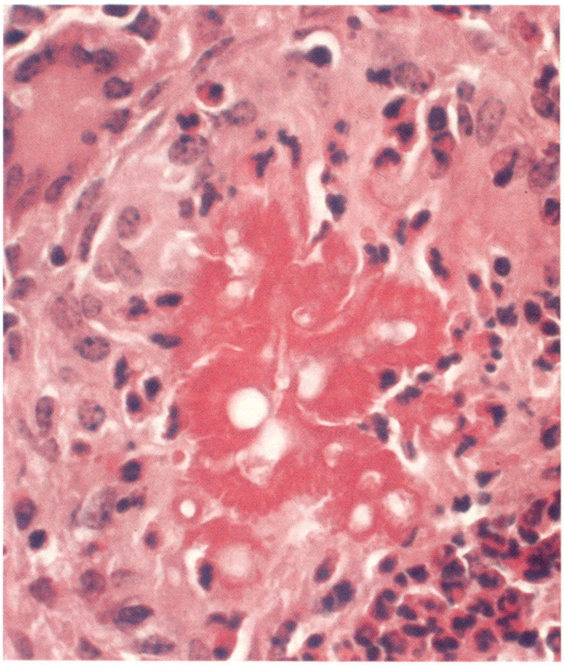

79

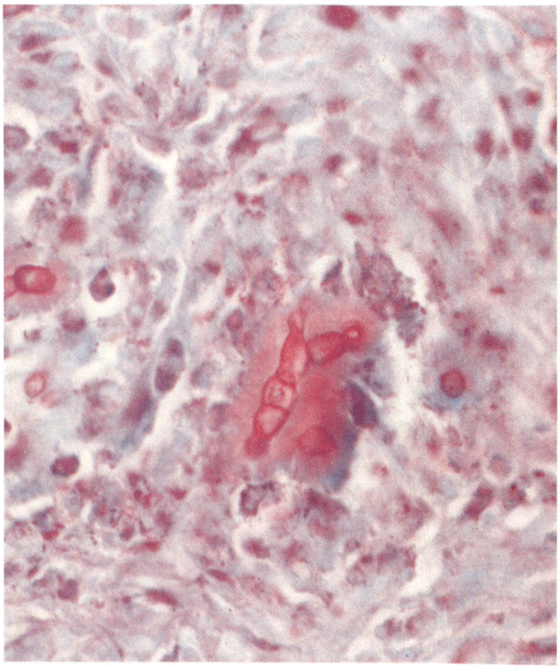

78 Chronic aspergillosis of bovine lung. Clusters of *Aspergillus* elements are surrounded by a radial corona of Splendore–Hoeppli material. Note the mixed purulent and granulomatous inflammatory reaction. (H&E, ×200)

79 Chronic aspergillosis Replicate section of **78**. Note the well stained *Aspergillus* hyphae surrounded by lightly stained Splendore–Hoeppli material. (PAS, ×200)

80

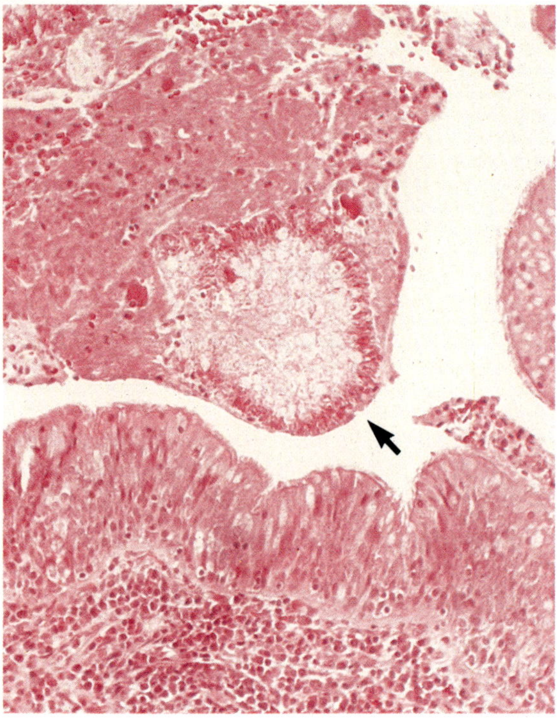

81

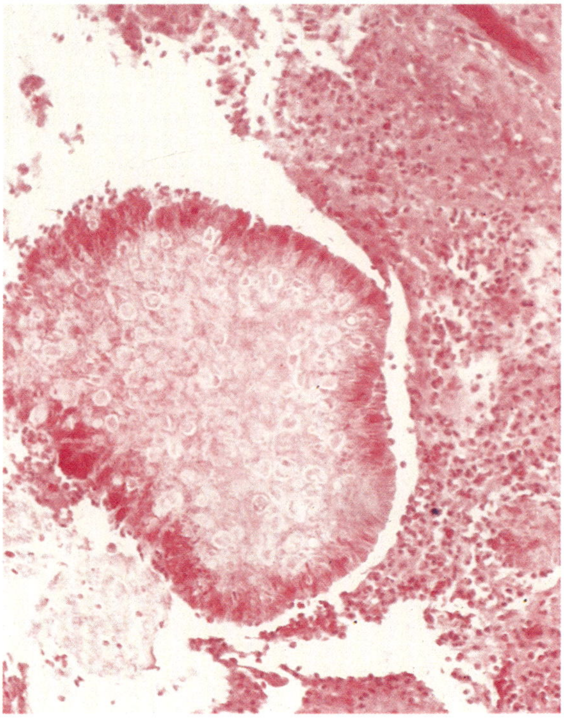

80 Aspergillosis A small fungus ball (arrow) surrounded by mucus and cellular debris is within the lumen of an ectatic bronchus. The bronchial mucosa is intact, and the submucosa contains mononuclear inflammatory cells. (H&E, ×50)

81 Aspergillosis Larger fungus ball in another ectatic bronchus in the same patient as **80**. The bronchial epithelium is eroded and the wall is infiltrated by mixed inflammatory cells. (H&E, ×50)

82

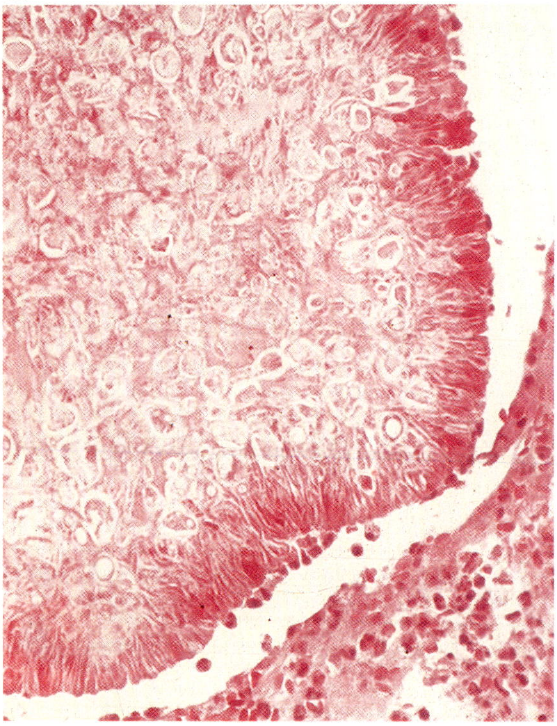

83

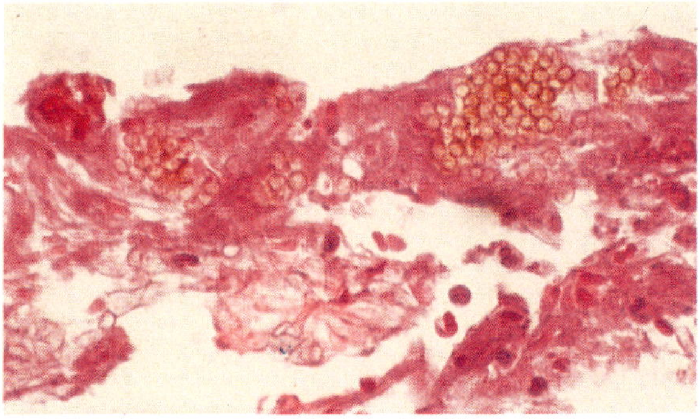

82 Aspergillosis Higher magnification of **81** to show details of the fungus ball. The periphery of the ball is deeply eosinophilic because of the deposition of Splendore–Hoeppli material. The fungal elements that make up the ball are poorly stained, but visible. (H&E, ×100)

83 Aspergillosis Another area in the bronchiectatic cavity shown in **81**. The numerous brown spores suggest that the aetiologic agent was *Aspergillus niger*. Conidial heads are not seen in this field. (H&E, ×200)

84

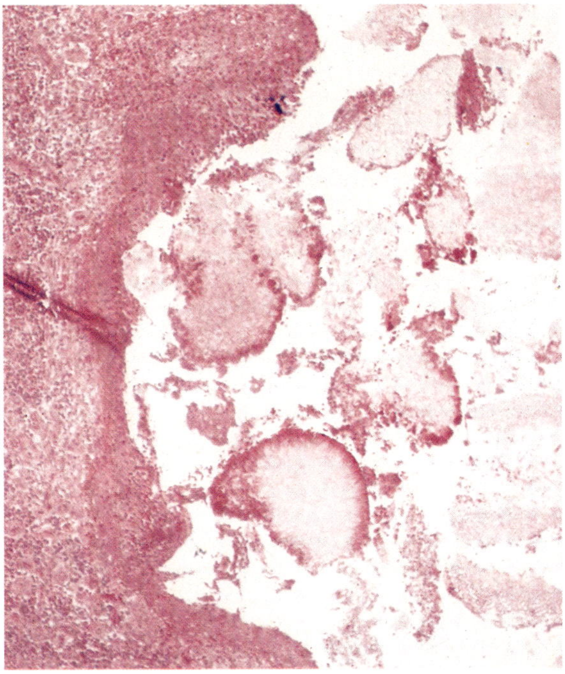

85

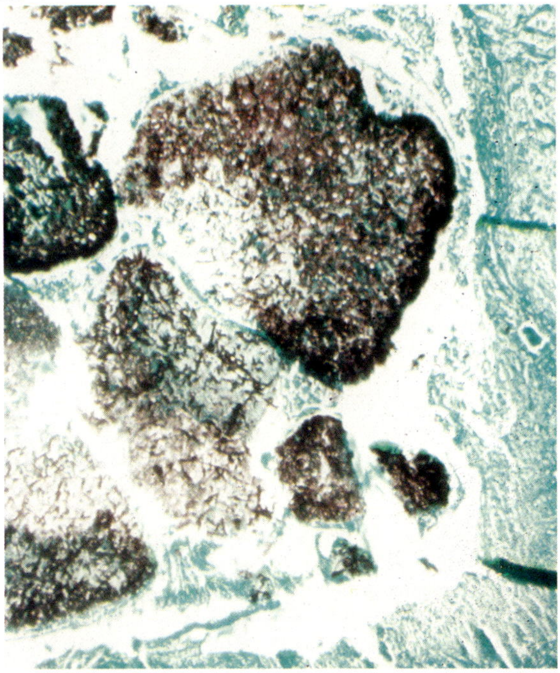

84 Aspergillosis Another example of a fungus ball within a bronchiectatic cavity. Note that the ball is broken up into discrete parts. (H&E, ×20)

85 Aspergillosis Replicate section of **84** but stained by GMS to show the abundant hyphae that make up the fungus ball. (GMS, ×20)

86

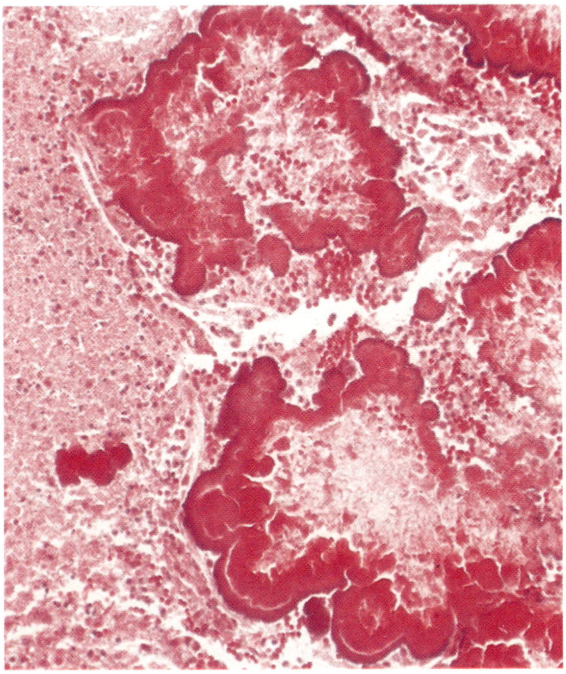

87

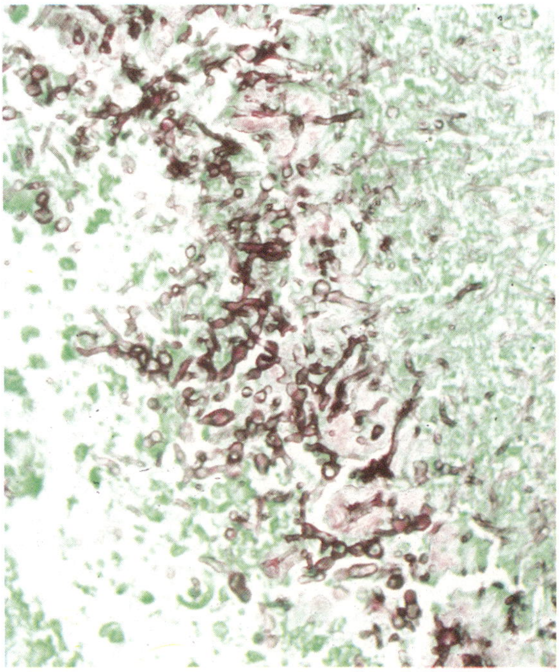

86 Aspergillus sp. fungus ball in a human lung cavity. The ball is broken up, and the periphery of each part is surrounded by abundant Splendore–Hoeppli material. The cavity also contains inflammatory cells and necrotic debris. (H&E, ×50)

87 Aspergillosis Replicate section of **86** but stained by GMS to reveal *Aspergillus sp.* hyphae within a fungus ball. Note that some hyphae are surrounded by and embedded in Splendore–Hoeppli material that is stained light brown. (GMS, ×100)

88

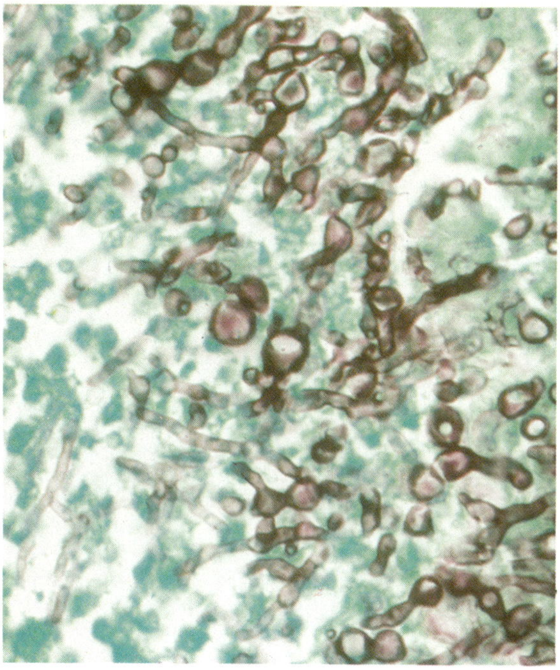

88 Aspergillosis Higher magnification of **87** showing details of the edge of the fungus ball. Note that the hyphae are septate and have vesicular swellings. (GMS, ×200)

89

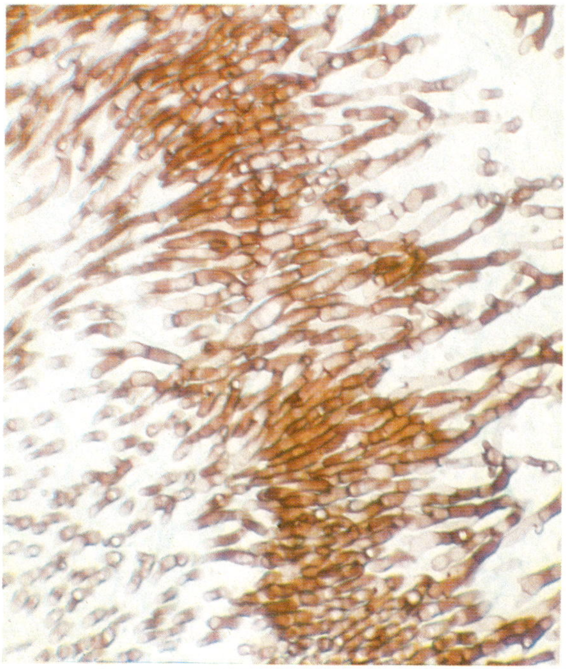

89 Aspergillosis Periphery of a large fungus ball in a human pulmonary cavity. Observe that the compact hyphae are septate and show the characteristic dichotomous branching. As illustrated here, the branches are often oriented in the same direction. (GMS, ×100)

90

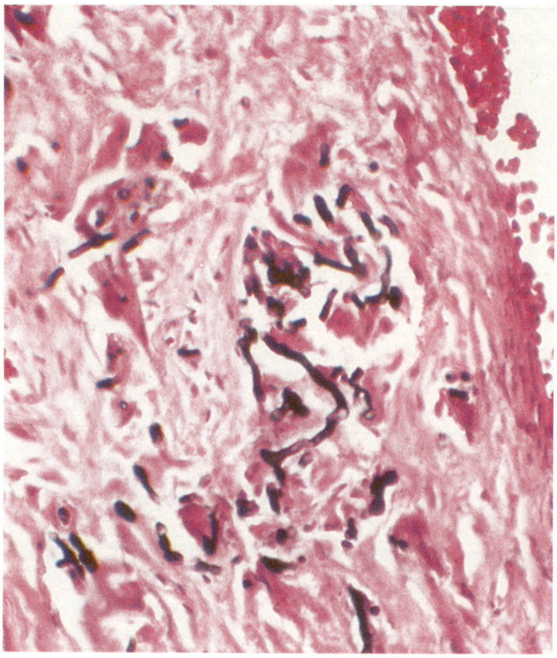

90 Chronic Aspergillus flavus infection of human paranasal sinus. Note short, bizarre hyphal elements embedded in fibrogranulomatous lesion of submucosa. (GMS–H&E, ×100)

91

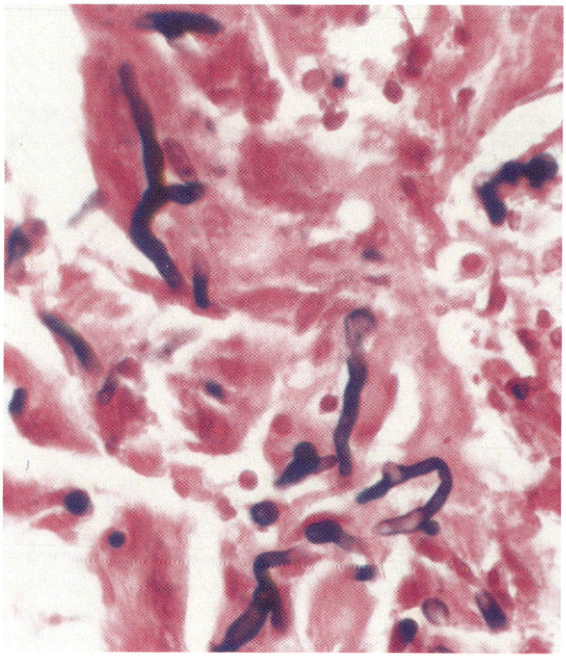

91 Aspergillus flavus Higher magnification of **90** to show details of bizarre hyphal forms within huge multinucleated giant cells. The latter are often distorted, as shown here, in an attempt to accommodate the fungus. (GMS–H&E, ×200)

92

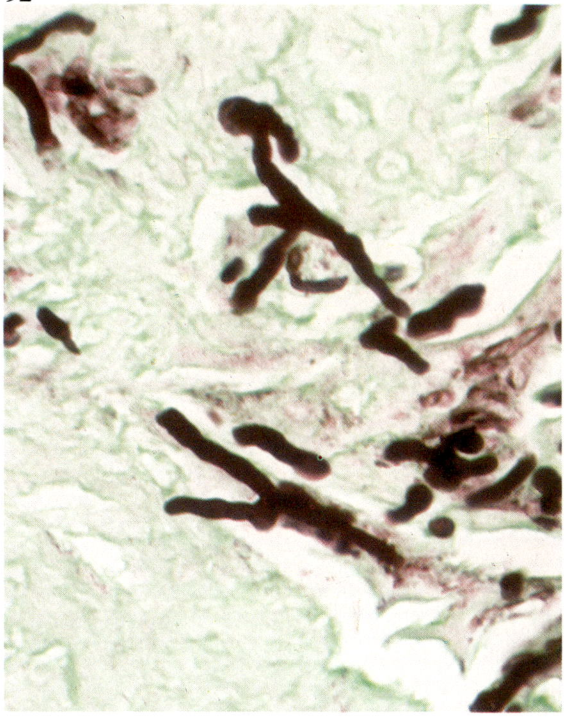

93

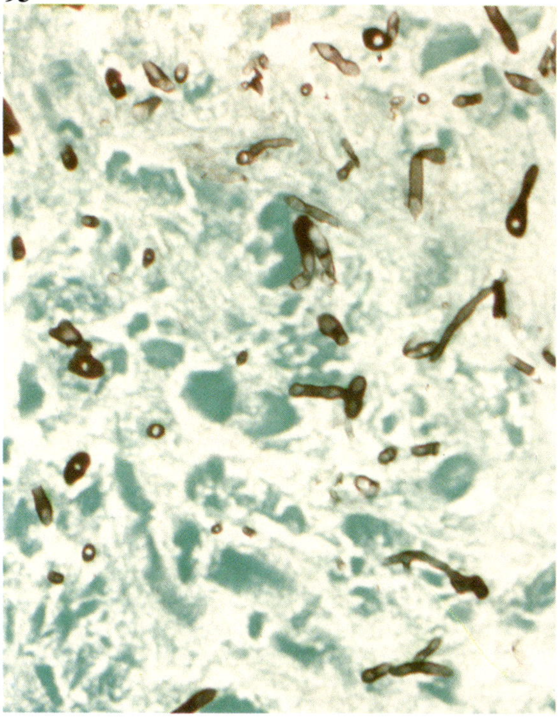

92 Chronic aspergillosis of human paranasal sinus. Observe short atypical *Aspergillus* hyphae. One hypha shows dichotomous branching. (GMS, ×200)

93 Chronic aspergillosis of human orbit. Short hyphal fragments, some of which are branched, are embedded in the granulomatous lesion. Such forms are commonly found in chronic infections. (GMS, ×100)

94

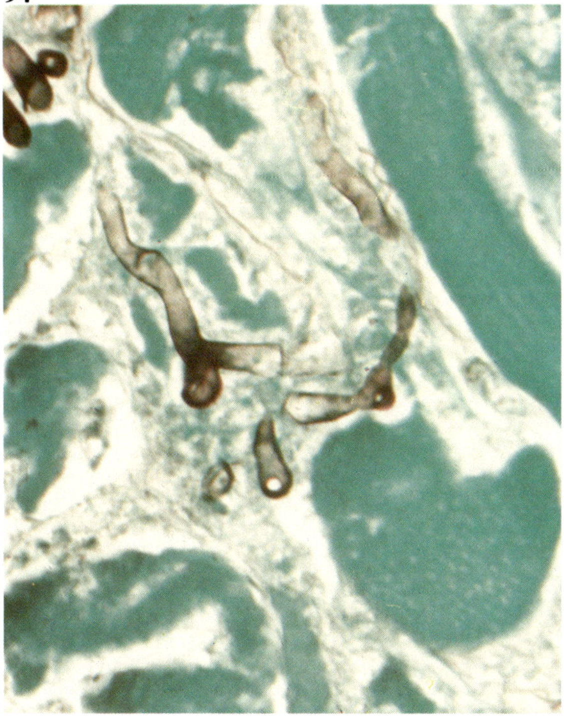

94 Aspergillosis Higher magnification of another field in **93** showing details of the short, branched, septate hyphae of the *Aspergillus sp.* invading the skeletal muscle of the orbit. (GMS, ×200)

95

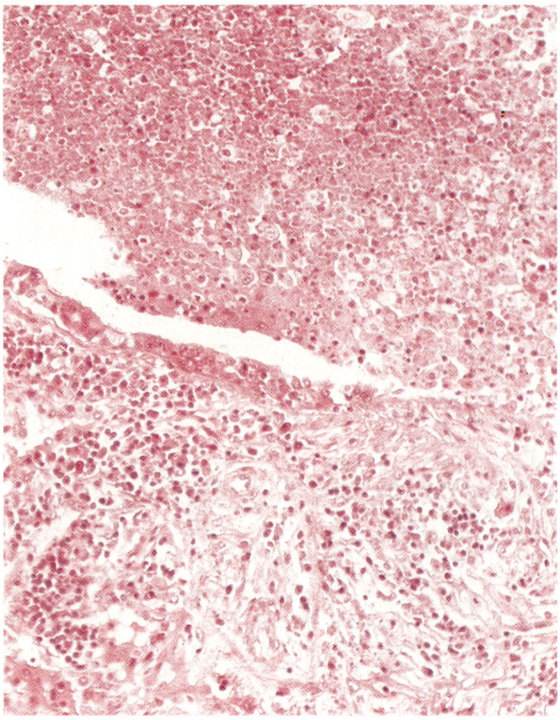

96

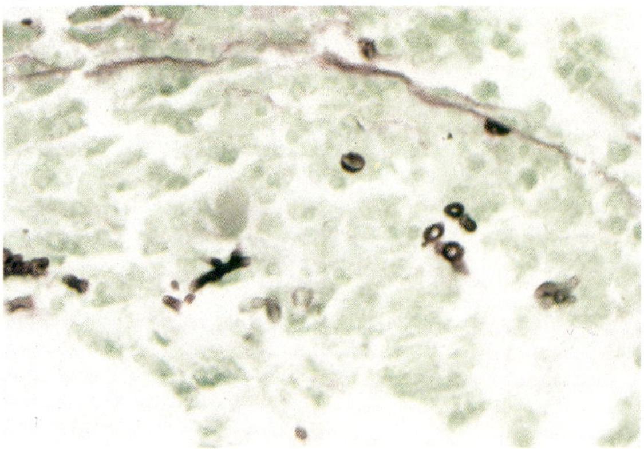

95 Allergic bronchopulmonary aspergillosis The mucous plug in the bronchial lumen contains inflammatory cells and necrotic debris. There is focal erosion of the bronchial mucosa and infiltration of the wall by mixed inflammatory cells. (H&E, ×50)

96 Allergic bronchopulmonary aspergillosis Replicate section of **95** stained by GMS to show short fragments of the hyphae of an *Aspergillus sp.* in a mucous plug. (GMS, ×200)

97

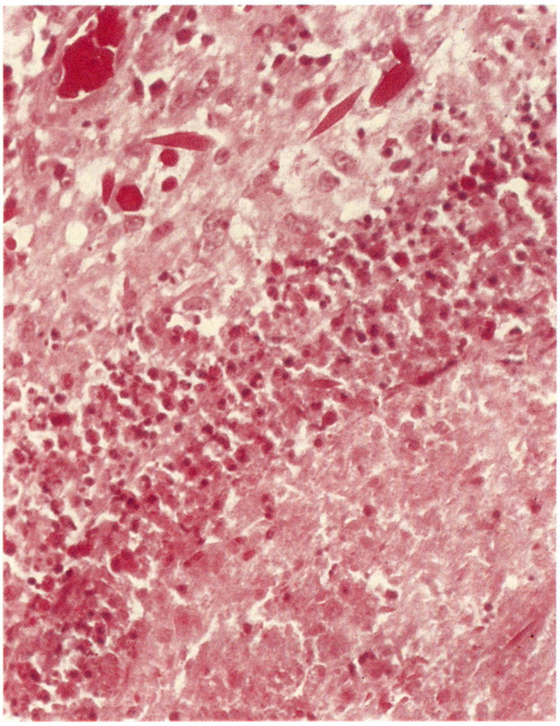

98

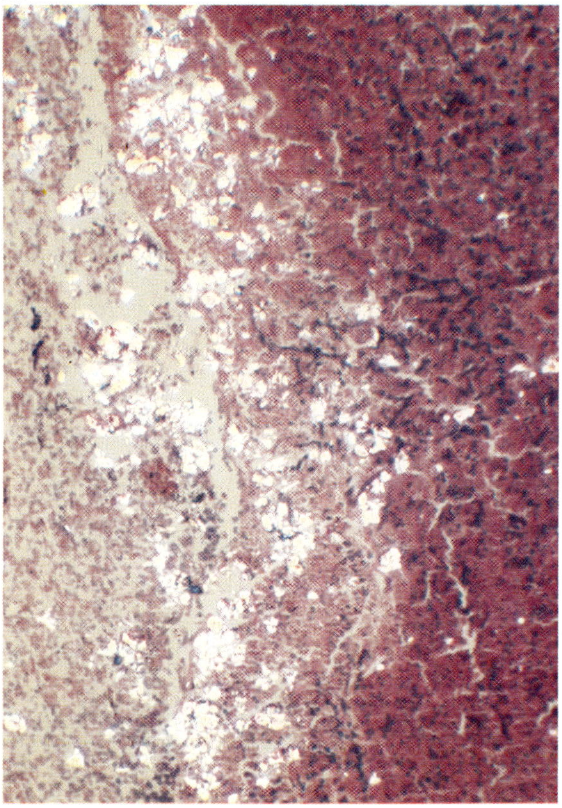

97 Allergic bronchopulmonary aspergillosis The necrotic bronchial wall is rimmed by epithelioid cells and eosinophils. Note the Charcot–Leyden crystals. Hyphal fragments are not visible. (H&E, ×100)

98 Pulmonary aspergillosis in a parrot. Masses of *Aspergillus flavus* hyphae in infected tissue are associated with numerous calcium oxalate crystals. Photograph taken under partially polarised light. (H&E, ×50)

99

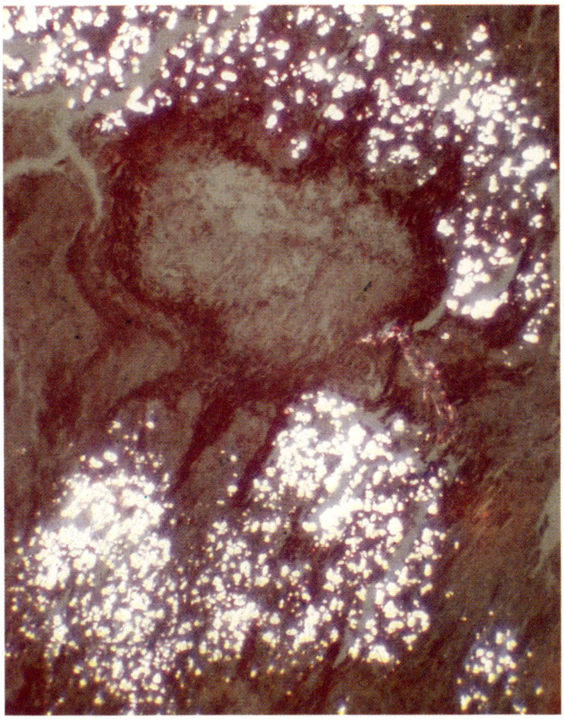

100

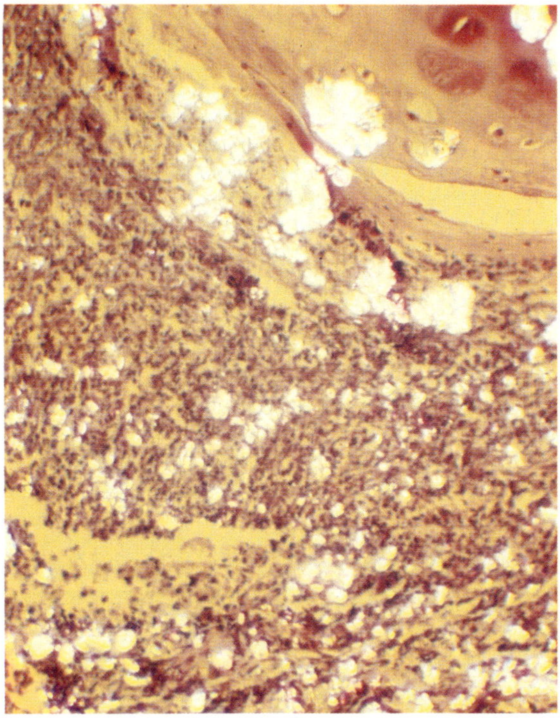

99 Aspergillus infection of parrot lung. A large area of necrotic tissue contains masses of poorly stained *Aspergillus flavus* hyphae. Abundant oxalate crystals are seen under partially polarised light. (H&E, ×50)

100 Aspergillosis of human lung. Note the peribronchial accumulation of inflammatory cells and many fan-shaped oxalate crystals. The fungal elements are not visible under the partially polarised light. (H&E, ×100)

101

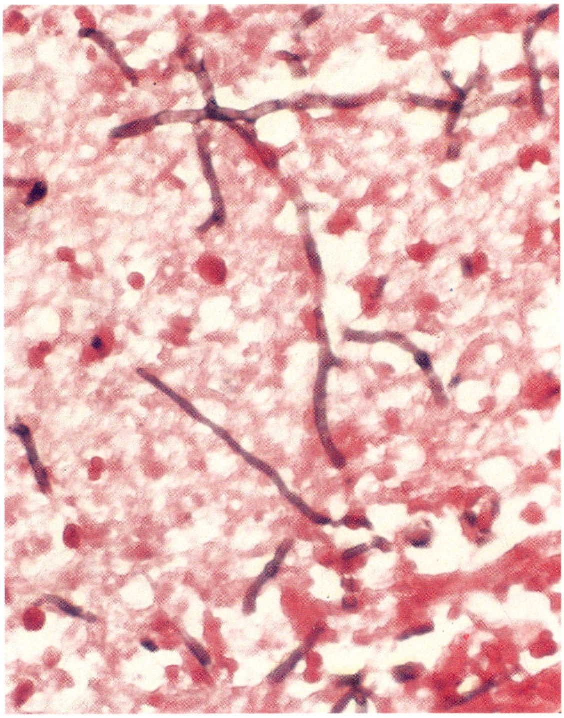

101 Petriellidium boydii hyphae in human brain. These hyphae resemble those of the aspergilli in tissue, although as a rule they are narrower and do not show the characteristic dichotomous branching (see also **514–518**). (GMS–H&E, ×200)

7 Blastomycosis

Text pages: 39–41

102

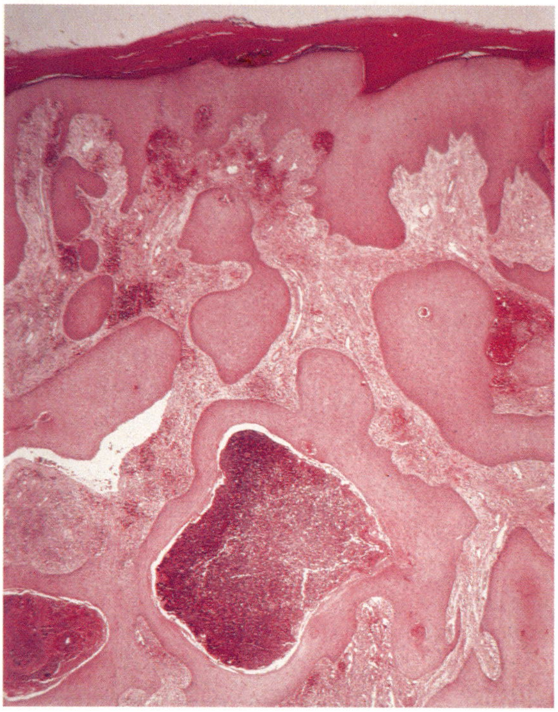

103

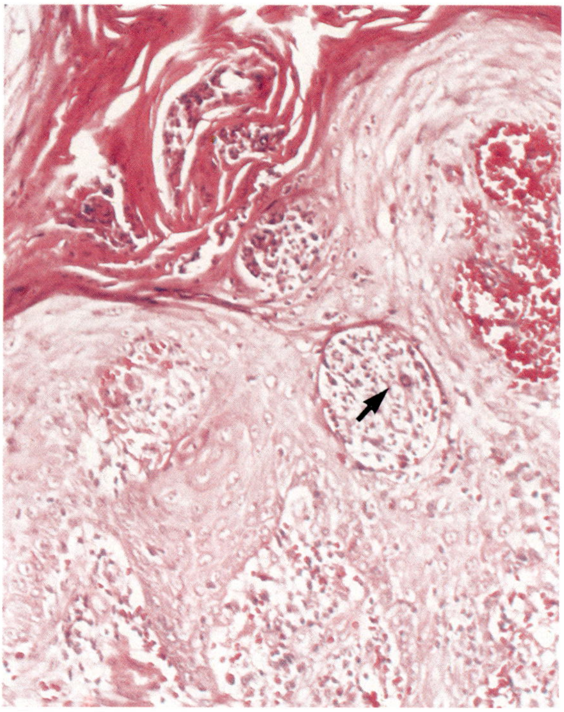

102 Cutaneous blastomycosis in a human. The lesion was clinically mistaken for a squamous cell carcinoma. Note the severe pseudoepitheliomatous hyperplasia of the epidermis and the mixed inflammatory reaction in the dermis. Histological examination established the true nature of the disease. (H&E, ×20)

103 Cutaneous blastomycosis in another human. There is hyperkeratosis and pseudoepitheliomatous hyperplasia of the epidermis, along with a mixed purulent and granulomatous inflammatory reaction in the dermis. Note the intraepidermal micro-abscess containing a faintly visible fungal cell (arrow). (GMS–H&E, ×50)

104

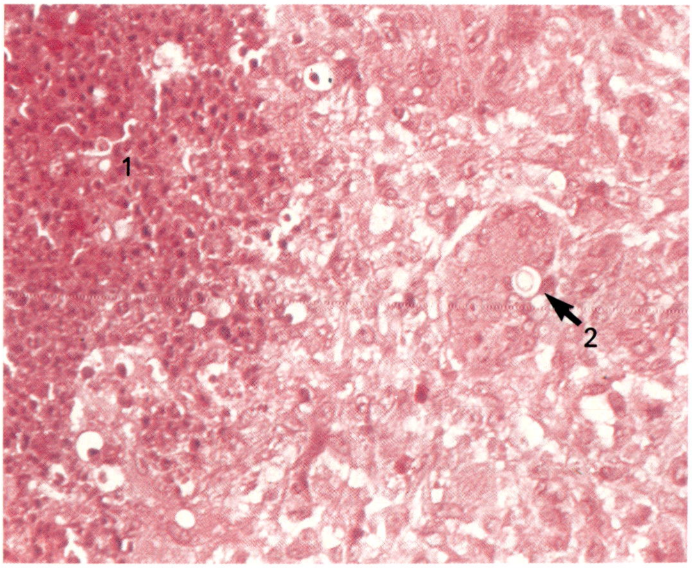

104 Cutaneous blastomycosis A large dermal abscess is present (**1**), bordered by a granulomatous reaction consisting of epithelioid and giant cells. A single faintly stained fungal cell (**2**) can be seen within a giant cell. (H&E, ×100)

105

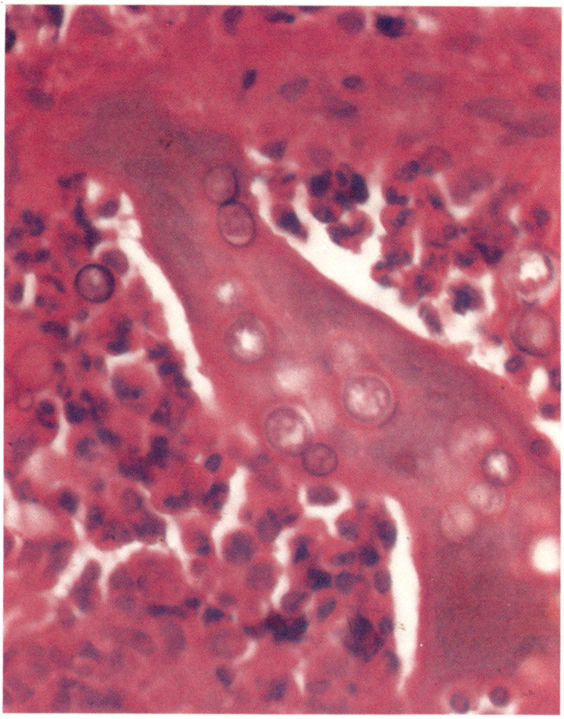

105 **Cutaneous blastomycosis** Observe single and budding *Blastomyces dermatitidis* tissue-form cells within a large giant cell that is embedded in a dermal micro-abscess. Fungal cells are also extracellular in the purulent exudate. (GMS–H&E, ×200)

106

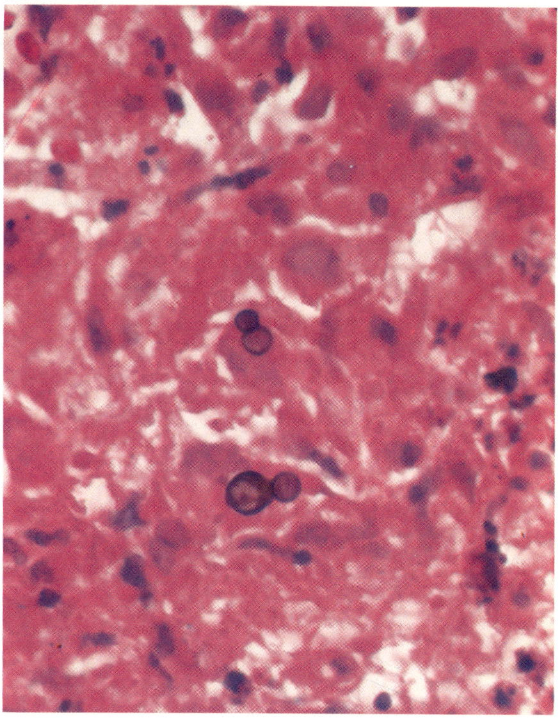

106 **Cutaneous blastomycosis** in a human Two budding yeast cells are within a granuloma. Observe that the buds have a broad basal attachment to the parent cells. (GMS–H&E, ×200)

107

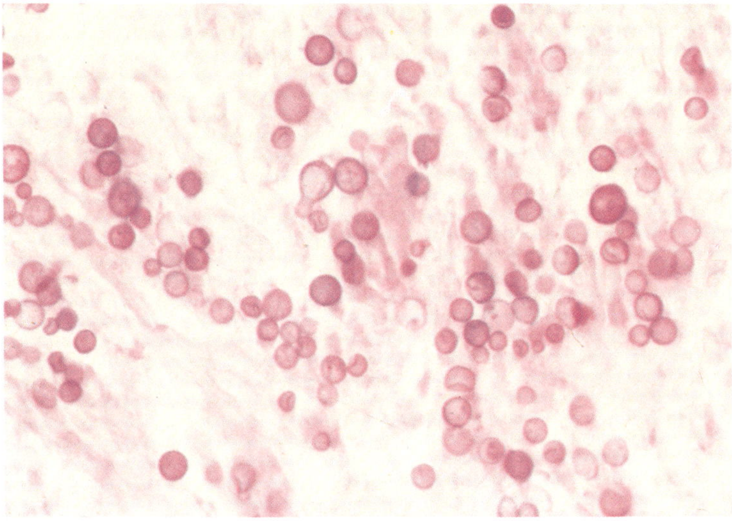

107 **Blastomyces dermatitidis** infection of human skin. Unusually large numbers of fungus cells are well demonstrated. (PAS, ×200)

108

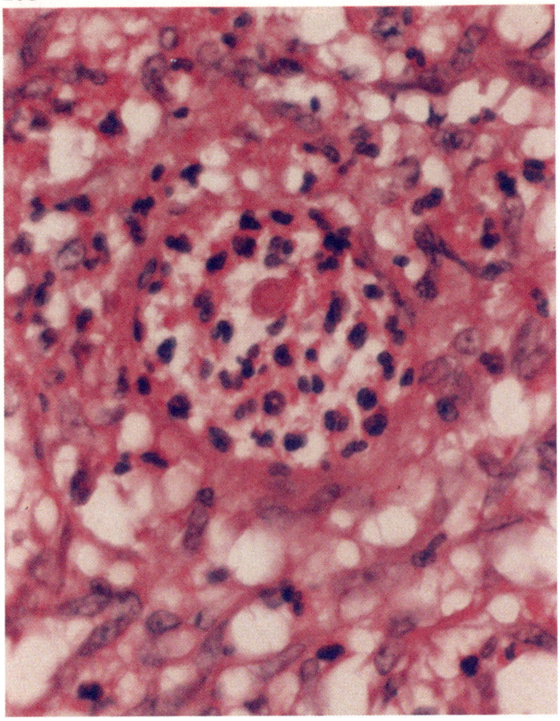

109

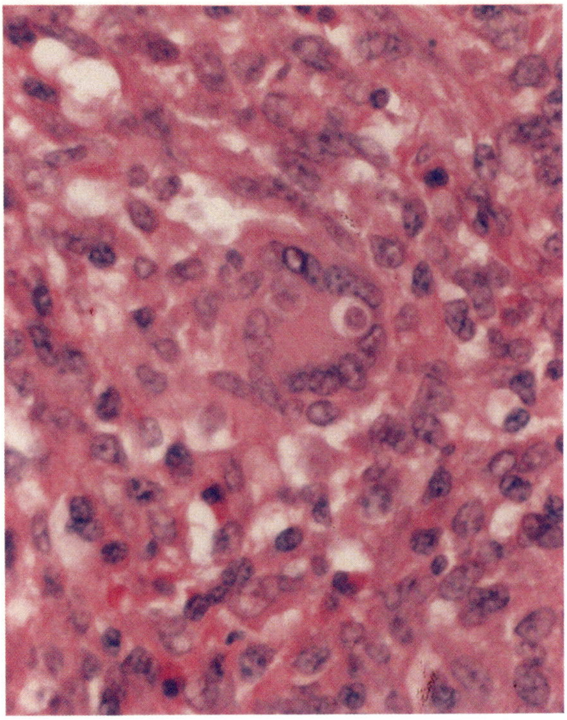

108 Blastomyces dermatitidis causing granulomatous lymphadenitis in a human. Note single, poorly stained yeast cell surrounded by neutrophils in the centre of a granuloma. (H&E, ×200)

109 Blastomyces dermatitidis Another field in **108**. Two yeast cells are contained within a Langhans' giant cell. (H&E, ×200)

110

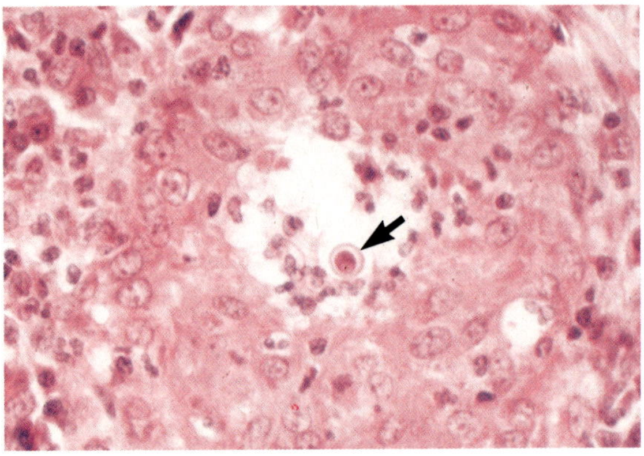

110 Canine pulmonary blastomycosis A single yeast cell (arrow) is seen in the centre of an epithelioid cell granuloma. The cytoplasm of the fungal cell is retracted from the wall because of shrinkage during fixation and processing. (H&E, ×200)

111 Canine pulmonary blastomycosis Two fungus cells (arrows) are seen in an epithelioid cell granuloma that contains a microabscess. The fungus cells' cytoplasm is well stained but their thick walls are not. (H&E, ×200)

111

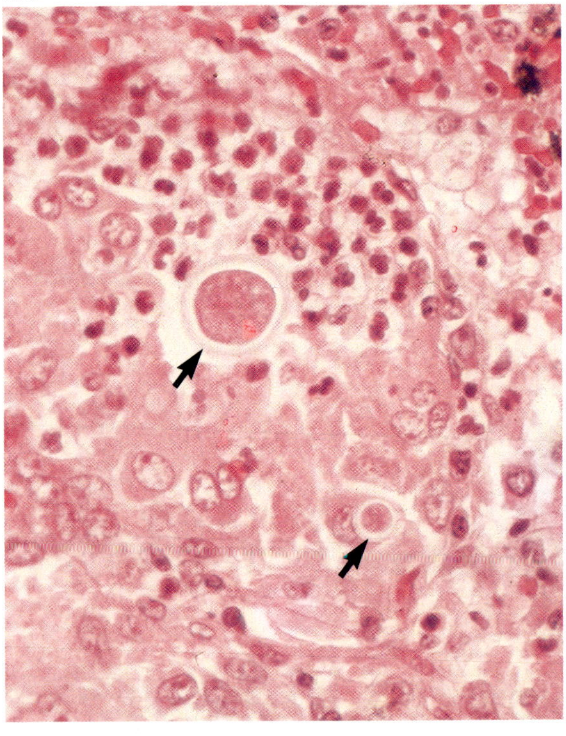

112

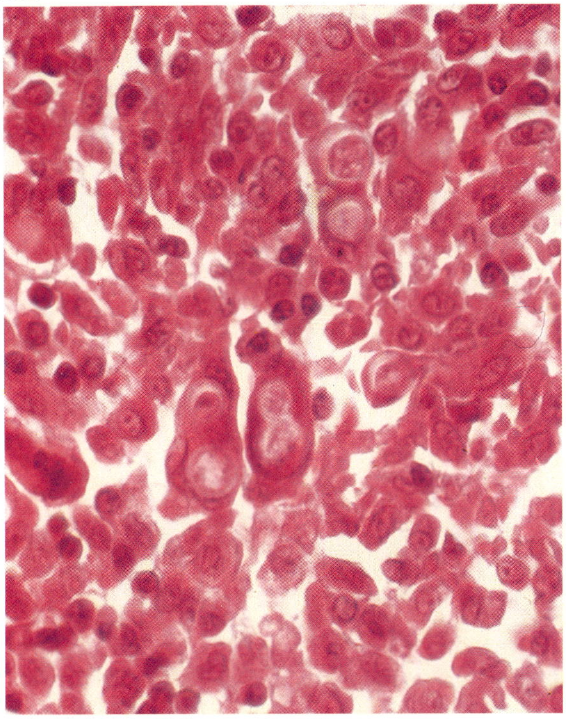

112 **Pulmonary blastomycosis** Another case showing single and budding *Blastomyces dermatitidis* cells in a granulomatous lesion. Note the diagnostically significant broad basal attachment of the buds to their parent cells. (H&E, ×200)

113

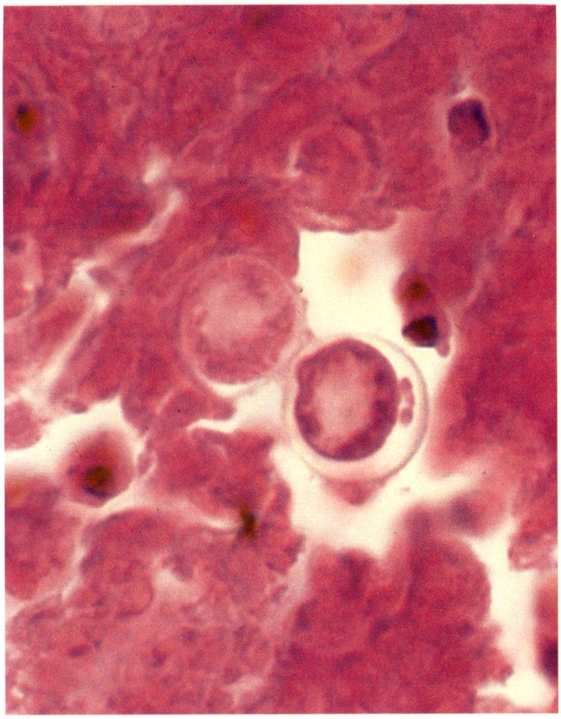

113 **Pulmonary blastomycosis** Another field in **112** showing the budding pattern of *Blastomyces dermatitidis* in greater detail. The characteristic broad basal attachment of the bud to the parent cell, and the multiple nuclei in both the parent and daughter cells, are clearly seen. (H&E, ×500)

114

114 **Pulmonary blastomycosis** Replicate section of **112** but stained by GMS to show the typical broad basal attachment of the bud to the parent cell. The cytoplasmic contents are unstained in these cells. (GMS, ×500)

115

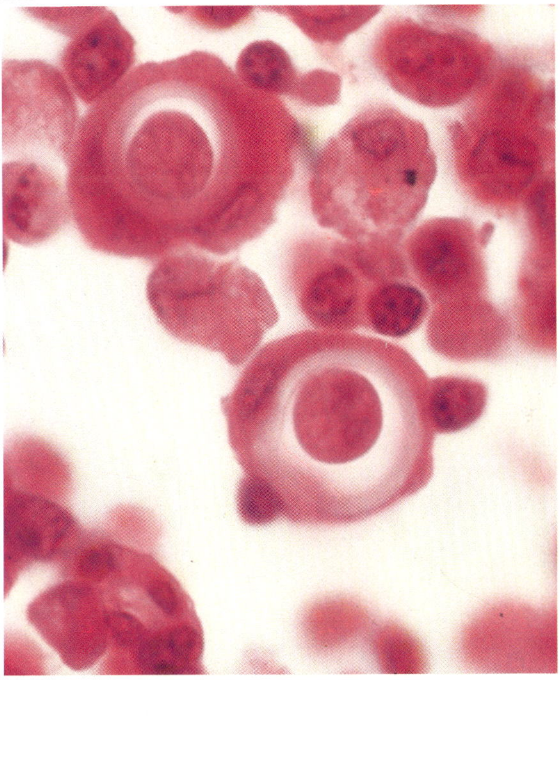

115 **Pulmonary blastomycosis** Another field in **112** that shows two single *Blastomyces dermatitidis* cells within alveolar macrophages. Note the thick walls and the cytoplasmic retraction within the fungal cells. (H&E, ×500)

116

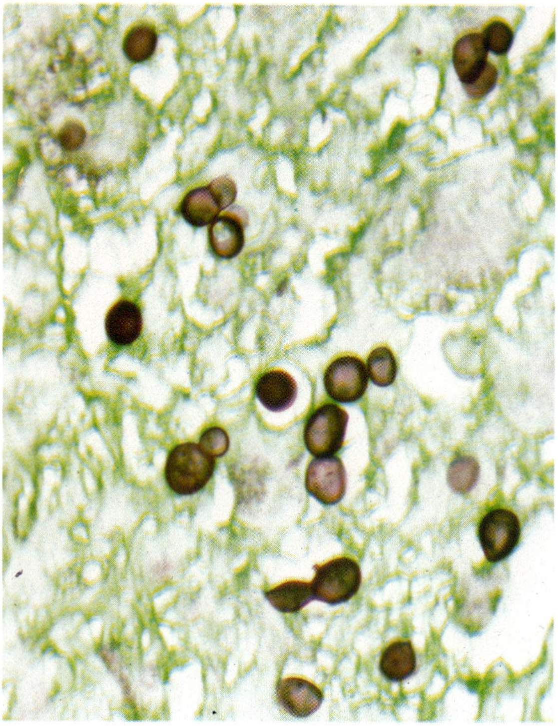

117

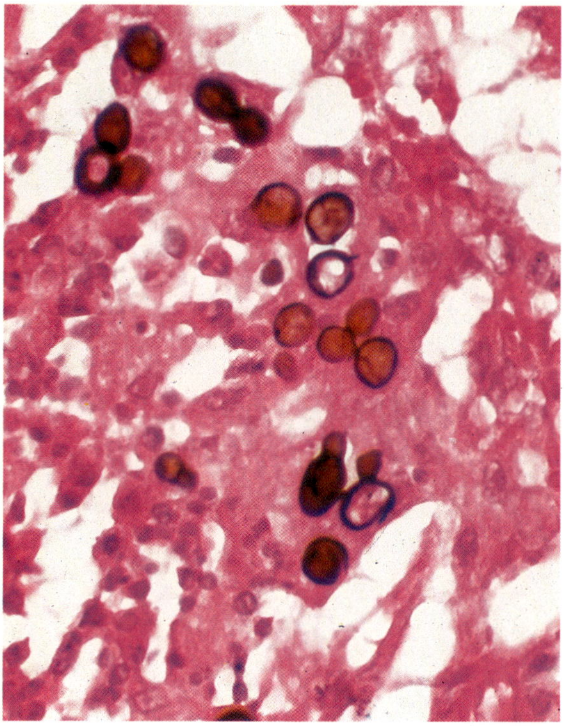

116 Feline pulmonary blastomycosis Single and budding yeast cells are well stained. (GMS, ×200)

117 Feline pulmonary blastomycosis Replicate section of **116** showing *Blastomyces dermatitidis* cells within a granulomatous lesion. Note that the combined GMS–H&E stain makes it possible to observe the fungus as well as the background inflammatory response. (GMS–H&E, ×200)

118

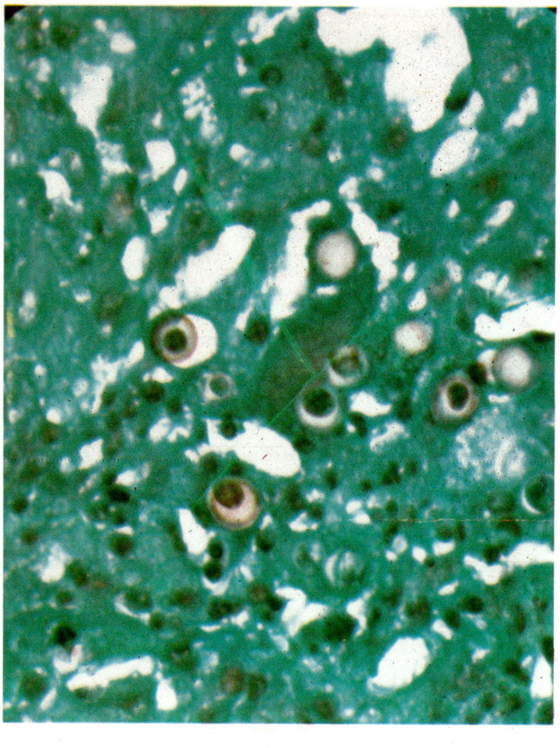

118 Feline pulmonary blastomycosis Replicate section of **116** but stained with Mayer's mucicarmine procedure. As shown here, the cell walls of *Blastomyces dermatitidis* are sometimes weakly carminophilic. (Mayer's mucicarmine, ×200)

119

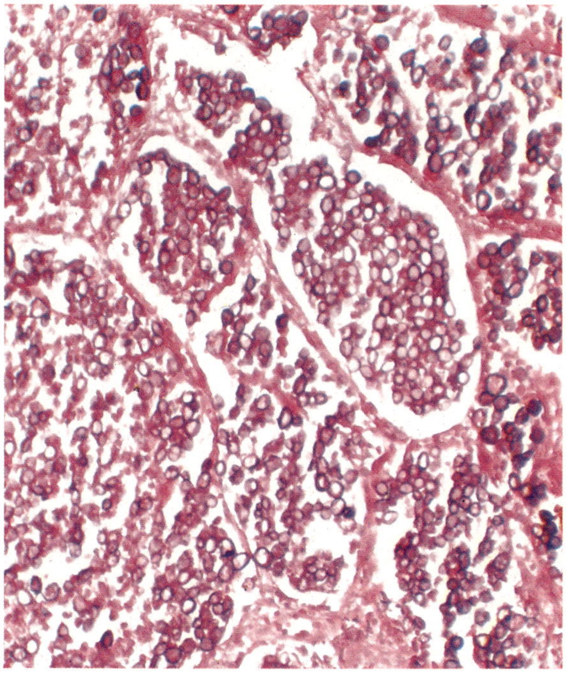

120

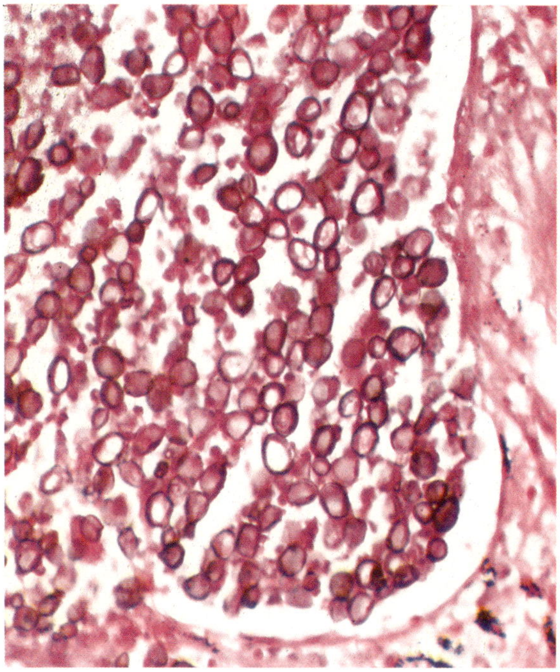

119 Pulmonary blastomycosis in an immunosuppressed human. Alveolar spaces are filled with unusually large numbers of *Blastomyces dermatitidis* cells. Inflammation is minimal. (GMS–H&E, ×100)

120 Pulmonary blastomycosis Higher magnification of **119** to show typical *Blastomyces dermatitidis* cells in greater detail. (GMS–H&E, ×200)

121

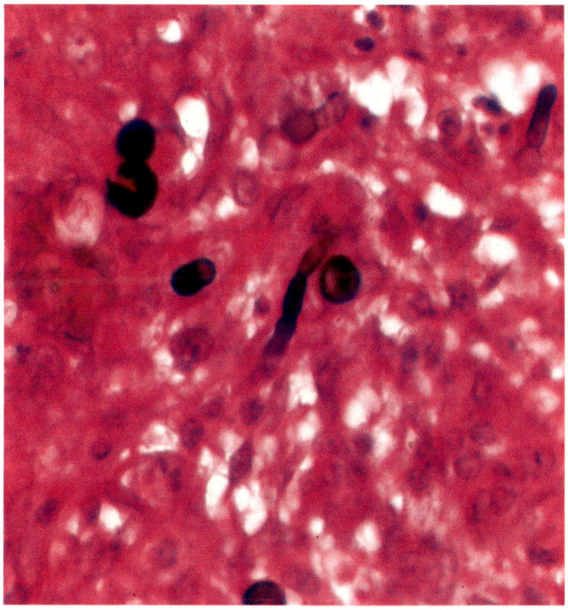

122

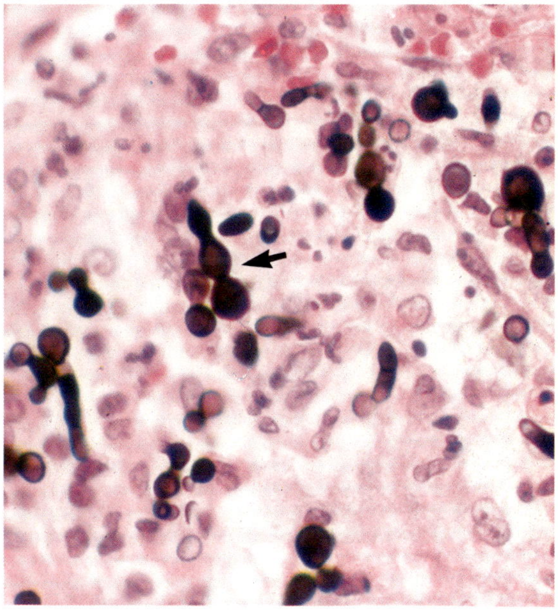

121 Cutaneous blastomycosis in a human. Budding yeast cells and short hyphal elements are seen in the granulomatous lesion. Hyphae of *Blastomyces dermatitidis* are rarely formed in tissue. (GMS–H&E, ×200)

122 Pulmonary blastomycosis in a human. This section shows a short chain of yeast cells (arrow), cells with single buds, and hyphal elements of *Blastomyces dermatitidis*. (GMS–H&E, ×200)

131

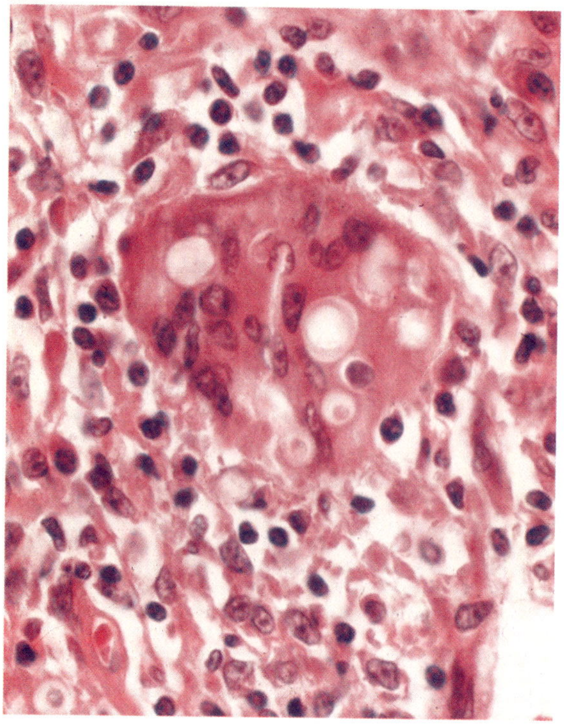

131 **Pulmonary blastomycosis** in a native African. Several large and poorly stained yeast cells of *Blastomyces dermatitidis* are contained within a foreign body giant cell. (H&E, ×200)

132

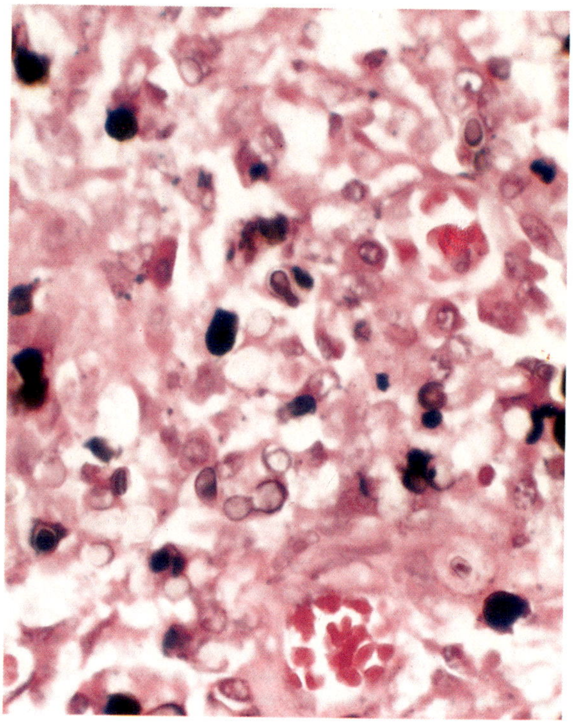

132 **Pulmonary blastomycosis** Replicate section of **131**. The yeast cells bud by a broad basal attachment to the parent cell and are morphologically similar to those found in New World cases of blastomycosis. Note the granulomatous inflammatory response. (GMS–H&E, ×200)

133

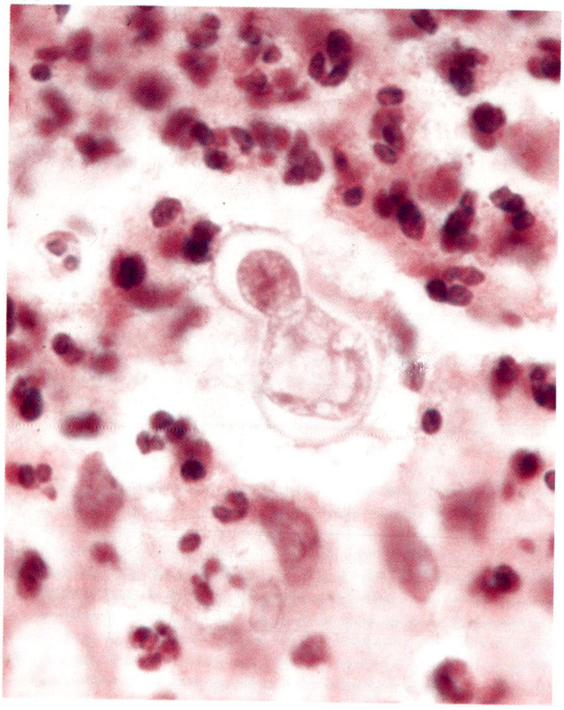

133 **Blastomycosis** in an African. Details of a budding cell of *Blastomyces dermatitidis* embedded in neutrophils. The bud has a broad basal attachment to its parent cell. (H&E, ×400)

134

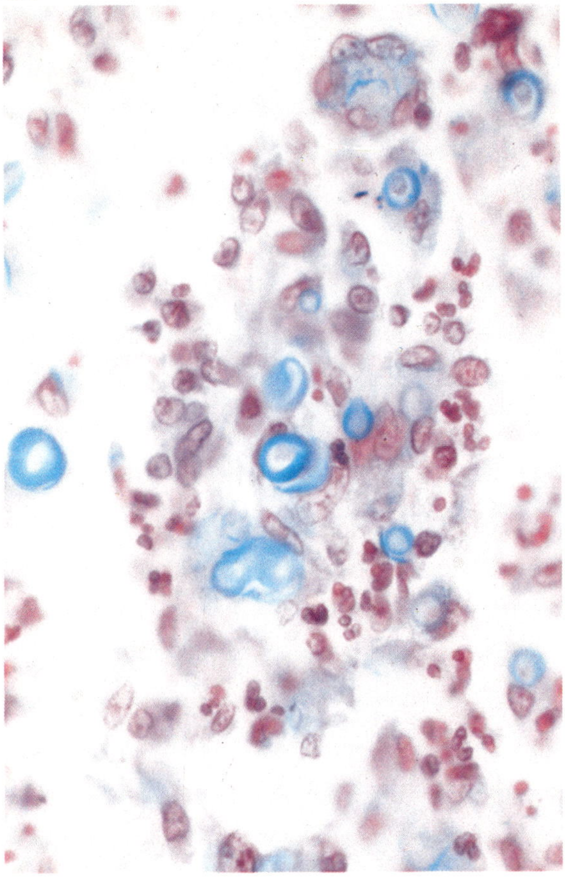

135

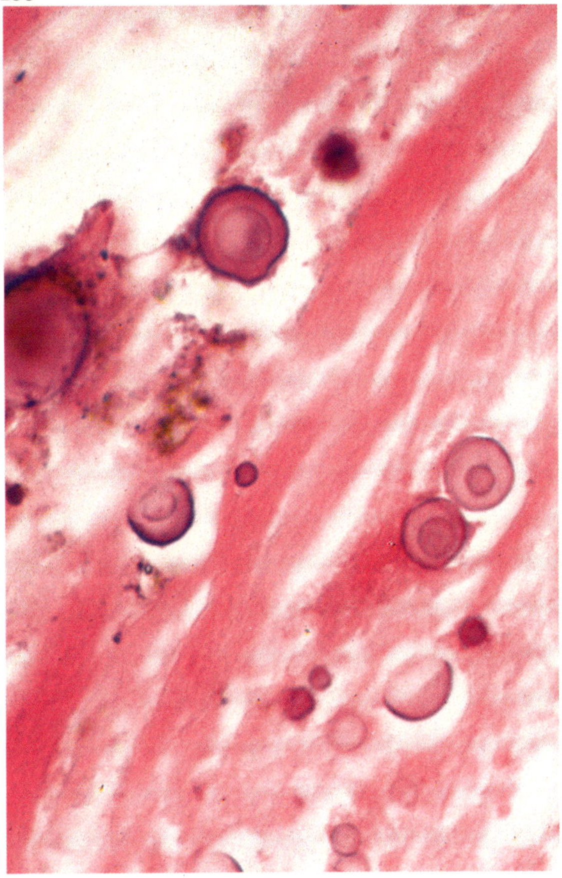

134 Blastomycosis Replicate section of **131** except that it is stained by the alcian blue procedure, a mucopolysaccharide stain. The fungal cell walls may react positively to this stain. (Alcian blue, ×200)

135 Calcific bodies within a fibrocaseous nodule. Note their superficial resemblance to *Blastomyces dermatitidis* cells in H&E stained sections. (H&E, ×200)

8 Candidiasis (including Torulopsosis)

Text pages: 42–46

136

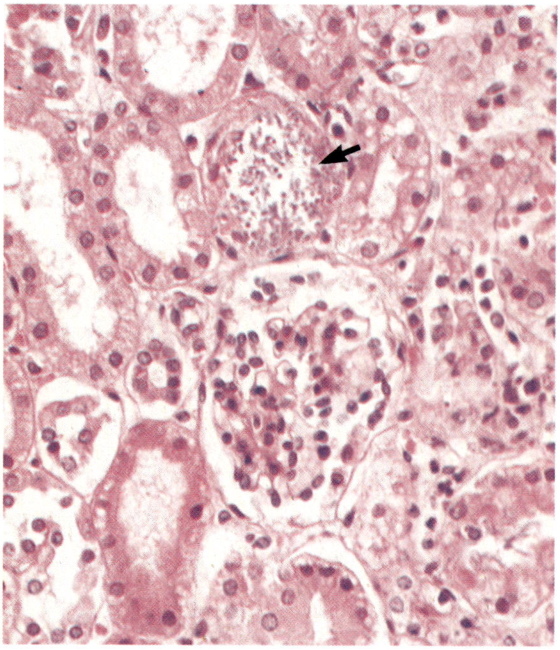

137

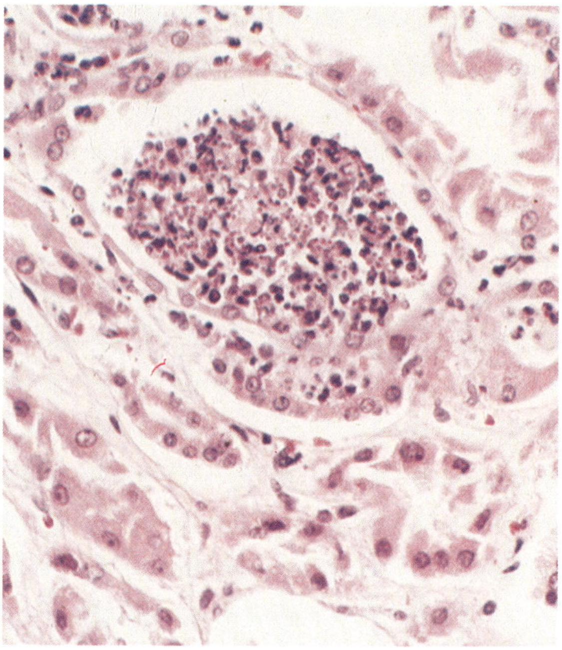

136 Candida sp. Renal candidiasis in a human. A renal tubule (arrow) contains poorly stained blastospores. At this early stage of infection, inflammation is minimal. (H&E, ×100)

137 Candida albicans Renal candidiasis in another human. A kidney tubule is distended by inflammatory cells and poorly stained blastospores. Interstitial inflammation is minimal. (H&E, ×100)

138

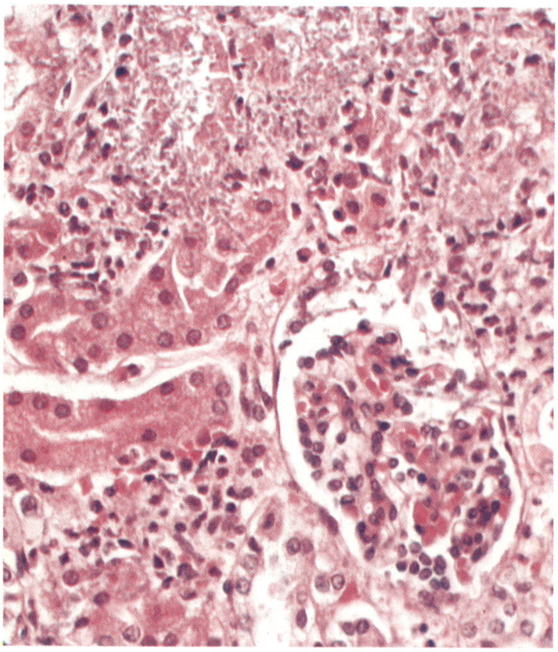

138 Disseminated candidiasis Abscess in renal cortex of a human. Masses of lightly basophilic blastospores are surrounded by polymorphonuclear leucocytes. (H&E, ×100)

139

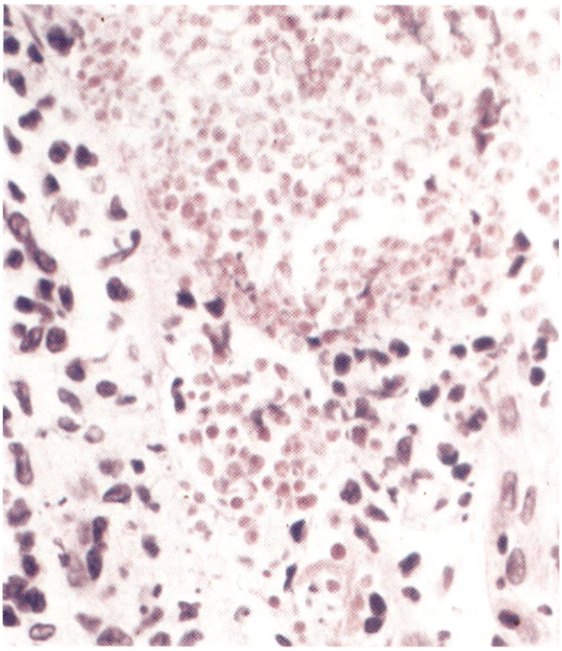

139 Disseminated candidiasis Higher magnification of another field in **137** showing details of the numerous lightly stained but clearly visible blastospores of *Candida albicans*. Pseudohyphae or hyphae are not visible at this early stage of infection. (H&E, ×200)

140

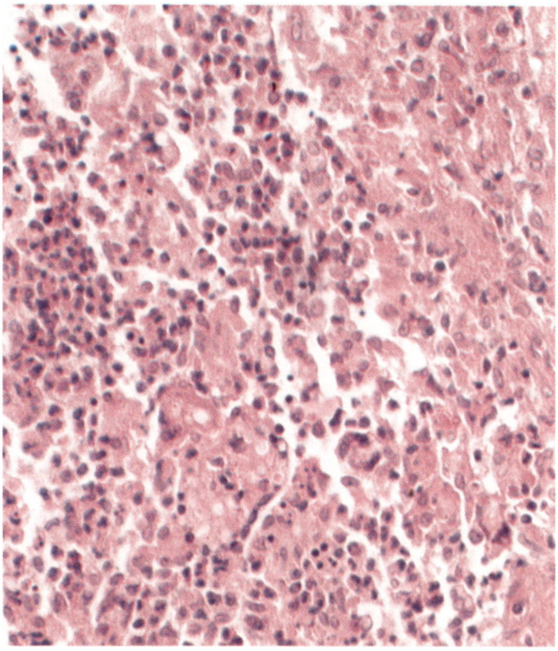

140 Chronic renal candidiasis in a human. A granulomatous lesion contains epithelioid cells, giant cells, and neutrophils. Poorly stained fungal cells are within giant cells. (H&E, ×100)

141

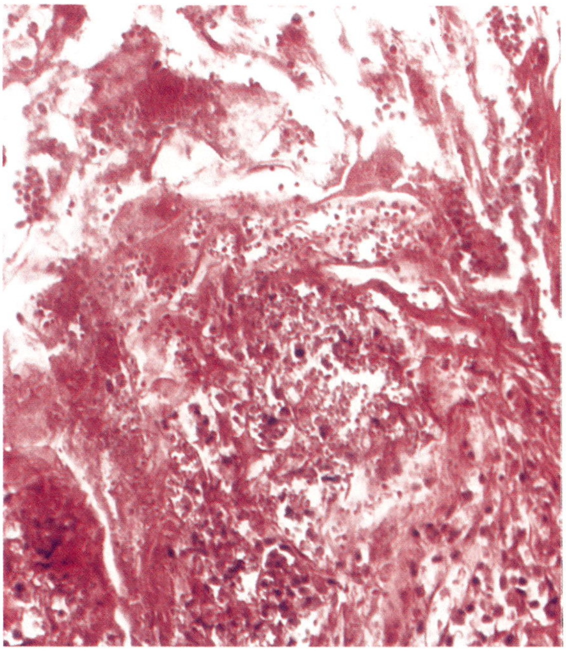

141 Candida albicans infecting bovine rumen. There is focal necrosis of the epithelium and infiltration of mixed inflammatory cells in the underlying tissues. The fungal cells are not well demonstrated with this stain. (H&E, ×100)

142

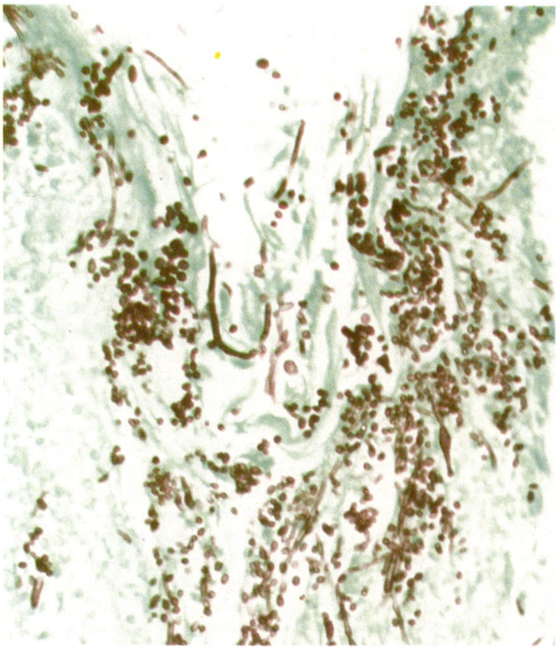

142 Candida albicans Replicate section of **141** but stained by GMS to show invasion of the rumen wall. Numerous fungal elements are clearly demonstrated by this stain. (GMS, ×100)

143

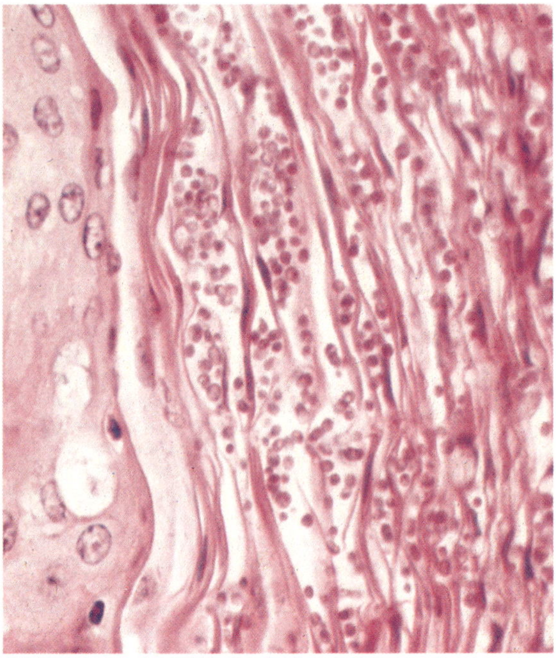

143 Candida albicans Preterminal infection of the oesophagus. Numerous blastospores are in the hyperkeratotic layer. Pseudohyphae are not evident. (H&E, ×200)

144

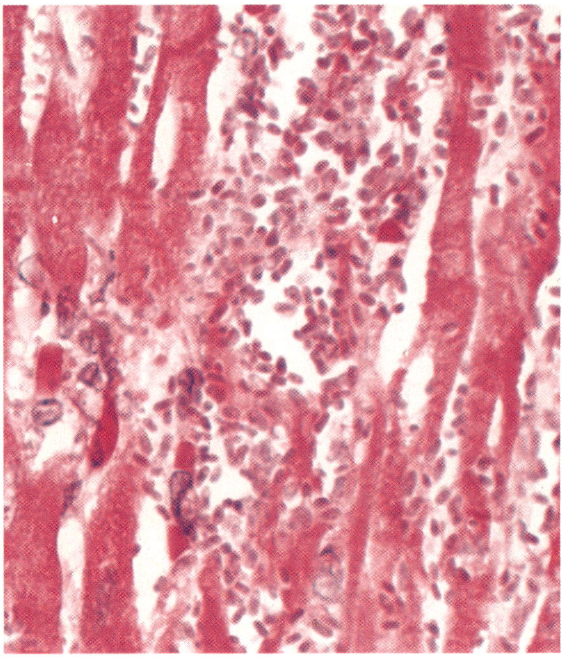

144 Candida sp. in the myocardium of a patient who died of leukaemia. Although numerous fungal elements are present, there is little or no inflammation. (H&E, ×200)

145

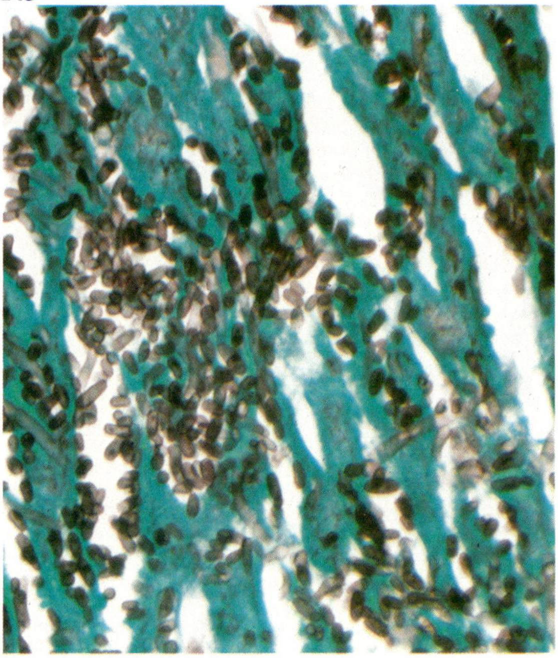

145 Candida sp. Replicate section of **144** but stained by GMS. The myocardium is invaded by both blastospores and hyphae. (GMS, ×200)

146

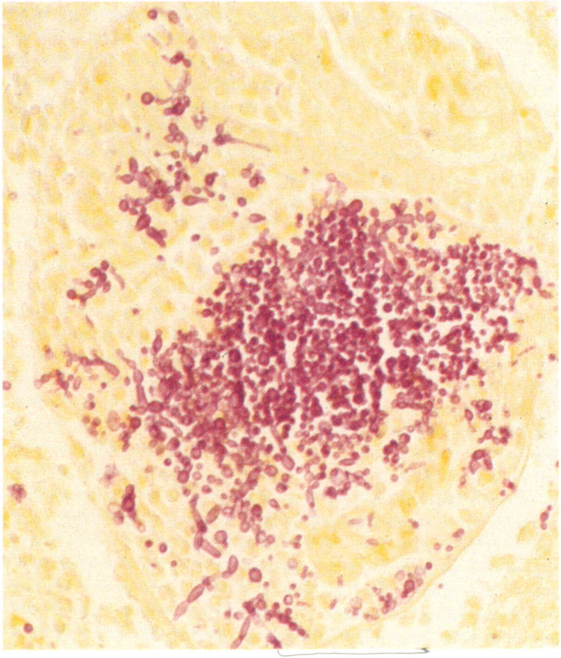

146 Candida albicans Early infection of human kidney. Masses of blastospores and few pseudohyphae are present. (GF, ×100)

147

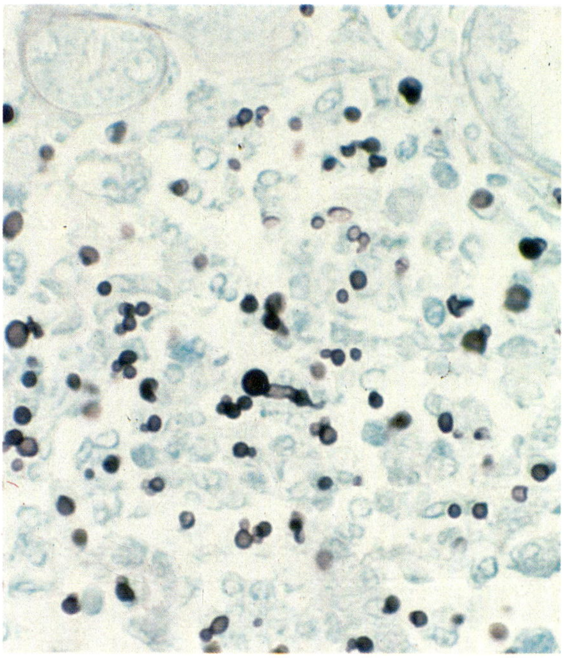

148

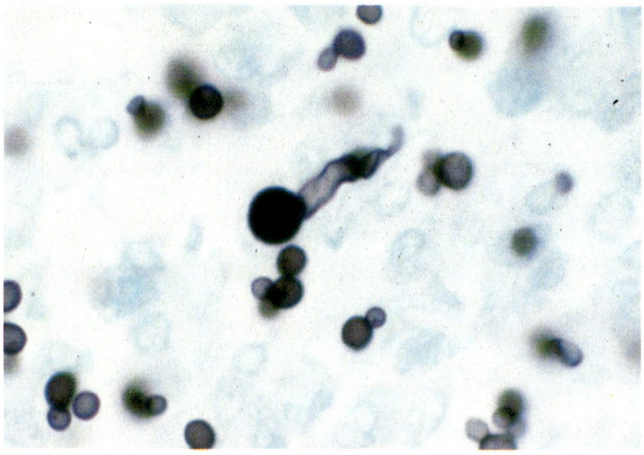

148 Acute renal candidiasis Higher magnification of **147** showing details of the germinating blastospore of *Candida albicans*. The germ tube is tapered and folded because its wall lacks rigidity. This pattern of tapering and folding of germ tubes is frequently seen in early lesions. (GMS, ×500)

147 Acute renal candidiasis in a human. Scattered single and budding blastospores are seen in an abscess. One blastospore has formed a short germ tube. (GMS, ×200)

149

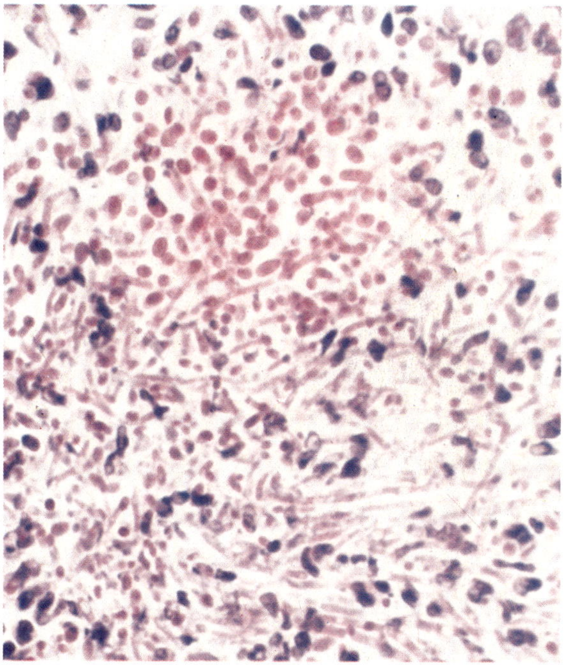

150

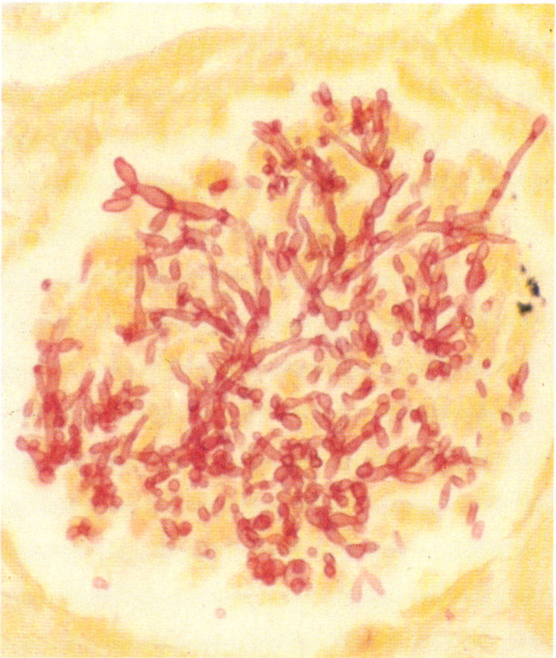

149 Candida albicans Human renal abscess containing masses of poorly stained but plainly visible blastospores and pseudohyphae. (H&E, ×200)

150 Renal candidiasis in another patient. Blastospores and numerous pseudohyphae are seen within a glomerular tuft. The combination of blastospores and pseudohyphae is characteristic of the *Candida spp.* in tissue. (GF, ×*200)*

151

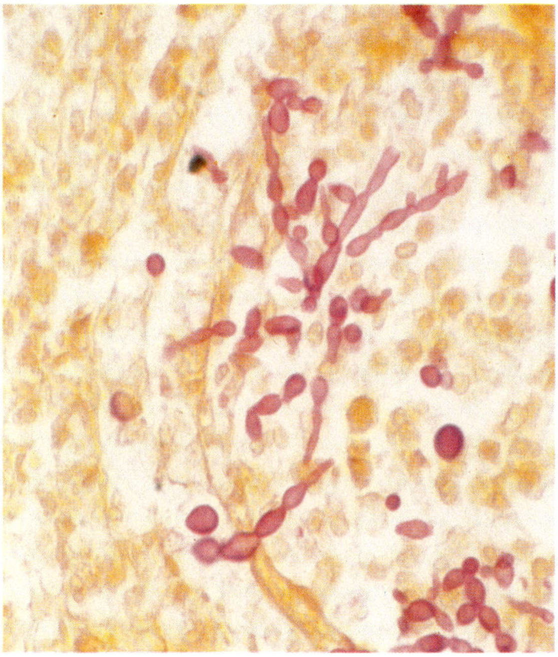

152

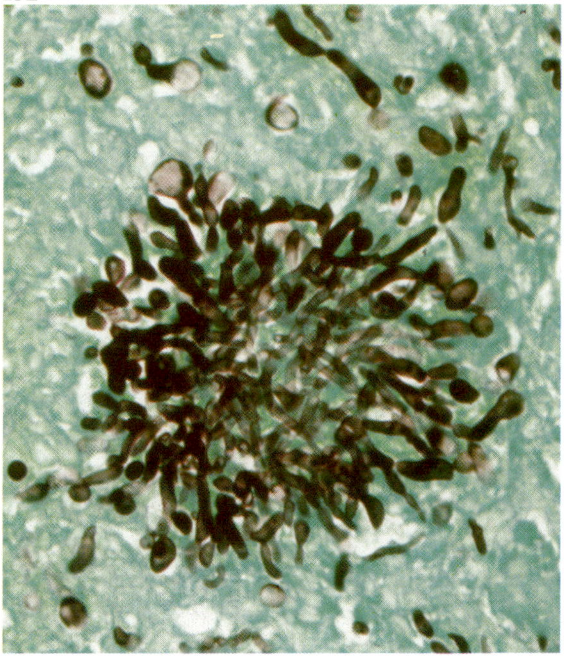

151 **Candida albicans** causing abscess of renal cortex. Pseudohyphae, individual blastospores, and chains of blastospores are present. Only the outlines of the inflammatory cells can be seen. (GF, ×200)

152 **Renal candidiasis** in a patient with fatal Legionnaires' disease. The opportunistic fungus appears as a tangled mass of hyphae, pseudohyphae, and blastospores. A few budding cells are seen outside the mycelial mass. (GMS, ×200)

153

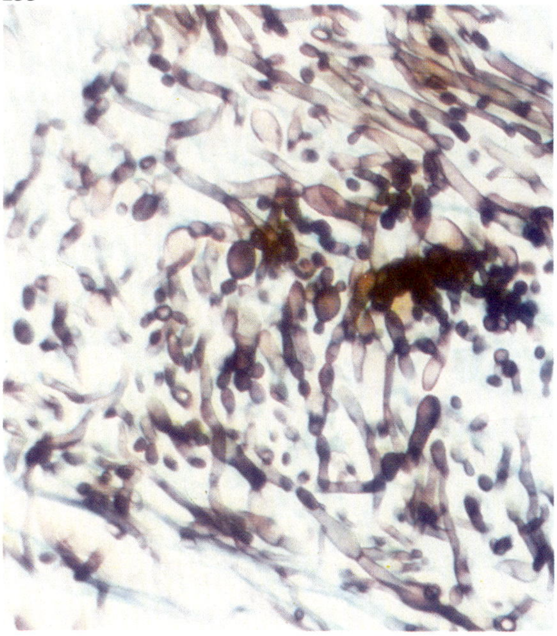

154

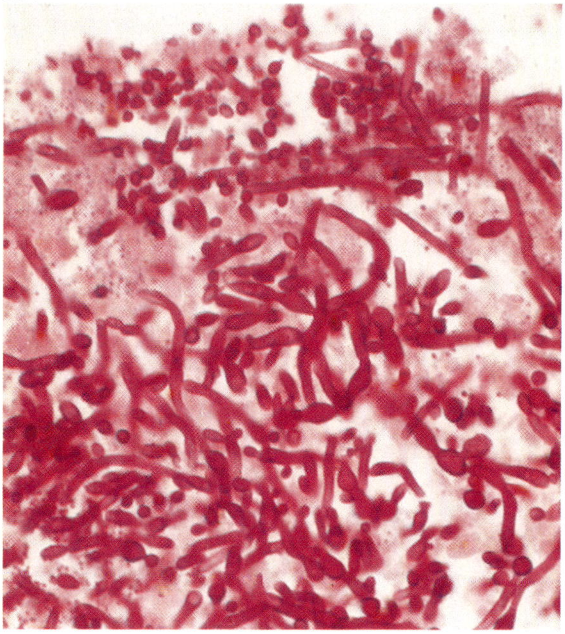

153 **Preterminal candidiasis** of human oesophagus. Numerous pseudohyphae and a few blastospores have invaded the submucosa. (GMS, ×200)

154 **Superficial candidiasis** in the colon of a child. Blastospores predominate at the surface, and pseudohyphae and hyphae infiltrate the deeper layers. (PAS, ×200)

155

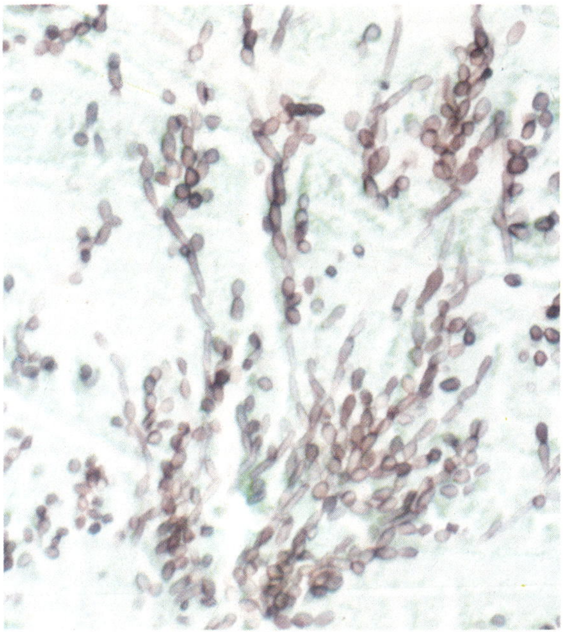

155 Candida albicans causing valvular endocarditis in a human. Pseudohyphae and blastospores have infiltrated the stroma of the heart valve. (GMS, ×200)

156

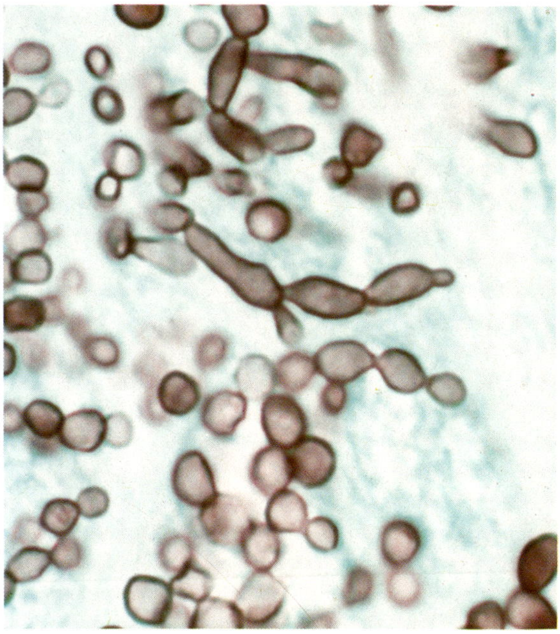

156 Candida albicans Higher magnification of **155** to show details of the fungus. Note pseudohyphae and blastospores – a combination that is characteristic of the *Candida spp.* in acute lesions. (GMS, ×500)

157

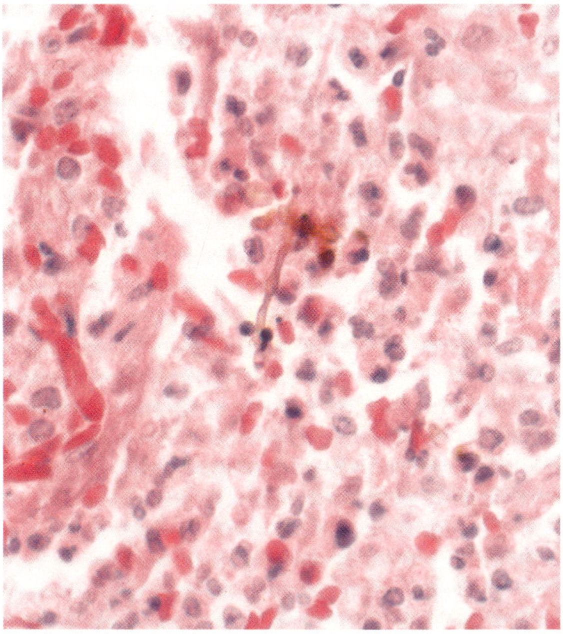

157 Pulmonary phaeohyphomycosis in a human. A dematiaceous fungus morphologically suggestive of a *Cladosporium sp.* was the aetiologic agent. There is a mixed inflammatory reaction similar to that seen in other acute fungus infections. This case was submitted to us with a presumptive diagnosis of candidiasis. (H&E, ×200)

158

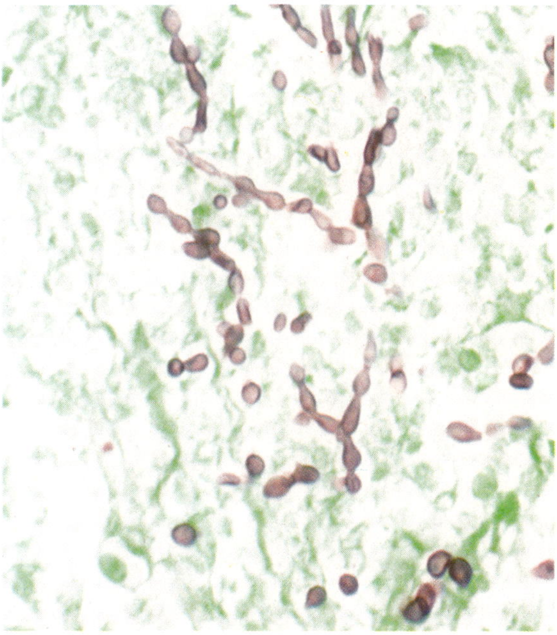

158 Pulmonary phaeohyphomycosis Replicate section of **157**, but stained by GMS to show details of the fungal elements. Observe single and branched moniliform hyphae. The dematiaceous nature of the aetiological agents of phaeohyphomycosis is not evident when they are stained by GMS. Note resemblance of the hyphae of this fungus to the *Candida sp.* in **151**. (GMS, ×200)

159

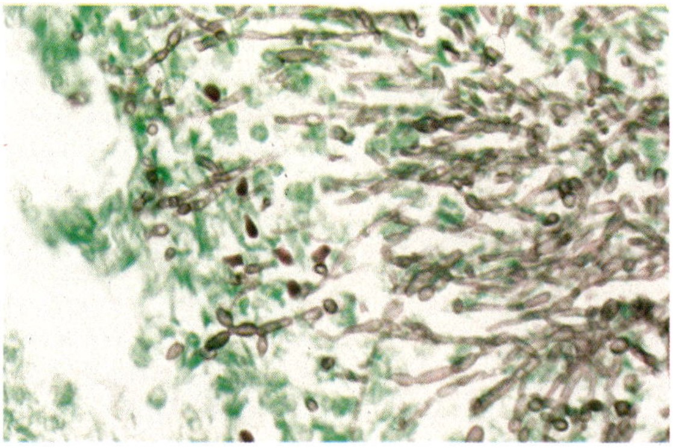

160

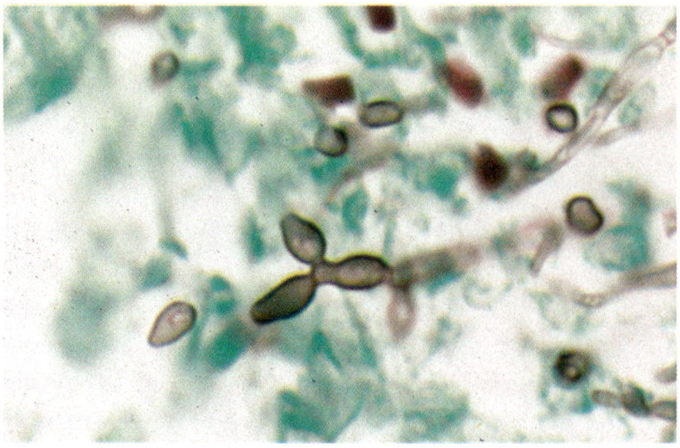

161

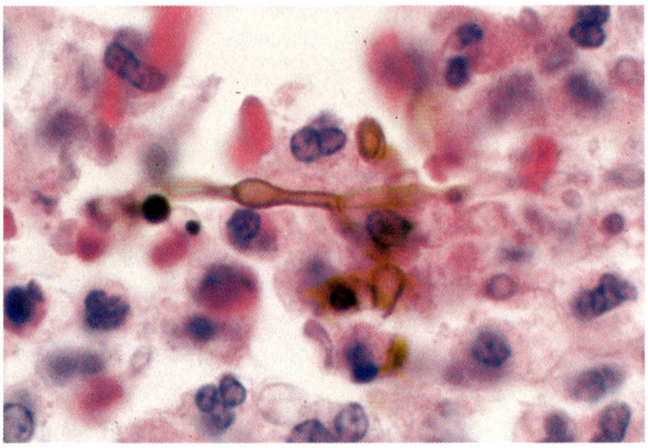

159 Pulmonary phaeohyphomycosis Another field in **158** showing masses of hyphae morphologically resembling the *Candida sp*. in **150**. (GMS, ×200)

160 Pulmonary phaeohyphomycosis Higher magnification of **159** to illustrate detailed morphology of the dematiaceous pathogen. (GMS, ×500)

161 Pulmonary phaeohyphomycosis Higher magnification of **157** to show detailed appearance of this unknown fungus when stained by H&E. Since its mycelium is dematiaceous, it is obviously not a *Candida sp*. (H&E, ×500)

162

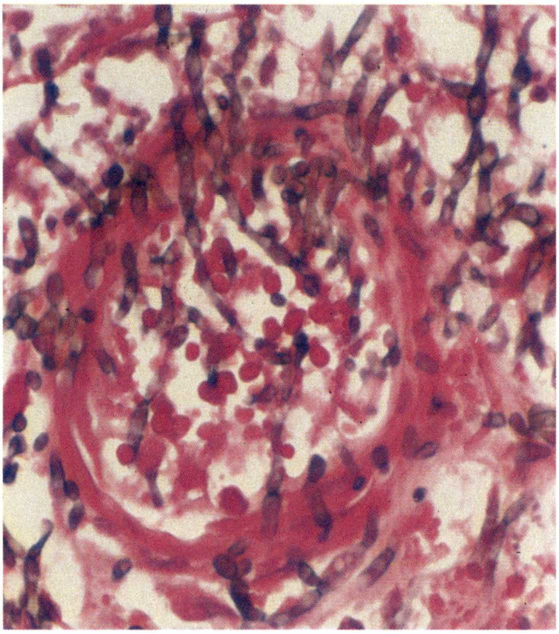

162 Candida albicans causing preterminal oesophagitis in a human. Note invasion of a blood vessel in the submucosa. Angioinvasion may lead to thrombosis and widespread dissemination of the infection. (GMS–H&E, ×200)

163

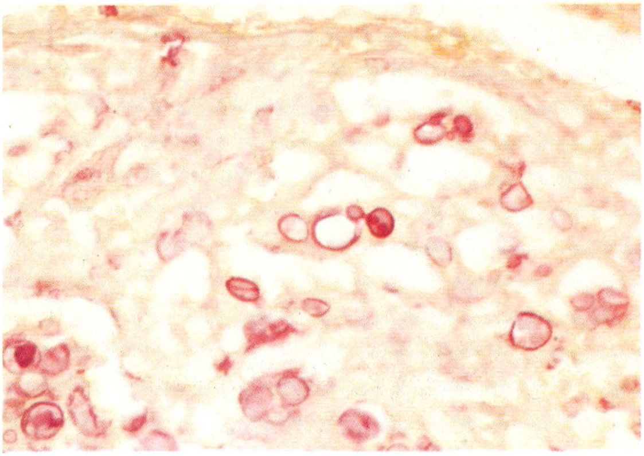

163 Candida sp. causing canine granulomatous splenitis. The distorted blastospores are variably stained. Morphologically, it would be difficult to identify this fungus as a *Candida sp*. (GF, ×200)

164

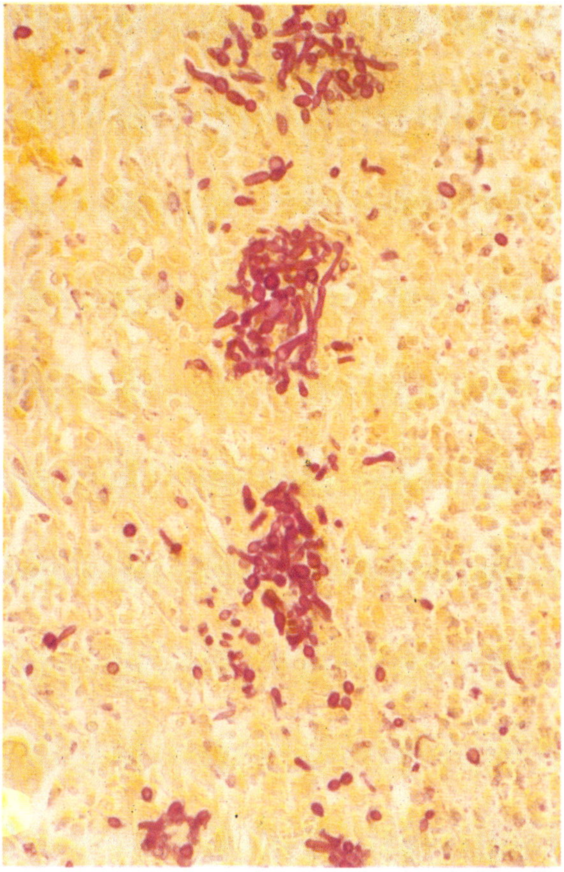

165

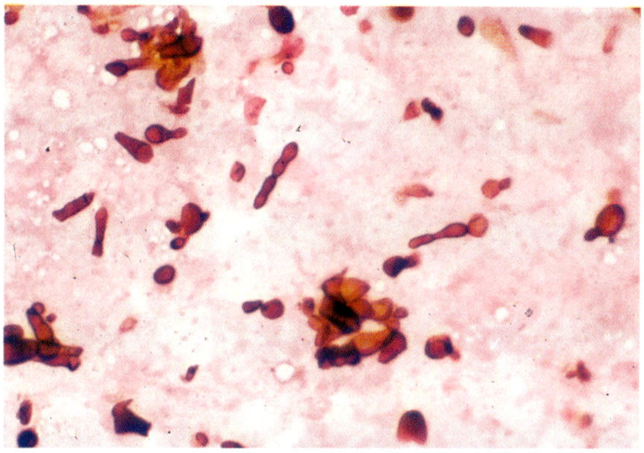

164 Chronic renal candidiasis Aggregates of *Candida albicans* cells within large giant cells in the granulomatous wall of a renal abscess. Although most of the fungal elements are intracellular, typical forms can still be identified. (GF, ×100)

165 Chronic renal candidiasis Another area in **164** with budding cells, short chains of blastospores, and pseudohyphal fragments of *Candida albicans* in the necrotic centre of a renal abscess. (GMS–H&E, ×200)

166

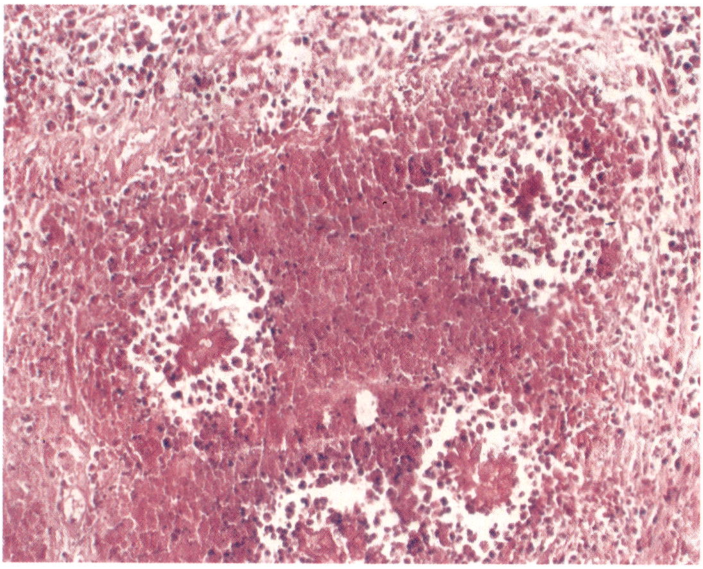

166 Candida albicans causing chronic granulomatous hepatitis in a human. The necrotic and purulent exudate in the centre of a large granuloma contains clusters of fungus cells that are surrounded by abundant Splendore–Hoeppli material. (H&E, ×50)

167

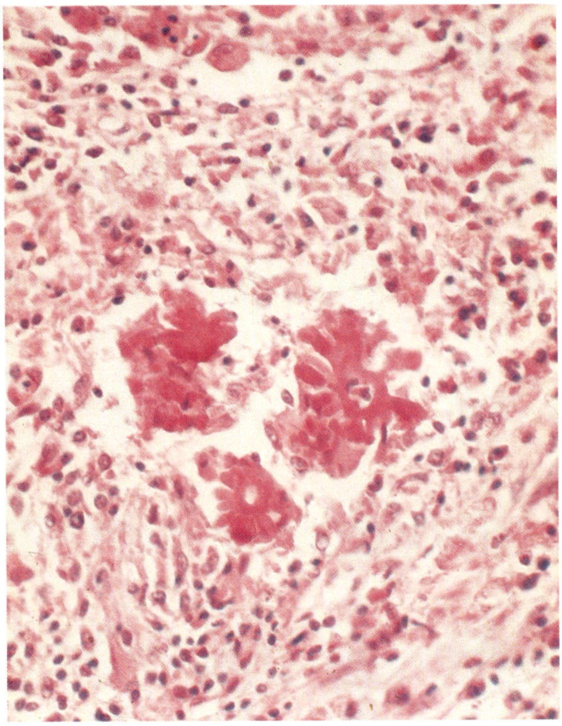

168

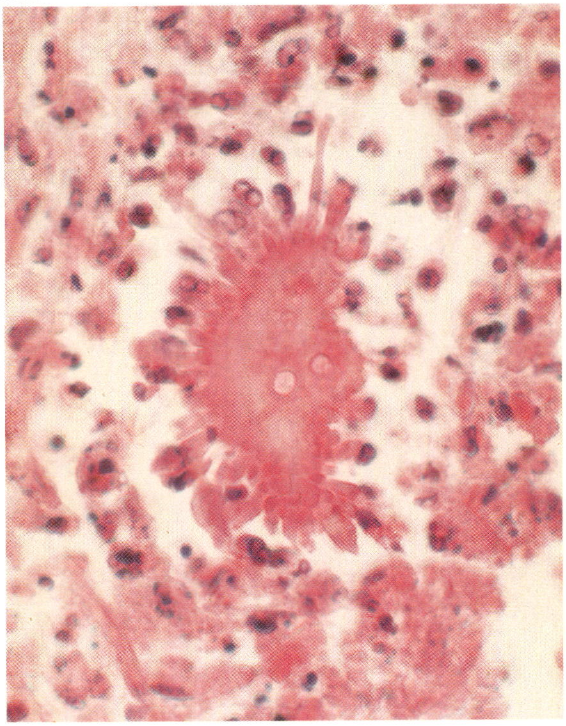

167 Candida albicans Another field in **166** showing several fungal cells surrounded by deeply eosinophilic Splendore–Hoeppli material. The granuloma, composed of histiocytes and giant cells, is enveloped by a fibrotic wall. (H&E, ×100)

168 Candida albicans Higher magnification of another field in **166** to show details of abundant Splendore–Hoeppli material around two *Candida albicans* cells. The asteroid body has eosinophilic peripheral rays of uneven length. It is unusual to find asteroid formation in candidiasis. (H&E, ×200)

169

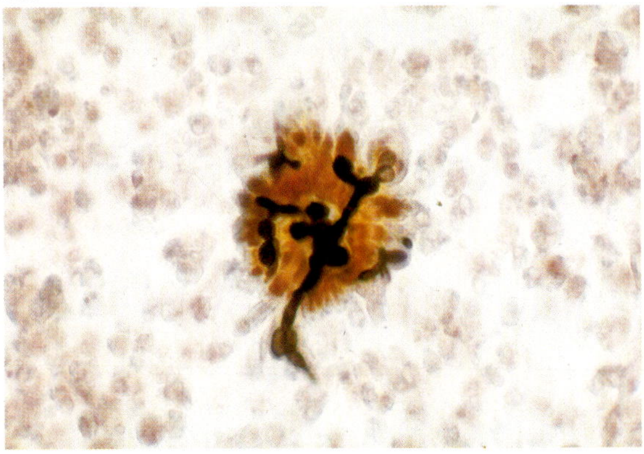

170

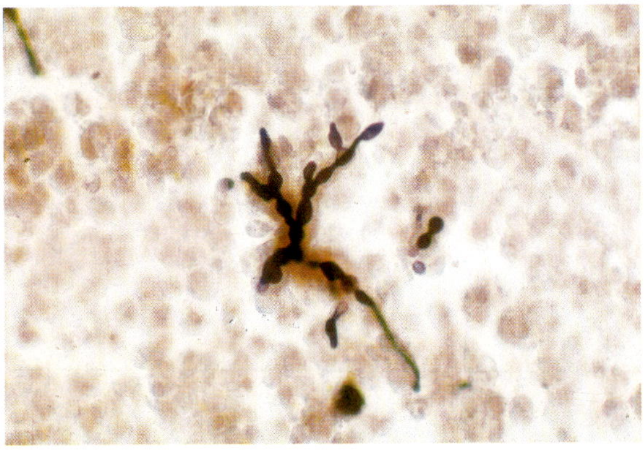

169 Candida albicans Replicate section of **168**. Portions of the deeply stained pseudohyphae and blastospores of *Candida albicans* are embedded in lightly stained Splendore–Hoeppli material. (GMS, ×200)

170 Candida albicans Another field in **169** showing branched chains of pseudohyphae and a few blastospores that are partially surrounded by poorly stained Splendore–Hoeppli material. (GMS, ×200)

171

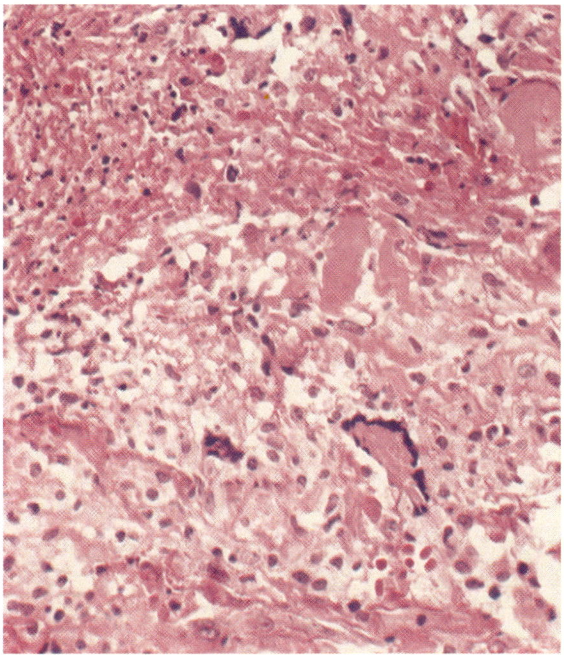

172

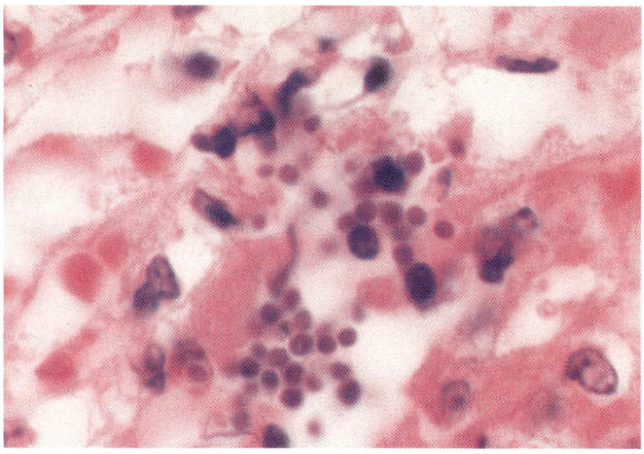

172 Candida (Torulopsis) glabrata Necrotic lesion in subcutaneous tissue of human. The lesion contains clusters of *Candida (Torulopsis) glabrata* cells. Note that the yeast cells are both intracellular and extracellular, and that their basophilic cytoplasm is readily visible. (H&E, ×500)

171 Candida (Torulopsis) glabrata causing granulomatous pneumonia in a human. Note the giant cells and areas of necrosis. Fungus cells are not visible at this magnification. (H&E, ×100)

173

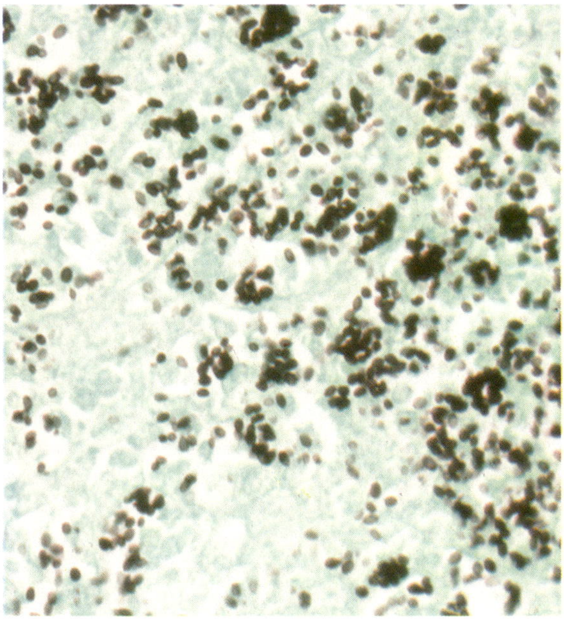

174

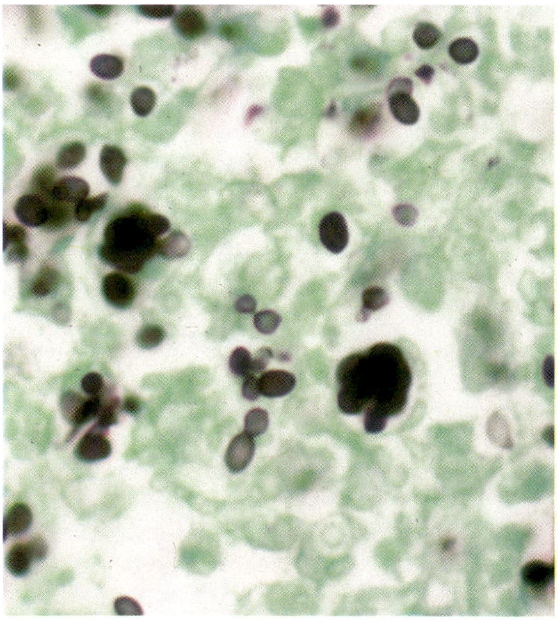

173 Candida (Torulopsis) glabrata Replicate section of **171**. Numerous yeast cells are seen, some of which appear in clusters while others are scattered in the lesion. Note their close resemblance to *Histoplasma capsulatum* var. *capsulatum*. The fluorescent antibody technique can be used to differentiate these two fungi in tissue. (GMS, ×200)

174 Candida (Torulopsis) glabrata Higher magnification of **173** to show details of cells. Again, note the clustering of fungal cells within phagocytes, as well as individual fungal cells, some of which are budding. This histological picture closely resembles that of acute histoplasmosis capsulati. (GMS, ×500)

9 Chromoblastomycosis

Text pages: 47–49

175

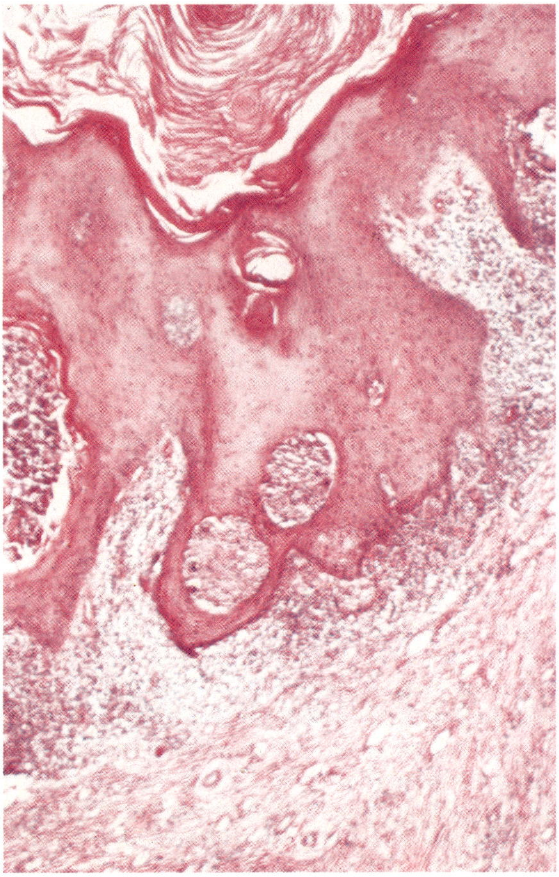

176

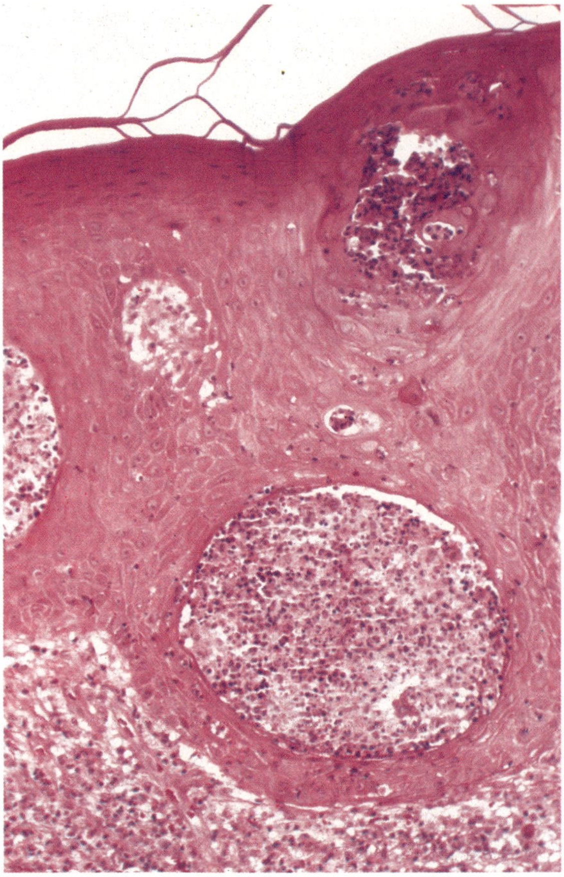

175 Cutaneous chromoblastomycosis in a human. Note the hyperkeratosis, pseudoepitheliomatous hyperplasia, and intraepidermal microabscesses. There is a mixed granulomatous and purulent inflammatory reaction in the dermis. (H&E, ×20)

176 Cutaneous chromoblastomycosis in another human. There are microabscesses in the acanthotic epidermis and a mixed inflammatory reaction in the underlying dermis. (H&E, ×50)

177

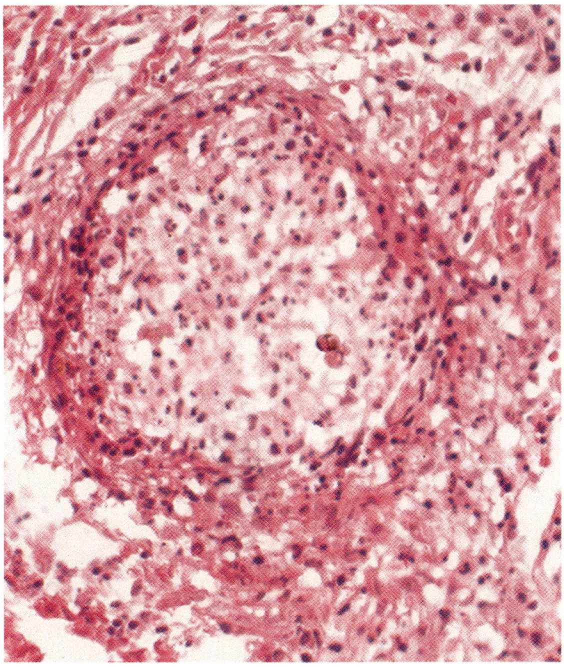

177 Cutaneous chromoblastomycosis Another field in **176** that shows a dermal abscess containing brown sclerotic bodies. The abscess is surrounded by a concentric zone of granulation tissue. (H&E, ×100)

178

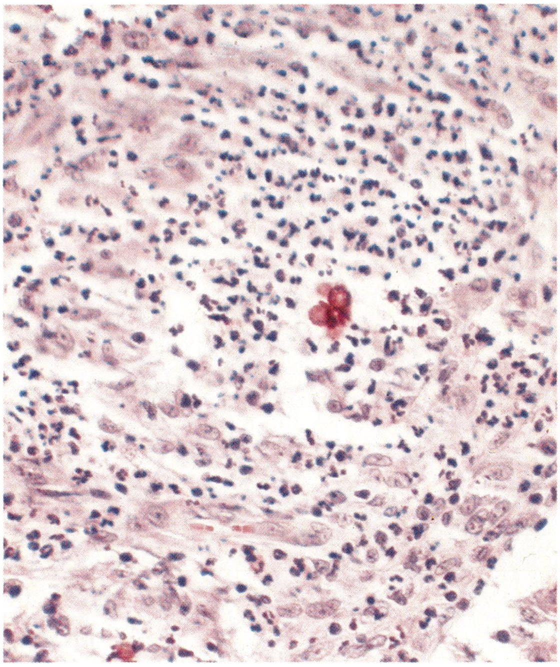

178 Phialophora verrucosa causing chromoblastomycosis of the skin of the elbow. A dermal microabscess contains a cluster of dematiaceous sclerotic bodies and is surrounded by a granulomatous reaction. (H&E, ×100)

179

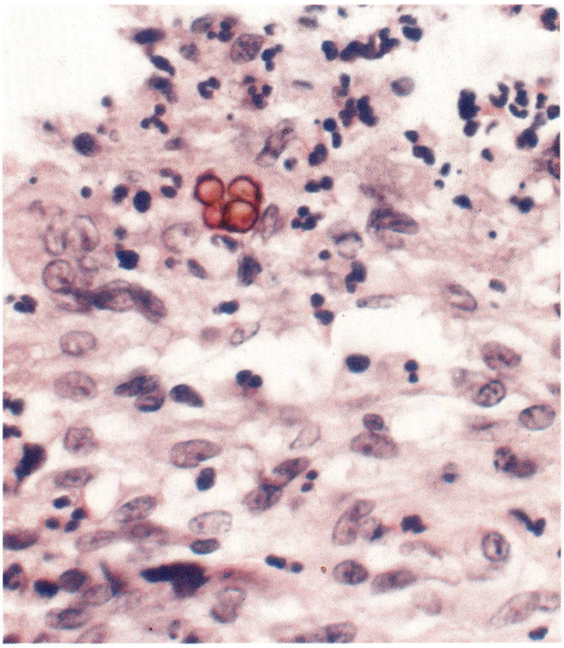

179 Phialophora verrucosa Higher magnification of **178** showing a cluster of dematiaceous sclerotic bodies intimately surrounded by neutrophils in the centre of a granuloma. The innate brown colour of the fungus makes special stains unnecessary. (H&E, ×200)

180

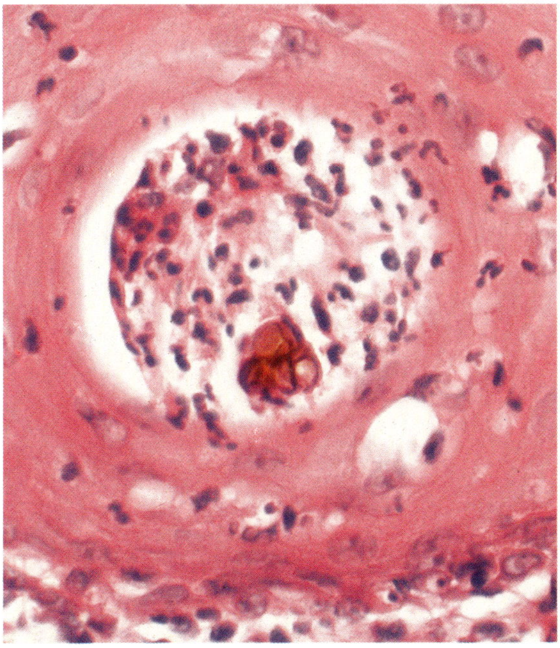

180 Chromoblastomycosis in a Brazilian. An intra-epidermal microabscess contains a cluster of sclerotic bodies. There is a mixed inflammatory reaction in the underlying dermis. (H&E, ×200)

181

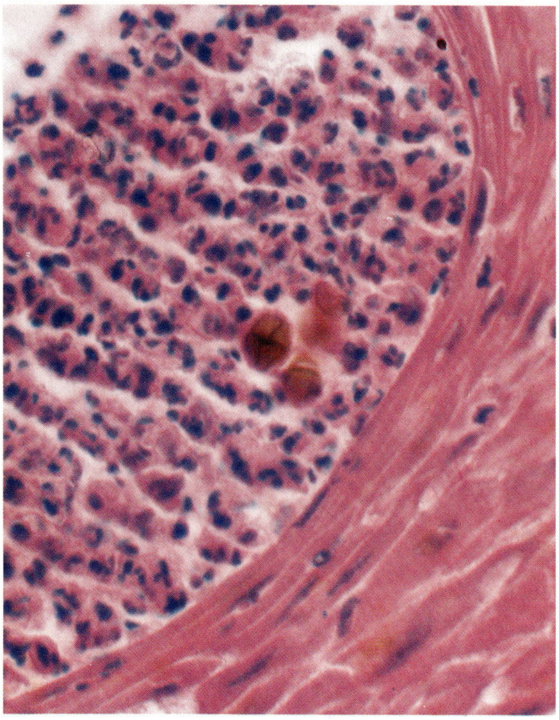

182

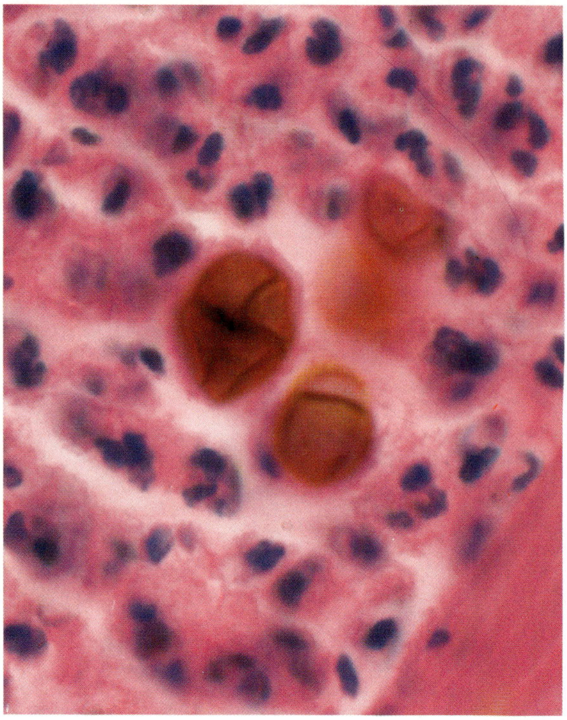

181 Cutaneous chromoblastomycosis in a Cuban. A large intraepidermal abscess contains the diagnostic brown sclerotic bodies. One of the sclerotic bodies is septate in two planes. (H&E, ×200)

182 Cutaneous chromoblastomycosis Higher magnification of **181** to show details of the muriform tissue-form cells characteristic of chromoblastomycosis. The brown colour of the sclerotic bodies is clearly seen. (H&E, ×500)

183

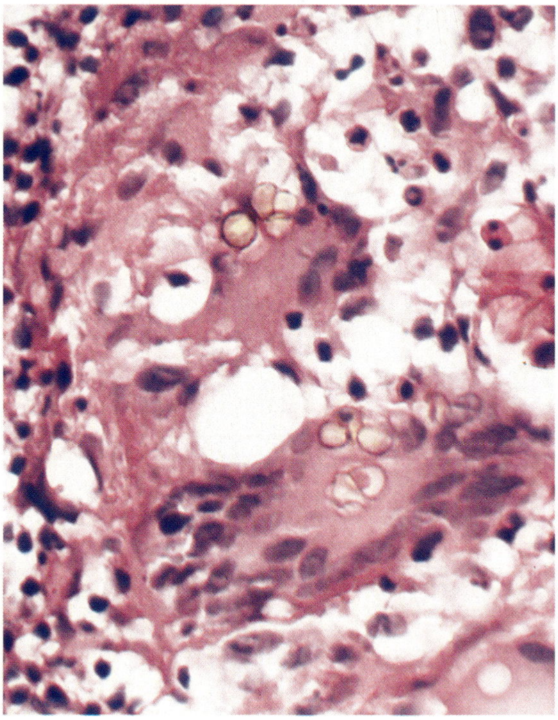

183 Chromoblastomycosis in a human. Note the groups of dematiaceous fungus cells within Langhans' giant cells in the dermis. Septations are not evident in these sclerotic cells. (H&E, ×200)

184

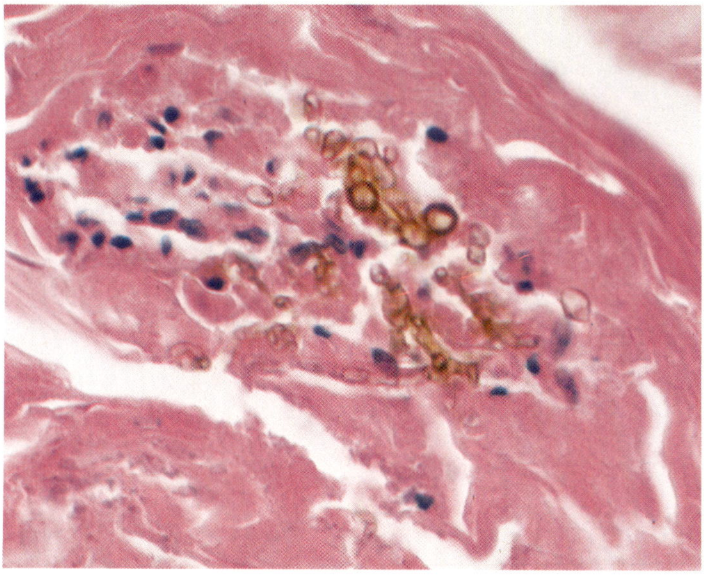

184 Cutaneous chromoblastomycosis in a Cuban. Branched, septate, dematiaceous hyphae and a few thick-walled sclerotic cells are seen in the superficial hyperkeratotic layer of the skin. (H&E, ×200)

185

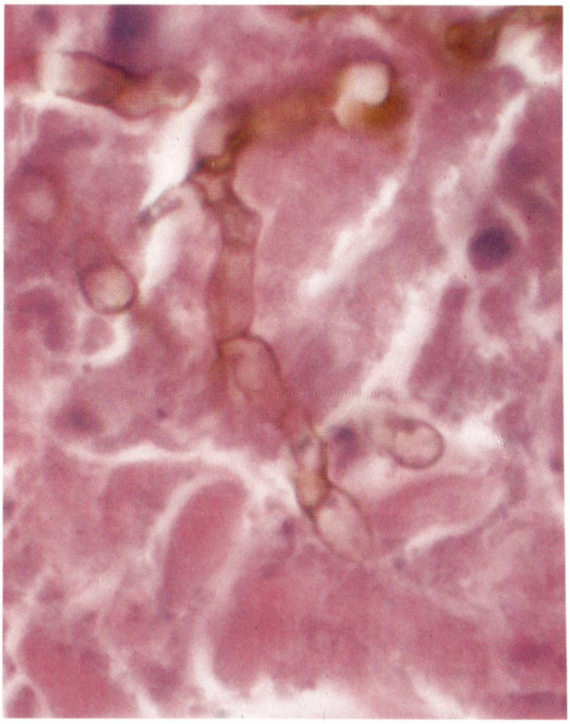

185 Cutaneous chromoblastomycosis Higher magnification of another field in **184** showing details of the branched, septate, dematiaceous hyphae embedded in the keratin layer of the skin. (H&E, ×500)

10 Coccidioidomycosis

Text pages: 50–53

186

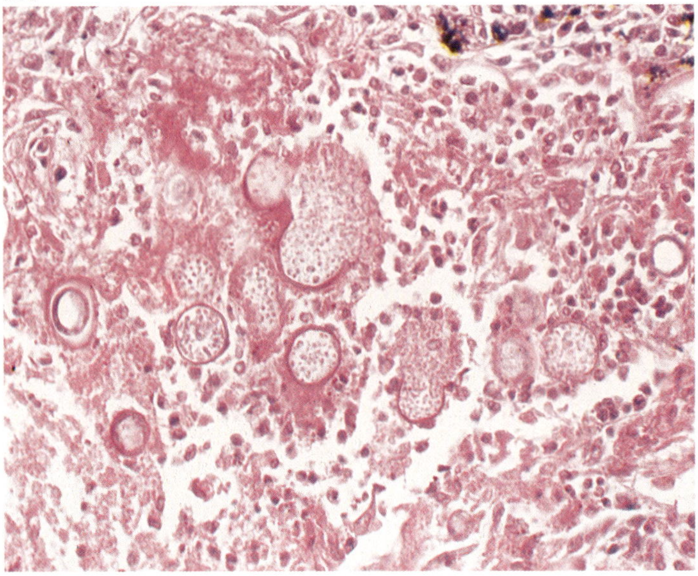

186 Coccidioides immitis causing granulomatous pneumonia in a human. Numerous spherules, many of which contain endospores, are seen. The walls of some of the spherules are ruptured, and endospores have been released. The H&E stain is generally adequate for demonstrating *Coccidioides immitis* in tissue. (H&E, ×50)

187

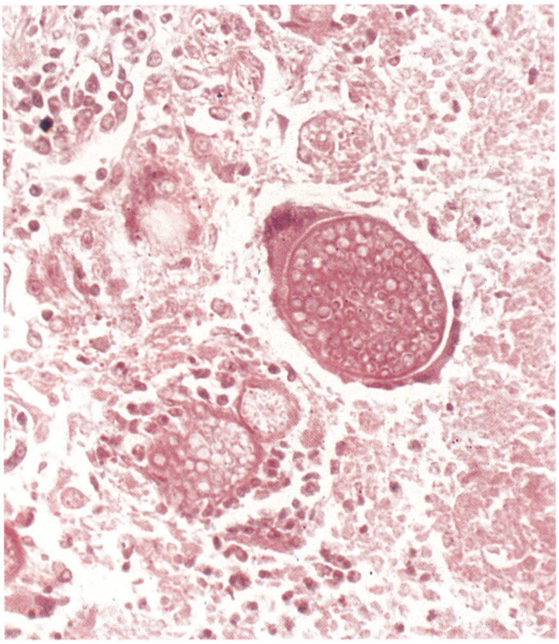

188

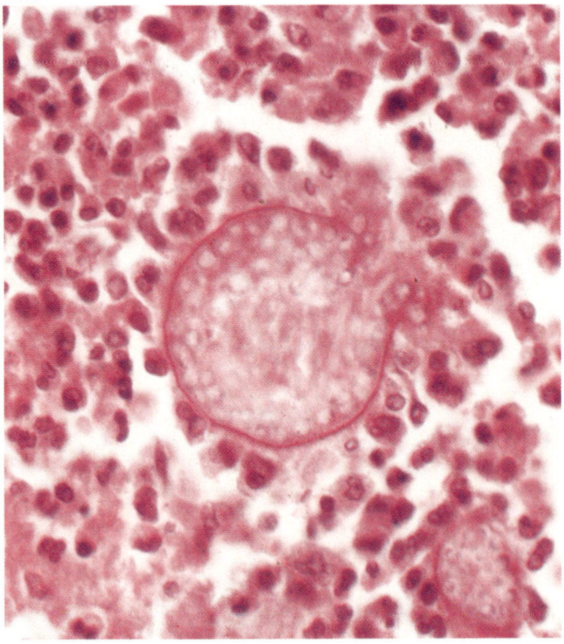

187 Coccidioides immitis Higher magnification of another field in **186** showing the diagnostic endosporulating spherules in greater detail. The larger intact spherule is being phagocytised by a giant cell. The wall of another spherule is ruptured and endospores are in the process of being released. (H&E, ×100)

188 Coccidioides immitis was the infectious agent in this acute inflammation of the human lung. A typical mature spherule surrounded by neutrophils is present. The eosinophilic wall of the spherule is broken, and several endospores have been released. (H&E, ×200)

189

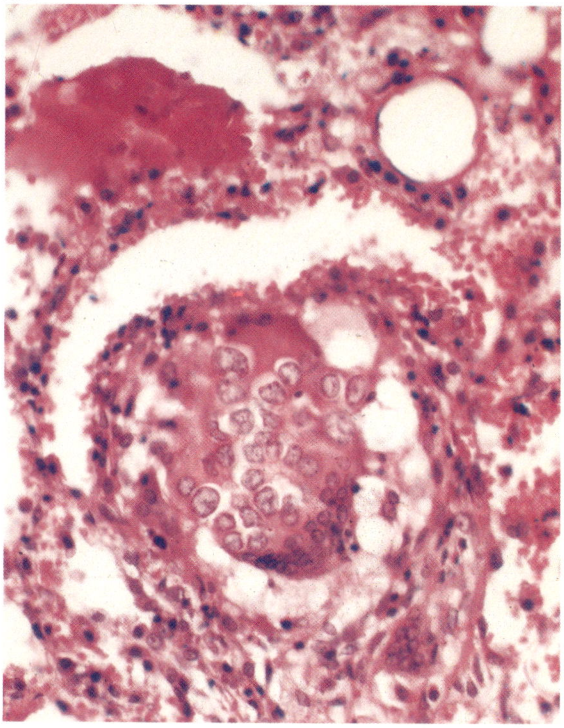

190

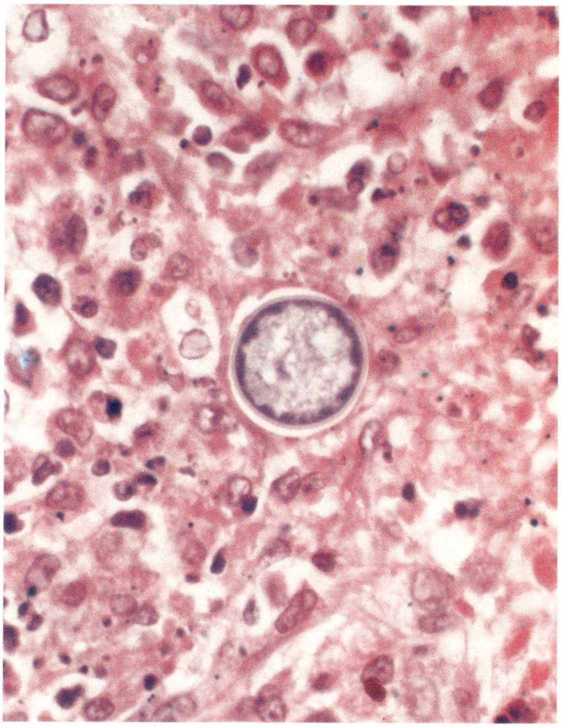

189 Coccidioides immitis causing granulomatous pneumonia in another human. A cluster of immature spherules is within a huge giant cell. Demonstration of immature spherules alone is not a sufficient basis for making a histological diagnosis of coccidioidomycosis. (H&E, ×100)

190 Coccidioides immitis causing granulomatous lymphadenitis in a human. Present is a single immature spherule whose granular basophilic cytoplasm is slightly retracted from the cell wall. At this stage of development, the morphology is not diagnostic for *Coccidioides immitis*. (H&E, ×200)

191

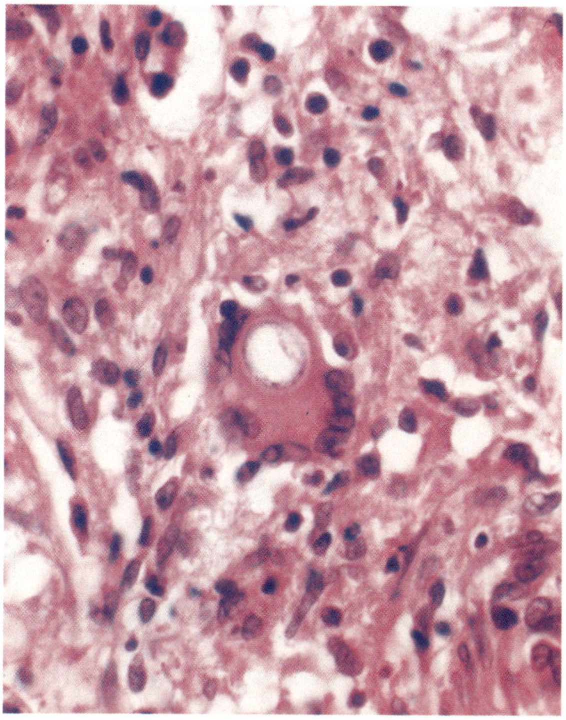

191 Pulmonary coccidioidomycosis in a human. A single immature spherule is seen within a Langhans' giant cell in an area of granulomatous pneumonia. (H&E, ×200)

192

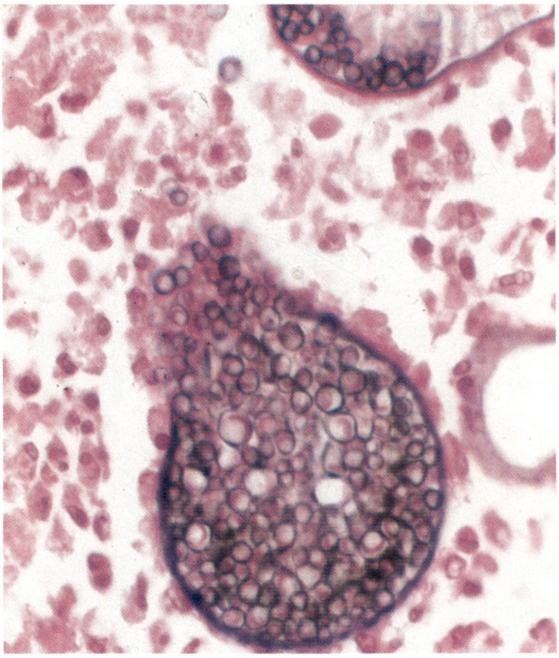

193

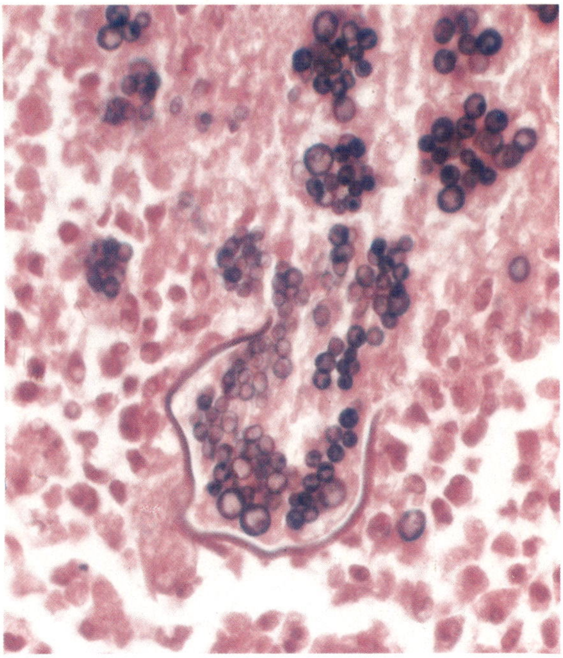

192 Coccidioides immitis causing acute inflammation of human lung. The wall of the spherule, its endospores, and the background tissue response are well demonstrated. (GMS–H&E, ×200)

193 Coccidioides immitis Another field in **192** showing released endospores from a ruptured, partially collapsed spherule. Fungal elements are embedded in purulent and necrotic exudate. (GMS–H&E, ×200)

194

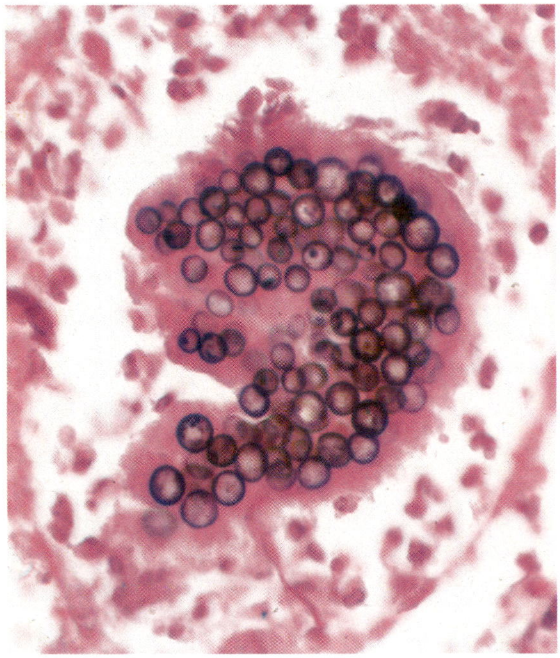

195

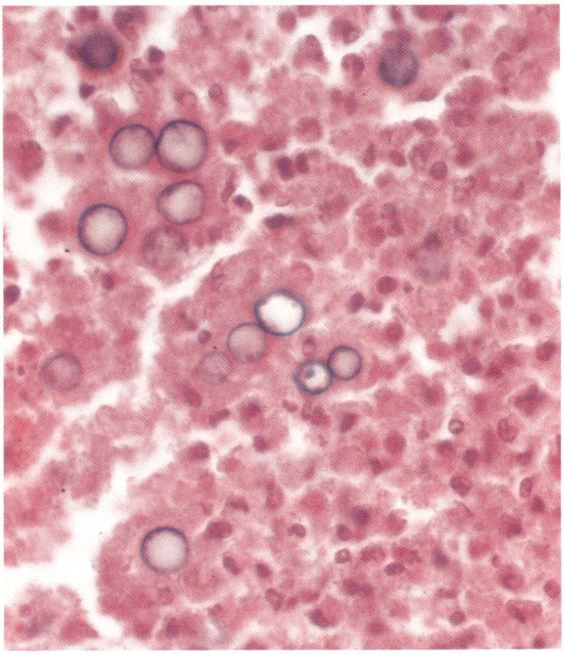

194 Coccidioides immitis Another field in **192** reveals a cluster of well stained immature spherules embedded in and surrounded by Splendore–Hoeppli material. (GMS–H&E, ×200)

195 Coccidioides immitis Large pulmonary abscess containing scattered immature spherules in a human. At this stage of their development, the spherules are not diagnostic for *Coccidioides immitis*. (GMS–H&E, ×200)

196

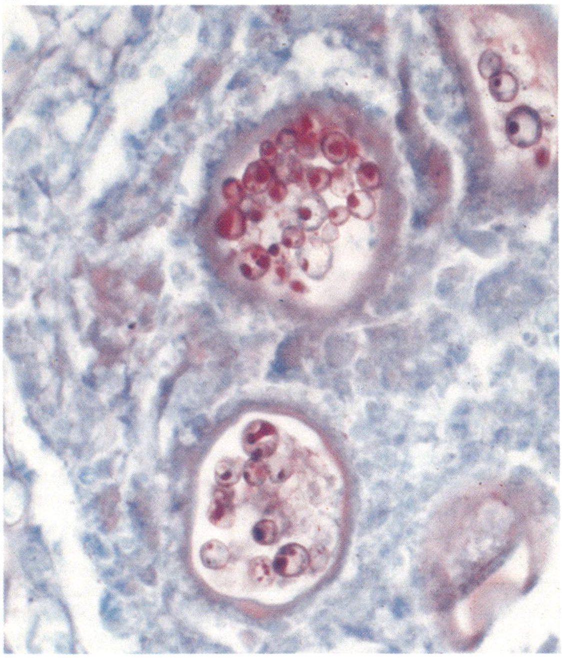

196 Coccidioides immitis Replicate section of **192**. The endospores are well stained but the wall of the spherule is not. (PAS, ×200)

197

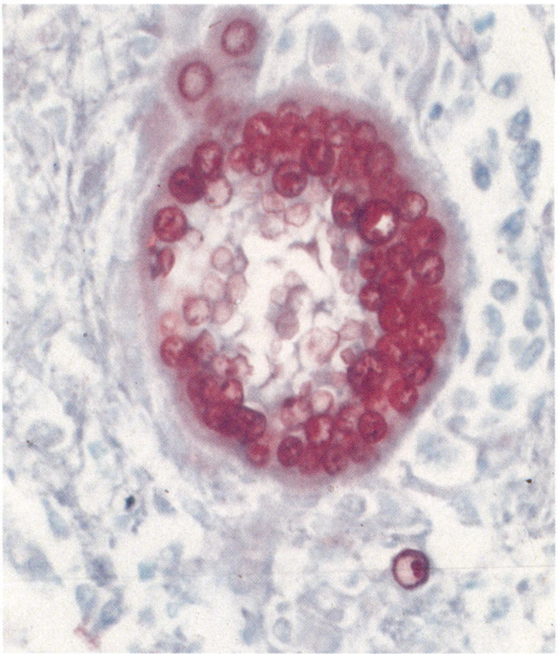

197 Coccidioides immitis Another field in **196**. Here, the wall and internal contents of endospores are well stained. By contrast, the wall of the mature spherule is not stained. PAS is excellent for demonstrating *Coccidioides immitis* in tissue; a limitation is that it does not stain the wall of the mature spherule. (PAS, ×200)

198

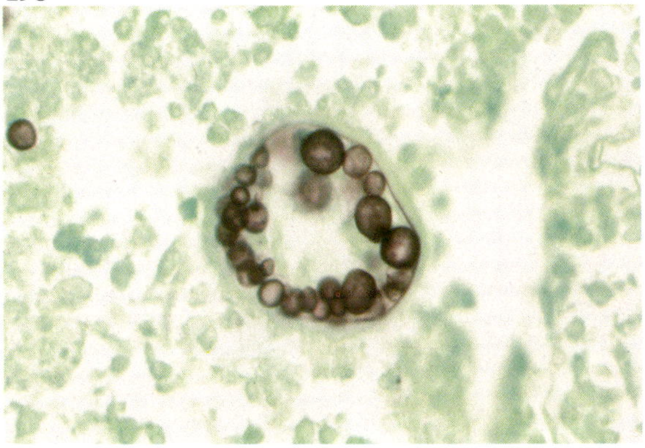

198 Coccidioides immitis Replicate section of **192** showing that both the wall of the mature spherule and its endospores stain well by GMS. However, the contents of the endospores are not as clearly defined as those stained by PAS in **197**. (GMS, ×200)

199

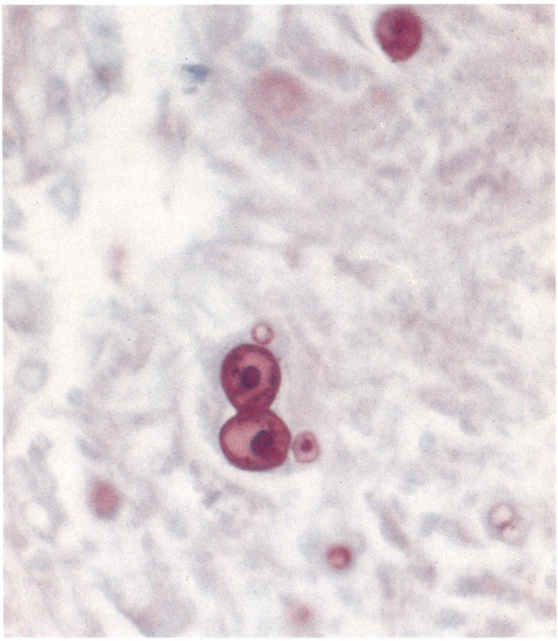

199 Coccidioides immitis Another field in **196** containing immature spherules whose walls and internal contents are well delineated. *Coccidioides immitis* in tissue does not reproduce by budding. However, when spherules are in apposition as shown in this photomicrograph, they may mimic budding yeasts. (PAS, ×200)

200

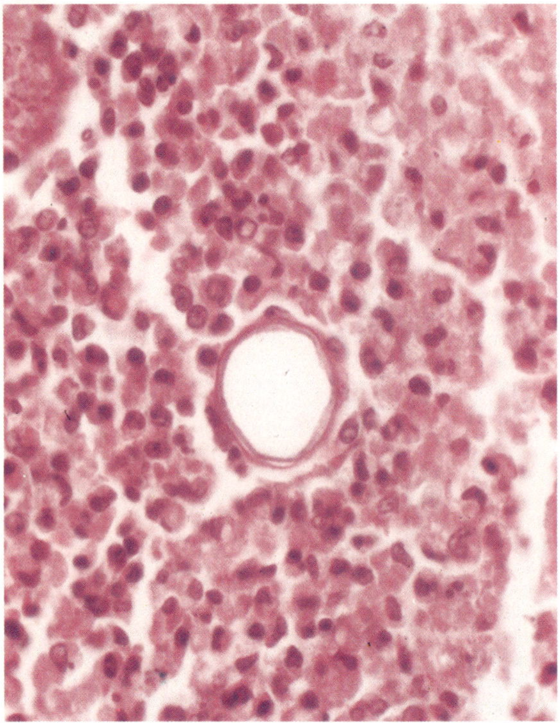

201

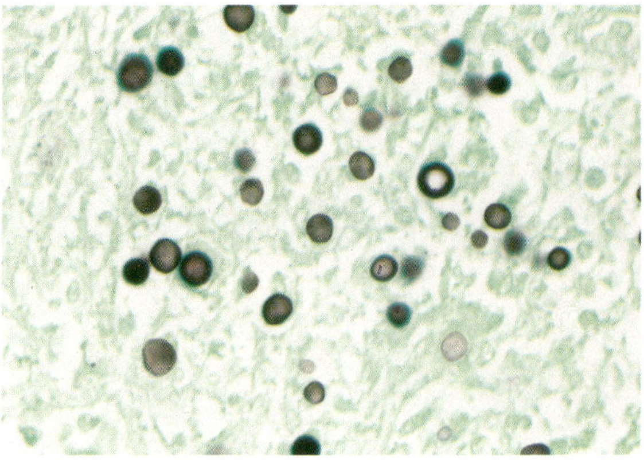

200 Pulmonary coccidioidomycosis in a human. At times, empty spherules are encountered in lesions. Such structures are not diagnostic for *Coccidioides immitis* since they may be confused with other fungi. A histopathological diagnosis is not possible if only empty spherules are present. (H&E, ×200)

201 Pulmonary coccidioidomycosis Replicate section of **200** reveals numerous immature spherules of *Coccidioides immitis* within a granulomatous lesion. (GMS, ×200)

202

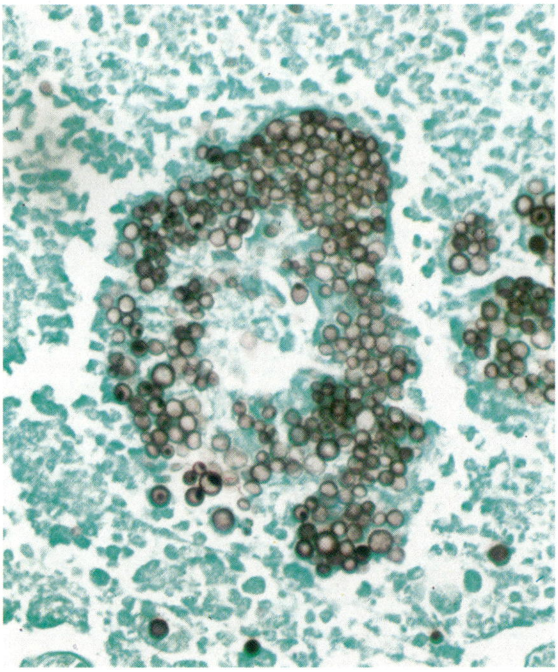

203

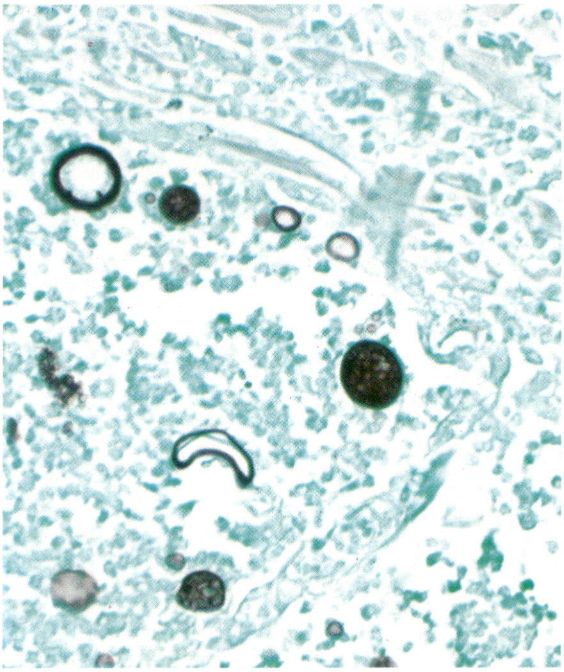

202 Pulmonary coccidioidomycosis Another field in **201** which shows masses of endospores that are not enclosed by an intact spherule wall or a fragment of one. Other fields should be searched for the presence of mature spherules in an effort to make a diagnosis. (GMS, ×100)

203 Coccidioides immitis in a human pulmonary granuloma. The variety of forms that spherules can take in tissue is well demonstrated. (GMS, ×100)

204

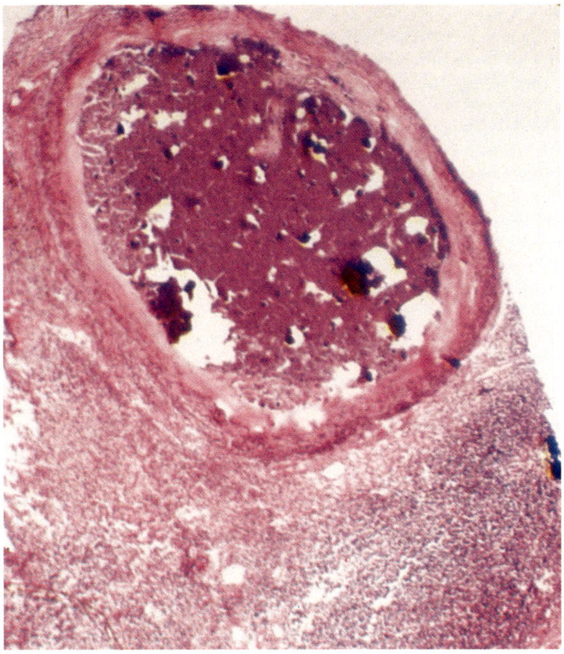

205

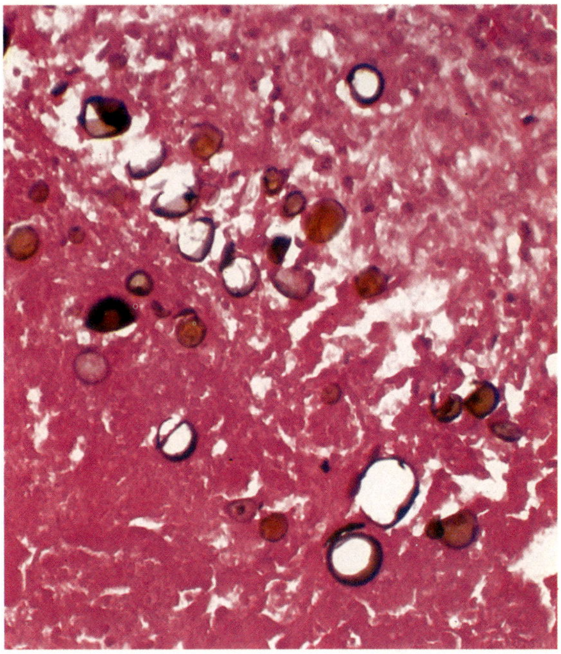

204 Coccidioidomycosis in a dog. A fibrocaseous nodule is seen in a mediastinal lymph node. Calcification of the central caseous material, as shown here, is not commonly encountered in this disease. (H&E, ×20)

205 Coccidioides immitis Fibrocaseous pulmonary nodule in a human. Distorted and empty spherules of *Coccidioides immitis* are present within the caseous material, especially near the interface of necrotic and viable tissues. (GMS–H&E, ×100)

206

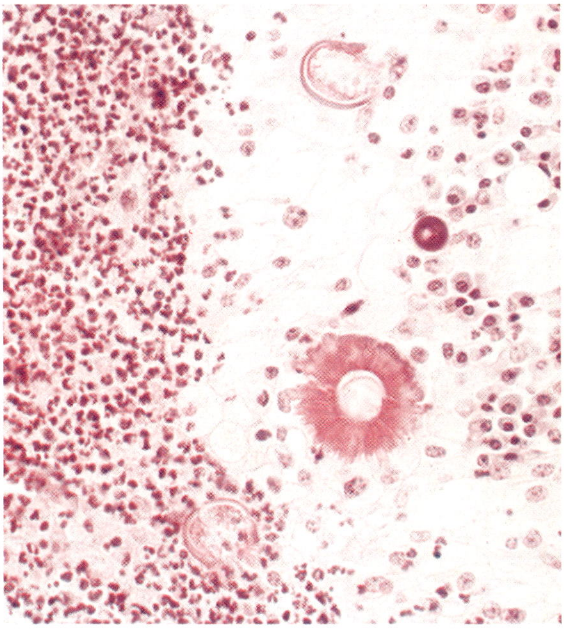

207

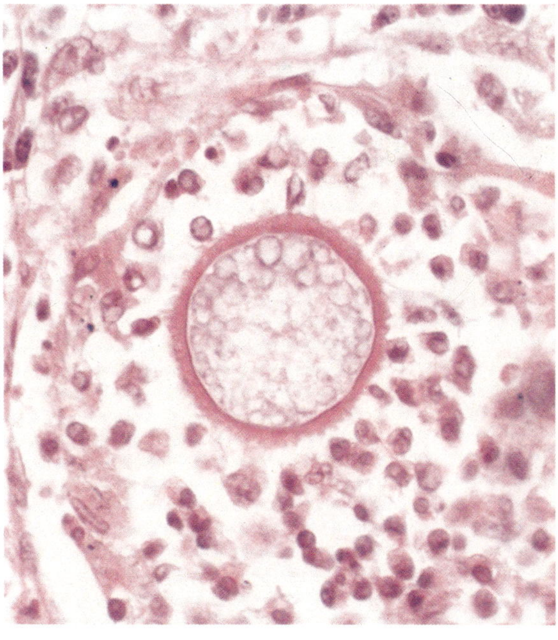

206 Coccidioides immitis causing bovine granulomatous lymphadenitis. Note the radial corona of Splendore–Hoeppli material surrounding one of the spherules. The formation of asteroid bodies is sometimes observed with *Coccidioides immitis*. (H&E, ×100)

207 Coccidioidomycosis of the human lung. Note the thin eosinophilic layer of Splendore–Hoeppli material surrounding a mature spherule. The mixed inflammatory reaction is also well demonstrated. (H&E, ×200)

208

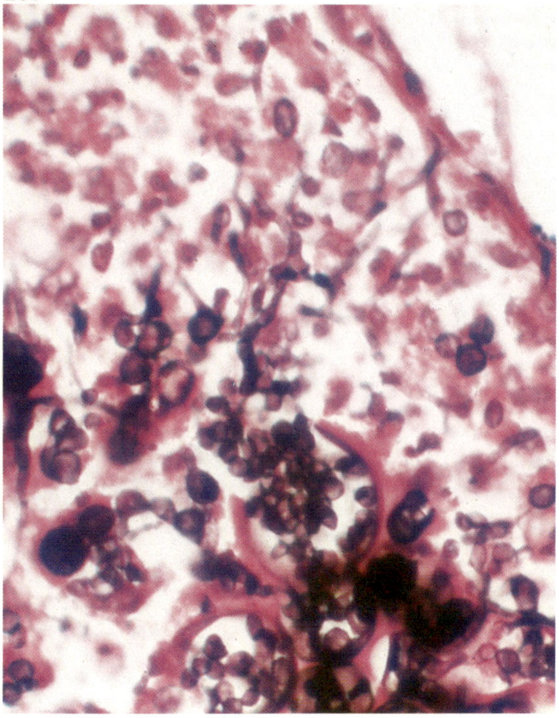

209

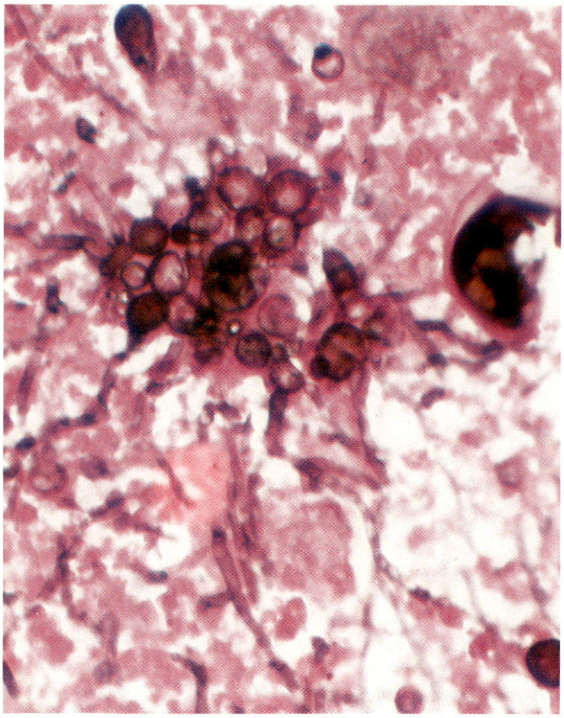

208 Coccidioides immitis Subpleural focus of granulomatous inflammation in human lung. Note that the mature spherules of *Coccidioides immitis* are ruptured and that endospores are being released. In addition, numerous endospores have germinated to form mycelium. (GMS–H&E, ×200)

209 Coccidioides immitis Another field in **208** that shows a cluster of endospores embedded in necrotic tissue. Many of the endospores have germinated to form hyphae. (GMS–H&E, ×200)

210

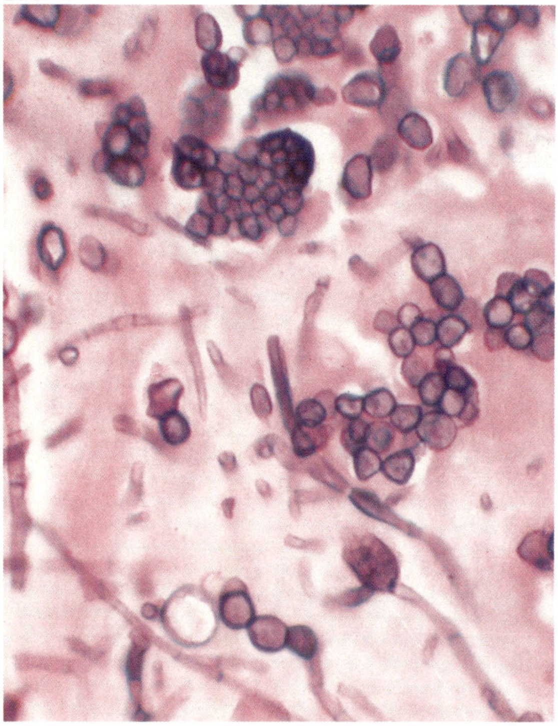

210 Coccidioides immitis in the lung of another human. Note spherules and branched, septate hyphae of *C. immitis*. Hyphal formation by this fungus is uncommon, but it is sometimes observed in cavitary and necrotic lesions. (GMS–H&E, ×200)

211

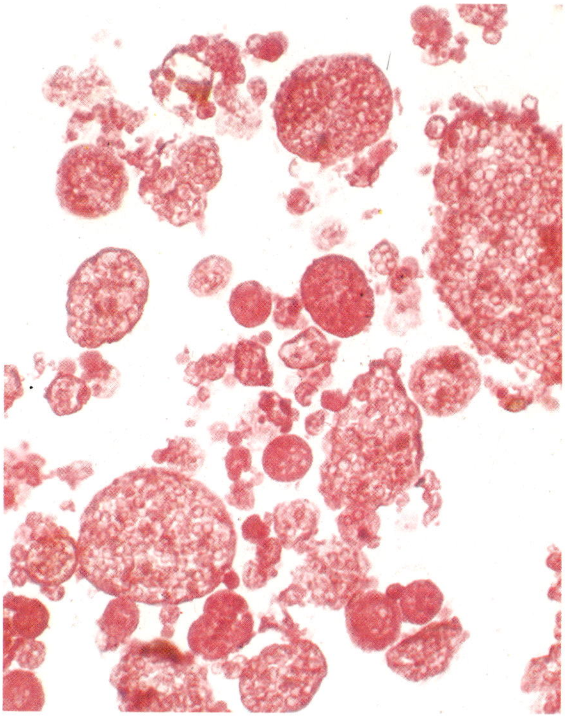

211 Myospherulosis Material curetted from surgical site in paranasal sinus of human. The structures that resemble endosporulating spherules of *Coccidioides immitis* are actually modified, degenerated red blood cells within a pseudomembrane in the phenomenon known as myospherulosis. (H&E, ×100)

212

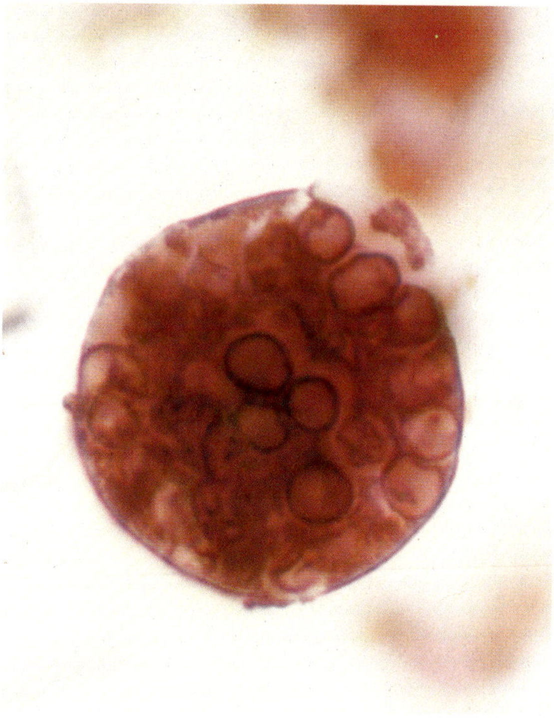

212 Myospherulosis Higher magnification of **211** showing details of the reddish-brown structures (altered red blood cells) observed in myospherulosis. (H&E, ×500)

213

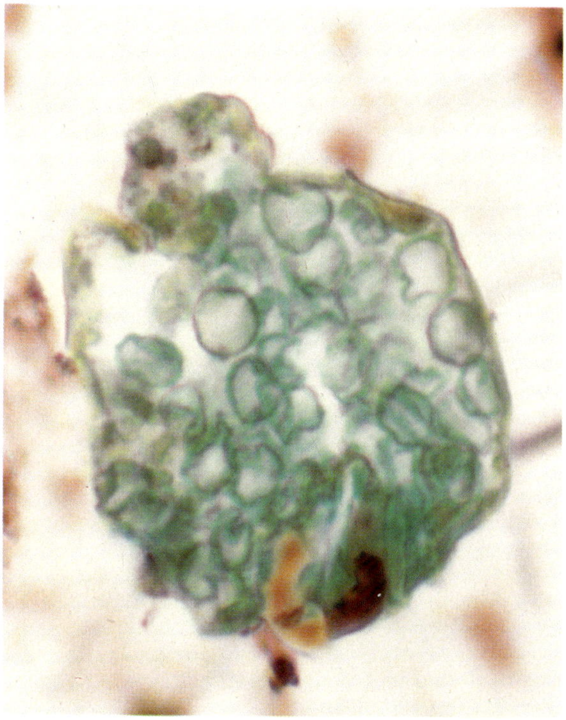

213 Myospherulosis Replicate section of **211**. Although the structures seen in myospherulosis may resemble *Coccidioides immitis* spherules when stained by H&E, they can be clearly differentiated by their failure to stain by GMS as shown in this photomicrograph. (GMS, ×500)

11 Cryptococcosis

Text pages: 54–58

214

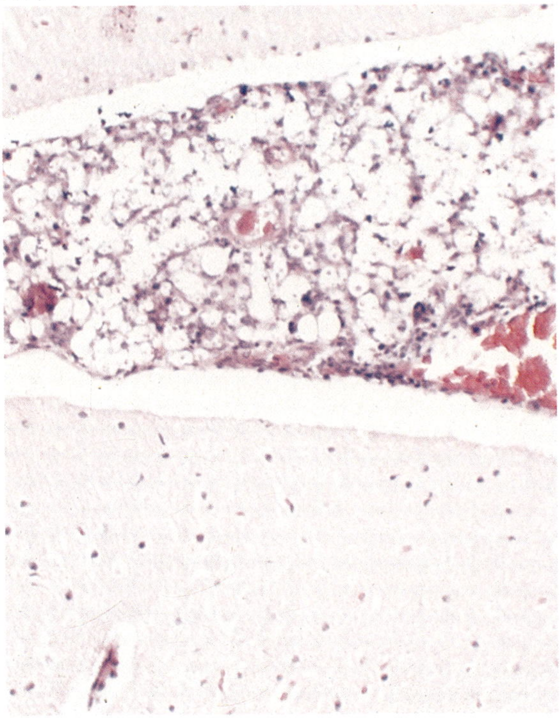

214 Cryptococcus neoformans causing feline cryptococcal meningitis. The clear spaces in the leptomeninges are masses of encapsulated *C. neoformans* cells. Inflammation is minimal, and the underlying brain parenchyma is not involved. (H&E, ×50)

215

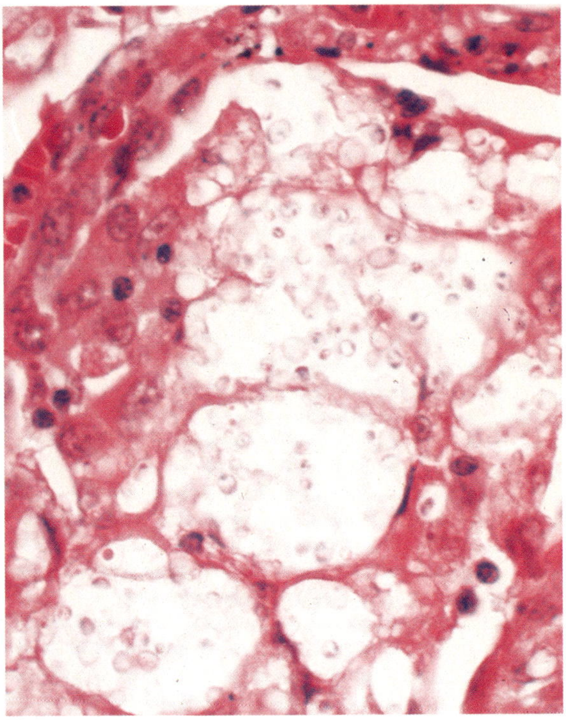

215 Cryptococcus neoformans causing cryptococcal pneumonia in a cat. Clusters of *C. neoformans* cells that are lightly basophilic fill an alveolar space and are surrounded by alveolar macrophages. There is little or no cellular reaction in the alveolar septum. (H&E, ×200)

216

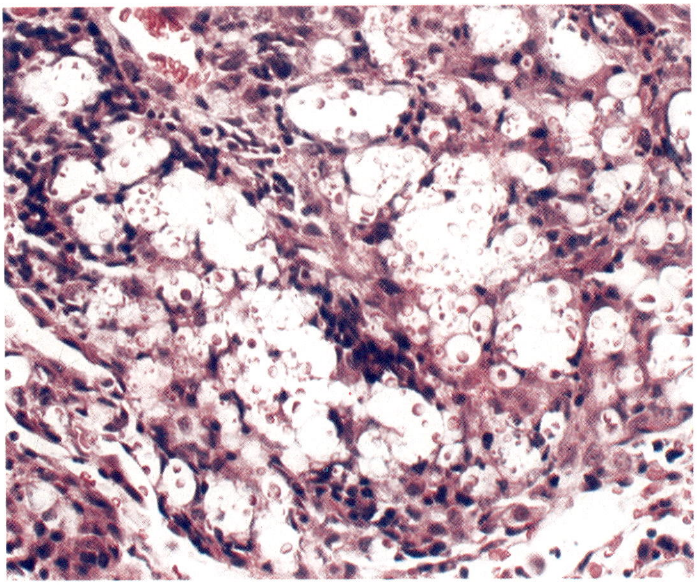

216 Cryptococcus neoformans causing granulomatous pneumonia in a dog. The clear spaces within the granulomatous lesion are masses of encapsulated fungal cells. (H&E, ×100)

217

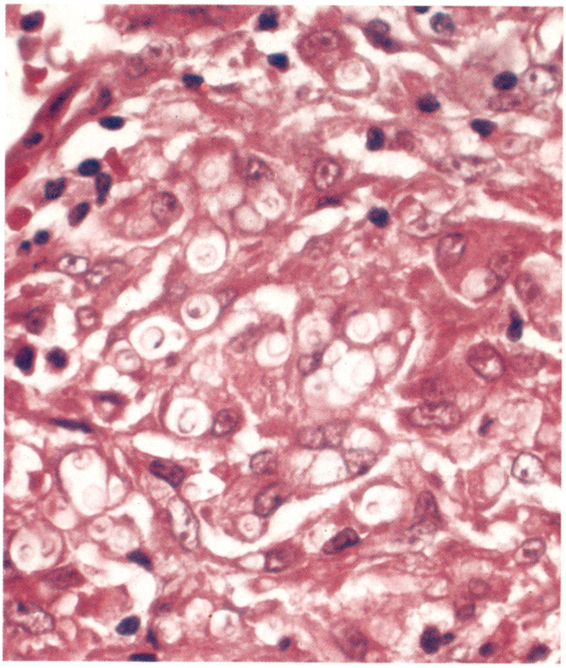

217 Cryptococcus neoformans cells within a feline pulmonary granuloma. The encapsulated yeast cells are within macrophages and giant cells. (H&E, ×200)

218

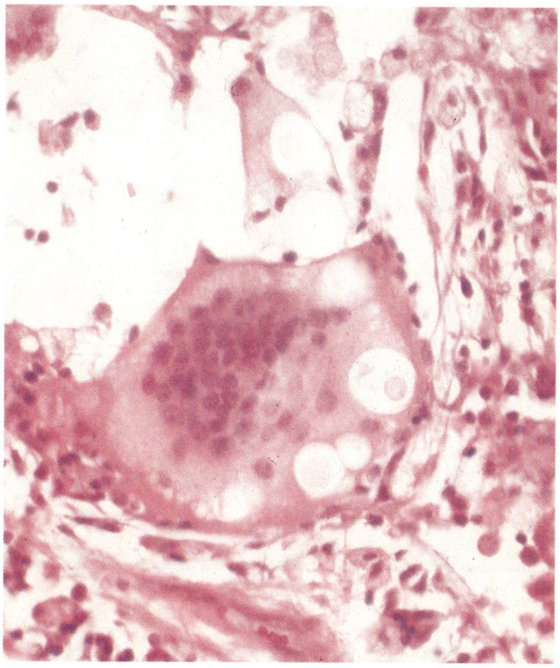

218 Cryptococcus neoformans causing granulomatous pneumonia in a human. The encapsulated fungus cells are within a huge foreign body giant cell located in an alveolar space. Alveolar septa contain mixed inflammatory cells. (H&E, ×100)

219

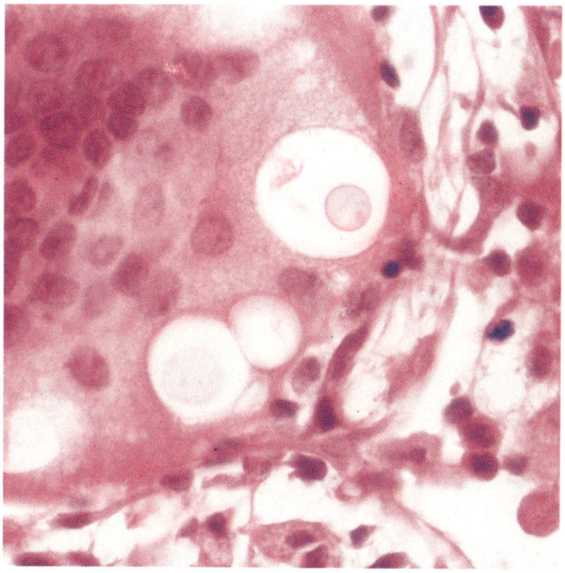

219 Cryptococcus neoformans Higher magnification of **218** showing details of the intracellular cryptococci. The fungal cells in this section are lightly eosinophilic. They are surrounded by a clear space which represents the capsular material. (H&E, ×200)

220

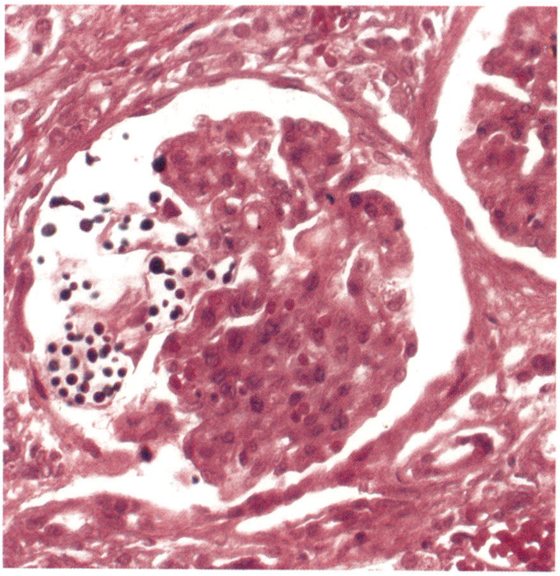

220 Cryptococcus neoformans Disseminated cryptococcosis in an immunosuppressed patient. A glomerular tuft contains numerous GMS-positive *Cryptococcus neoformans* cells. Inflammation is absent, and some fungal cells have entered the urinary space. (GMS–H&E, ×100)

221

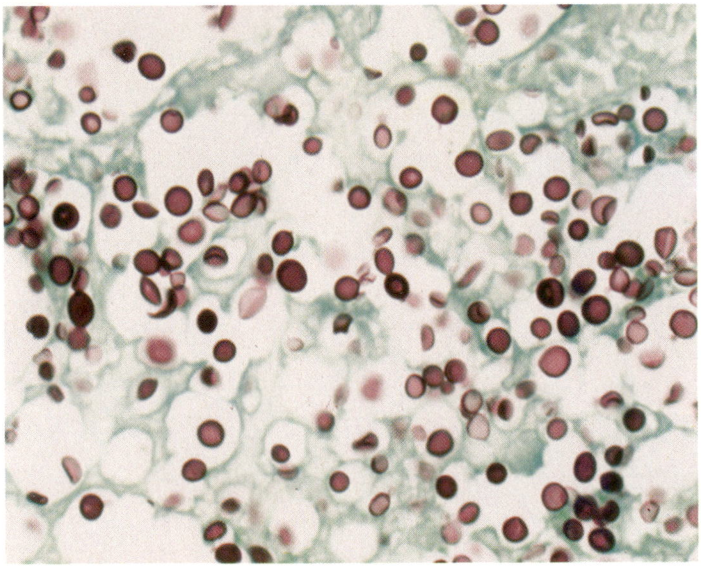

221 Cryptococcus neoformans causing cutaneous cryptococcosis in a cat. The yeast cells are deeply stained and well delineated by GMS. The clear zones represent the space occupied by their capsules. (GMS, ×200)

222

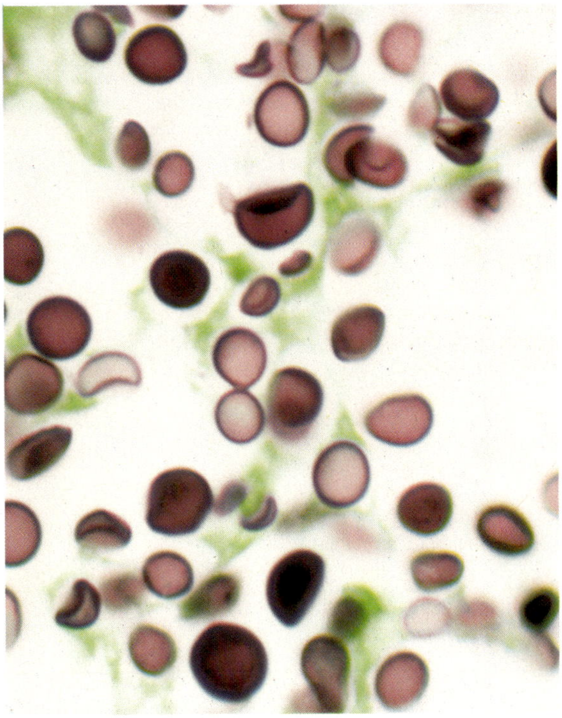

223

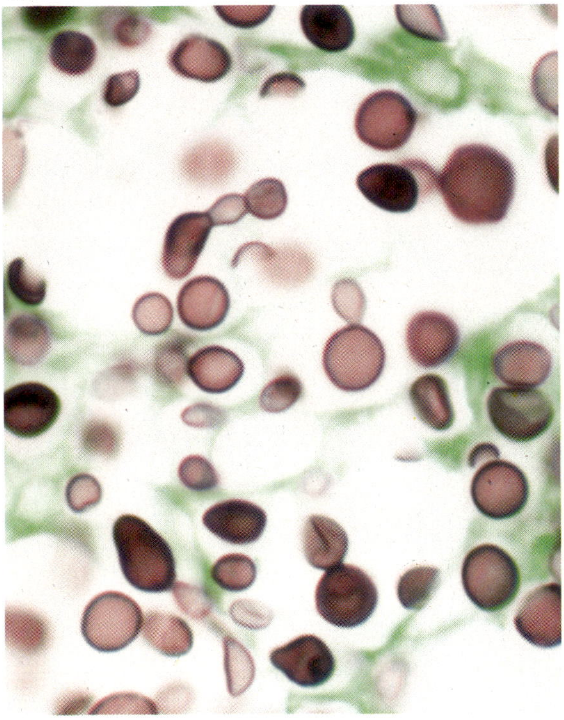

222 Cryptococcus neoformans Higher magnification of **221** showing details of the fungal cells. Note their variability in size and shape. Pleomorphic cryptococci in tissues can resemble other yeasts. (GMS, ×500)

223 Cryptococcus neoformans Another field in **222** showing cells with single buds and a narrow basal attachment to the parent cell. A chain of budding cells is also seen. (GMS, ×500)

224

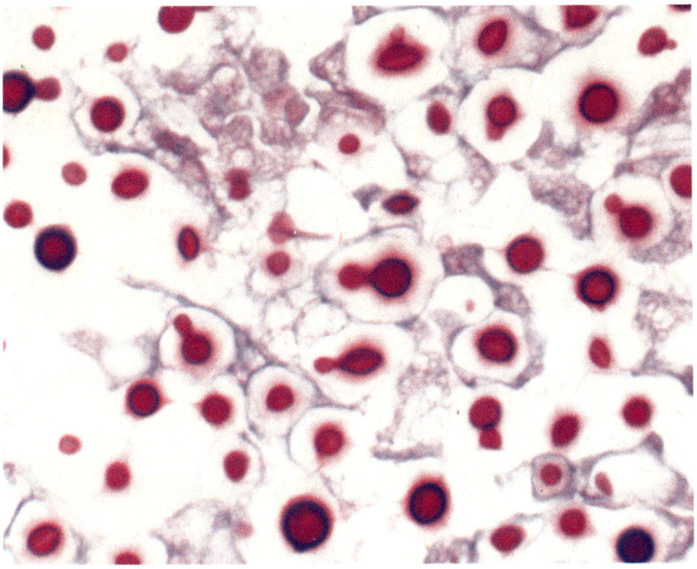

224 Cryptococcus neoformans Numerous yeast cells in a dog lung. When stained by PAS, the cryptococci are intensely coloured and some of the capsular material surrounding the cells is also stained. Note the characteristic budding. (PAS, ×200)

225

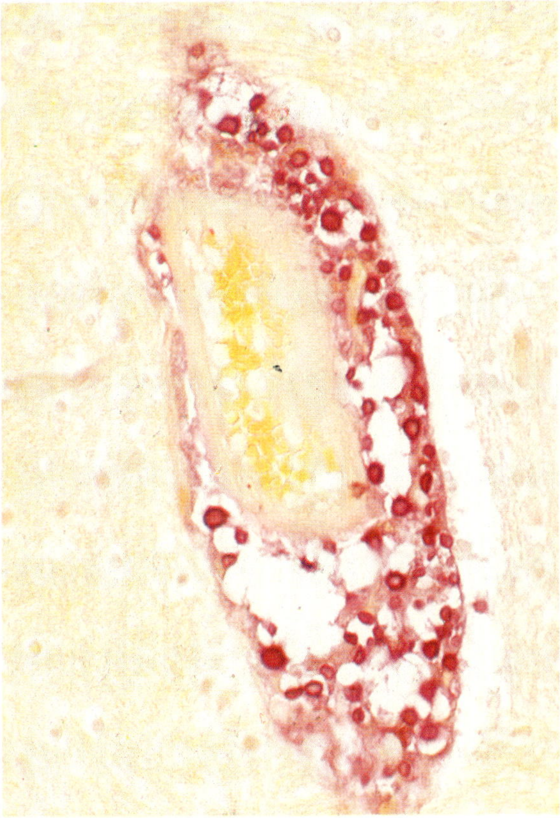

225 Cryptococci distending a perivascular space in the brain of a human. The fungal cells are well demonstrated with the mucicarmine stain. Note that the brain parenchyma is not involved. (Mayer's mucicarmine, ×100)

226

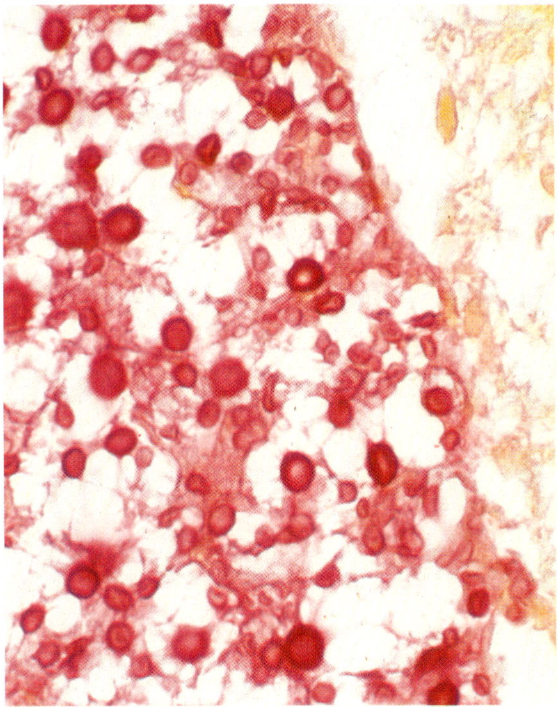

226 Cryptococcal meningitis in a human. The numerous fungal cells in the leptomeninges are well demonstrated by the mucicarmine stain. They are confined to the meninges. (Mayer's mucicarmine, ×200)

227

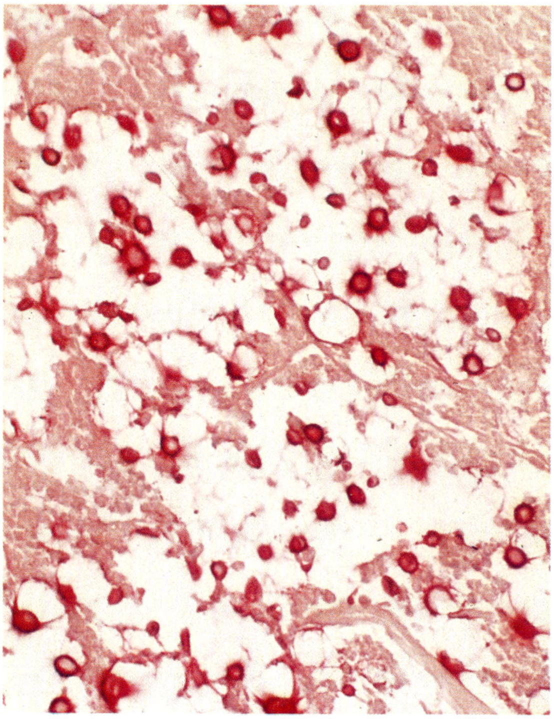

228

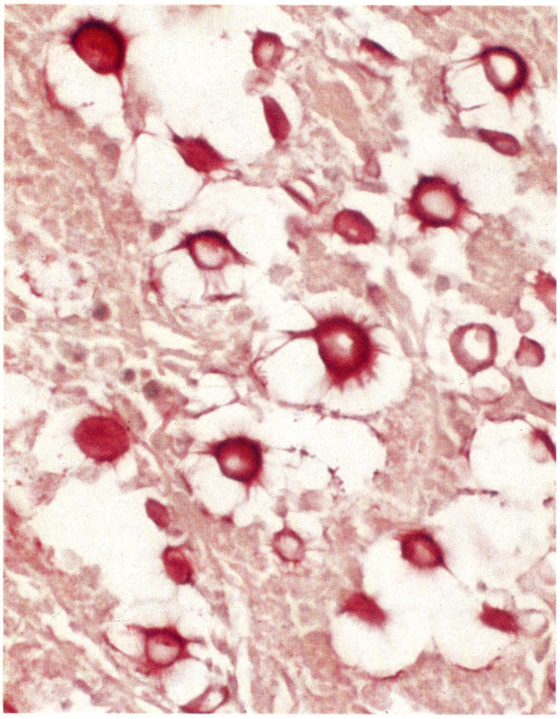

227 Cryptococcal encephalitis in a human. Note numerous fungal cells embedded in the brain parenchyma and the absence of an inflammatory response. The clear spaces surrounding the yeast cells are apparently due to shrinkage and loss of capsular material during processing. (Mayer's mucicarmine, ×100)

228 Cryptococcal encephalitis Higher magnification of **227** showing details of the cryptococci. The radiate or spiny appearance of the mucicarmine-positive capsular material is the result of shrinkage during processing of the tissue. (Mayer's mucicarmine, ×200)

229

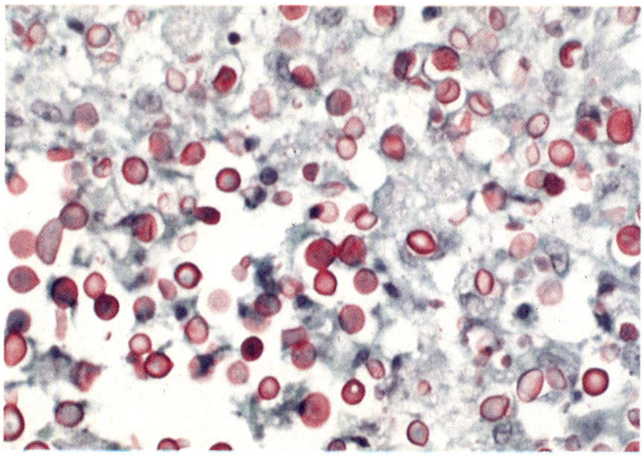

230

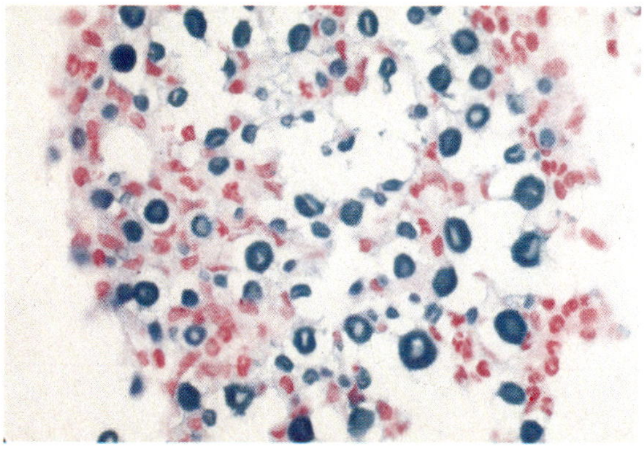

229 Cryptococcal encephalitis in a cat. Frequently, the mucicarmine-positive capsular material does not have a spiny appearance as shown in this photomicrograph. (Mayer's mucicarmine, ×200)

230 Cryptococcal encephalitis in a human. The alcian blue mucopolysaccharide stain also reacts with the capsular material of *Cryptococcus neoformans*. It can therefore be used in lieu of the mucicarmine procedure to demonstrate the encapsulated form of this fungus in tissue. (Alcian blue, ×200)

231

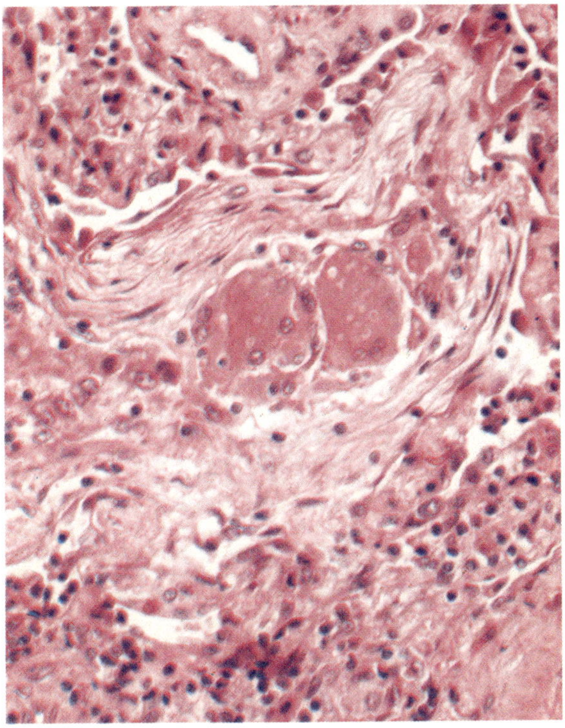

232

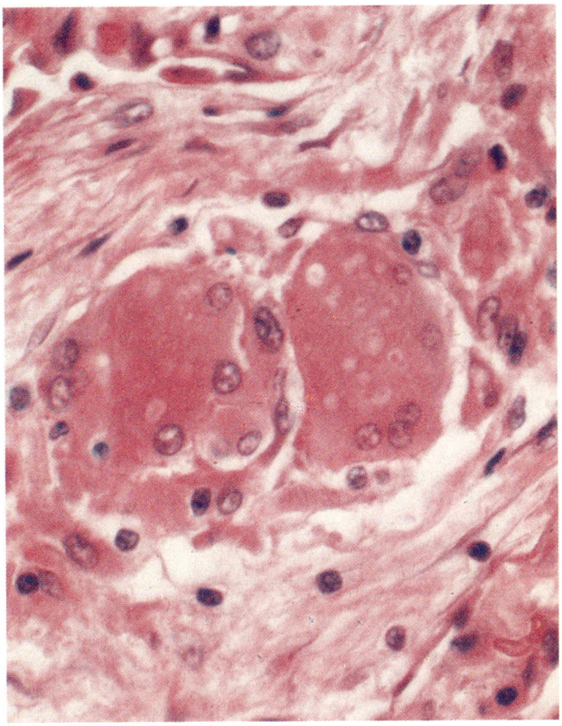

231 Cryptococcus neoformans Granulomatous pneumonia in a human. The infection was caused by a lightly encapsulated isolate of *C. neoformans*. Poorly stained cryptococci are within giant cells. (H&E, ×100)

232 Cryptococcus neoformans Higher magnification of **231** revealing the intracellular cryptococci in greater detail. No apparent capsule is seen. The clear zones surrounding the small central eosinophilic bodies resulted from retraction of the cytoplasm from the fungus cell wall. (H&E, ×200)

233

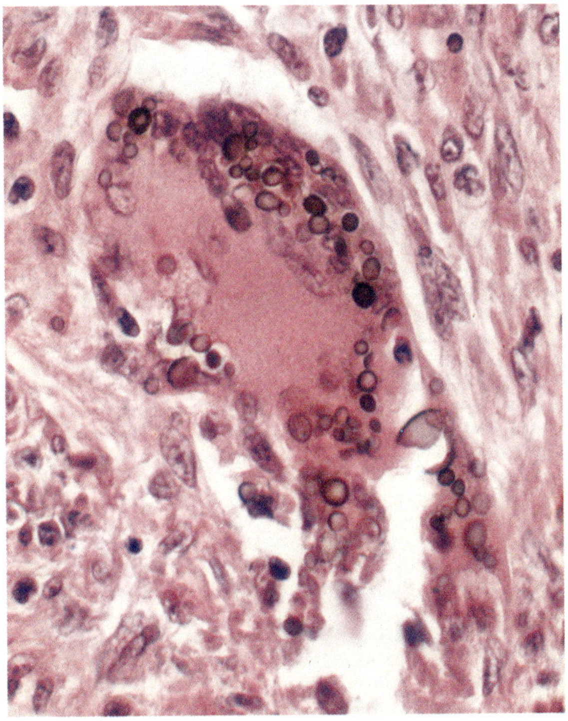

233 Cryptococcus neoformans Granulomatous pneumonia in a human caused by a lightly encapsulated *C. neoformans* isolate. Numerous intracellular yeast cells without a capsule are well demonstrated. (GMS–H&E, ×200)

234

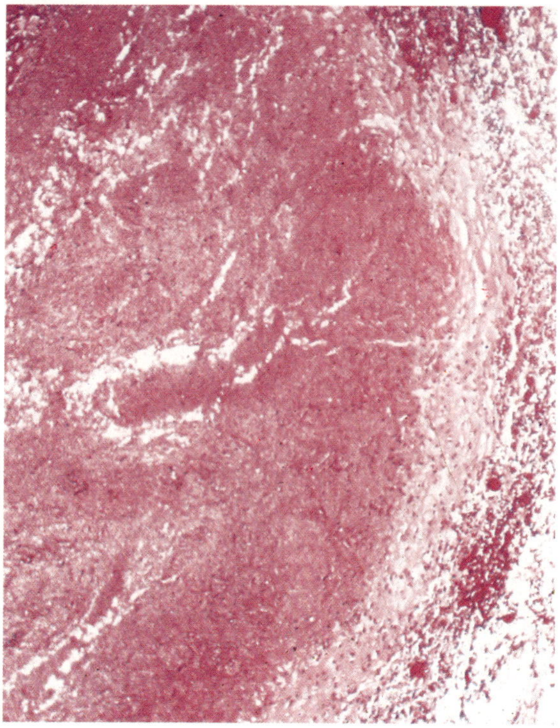

235

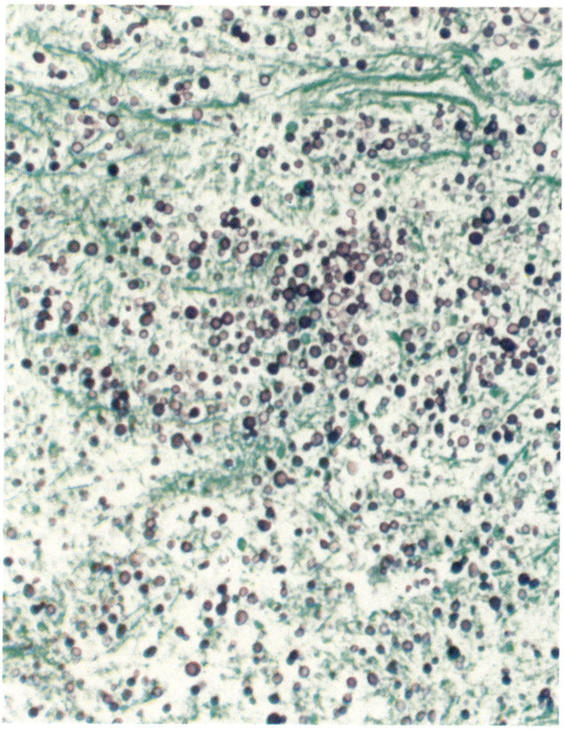

234 Cryptococcus neoformans Portion of a solitary pulmonary cryptococcal granuloma in a human. A central zone of caseous necrosis is surrounded by a thin fibrous wall that clearly demarcates the nodule from contiguous normal lung tissue. (H&E, ×20)

235 Cryptococcus neoformans Replicate section of **234.** Numerous lightly encapsulated fungal cells are seen within the central caseous zone of the pulmonary nodule. (GMS, ×100)

236

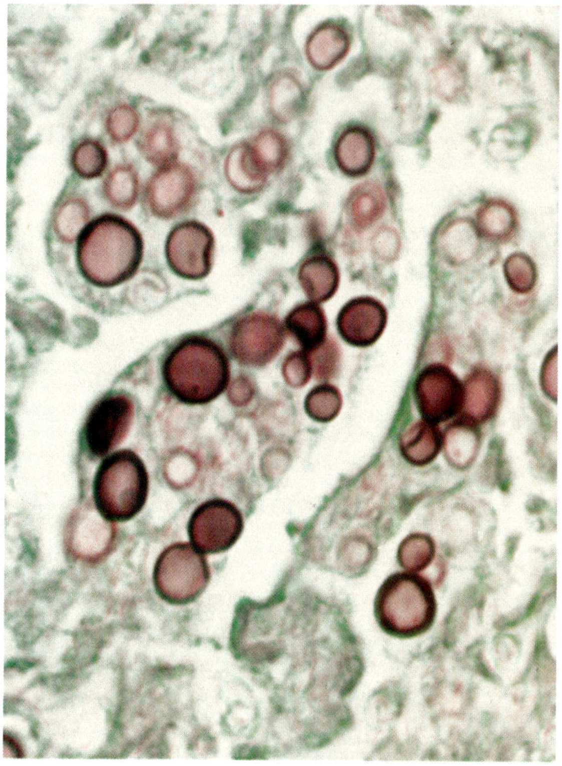

237

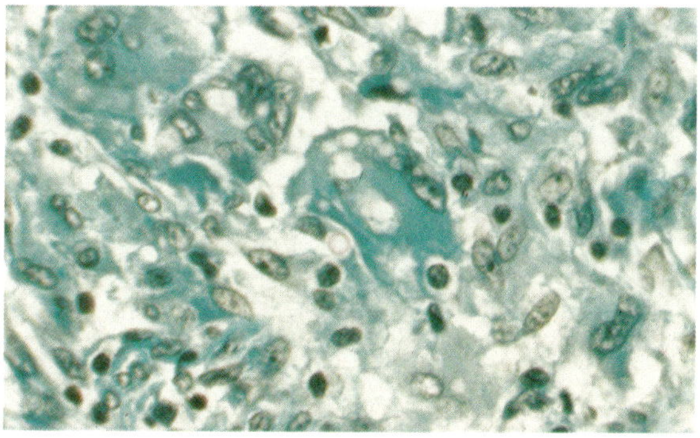

236 Cryptococcus neoformans Pulmonary cryptococcosis caused by lightly encapsulated *Cryptococcus neoformans* in a human. Compare the yeast cells in this photomicrograph to those in **222** and **223** which show wide clear spaces surrounding the fungal cells. (GMS, ×500)

237 Pulmonary granuloma containing very lightly encapsulated cryptococci stained by the mucicarmine procedure. All of the yeast cells are unstained with the exception of one faintly stained cell. (Mayer's mucicarmine, ×200)

238

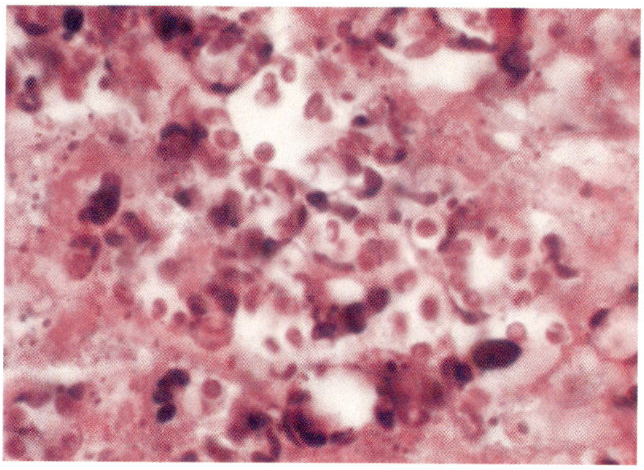

239

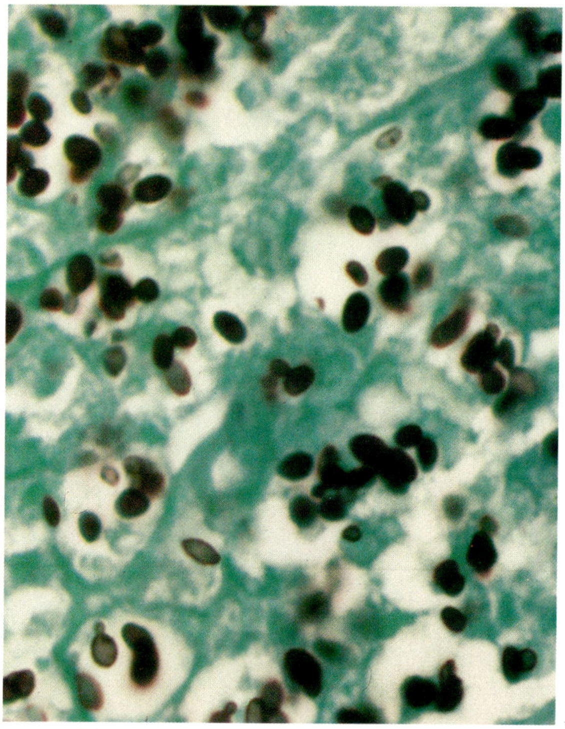

238 Candida (Torulopsis) glabrata causing pneumonia in a human. Note the superficial resemblance to *Cryptococcus neoformans* cells. (H&E, ×500)

239 Candida (Torulopsis) glabrata Replicate section of **238** stained by GMS. *Candida glabrata* cells may resemble small, lightly encapsulated cryptococci. If the mucicarmine reaction is equivocal, cultural and FA studies are useful to differentiate the two. (GMS, ×500)

240

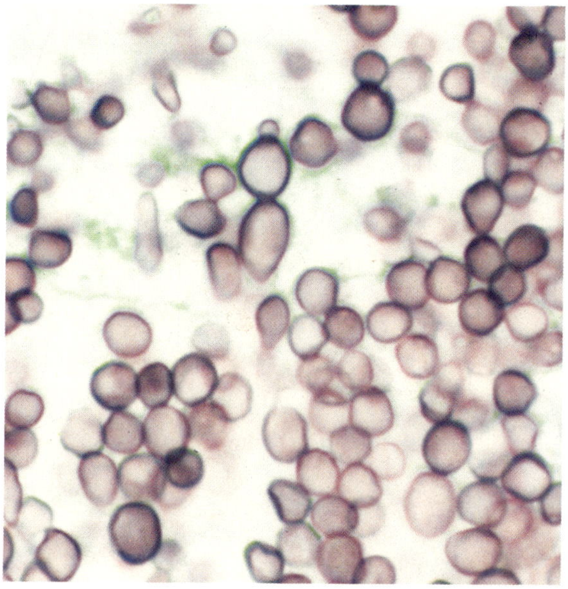

241

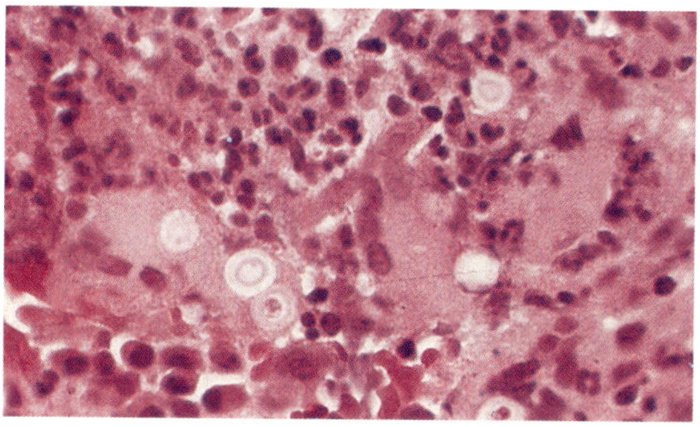

242

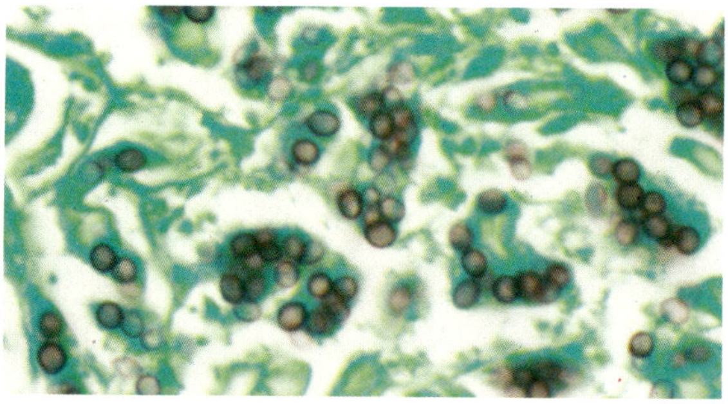

240 Candida albicans Masses of unicellular forms in a human heart valve. In the absence of hyphae or pseudohyphae these cells can be confused with lightly encapsulated cells of *Cryptococcus neoformans*. (GMS, ×500)

241 Blastomyces dermatitidis infection of human prostate gland. In some instances, as illustrated here, retraction of host cell cytoplasm away from the rigid fungal cell wall gives a false impression of a capsule. This appearance could possibly result in a misdiagnosis of cryptococcosis. (H&E, ×200)

242 Histoplasmosis capsulati of the adrenal gland in a human. Yeast cells of *Histoplasma capsulatum* var. *capsulatum* may also resemble small, intracellular, lightly encapsulated cryptococci. Generally, cryptococci show a greater variation in size and shape. (GMS, ×500)

243

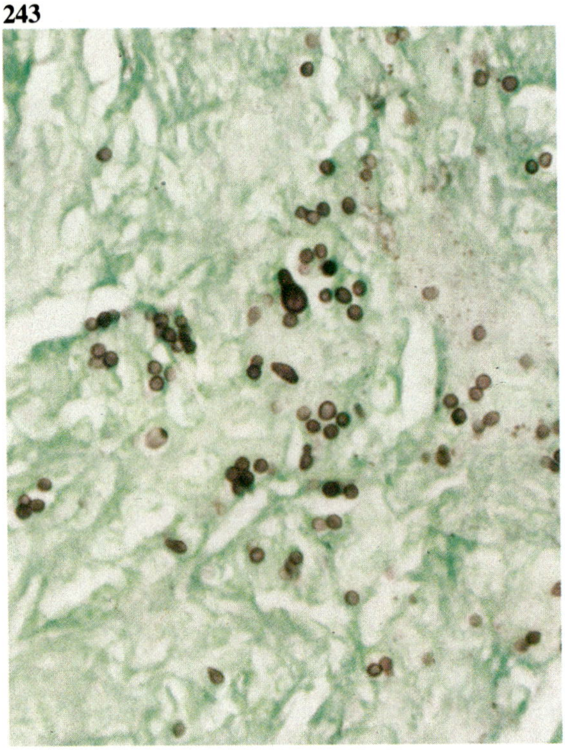

244

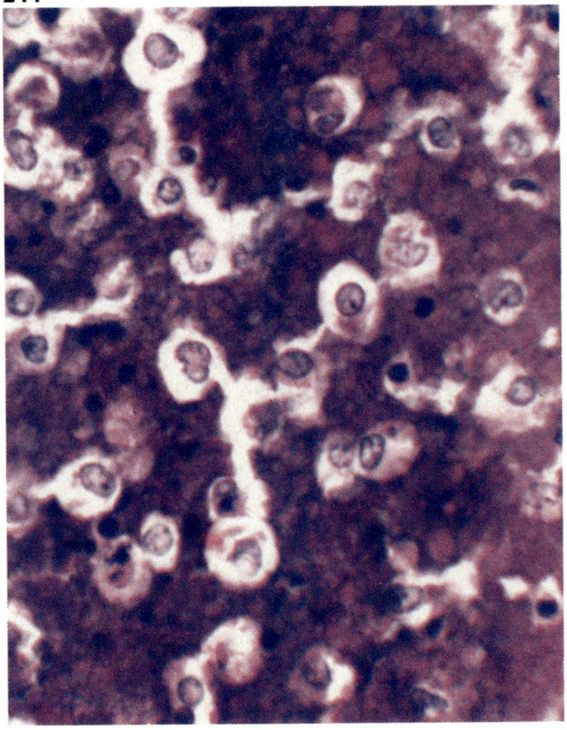

243 Blastomyces dermatitidis Pulmonary granuloma containing small tissue-form cells of *Blastomyces dermatitidis* in a human. They closely resemble the lightly encapsulated *Cryptococcus neoformans* cells in **233**. Careful examination of a section will usually reveal the larger typical forms of *B. dermatitidis*. (GMS, ×200)

244 Acute necrotising and purulent pneumonia in a human. As illustrated here, retraction of necrotic exudate away from intact inflammatory cells may give the false impression of a capsule in H&E stained tissue sections, suggesting that the inflammatory cells might be cryptococci. Careful examination of the nuclear morphology of these 'encapsulated' cells will lead to their correct identification. (H&E, ×200)

245

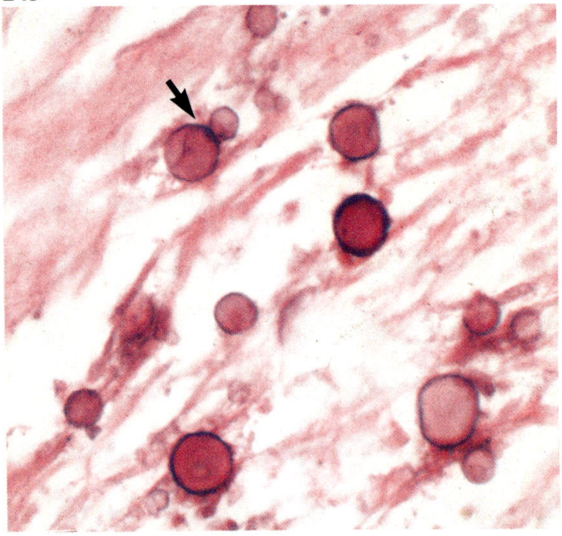

246

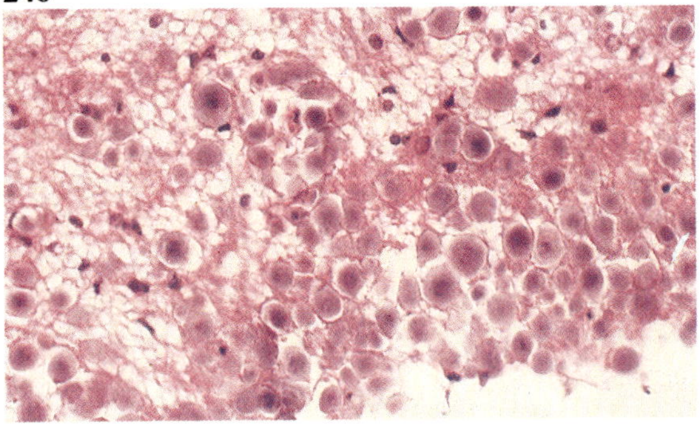

245 Calcific bodies in a fibrocaseous nodule of a human lung. In H&E-stained tissue sections, these bodies may resemble the cells of *Cryptococcus neoformans* or other yeasts. When in apposition (arrow), they may mimic budding yeasts. Calcific bodies can usually be distinguished from fungi by their failure to stain by GMS. (H&E, ×200)

246 Corpora amylaceae in a human brain. When stained by H&E, these structures are spherical and lightly basophilic with a deeply basophilic central core. They may superficially resemble cryptococci. (H&E, ×100)

247

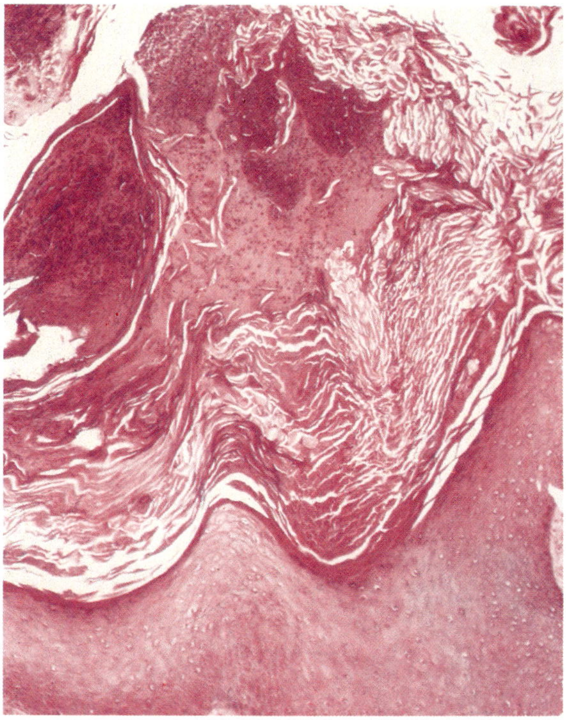

12 Dermatophilosis

Text pages: 59–62

247 Cutaneous dermatophilosis in a bovine. Note the marked hyperkeratosis and the presence of inflammatory cell debris within the keratin layers of the epidermis. There was a mild inflammatory cell infiltrate in the papillary dermis. (H&E, ×50)

248

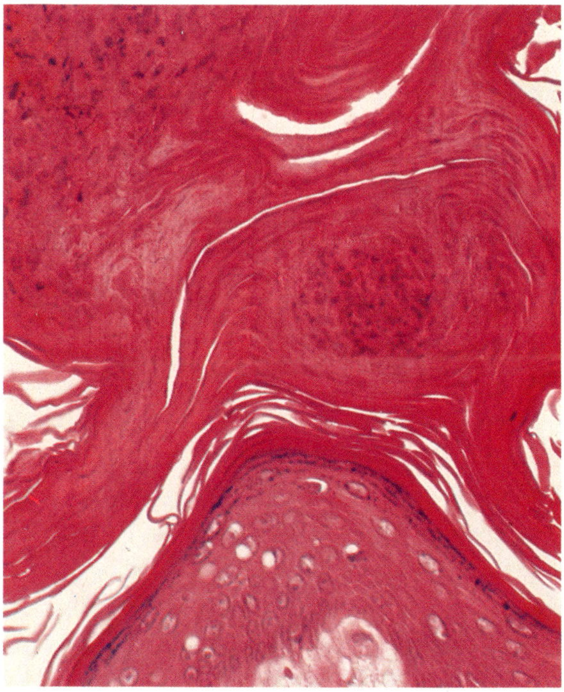

249

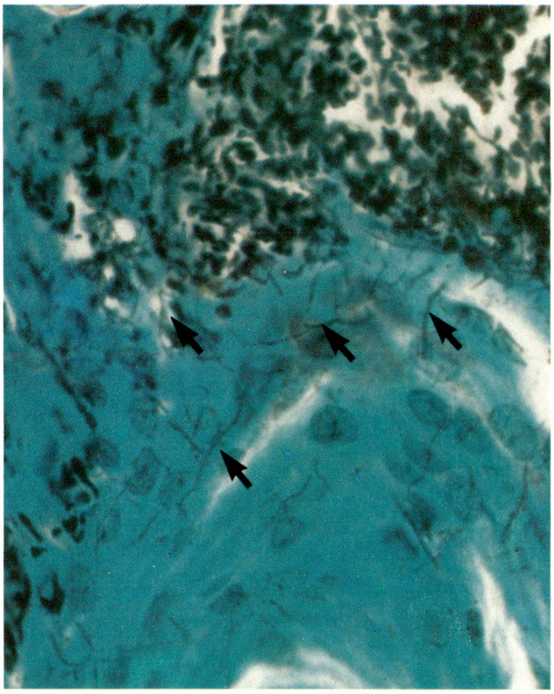

248 Cutaneous dermatophilosis in an owl monkey. Observe the extensive hyperkeratosis and the numerous inflammatory cells within the keratin layers of the epidermis. (H&E, ×100)

249 Dermatophilus congolensis Replicate section of **248** stained with Giemsa to show invasion of the epidermis by filaments of *D. congolensis* (arrows). Neutrophils and cellular debris are seen in the superficial layers. (Giemsa, ×200)

250

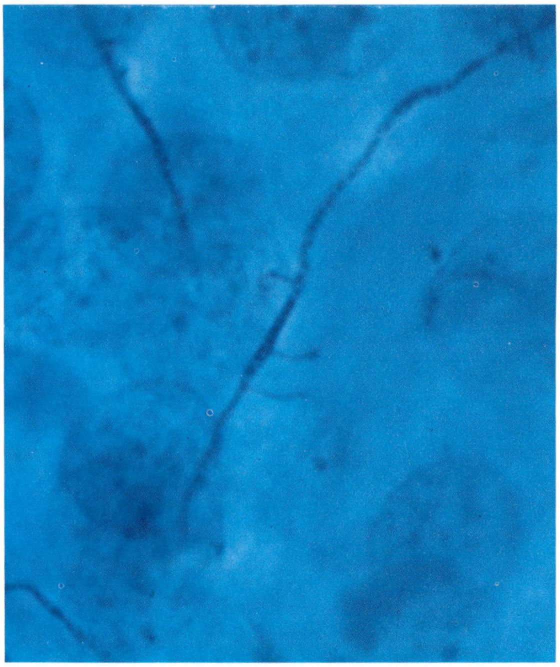

250 Dermatophilus congolensis Higher magnification of **249** that shows details of the branched, closely septate filaments within the stratum spinosum. (Giemsa, ×500)

251

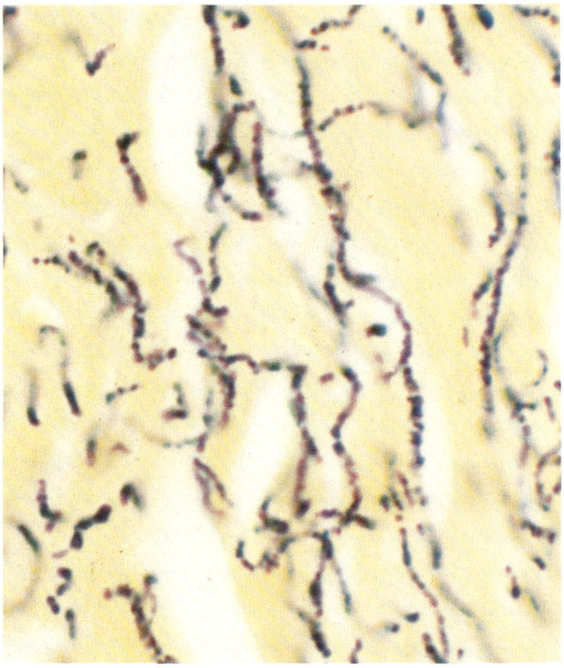

251 Dermatophilus congolensis causing cutaneous dermatophilosis. The branched, closely septate filaments are well demonstrated by the tissue Gram stains. The organisms are gram-positive. (B&B, ×500)

252

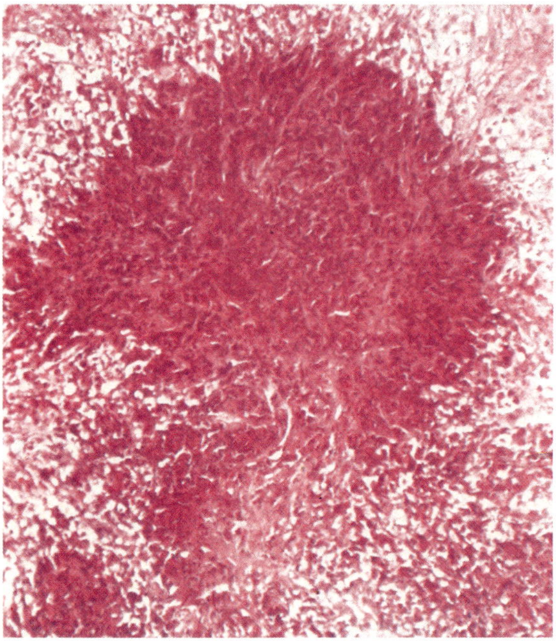

252 Dermatophilus congolensis infection of the glossal muscle of a cat. A central zone of necrosis is rimmed by granulomatous inflammation. (H&E, ×50)

253

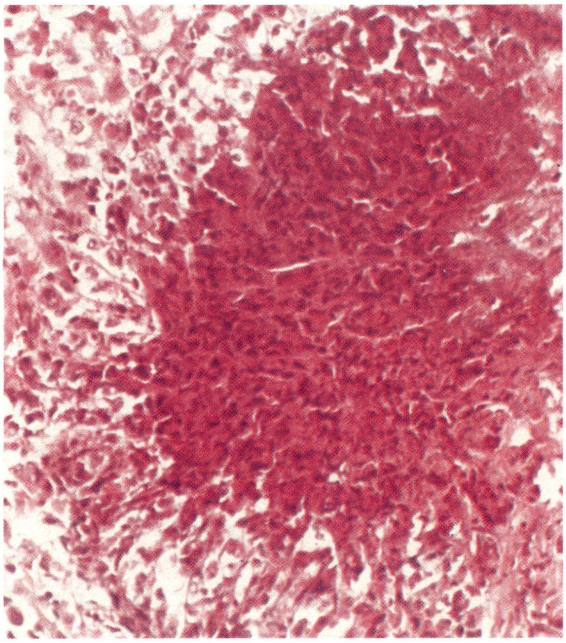

253 Dermatophilus congolensis Another area in **252** that shows details of the inflammatory response to invasion of the glossal muscle by *D. congolensis*. The filaments are not discernible. (H&E, ×100)

254

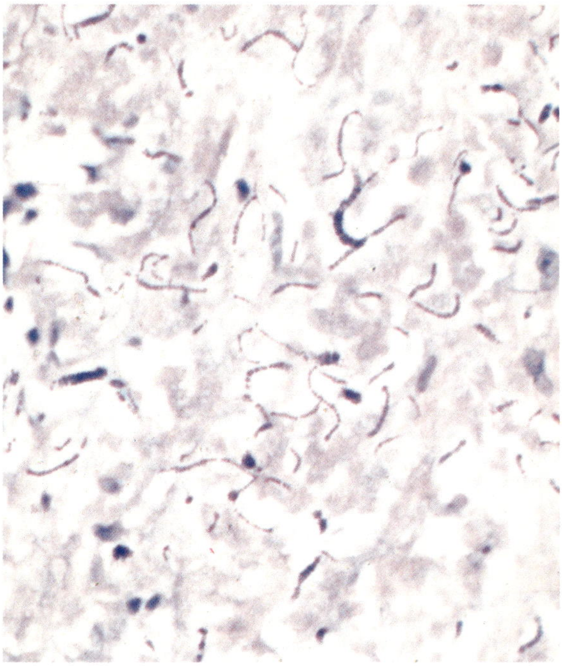

254 Dermatophilus congolensis Replicate section of **252**, but stained with Giemsa. Numerous filaments are revealed within the necrotic lesion. (Giemsa, ×200)

255

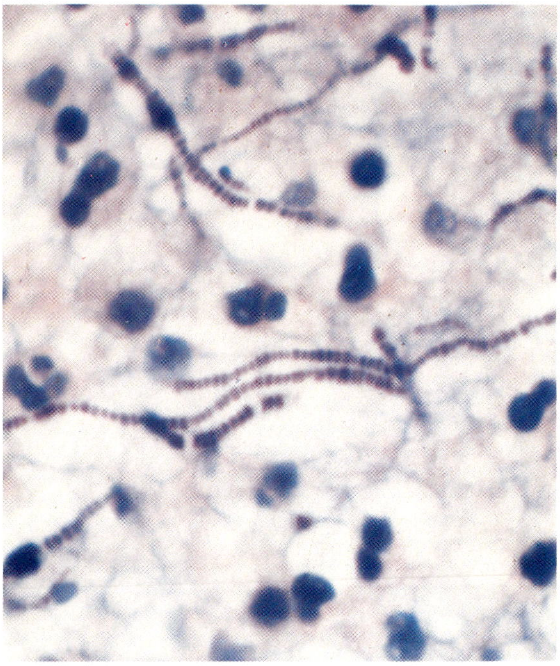

255 Dermatophilus congolensis Higher magnification of **254** to show the branched, closely septate filaments within the lesion. (Giemsa, ×500)

256

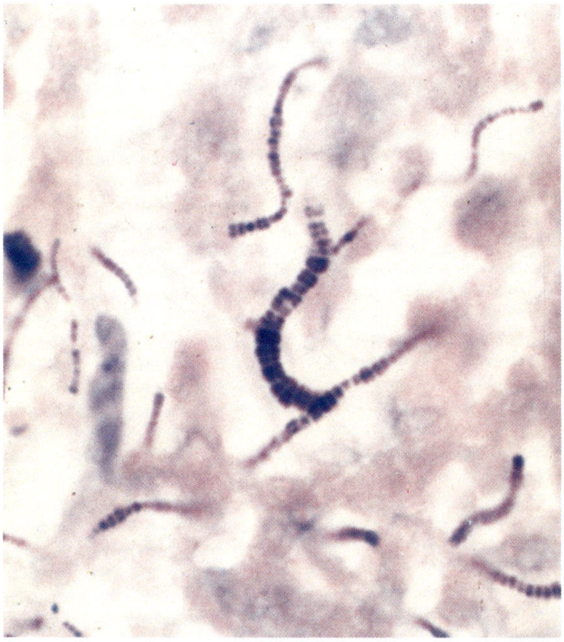

256 Dermatophilus congolensis Same area as **254** enlarged to illustrate the division of a filament in both transverse and longitudinal planes. (Giemsa, ×500)

257

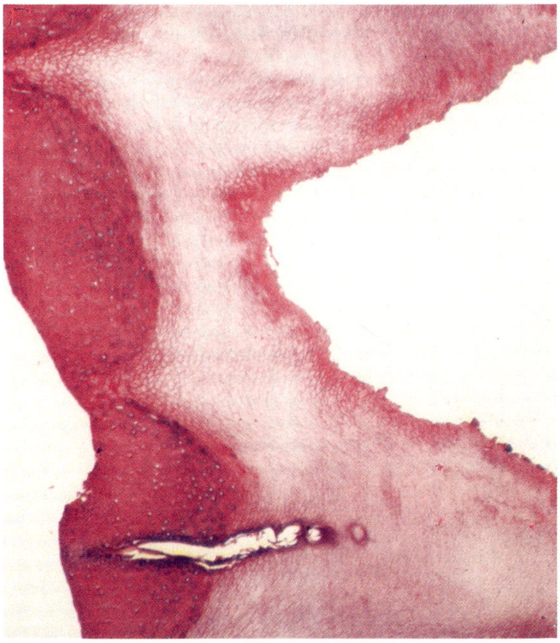

257 Pitted keratolysis of the sole of a young girl's foot. The characteristic appearance of a crateriform pit is clearly shown. As illustrated here, the pit does not usually extend beyond the keratin layer of the epidermis. (H&E, ×20)

258

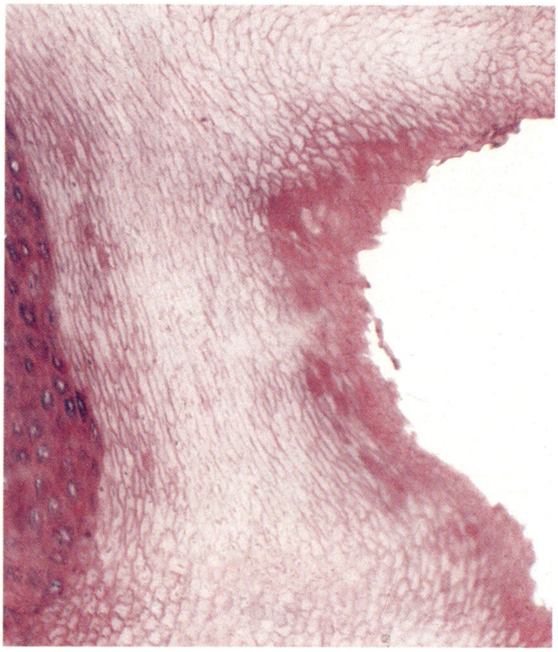

259

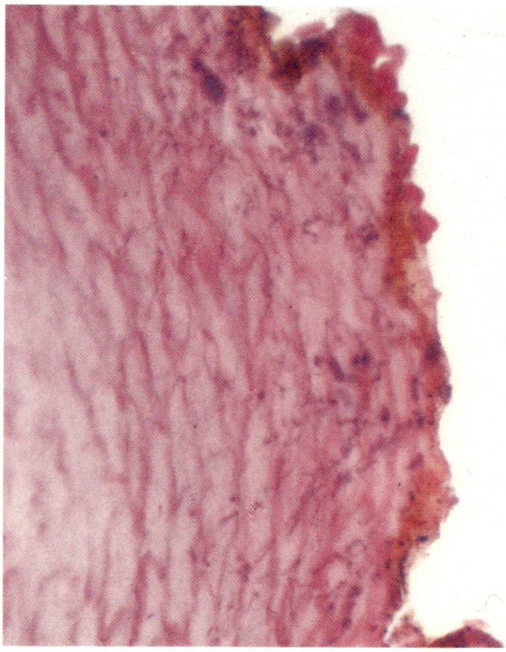

258 Pitted keratolysis Higher magnification of **257** depicting the deeply eosinophilic keratinolytic zone lining the base and adjacent walls of the pit. (H&E, ×50)

259 Pitted keratolysis of the sole in another human. Note invasion of the keratin layer by faintly basophilic filaments in the base of a pit. The brown, granular material on the surface of the pit is probably soil. (H&E, ×200)

260

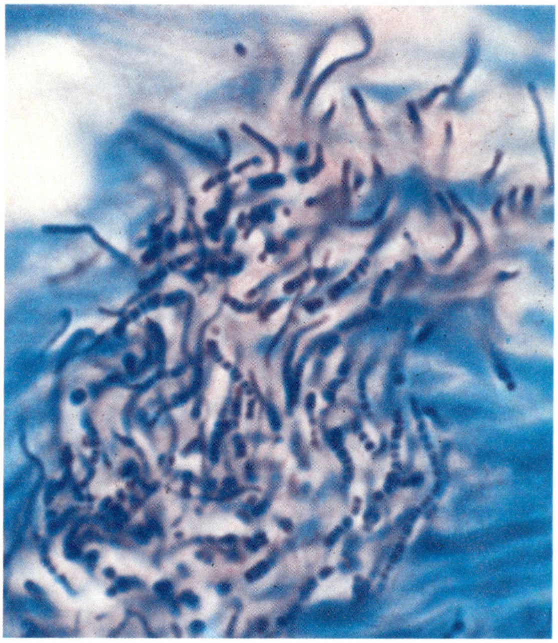

261

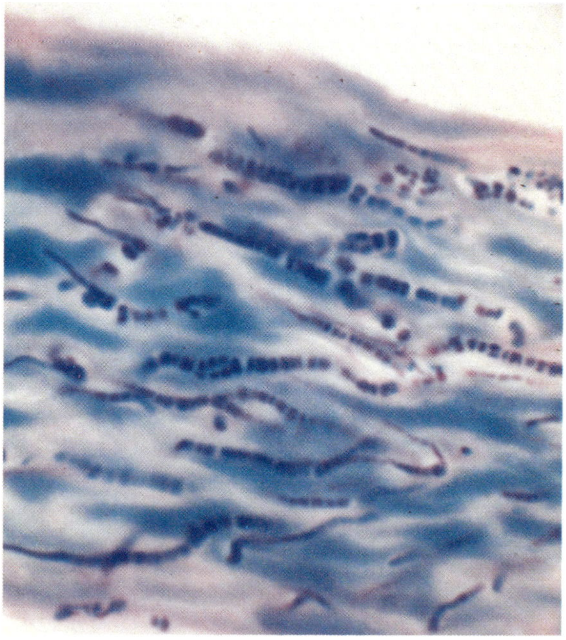

260 Pitted keratolysis Replicate section of **259** stained with Giemsa to show numerous, closely-septate filaments in the base of a pit. (Giemsa, ×500)

261 Pitted keratolysis Another field in **260** revealing the septation of filaments along transverse and longitudinal planes. These filaments have a striking morphological similarity to those in the lesions of animals with dermatophilosis. (Giemsa, ×500)

13 Histoplasmosis capsulati

Text pages: 63–66

262

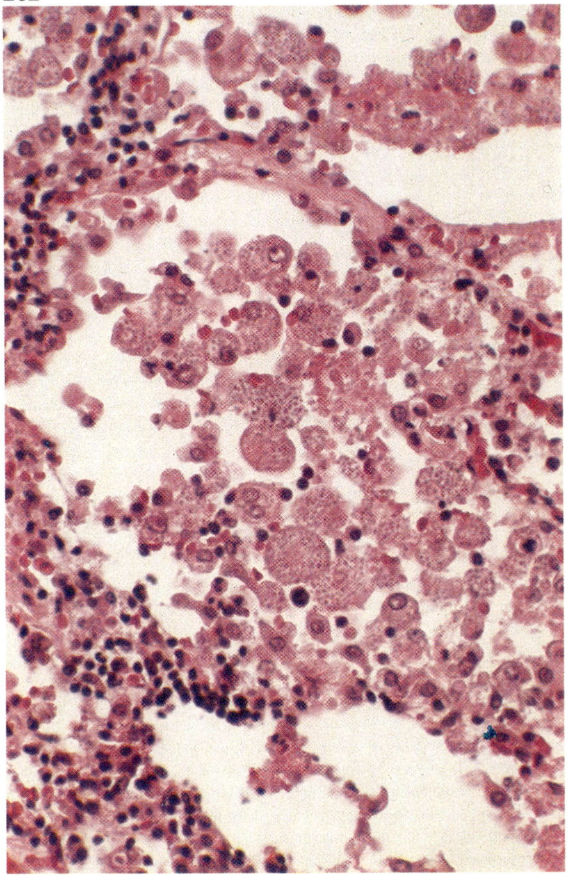

263

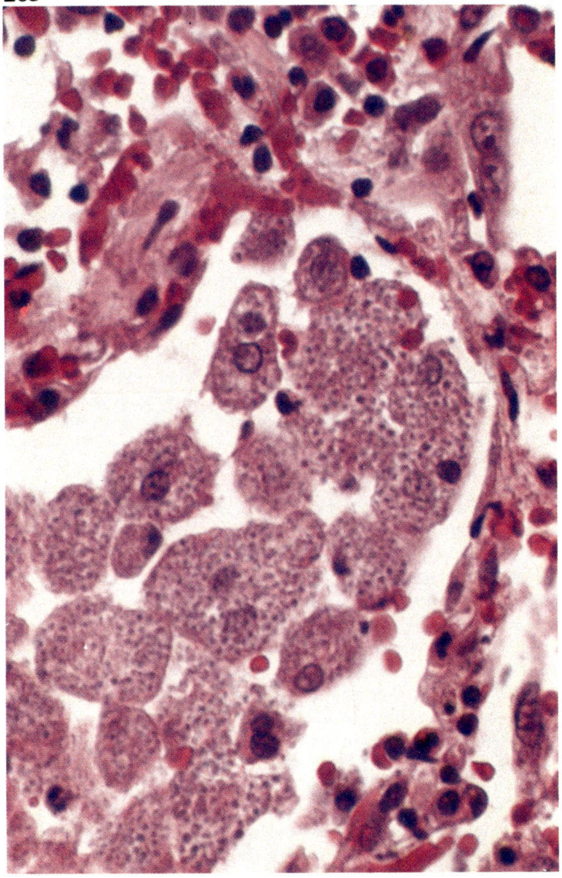

262 Histoplasma capsulatum var. **capsulatum** Acute pulmonary histoplasmosis in a human. Alveolar spaces contain macrophages that are filled with numerous tissue-form cells of the fungus. Alveolar septa contain mononuclear inflammatory cells. (H&E, ×100)

263 Histoplasma capsulatum var. **capsulatum** Higher magnification of **262** to show details of yeast cells within the alveolar macrophages. The basophilic cytoplasm of the fungi is retracted from the cell wall, giving the appearance of an unstained capsule. (H&E, ×200)

264

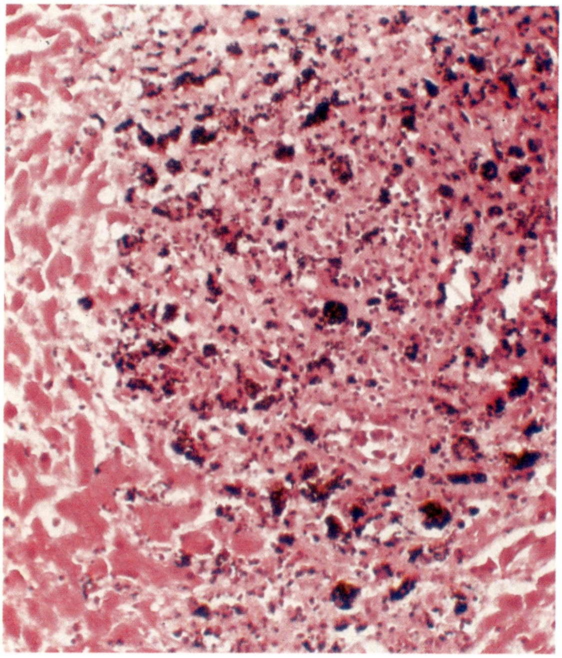

264 Acute disseminated histoplasmosis in a human. This photomicrograph of the liver shows one of many lesions containing myriads of fungal cells. The small dark masses represent aggregates of GMS-positive yeast cells within Kupffer cells and histiocytes. (GMS–H&E, ×50)

265

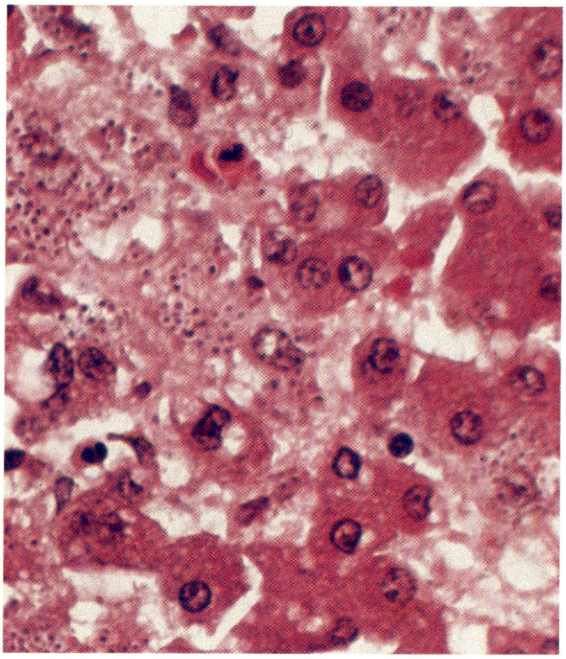

265 Histoplasma capsulatum var. **capsulatum** Higher magnification of **264** that shows Kupffer cells laden with tissue-form cells of the fungus. At this stage of infection, the lesion does not contain any other inflammatory cells except for occasional neutrophils in the hepatic sinusoids. (H&E, ×200)

266

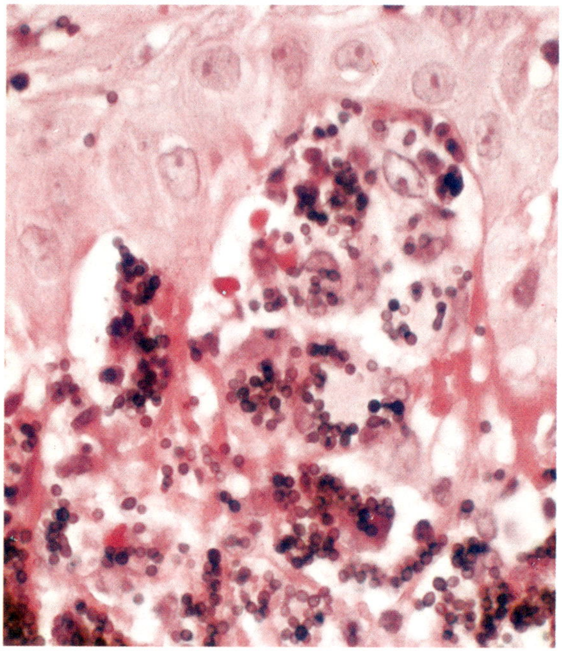

266 Disseminated histoplasmosis involving the larynx in a human. The submucosa contains many yeast cells, most of which are within giant cells and histiocytes. The overlying mucosa in this case is intact. (GMS–H&E, ×200)

267

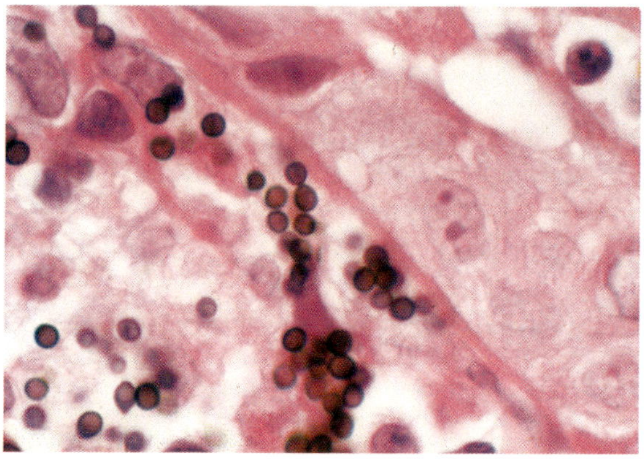

267 Histoplasma capsulatum var. **capsulatum** Higher magnification of **266** showing single and budding yeast cells beneath the laryngeal mucosa. The yeast cells are both intracellular and extracellular, and they have not penetrated the epithelial basement membrane. (GMS–H&E, ×500)

268

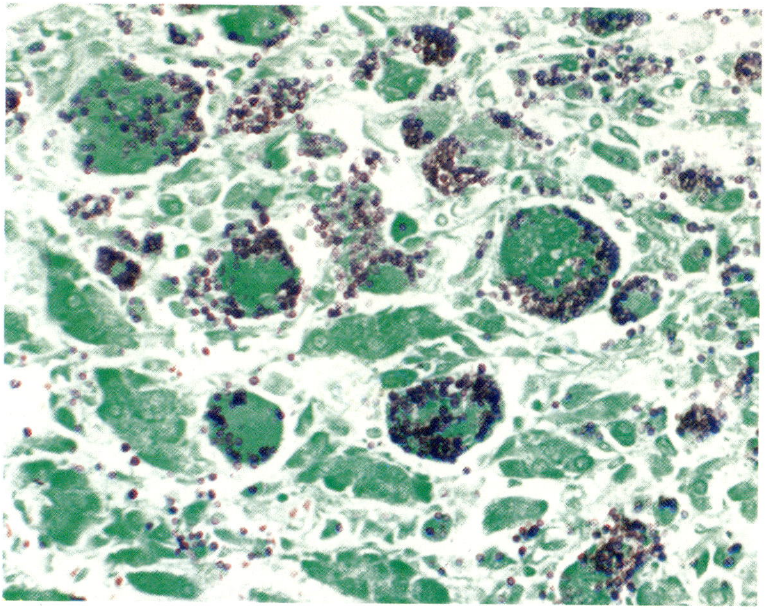

268 Disseminated histoplasmosis involving the adrenal gland in a human. Large aggregates of yeast cells are within giant cells and histiocytes. The adrenal gland is one of the target organs of disseminated histoplasmosis, and infection can lead to symptoms of Addison's disease. (GMS, ×100)

269

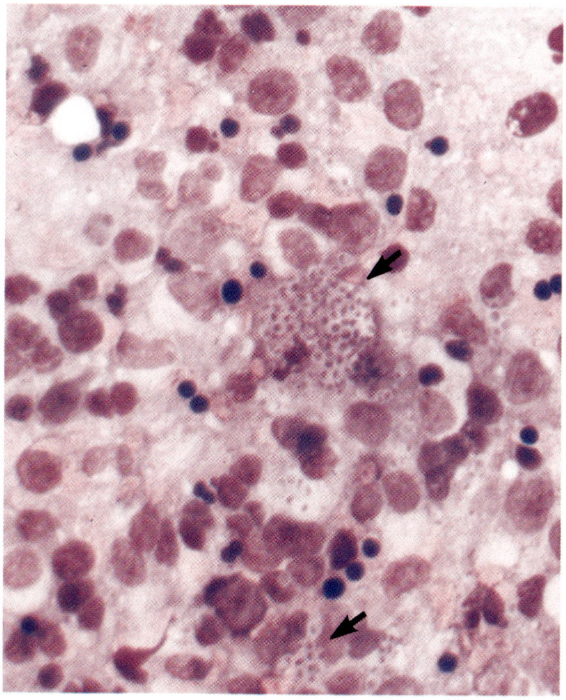

269 Acute disseminated histoplasmosis involving the bone marrow in a human. The yeast cells within the histiocytes are well demonstrated (arrows). (Wright's stain, ×200)

270

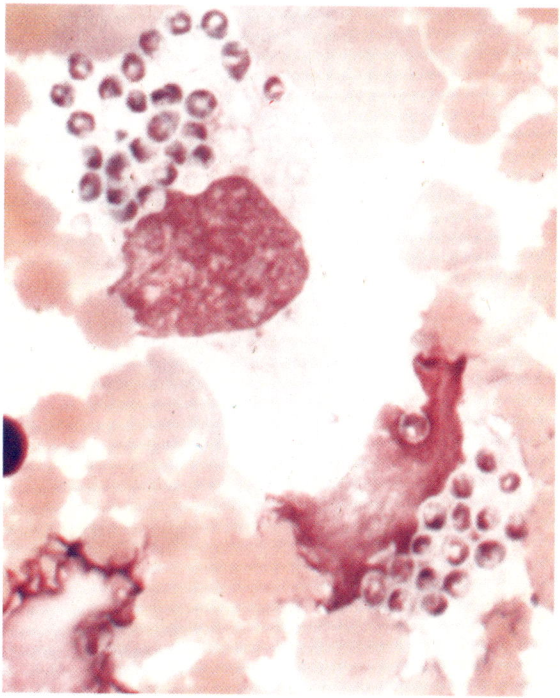

270 Disseminated histoplasmosis Peripheral blood smear from a human. Two monocytes contain numerous yeast cells. With Wright's stain, the darker violet chromatin of the yeast cells appears as an oval, half-moon to crescent-shaped mass within the clear cytoplasm. The cytoplasm is retracted from the unstained wall, giving the false impression of a capsule. (Wright's stain, ×500)

271

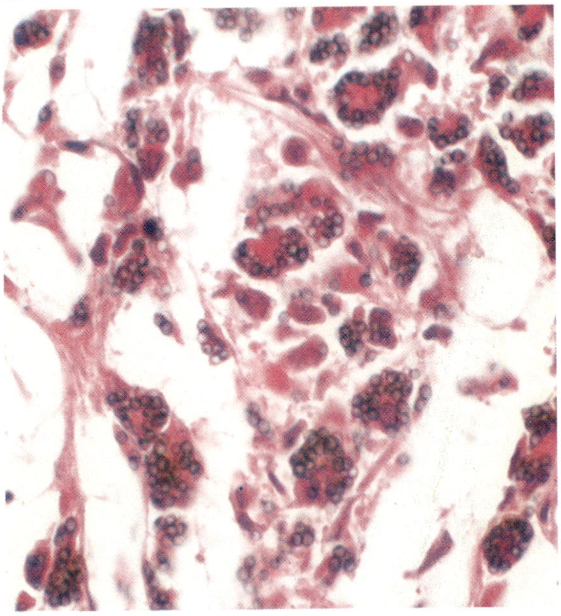

271 Histoplasma capsulatum var. **capsulatum** Granulomatous adrenalitis in another human with disseminated histoplasmosis. The normal histologic architecture is effaced by histiocytes and giant cells that contain many yeast cells of *H. capsulatum* var. *capsulatum*. (GMS–H&E, ×200)

272

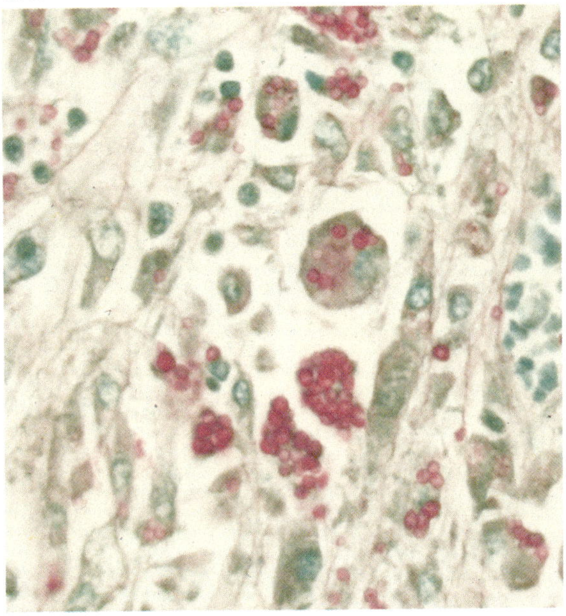

272 Histoplasma capsulatum var. **capsulatum** Replicate section of **271** that shows the appearance of fungal cells when stained by PAS. (PAS, ×200)

273

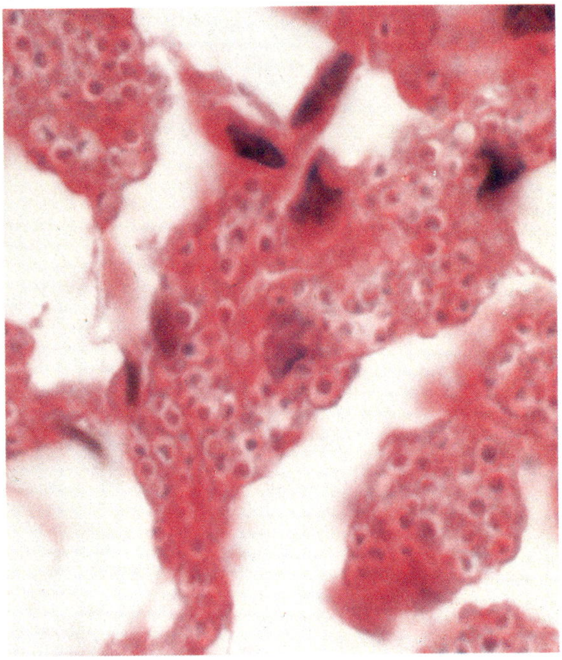

273 Histoplasma capsulatum var. **capsulatum** Replicate section of **271** showing the appearance of yeast cells when stained by H&E. The basophilic cytoplasm of the fungal cells is retracted from the poorly stained cell wall, giving the false impression of a capsule. (H&E, ×500)

274

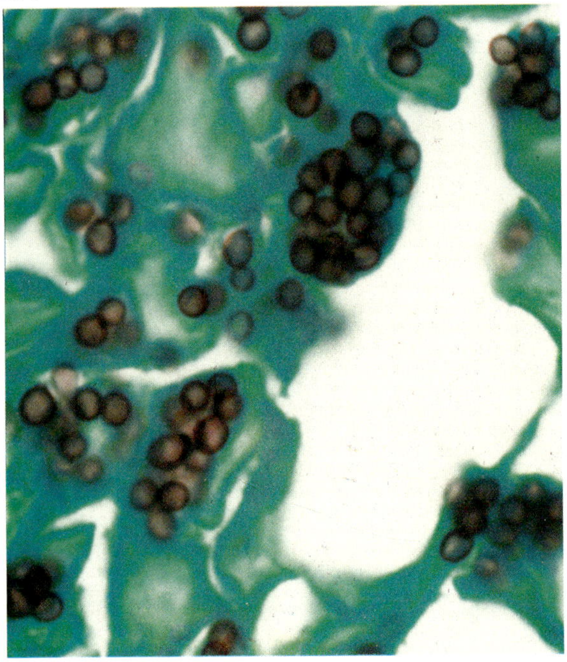

274 Histoplasma capsulatum var. **capsulatum** Replicate section of **271** stained by GMS. In contrast to the fungal cells in **273**, the cell wall stains intensely, indicating the full size of the organisms. There is no 'capsule' effect. (GMS, ×500)

275

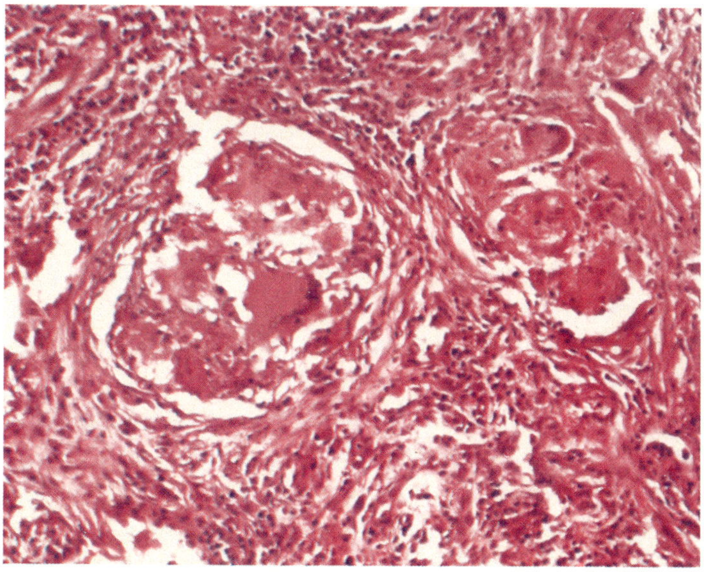

275 Histoplasma capsulatum var. **capsulatum** causing granulomatous pneumonia. The pulmonary parenchyma is replaced by numerous giant cells embedded in a fibrous connective tissue stroma that contains mixed inflammatory cells. (H&E, ×50)

276

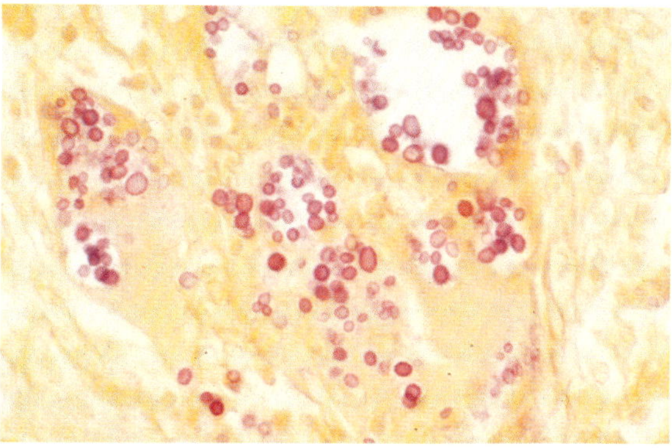

276 Histoplasma capsulatum var. **capsulatum** Replicate section of **275** clearly demonstrates many *H. capsulatum* var. *capsulatum* cells within poorly defined giant cells. The entire fungal cell wall is stained. (GF, ×200)

277

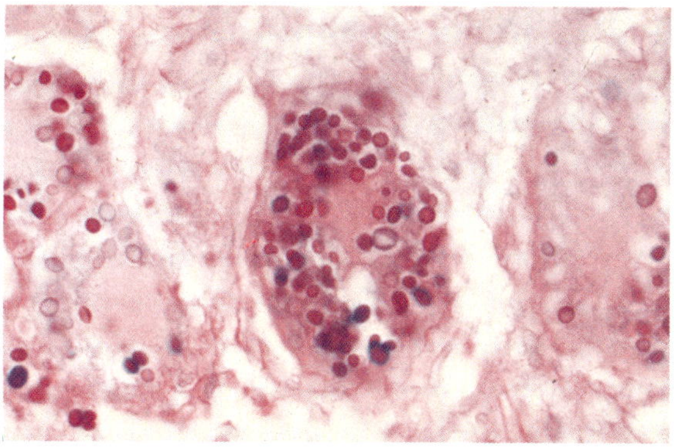

277 Histoplasma capsulatum var. **capsulatum** Replicate section of **275** stained by PAS. The inflammatory cells are better delineated by this stain than by the GF and GMS procedures. The yeast cells of *H. capsulatum* var. *capsulatum* are also well demonstrated. (PAS, ×200)

278

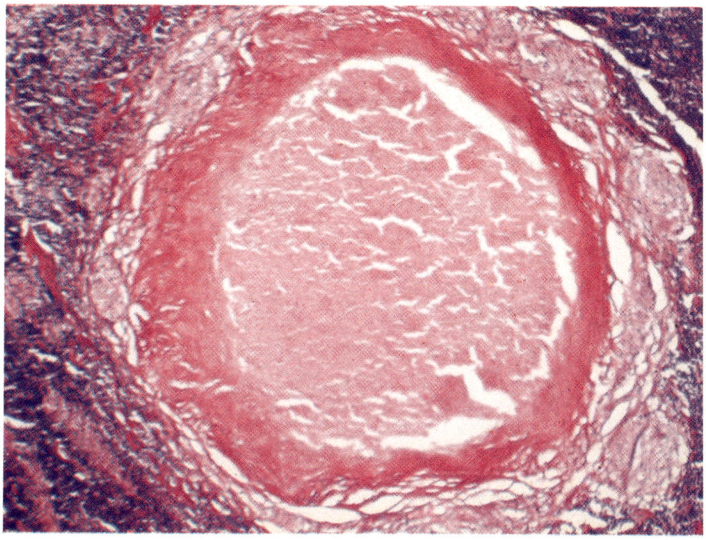

278 Histoplasma capsulatum var. **capsulatum** causing old fibrocaseous nodule in the hilar lymph node of a human. The central caseous zone is surrounded by a thick wall of dense collagenous connective tissue. The fungal cells in these old lesions are usually not seen when stained by H&E. (H&E, ×20)

279

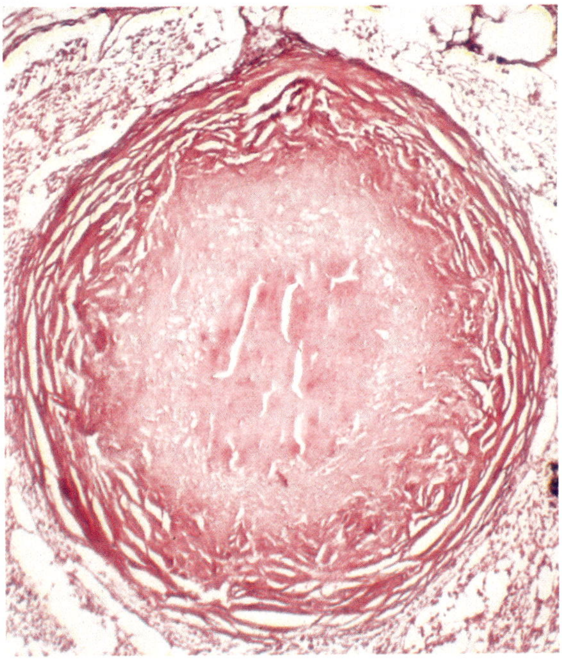

280

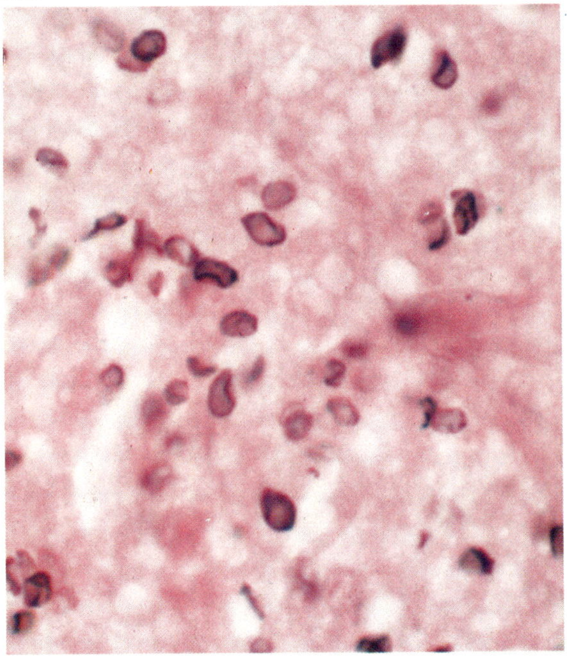

279 Histoplasma capsulatum var. **capsulatum** causing subpleural solitary nodule (histoplasmoma) in the lung of a human. Concentric layers of collagenous connective tissue enclose a central core of caseous material. A few yeast cells were found within the caseous centre when a GMS-stained replicate section was examined at higher magnification. The surrounding lung parenchyma appears normal. (H&E, ×50)

280 Histoplasma capsulatum var. **capsulatum** Replicate section of **279**, but stained by GMS–H&E to demonstrate yeast cells within the central caseous material. The organisms are distorted, unevenly stained and do not occur in clusters. Culture of the fungus from such lesions is usually not successful, and morphologically the tissue-form cells are frequently atypical. (GMS–H&E, ×500)

281

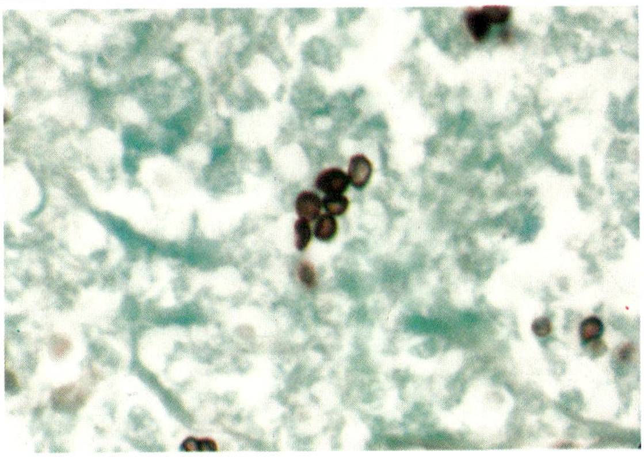

282

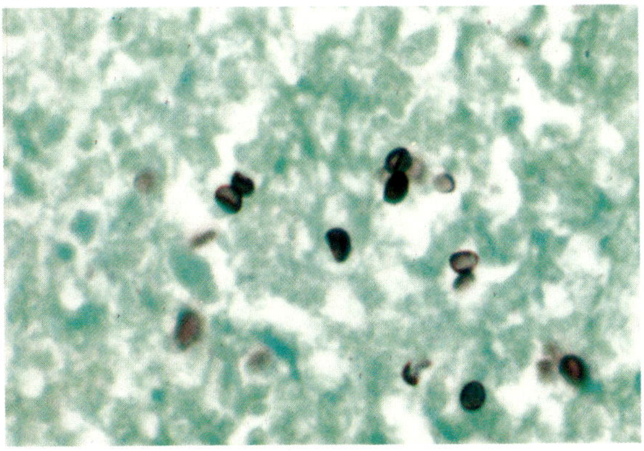

281 Histoplasma capsulatum var. **capsulatum** Central caseous zone in an old pulmonary fibrocaseous nodule (histoplasmoma) in a human. In this case, the yeast cells are more typical and better stained. Many are found in clusters. (GMS, ×500)

282 Histoplasma capsulatum var. **capsulatum** Another field in **281**. Here, the yeast cells are distorted and do not appear in prominent clusters. A budding cell is seen. Atypical forms of *H. capsulatum* var. *capsulatum* are frequently found in old fibrocaseous lesions. (GMS, ×500)

283

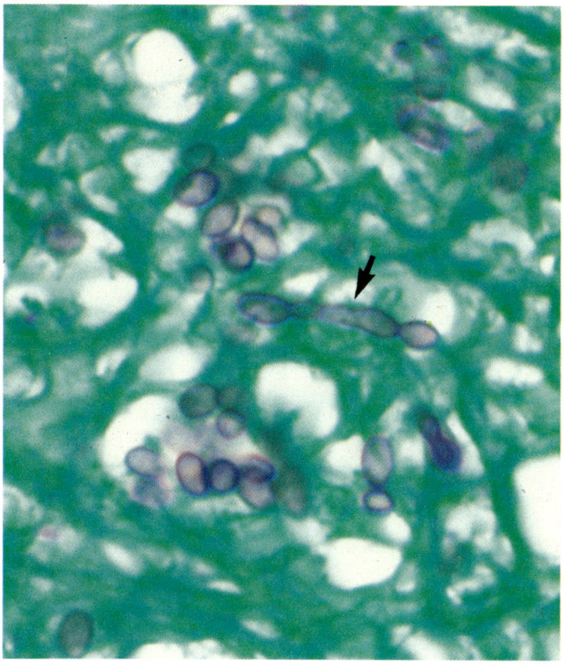

283 Disseminated histoplasmosis involving the vocal cord in a human. An atypical form (arrow) is seen together with typical yeast cells. (GMS, ×500)

284

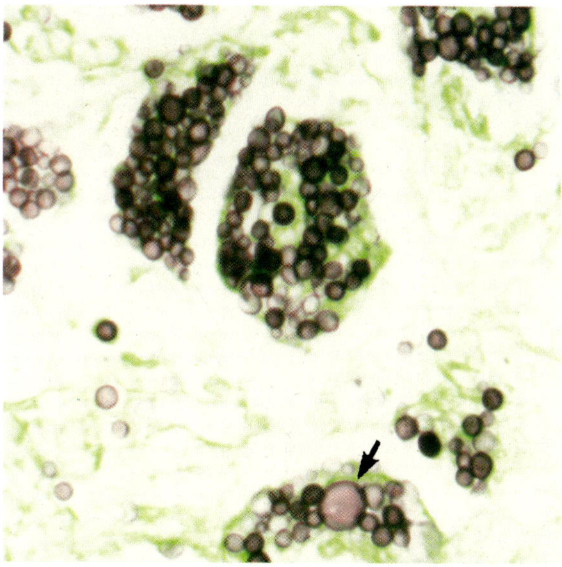

284 Paracoccidioides brasiliensis causing granulomatous pneumonia in a human. The clusters of small, densely packed blastospores within giant cells closely resemble *Histoplasma capsulatum* var. *capsulatum*. Careful examination of this field, however, reveals a typical large multiple budding cell of *P. brasiliensis* (arrow), enabling a histologic diagnosis of paracoccidioidomycosis to be made. (GMS, ×200)

285

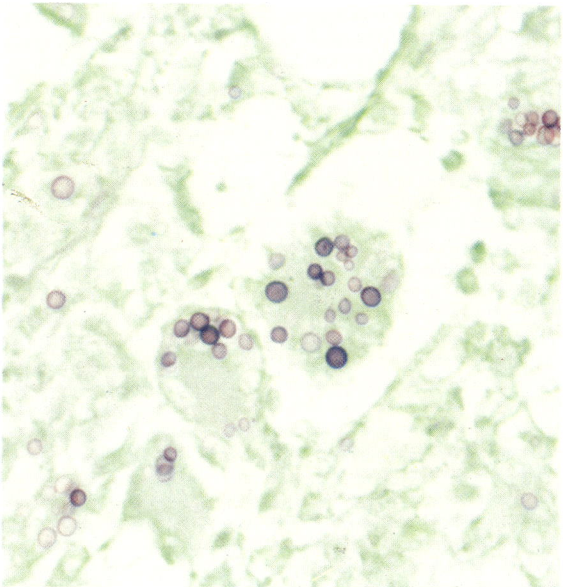

285 Cryptococcus neoformans yeast cells, poorly encapsulated, causing granulomatous pneumonia in a human. These yeast cells are predominantly intracellular and resemble yeast forms of *Histoplasma capsulatum* var. *capsulatum*. Generally, poorly encapsulated cryptococci show a greater variation in size, and at least some are carminophilic. (GMS, ×200)

286

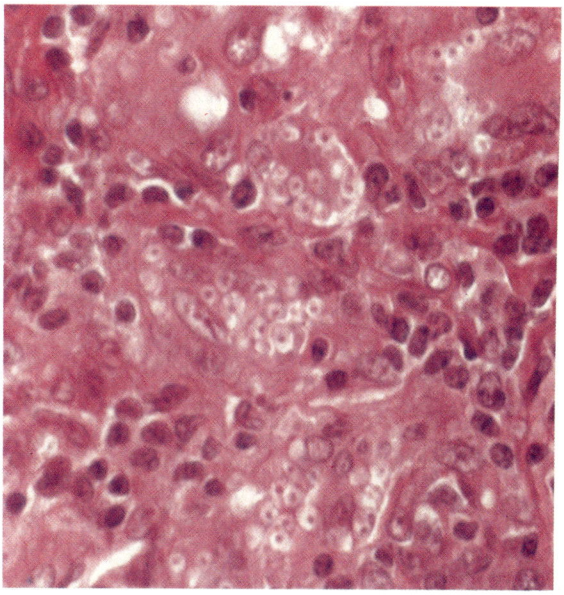

286 Blastomyces dermatitidis (small tissue forms) causing granulomatous pneumonia in a human. The clusters of densely-packed yeast cells within the phagocytes resemble *Histoplasma capsulatum* var. *capsulatum* cells as shown in **273**. (H&E, ×200)

287

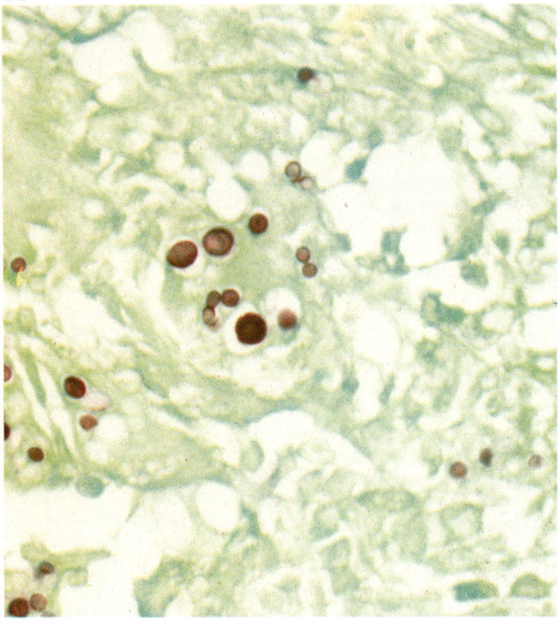

287 Blastomyces dermatitidis (small form isolate) causing pulmonary blastomycosis in a human. Here again, these intracellular yeast cells resemble those of *Histoplasma capsulatum* var. *capsulatum*. Careful examination of other fields will usually reveal *B. dermatitidis* forms of typical size. (GMS, ×200)

288

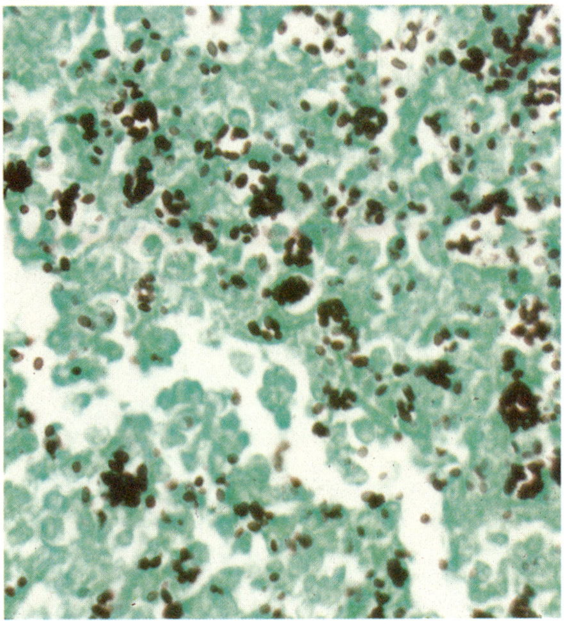

288 Candida (Torulopsis) glabrata causing pneumonia in a human. Numerous yeast cells which are similar in size and shape to those of *Histoplasma capsulatum* var. *capsulatum* are either free or clustered within phagocytes. These cells may be mistaken for those of *H. capsulatum* var. *capsulatum*, but the two can be readily differentiated by cultural or immunofluorescence studies. (GMS, ×200)

289

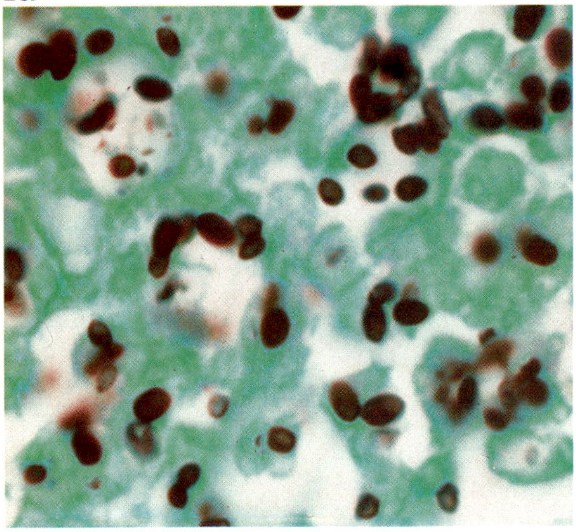

289 Candida (Torulopsis) glabrata Higher magnification of **288** showing in greater detail the similarity of *Candida glabrata* to *Histoplasma capsulatum* var. *capsulatum*. (GMS, ×500)

290

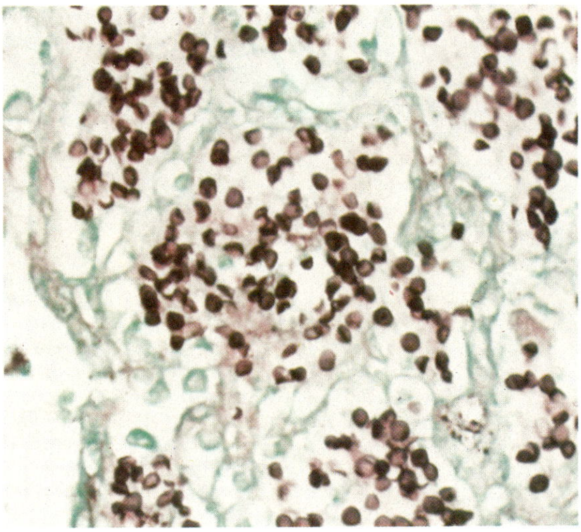

290 Pneumocystis sp. causing pulmonary pneumocystosis. Although this protozoan is not a fungus, its cyst forms stain intensely by GMS and thus may be mistaken for the yeast cells of *Histoplasma capsulatum* var. *capsulatum* and other fungi. *Pneumocystis spp.* do not bud, and they are nearly always extracellular. (GMS, ×200)

291

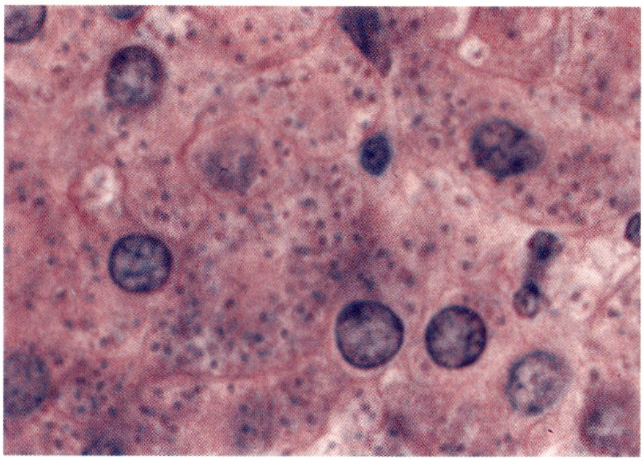

291 Leishmania donovani amastigotes within large reticuloendothelial cells of the spleen. These protozoans superficially resemble *Histoplasma capsulatum* var. *capsulatum* tissue-form cells in H&E-stained sections (see **265**). The *Leishmania* amastigotes can be differentiated from the latter by their failure to stain with the GMS, GF, or PAS procedures. Although this protozoan contains a kinetoplast, it may not be evident when stained by H&E. (H&E, ×500)

292

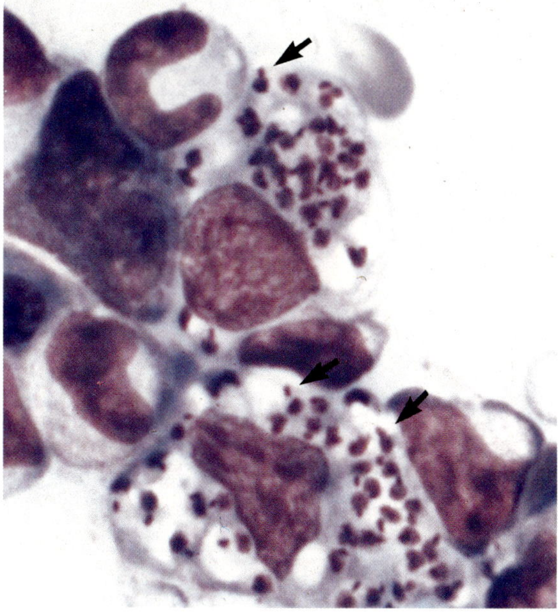

292 Leishmania sp. amastigotes within histiocytes in the bone marrow of a dog. When stained with Giemsa, these intracellular protozoans may also resemble *Histoplasma capsulatum* var. *capsulatum*, but they can be distinguished by the presence of a deeply stained bar-like kinetoplast (arrows) in their cytoplasm. (Giemsa, ×500)

293

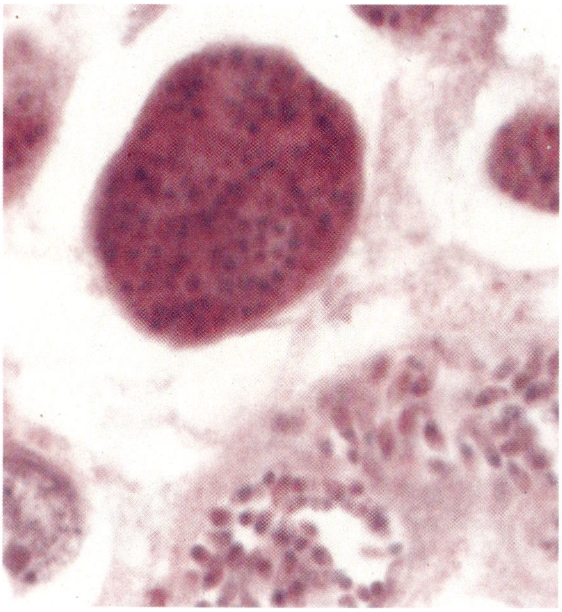

293 Toxoplasma gondii cell clusters in a human brain. When present in histiocytes, these protozoans may superficially resemble *Histoplasma capsulatum* var. *capsulatum* in H&E-stained sections. However, their smaller size, ability to parasitise host cells other than phagocytes, and failure to stain with the special fungus procedures differentiate them from *Histoplasma*. (H&E, ×500)

294

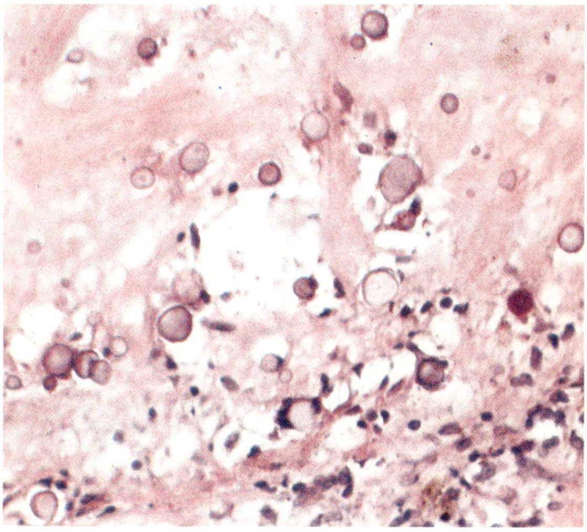

294 Calcific bodies within an old fibrocaseous pulmonary nodule. These bodies may superficially resemble the yeast cells of *Histoplasma capsulatum* var. *capsulatum* and when in apposition may even give the false impression of budding. Their pleomorphism and failure to stain by GMS clearly differentiate them from *H. capsulatum* var. *capsulatum*. (H&E, ×100)

14 Histoplasmosis duboisii

Text pages: 67–69

295

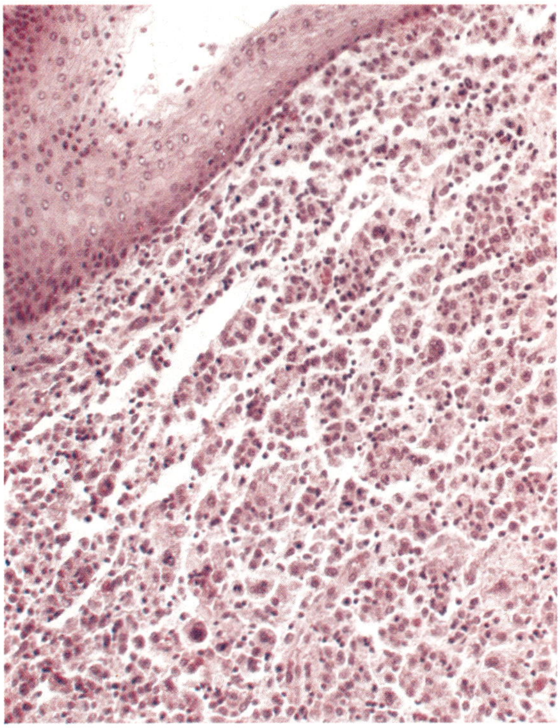

295 Histoplasma capsulatum var. **duboisii** causing cutaneous histoplasmosis in an African. The dermis is obliterated by densely packed histiocytes and giant cells. In this case, the overlying epidermis is intact. (H&E, ×50)

296

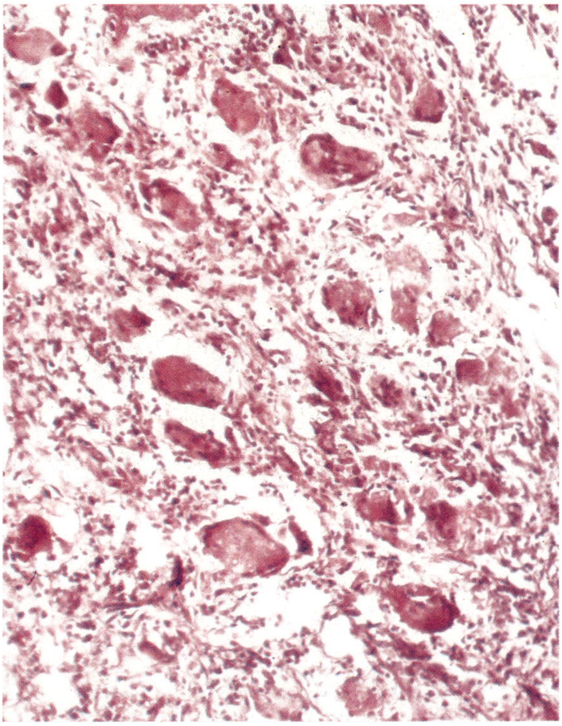

296 Pulmonary histoplasmosis duboisii in an African. The normal pulmonary architecture has been replaced by large numbers of huge giant cells embedded in a fibrous connective tissue stroma. Intracellular yeast forms of the fungus are not visible at this magnification. (H&E, ×50)

297

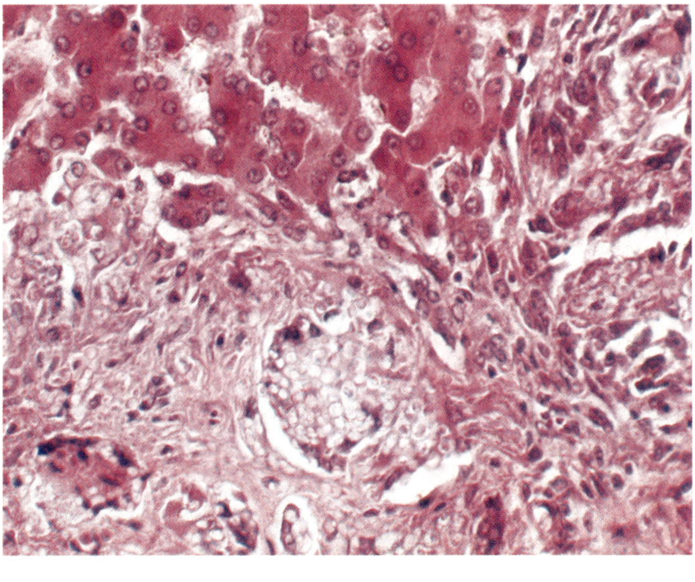

297 Histoplasma capsulatum var. **duboisii** causing granulomatous hepatitis in an African. Many intracellular yeast forms are present, but they are barely visible at this magnification. Note the extensive fibrosis. (H&E, ×100)

298

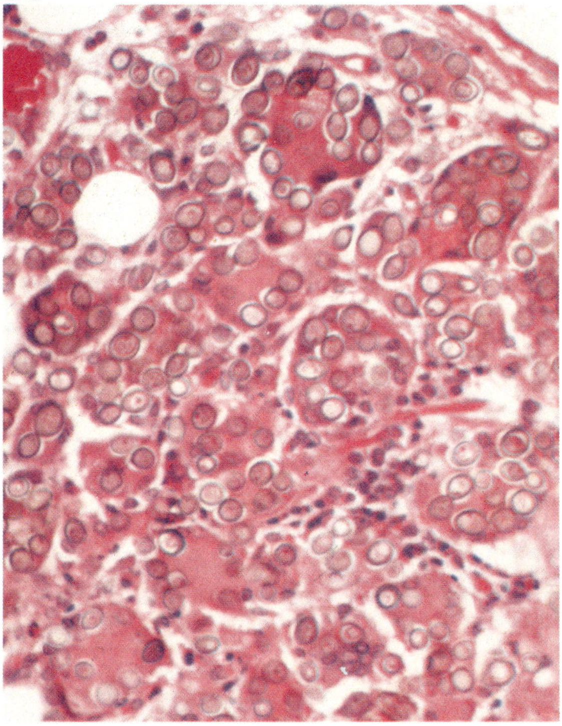

298 Histoplasma capsulatum var. **duboisii** in the spleen. The normal architecture has been effaced by solid sheets of giant cells. As illustrated here, the large yeast-like cells are found predominantly within huge Langhans' and foreign body giant cells. (GMS–H&E, ×100)

299

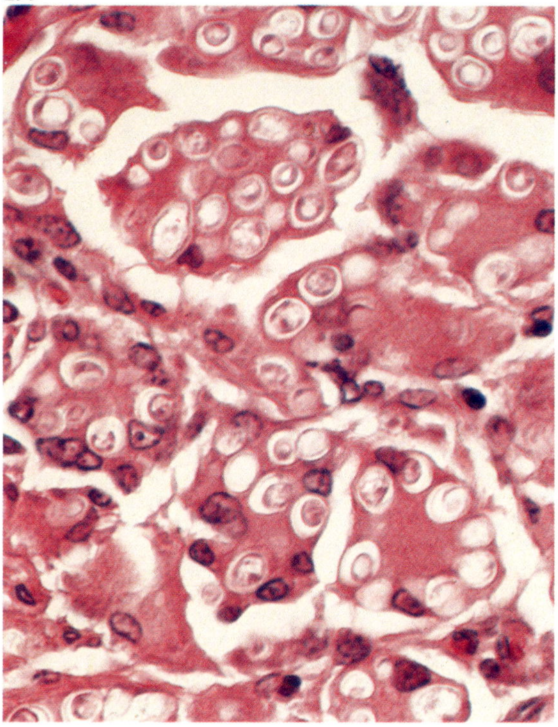

299 Cutaneous histoplasmosis duboisii in another African. Single and budding fungal cells are primarily within foreign body and Langhans' giant cells that fill the dermis. (H&E, ×200)

300

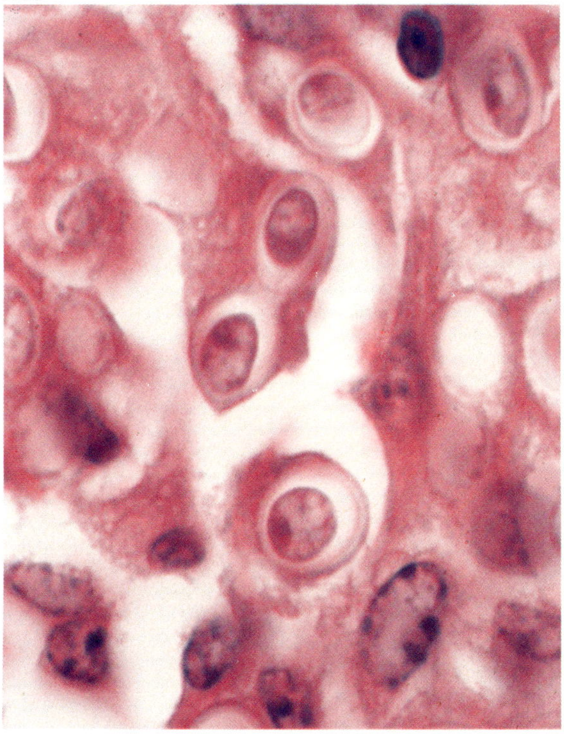

300 Cutaneous histoplasmosis duboisii Higher magnification of the lesion shown in **299**. The relatively thick wall of the fungus cells is unstained and the retracted cytoplasm is basophilic. Note that the fungal cells have a single nucleus whereas those of *Blastomyces dermatitidis* have multiple nuclei (see **113**). (H&E, ×500)

301

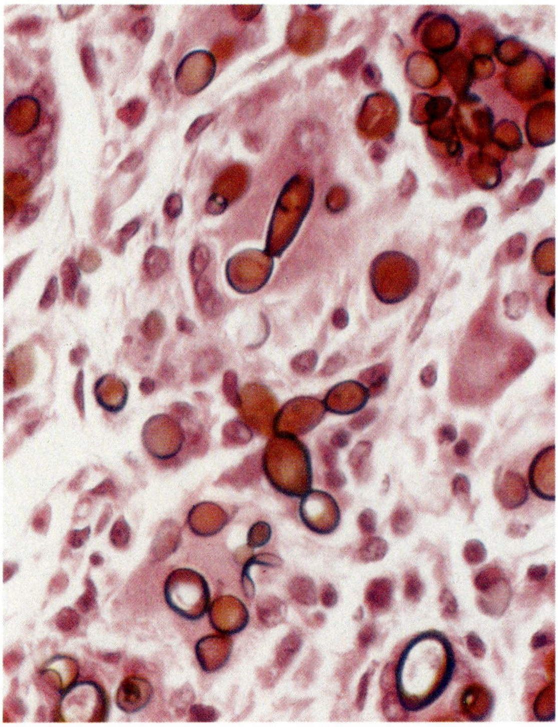

302

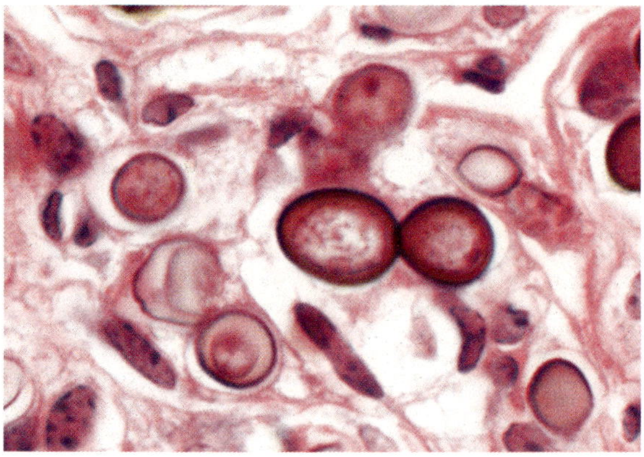

301 Histoplasma capsulatum var. **duboisii** in liver. The tissue-form cells of this fungus resemble those of *Blastomyces dermatitidis* in size and shape, but they differ from the latter in that, with few exceptions, their buds have a narrow basal attachment to the parent cells. Also, buds generally attain the same size as the parent cells before separation. (GMS–H&E, ×200)

302 Histoplasma capsulatum var. **duboisii** Another field in **301** revealing in detail the narrow basal attachment of the bud to the parent cell. (GMS–H&E, ×500)

303

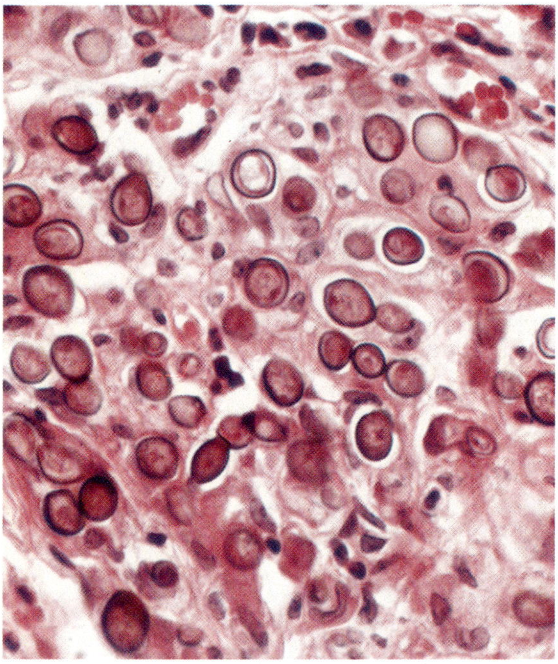

304

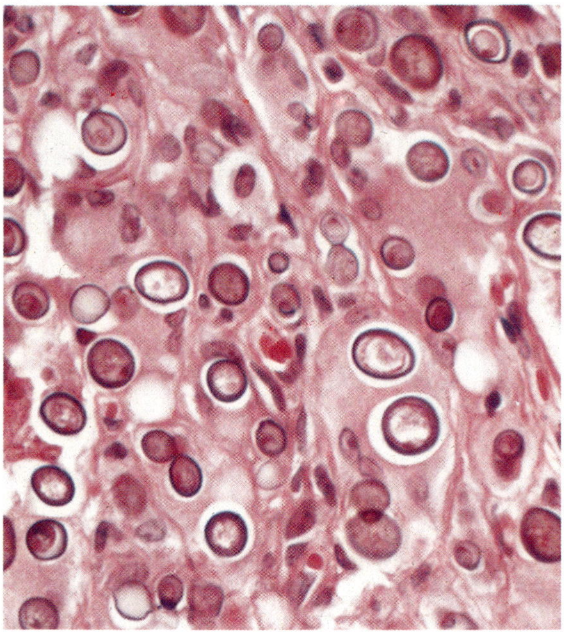

303 Histoplasma capsulatum var. **duboisii** Another field in **301** showing fungal cells with single buds as well as cells in short chains. (GMS–H&E, ×200)

304 Histoplasmosis duboisii of the skin in an African. The clear zone around some of the fungal cells is apparently due to retraction of the host cell's cytoplasm from the organisms. Some of the fungi are extracellular, probably because the phagocytes have disintegrated. (GMS–H&E, ×200)

305

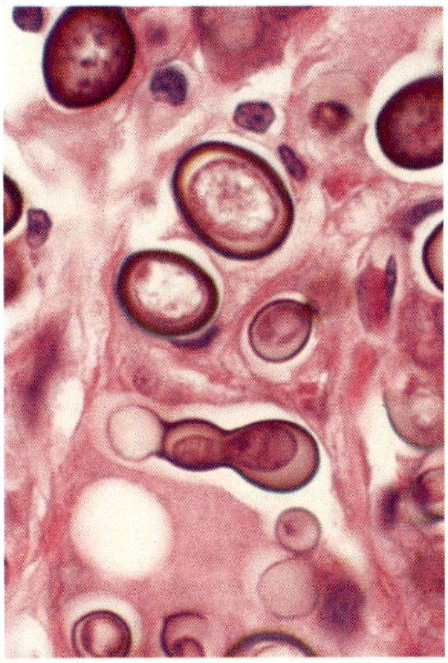

306

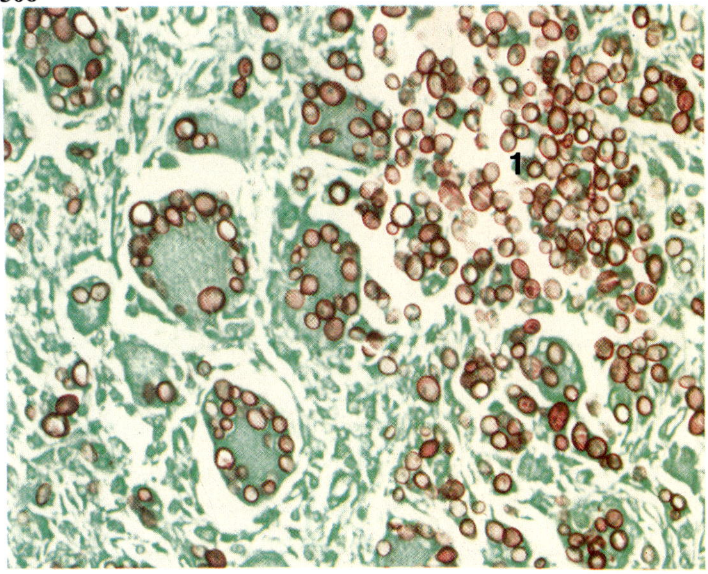

305 Histoplasmosis duboisii Another field in **301** showing details of several *Histoplasma capsulatum* var. *duboisii* cells within large giant cells. The cytoplasm of some of the fungal cells is vacuolated. A short chain of yeast cells is noted without the typical narrow basal attachments of daughter to mother cells. (GMS–H&E, ×500)

306 Histoplasma capsulatum var. **duboisii** Another field in **301**. Although most yeast-form cells are intracellular, clusters of these fungi are occasionally observed outside of cells, usually within foci of necrosis (1). (GMS, ×100)

307

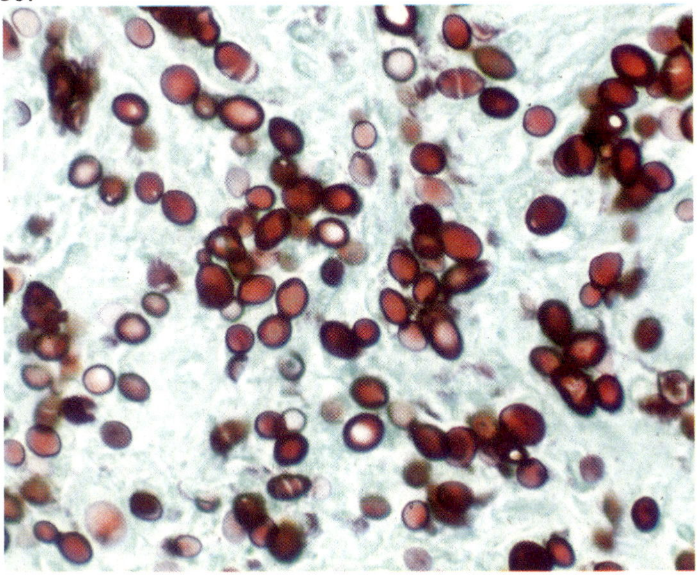

307 Cutaneous histoplasmosis duboisii Replicate section of **299**. The fungal cells are numerous and well demonstrated by GMS. Inflammatory cells are poorly delineated when the H&E counterstain is not used. (GMS, ×200)

15 Histoplasmosis farciminosi

Text pages: 70–72

308

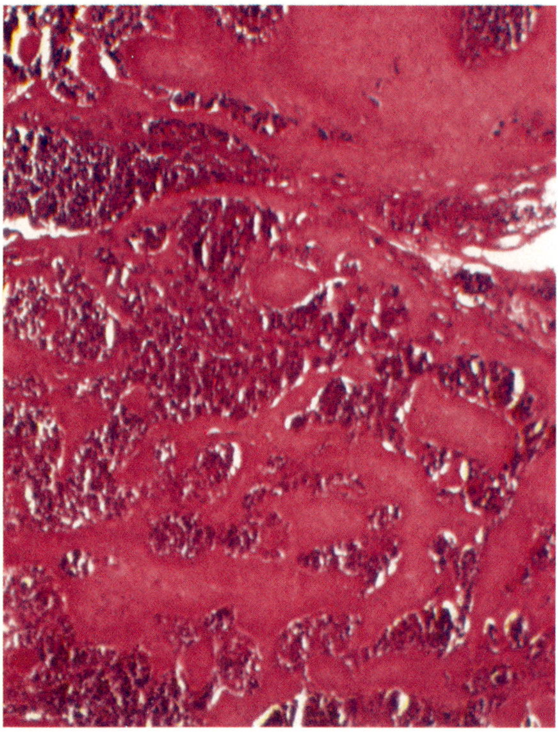

308 Histoplasma farciminosum in a horse. This section of skin shows marked pseudoepitheliomatous hyperplasia of the epidermis. The dark areas in the dermis are masses of GMS-positive *Histoplasma farciminosum* cells. (GMS–H&E, ×20)

309

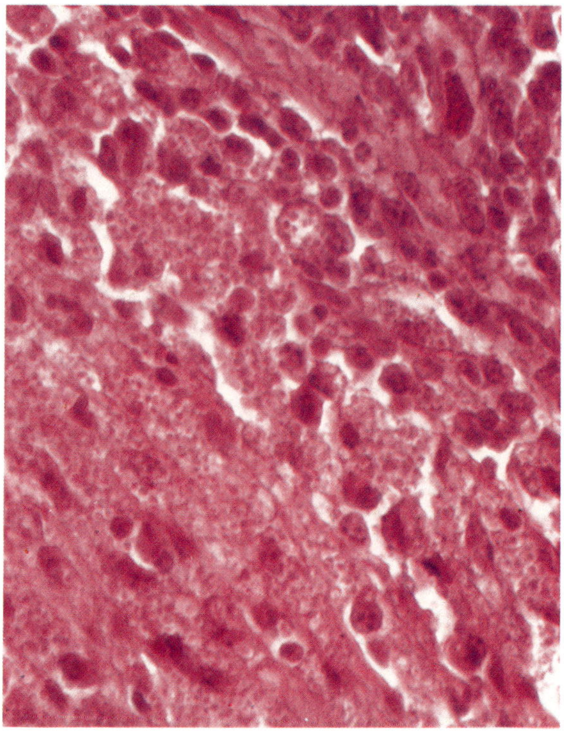

309 Histoplasmosis farciminosi in a mule. Large numbers of poorly stained yeast cells are within the granulomatous lesion. (H&E, ×200)

310

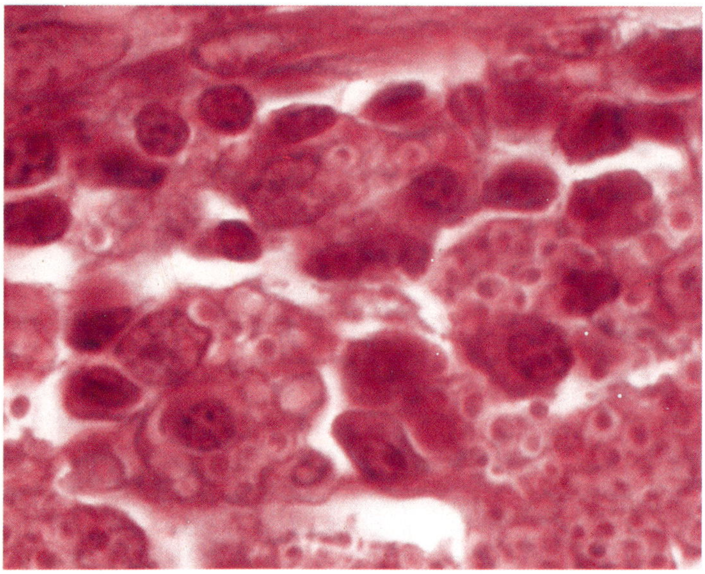

310 Histoplasmosis farciminosi Higher magnification of **309**. The fungal cells within the histiocytes and giant cells are morphologically and tinctorially identical to those of *Histoplasma capsulatum* var. *capsulatum* (see **273**). (H&E, ×500)

311

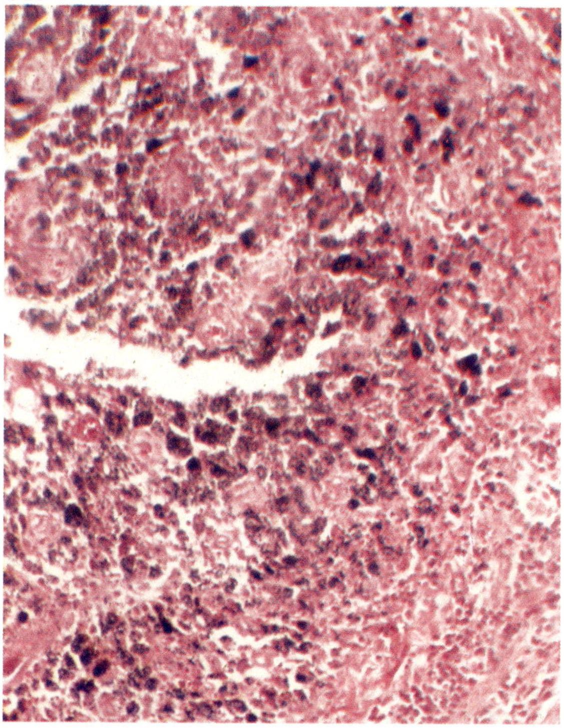

312

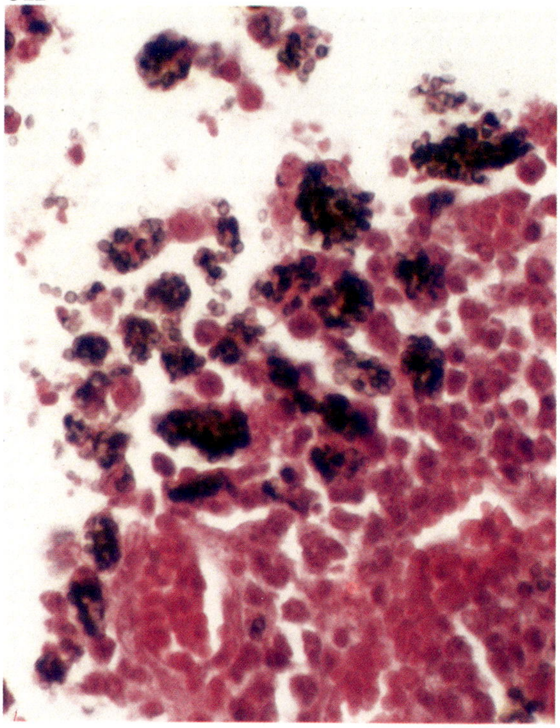

311 Histoplasmosis farciminosi in another horse. Note the presence of a sinus tract in the dermis. The dark masses within the surrounding fibrogranulomatous reaction are GMS-positive *Histoplasma farciminosum* cells. (GMS–H&E, ×50)

312 Histoplasma farciminosum Higher magnification of **311** showing clusters of yeast cells within histiocytes and giant cells that are located in the granulation tissue lining the sinus tract. (GMS–H&E, ×200)

313

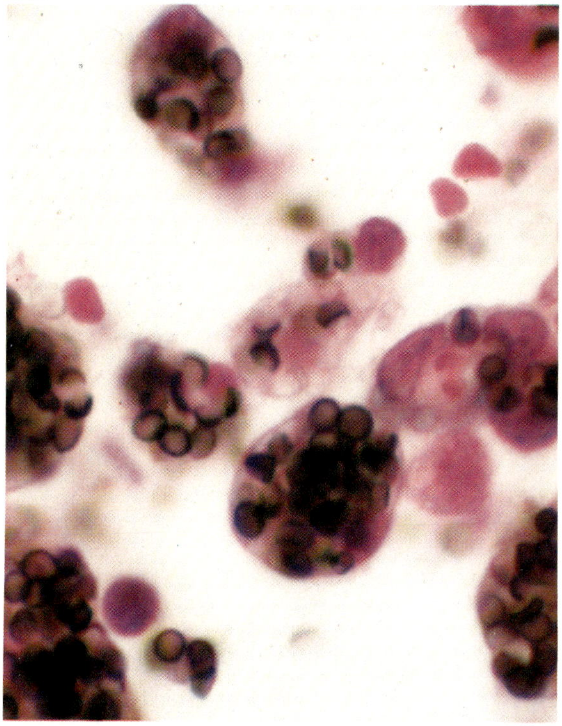

313 Histoplasma farciminosum Even higher magnification of **311** showing *Histoplasma farciminosum* cells within the phagocytes in greater detail. The yeast cells are well stained by GMS and appear identical to those of *Histoplasma capsulatum* var. *capsulatum* (see **274**). (GMS–H&E, ×500)

16 Lobomycosis

Text pages: 73–75

314

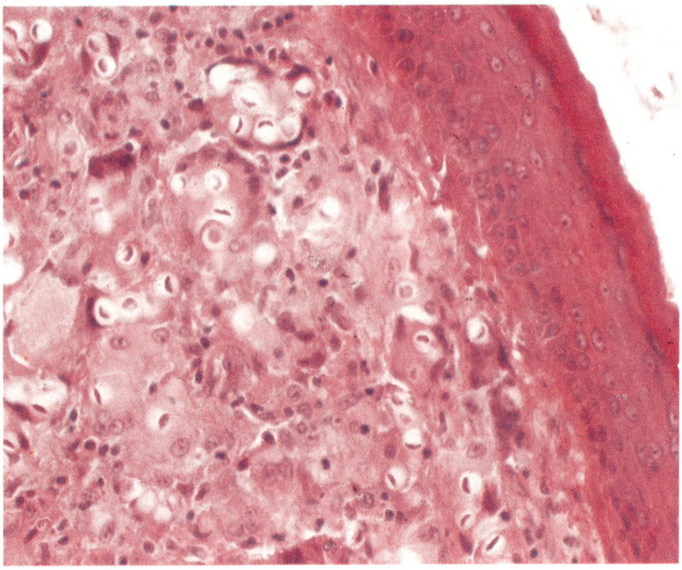

314 Loboa loboi causing lobomycosis in a Brazilian. The normal architecture of the dermis is effaced by a solid sheet of giant cells and histiocytes that contain numerous *Loboa loboi* cells. There is little or no dermal fibrosis. The overlying epidermis is unaffected. (H&E, ×100)

315

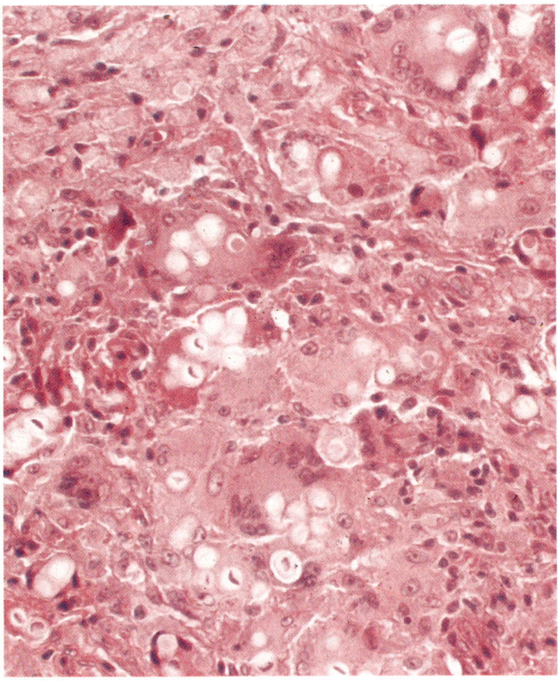

315 Loboa loboi Another field in **314** that shows poorly stained but clearly evident *Loboa loboi* cells within huge Langhans' and foreign body giant cells in the deep dermis. The basophilic cytoplasm of some fungal cells is retracted. (H&E, ×100)

316

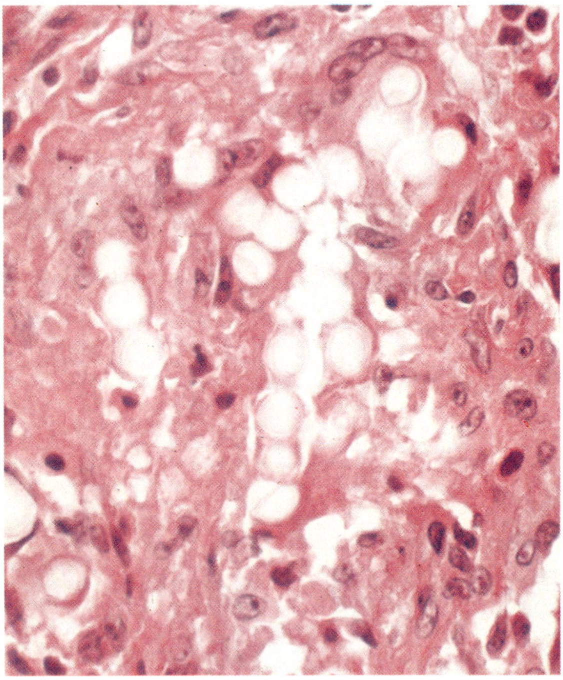

316 Loboa loboi Higher magnification of another field in **314** that shows chains of *Loboa loboi* cells within giant cells. Although the fungal cells are poorly stained by H&E, they are clearly visible. The cytoplasmic contents of most of the fungal cells in this field are not stained. (H&E, ×200)

317

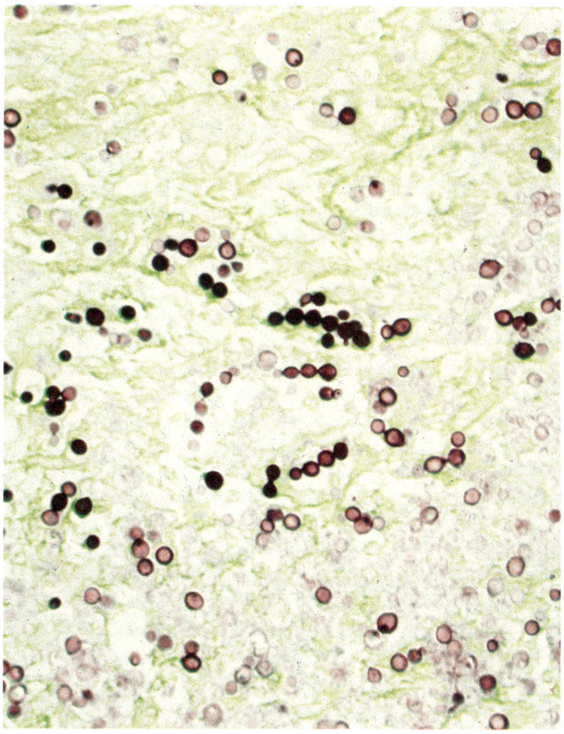

318

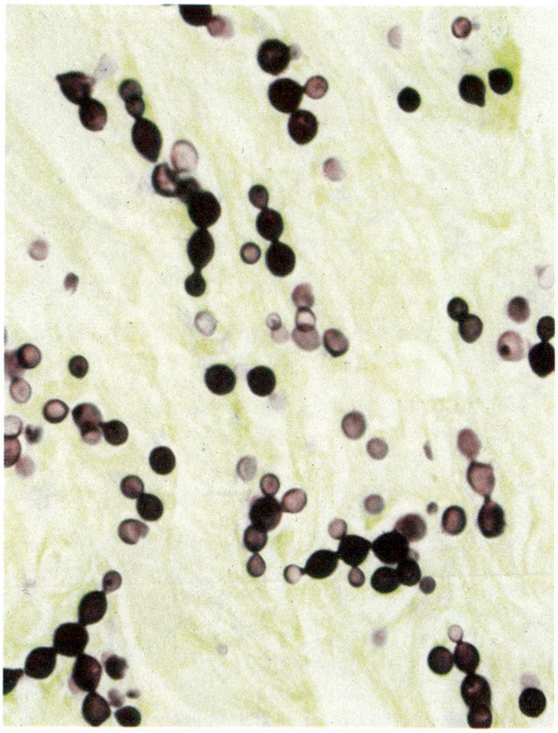

317 Loboa loboi Replicate section of **314** but stained by GMS to show the large numbers of *Loboa loboi* cells within the granulomatous lesion. (GMS, ×100)

318 Loboa loboi Higher magnification of **317**. The fungal cells are arranged in single and branched chains of varying lengths. Each fungal cell in the chain is connected to the other by a short, thick, tube-like structure. (GMS, ×200)

319

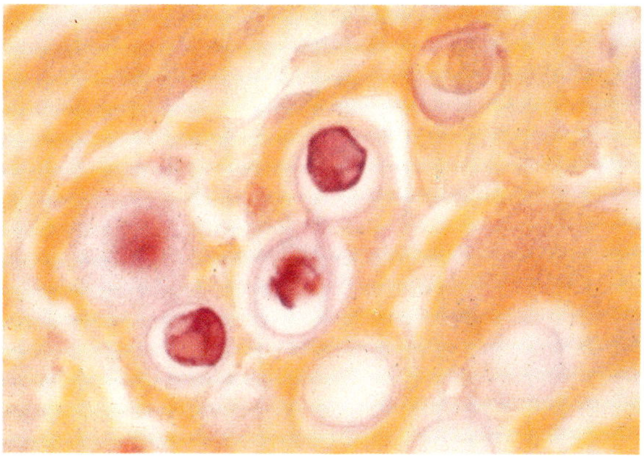

320

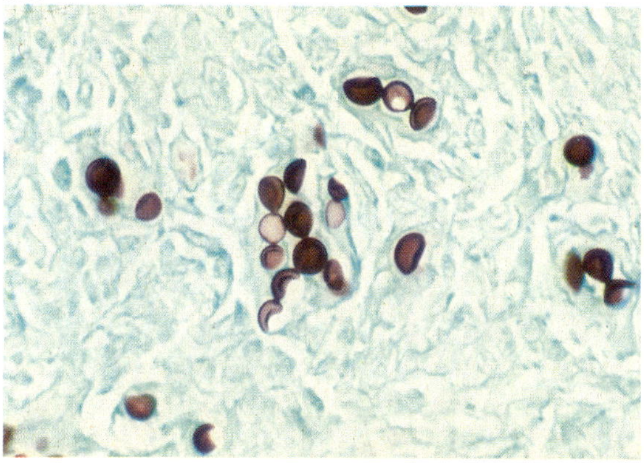

319 Loboa loboi Replicate section of **314** which shows in detail a tubular bridge connecting two cells. In this photomicrograph, the fungal cell wall is weakly stained and the retracted cytoplasmic contents are strongly GF-positive. (GF, ×500)

320 Loboa loboi Another field in **317** to show the appearance of distorted *Loboa loboi* cells within giant cells. In other fields, typical fungal cells in chain formation were seen. (GMS, ×200)

321

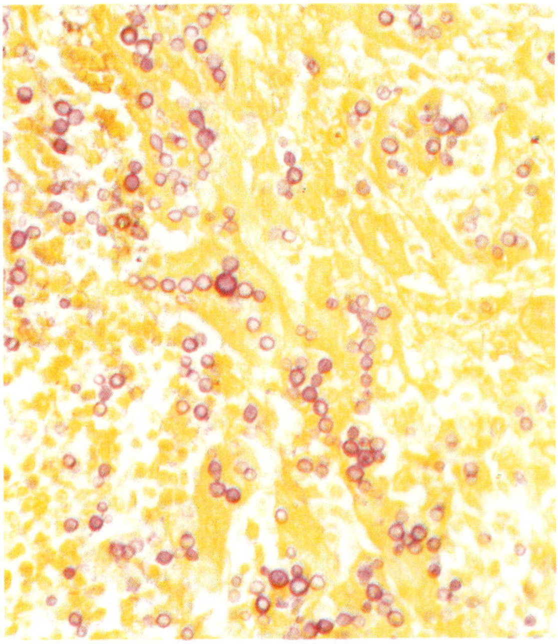

322

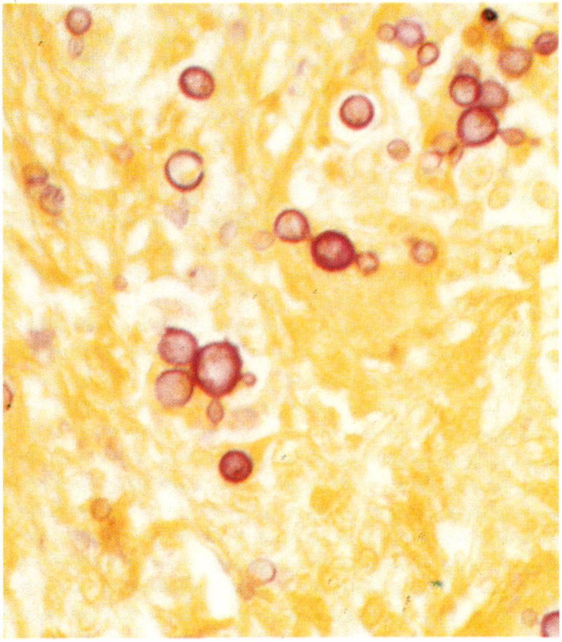

321 Lobomycosis in a dolphin. Note the large number of fungal cells, many of which are arranged in long chains. (GF, ×100)

322 Loboa loboi Higher magnification of **321** which shows single and multiple budding cells of *Loboa loboi* in the dermis. Note the intensely stained granular material on the surface of some fungal cells. (GF, ×200)

323

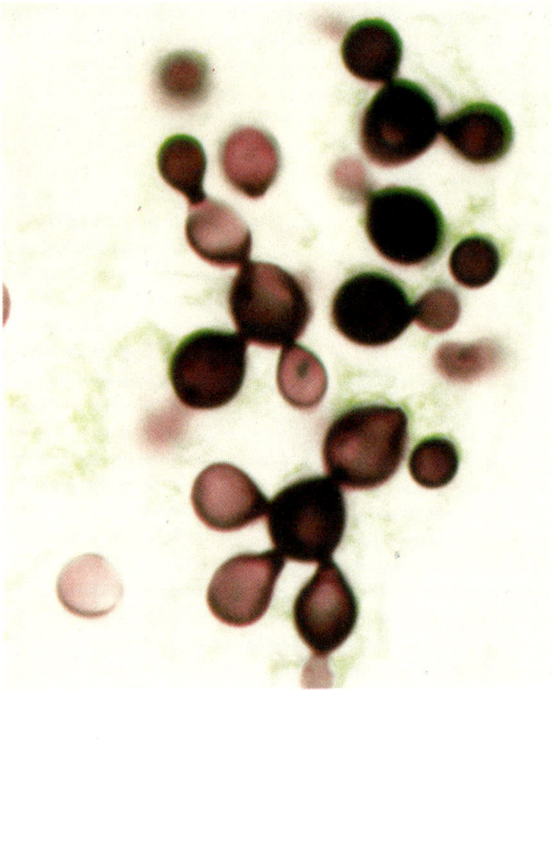

324

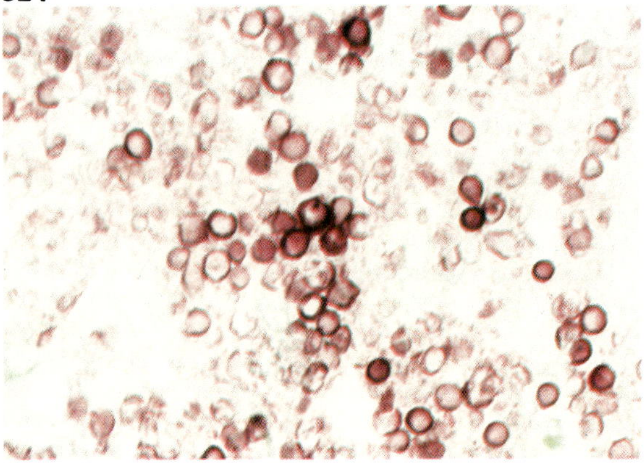

323 Loboa loboi Replicate section of **321** but stained by GMS to show details of single and multiple budding yeast cells and the tube-like processes that interconnect these cells. (GMS, ×500)

324 Loboa loboi Another area in **323** that shows degenerated and intact cells, and GMS-positive fungal cell debris within histiocytes and giant cells. (GMS, ×200)

325

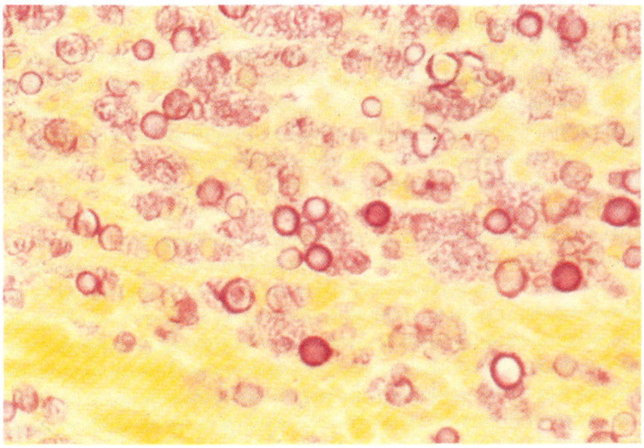

325 Loboa loboi Another field in **321** which shows abundant GF-positive fungal cell debris as well as distorted and typical *Loboa loboi* cells within phagocytes in the dermis. (GF, ×200)

326

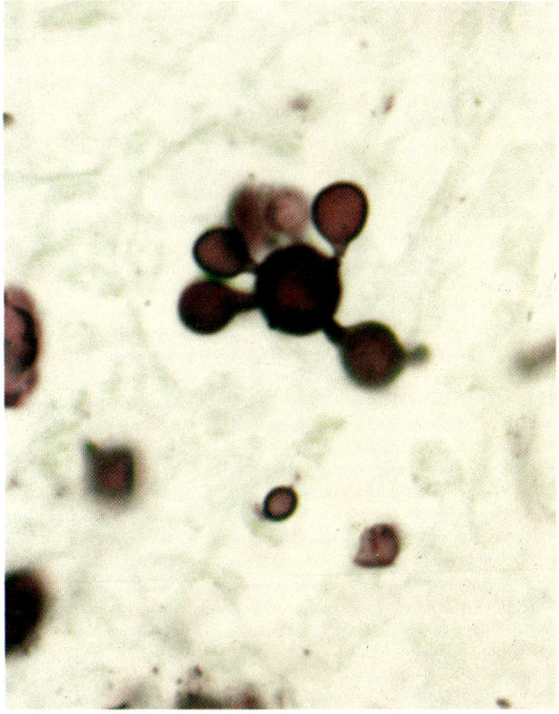

326 Cutaneous paracoccidioidomycosis in a human. Note the morphological resemblance of the multiple budding cell of *Paracoccidioides brasiliensis* to those of *Loboa loboi* in **323**. The latter can usually be differentiated from *P. brasiliensis* in tissue because they characteristically appear in long chains (see **318**) and are relatively uniform in size. (GMS, ×500)

17 Mycetomas

Text pages: 76–82

327

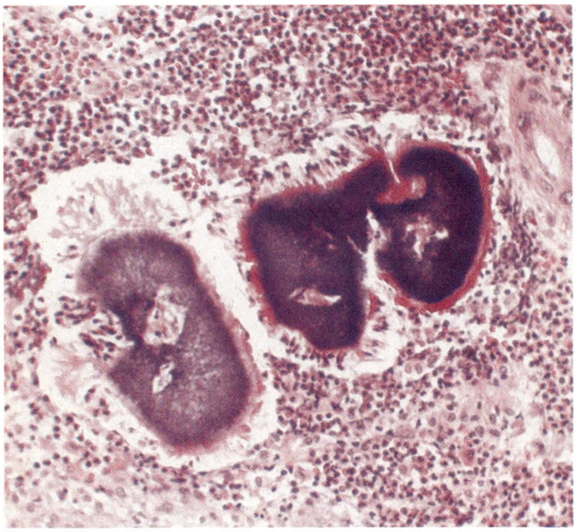

327 Actinomadura madurae causing mycetoma in a Mexican. Deeply basophilic granules with lighter eosinophilic central zones are present. The granules are bordered by brightly eosinophilic Splendore–Hoeppli material and are embedded in an abscess that is surrounded by granulation tissue. (H&E, ×50)

328

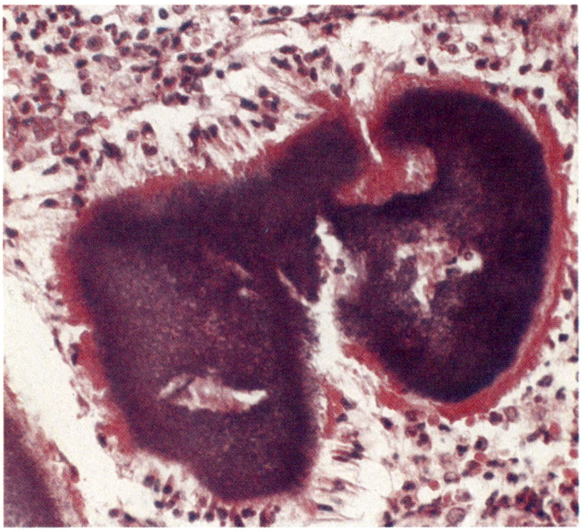

328 Actinomadura madurae Higher magnification of **327** showing one of the *Actinomadura madurae* granules and the surrounding inflammatory reaction in greater detail. The irregular periphery of the granule is more basophilic than the inner portions. Eosinophilic zones can be seen in its centre. A narrow zone of eosinophilic Splendore–Hoeppli material intimately surrounds the granule. (H&E, ×100)

329

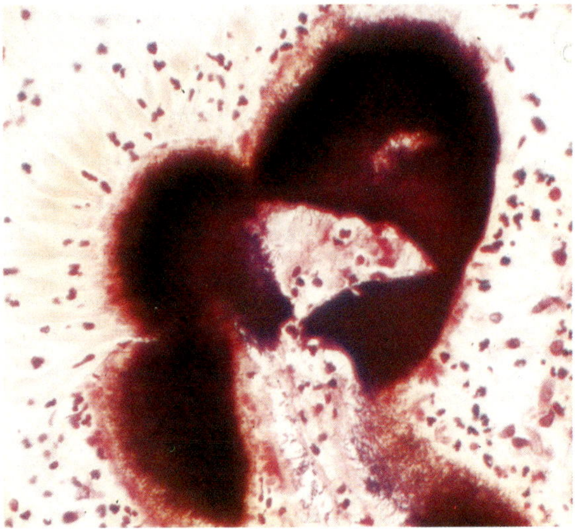

329 Actinomadura madurae Another granule stained by a tissue Gram stain. The granule proper is intensely gram-positive but the surrounding Splendore–Hoeppli material is gram-negative. (B&B, ×100)

330

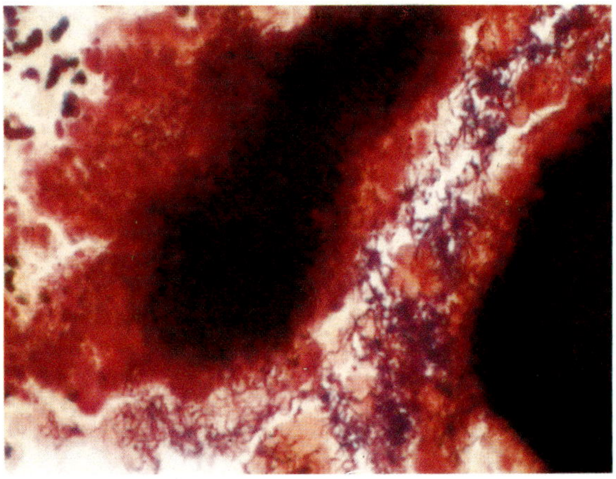

330 Actinomadura madurae Higher magnification of **329** revealing the numerous, delicate (≤1 μm) gram-positive filaments at the periphery of the granule. Some of the filaments are embedded in Splendore–Hoeppli material. The presence of delicate (≤1 μm) filaments within a granule immediately indicates that the patient has an actinomycotic mycetoma. (B&B, ×200)

331

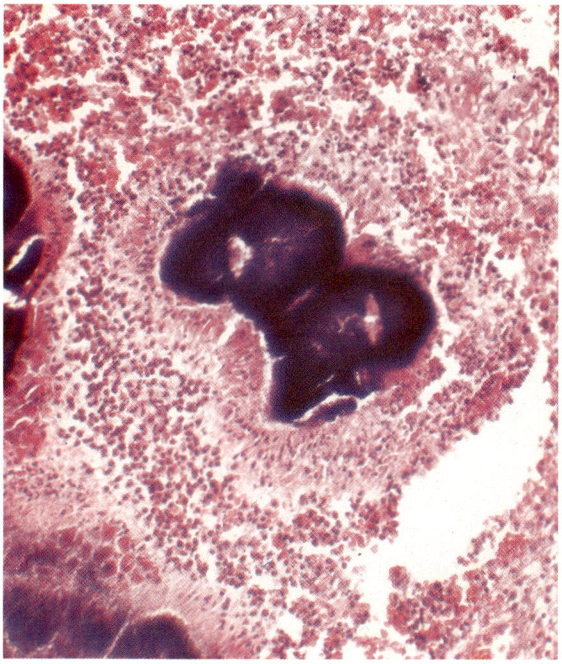

331 Actinomadura pelletieri causing a mycetoma. The deeply basophilic granules are embedded in a haemorrhagic abscess. (H&E, ×50)

332

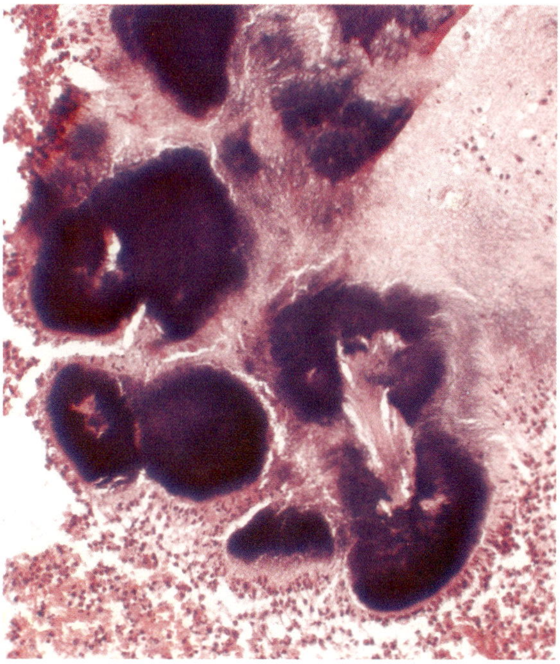

332 Actinomadura pelletieri Another field in **331** that shows several granules of *Actinomadura pelletieri*. In some of the granules, basophilic filaments radiate from the periphery into the surrounding tissues. (H&E, ×50)

333

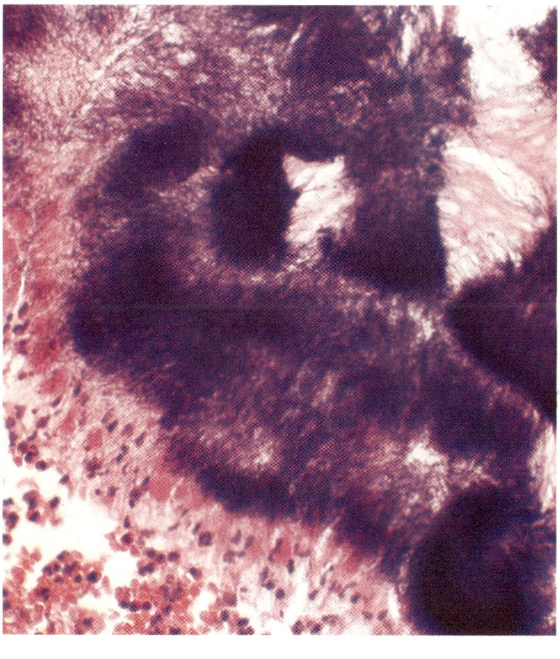

333 Actinomadura pelletieri Higher magnification of **332**. Numerous basophilic filaments radiate from the periphery of the granule into surrounding tissue. The advancing filaments are bordered by irregular deposits of eosinophilic material. (H&E, ×100)

334

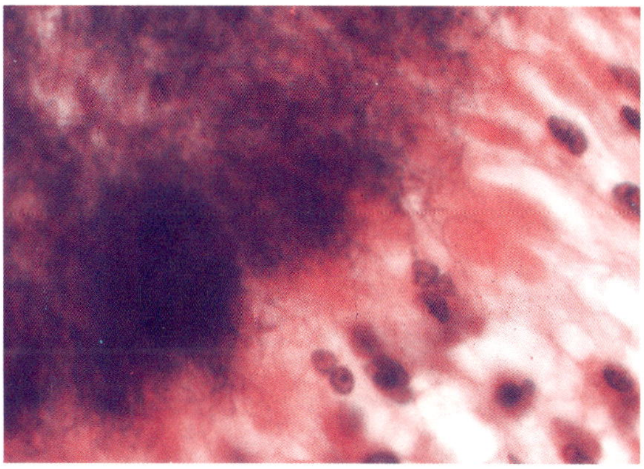

334 Actinomadura pelletieri An even higher magnification of **332** to show the advancing basophilic filaments and the border of Splendore–Hoeppli material in greater detail. Polymorphonuclear leucocytes are intimately associated with the eosinophilic material. (H&E, ×500)

335

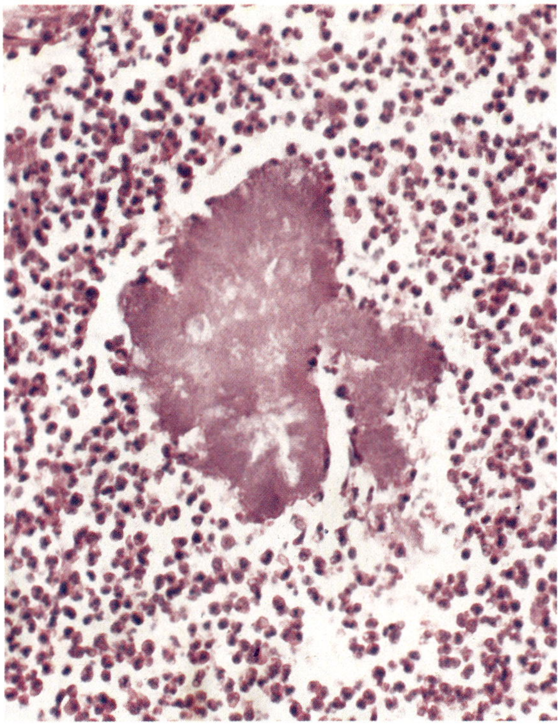

336

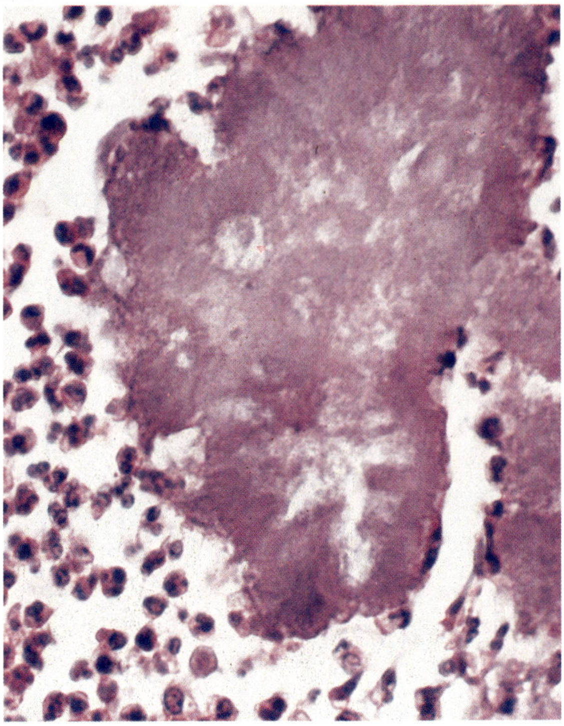

335 Nocardia asteroides granule in a pulmonary abscess in an orangutan. This lightly basophilic granule has an irregular border. Splendore–Hoeppli material is not evident in this case. (H&E, ×100)

336 Nocardia asteroides Higher magnification of **335** showing details of the granule embedded in purulent exudate. Although the entire granule is well stained, individual filaments of *Nocardia asteroides* are not discernible. (H&E, ×200)

337

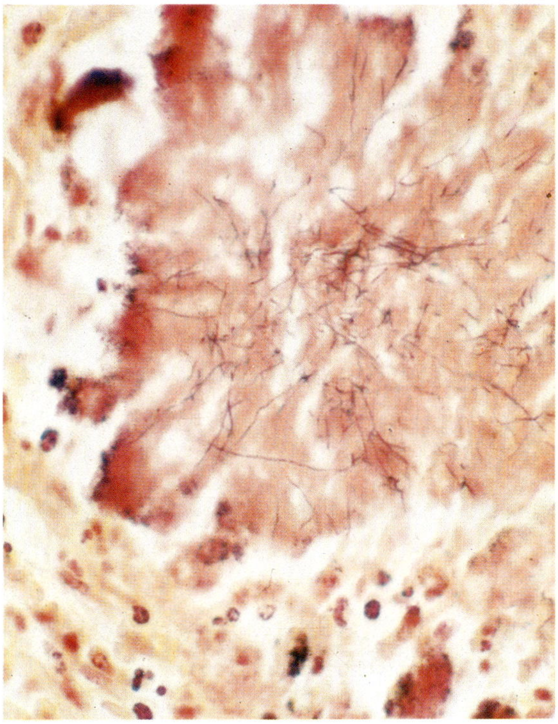

338

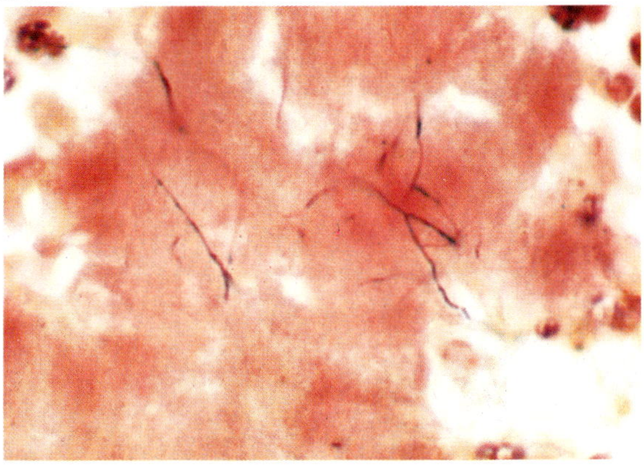

337 Nocardia asteroides Replicate section of **335** stained by a tissue Gram stain to show filaments of varying lengths within the matrix of the granule. (B&B, ×200)

338 Nocardia asteroides Higher magnification of **337** which shows the beaded appearance of the delicate (≤1 μm), branched filaments within the matrix of the granule. (B&B, ×500)

339

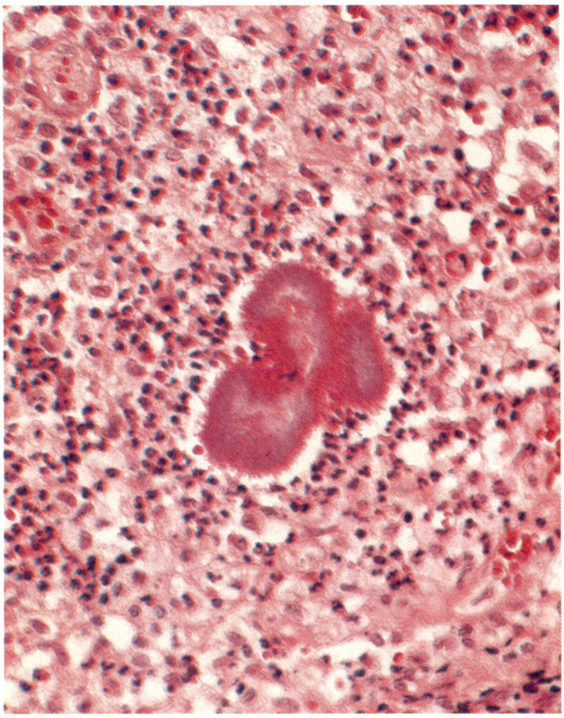

340

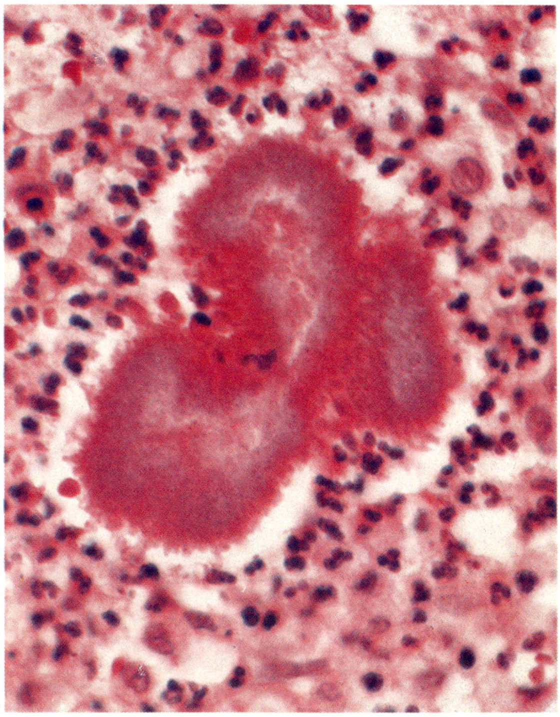

339 Nocardia brasiliensis causing mycetoma in a Mexican. The irregular granule is basophilic, bordered by deeply eosinophilic Splendore–Hoeppli material, and embedded in a mixed purulent and granulomatous lesion. (H&E, ×100)

340 Nocardia brasiliensis Higher magnification of **339**. Although the granule is well stained by haematoxylin, its individual filaments are not seen. Peripheral eosinophilic clubs are evident. (H&E, ×200)

341

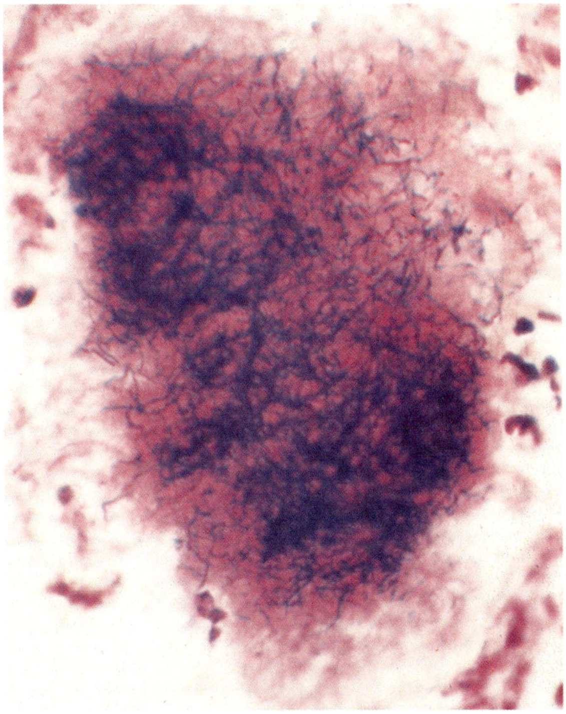

341 Nocardia brasiliensis causing mycetoma in another subject. A tissue Gram stain clearly demonstrates the numerous, delicate gram-positive filaments embedded in the matrix of the granule. Some of the filaments are fragmented. (B&B, ×200)

342

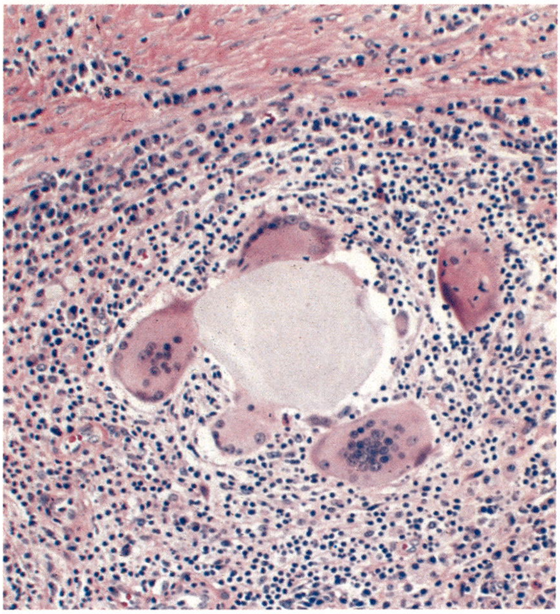

343

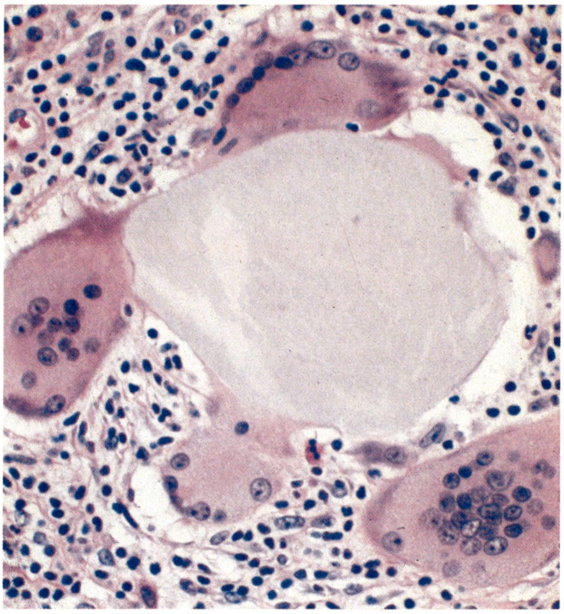

342 Streptomyces somaliensis causing actinomycotic mycetoma in a human. A poorly stained, homogeneous, oval granule is surrounded by a fibrogranulomatous reaction. Huge foreign body and Langhans' giant cells adhere to and are attempting to engulf this highly distinctive granule. (H&E, ×50)

343 Streptomyces somaliensis Higher magnification of **342** showing the intimate attachments of the huge giant cells to the surface of the granule. The distinctive appearance of the granules of *Streptomyces somaliensis* allows a specific aetiologic diagnosis to be made from histological sections. Large numbers of lymphocytes and plasma cells are seen in the surrounding granulation tissue. (H&E, ×100)

344

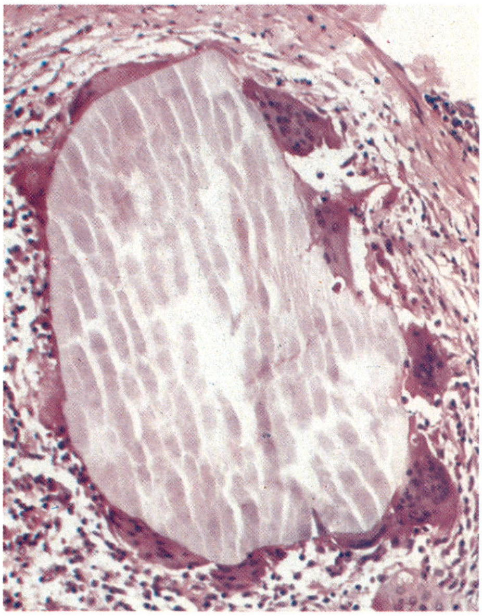

345

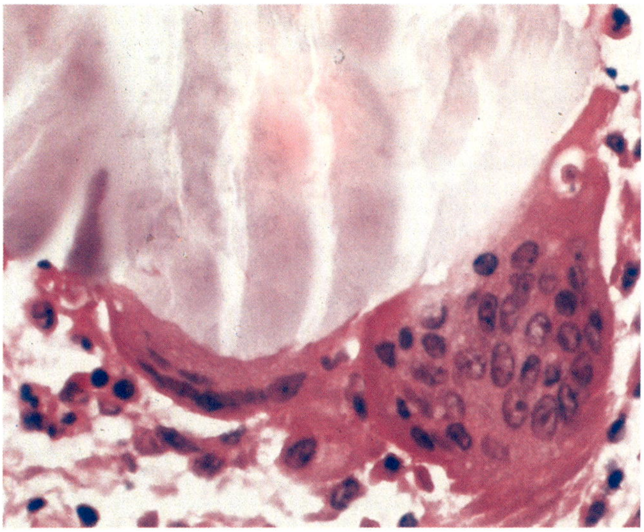

344 Streptomyces somaliensis causing mycetoma in another human. Here, the inflammatory response is similar to that in **342**. Because the cement material of the granule is hard, the granule is often fractured by the microtome knife. (H&E, ×50)

345 Streptomyces somaliensis Higher magnification of **344** shows a huge foreign body giant cell partially surrounding the granule in an attempt to engulf it. In this granule, filaments are not evident. The undulating fracture lines within the hard granule are clearly seen. (H&E, ×200)

346

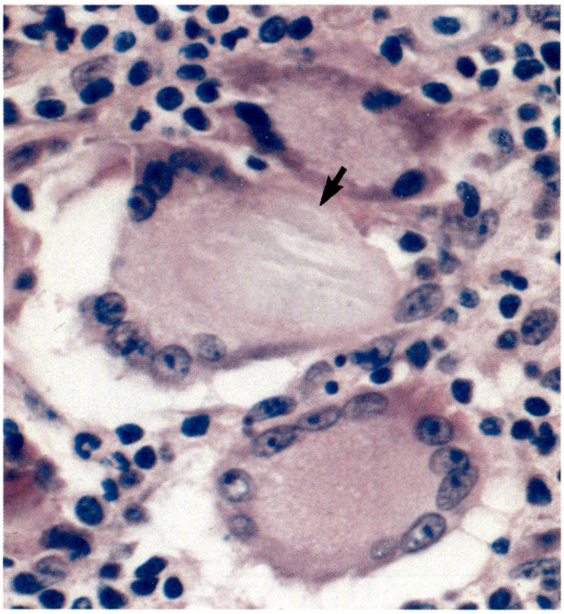

347

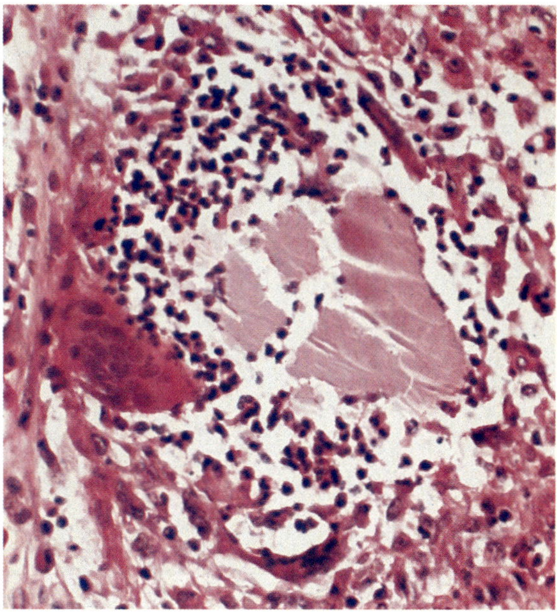

346 Streptomyces somaliensis Another field in **342** showing a small granule (arrow) engulfed by a Langhans' giant cell. (H&E, ×200)

347 Streptomyces somaliensis A disintegrated granule surrounded by a mixed purulent and granulomatous inflammatory reaction. (H&E, ×100)

348

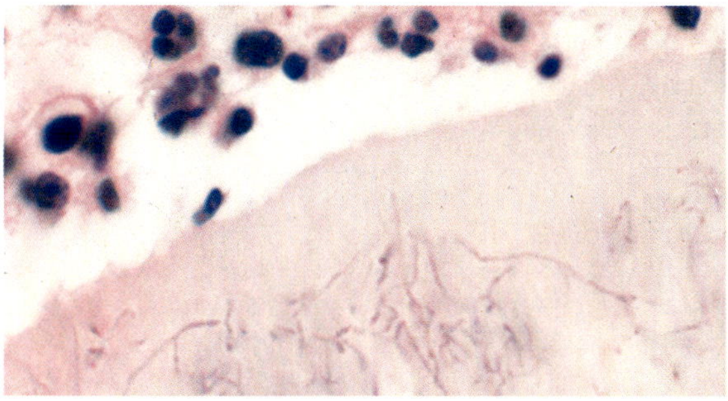

349

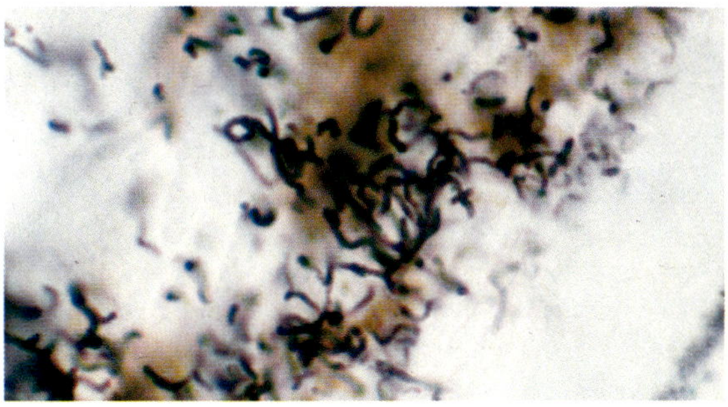

348 Streptomyces somaliensis Another field in **342** demonstrating that in some granules, the individual delicate filaments in the cement are faintly basophilic and visible when stained by H&E. (H&E, ×500)

349 Streptomyces somaliensis Replicate section of **348**. The delicate branched filaments that occur in the granule are GMS-positive and clearly visible. (GMS, ×500)

350

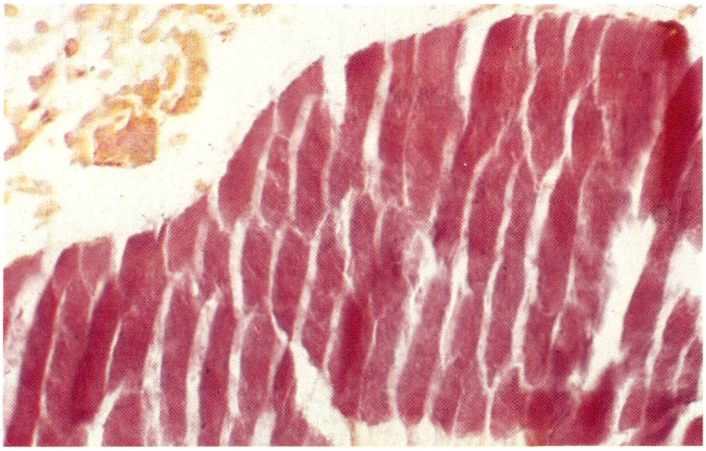

350 Streptomyces somaliensis Replicate section of **344** stained by the GF procedure. Although the entire granule is stained, individual filaments are not seen. (GF, ×100)

351

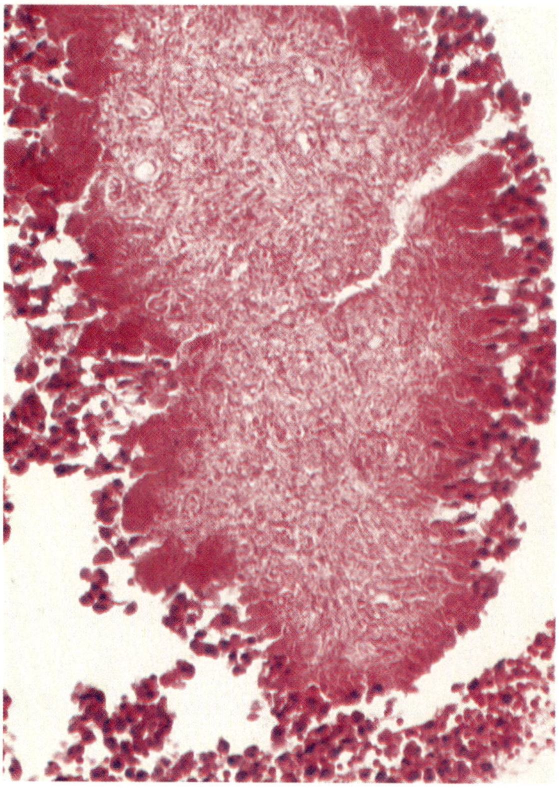

352

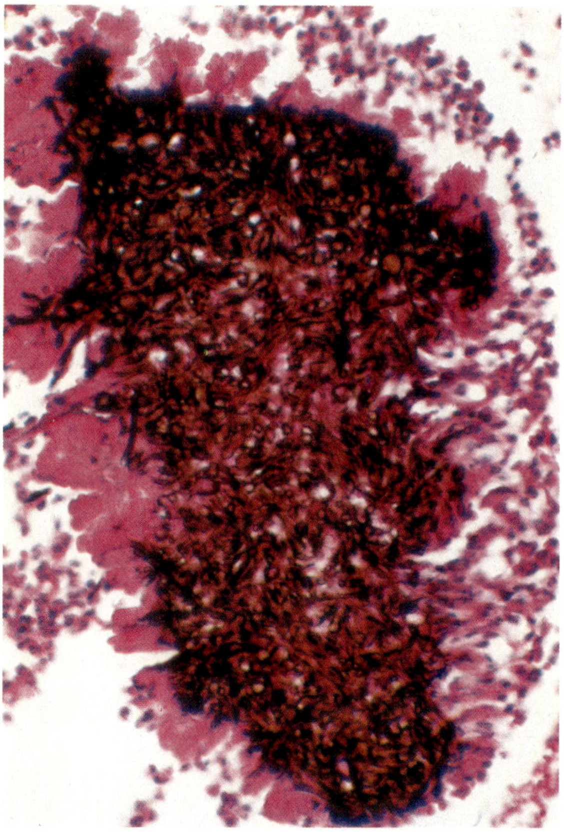

351 Acremonium falciforme causing white grain mycetoma in a human. This irregularly-shaped granule is made up of an intricate network of hyaline mycelium and small chlamydospores. It has a prominent eosinophilic border of Splendore–Hoeppli material, and closely resembles those of *Acremonium recifei* and *Petriellidium boydii*. (H&E, ×100)

352 Acremonium falciforme Replicate section of **351** but stained by GMS–H&E to better demonstrate the network of mycelium and small chlamydospores that form the granule. The Splendore–Hoeppli material that borders the granule is not stained by GMS, but the H&E counterstain colours it brightly eosinophilic. (GMS–H&E, ×100)

353

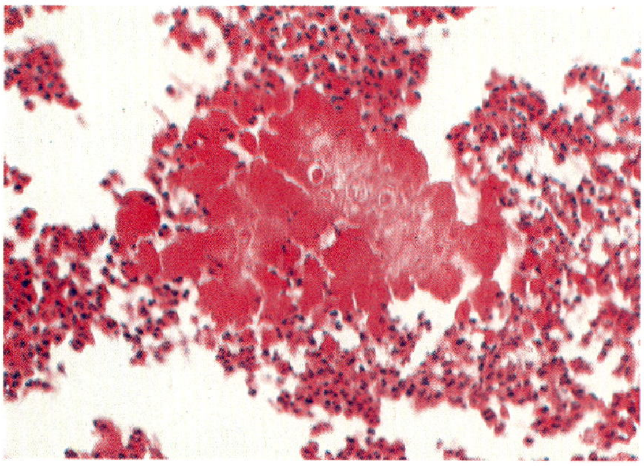

354

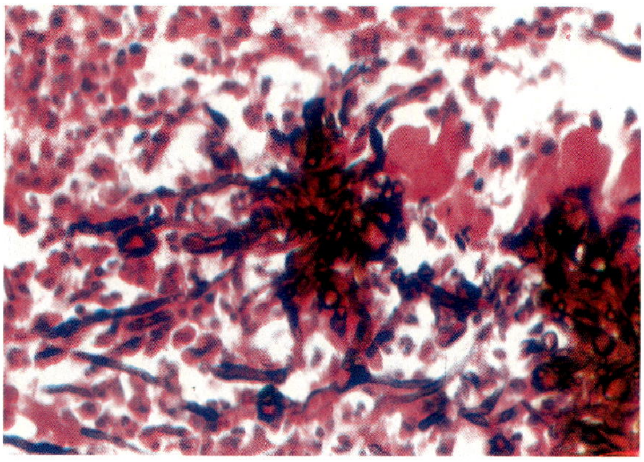

353 Acremonium falciforme (young granule). A few hyaline chlamydospores are surrounded by abundant Splendore–Hoeppli material. Note the purulent inflammatory reaction. (H&E, ×100)

354 Acremonium falciforme Another field in **352** which shows an early stage in granule formation. The network of mycelium and small chlamydospores are clearly indicated, as are the individual hyphae outside the granule. (GMS–H&E, ×200)

355

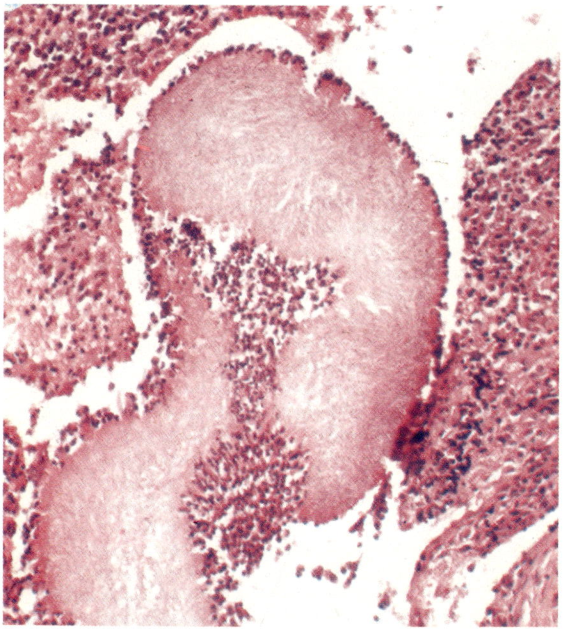

356

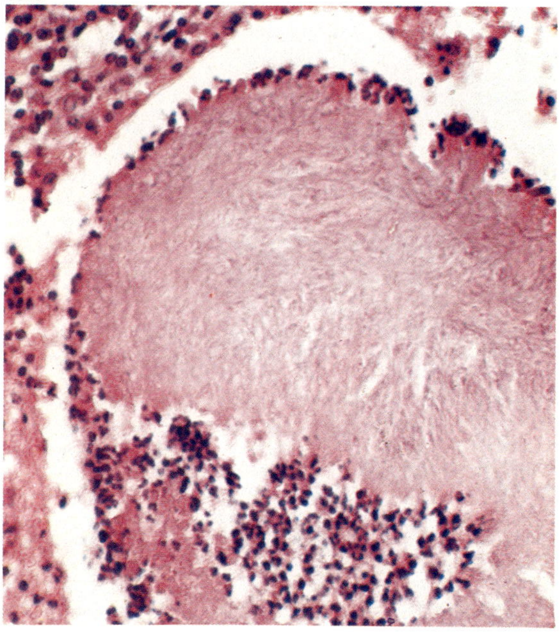

355 Acremonium recifei causing white grain mycetoma in an East Indian. This granule, like the one shown in **351**, is composed of an intricate network of hyaline mycelium and small chlamydospores. In this case, an eosinophilic border is present but not prominent. The granules of the *Acremonium spp*. are very similar in tissues and their differentiation requires cultural studies. (H&E, ×50)

356 Acremonium recifei Higher magnification of **355** that shows in greater detail the mycelium and small chlamydospores that form the granule. A mixed inflammatory reaction surrounds the granule. (H&E, ×100)

357

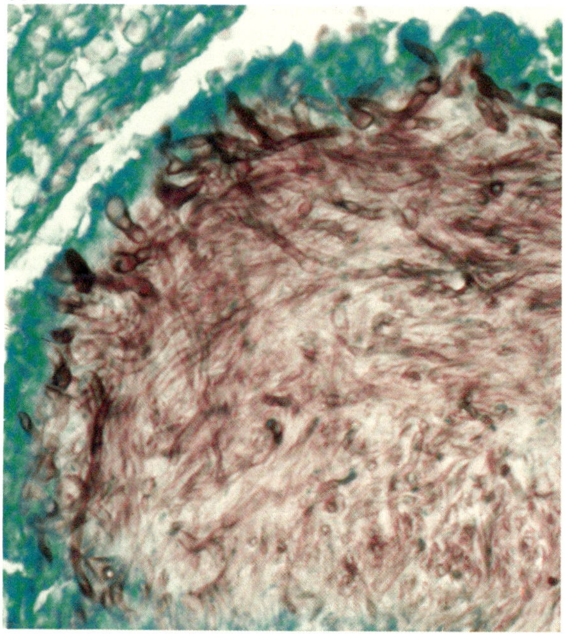

358

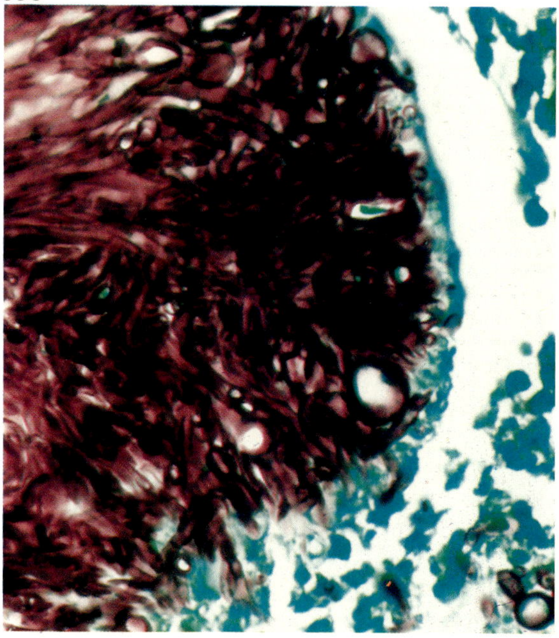

357 Acremonium recifei Replicate section of **355** but stained by GMS to show the fungal elements that make up the granule. (GMS, ×100)

358 Acremonium recifei Higher magnification of a granule shows that it is composed of a dense network of mycelium and a few peripheral chlamydospores. (GMS, ×200)

359

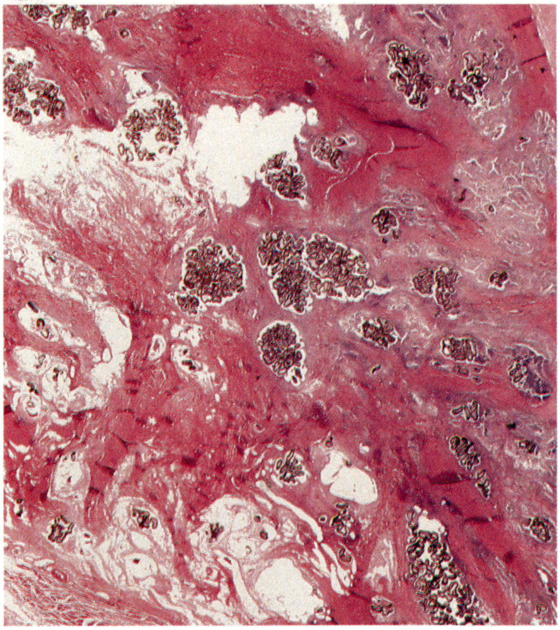

359 Curvularia geniculata causing black grain mycetoma in a dog. The dark masses represent clusters of pigmented granules in soft tissue and bone. Note the extensive fibrosis. This subgross photomicrograph illustrates the extensive fungus involvement that may occur in a mycetoma. (H&E, ×1)

360

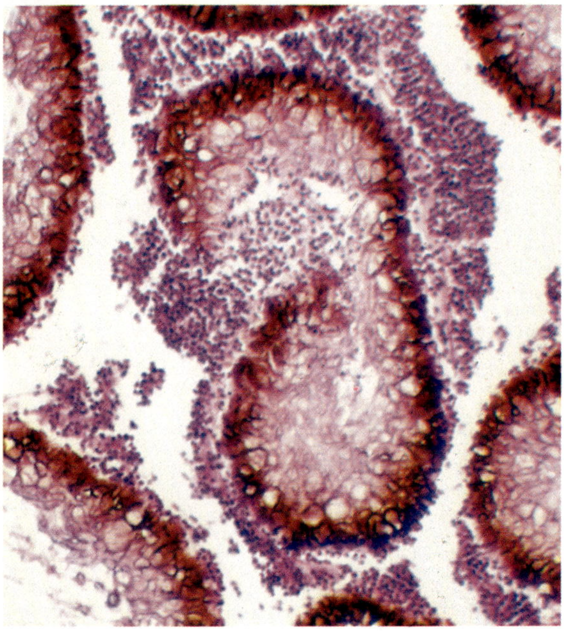

360 Curvularia geniculata Higher magnification of **359** to show the individual granules. Note the dark periphery of compact dematiaceous hyphae and chlamydospores, and the loose network of mycelium in the interior of the granule. Some of the granules appear to be hollow and thus resemble those of *Leptospheria senegalensis*. (H&E, ×20)

361

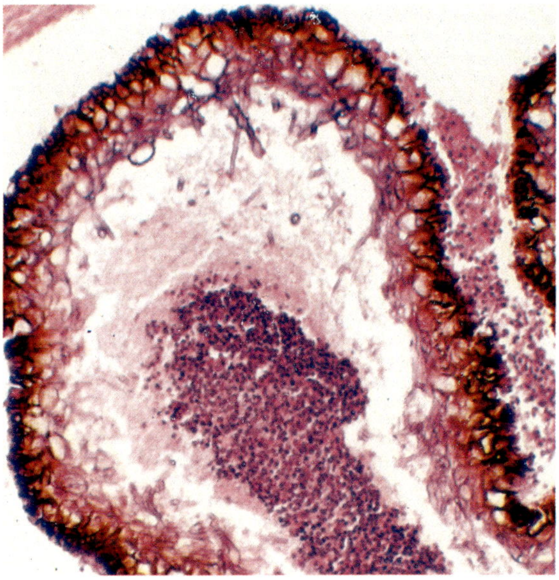

361 Curvularia geniculata Another granule that shows in detail the peripheral dematiaceous mycelium and chlamydospores. In the inner parts of the granule, the mycelium is not pigmented. The hollow centre of the granule contains neutrophils and cellular debris. (H&E, ×50)

362

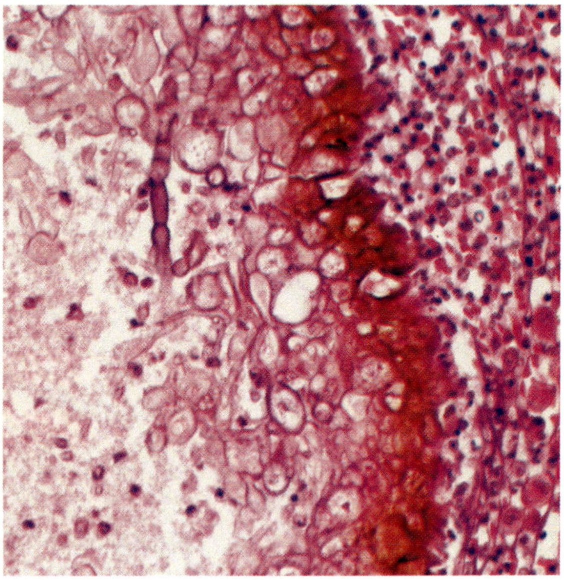

362 Curvularia geniculata Higher magnification of **361**. The dematiaceous mycelium and chlamydospores that make up the periphery of the granule are embedded in a cement-like material. The fungal elements towards the interior are nonpigmented. (H&E, ×100)

363

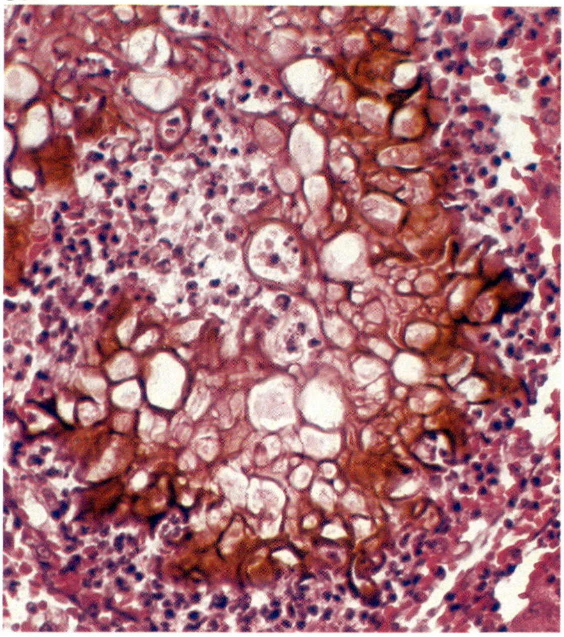

364

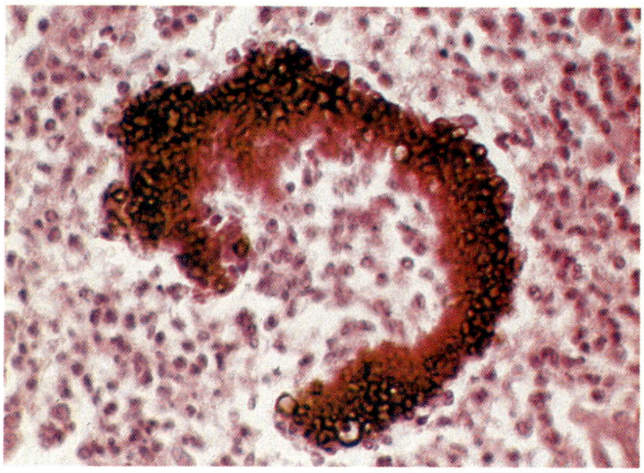

364 Exophiala jeanselmei causing black grain mycetoma in a human. The distinctive crescent-shaped granule is composed of dematiaceous chlamydospores and hyphae. A mixed purulent and granulomatous reaction surrounds the granule. (H&E, ×100)

363 Curvularia geniculata A young granule embedded in a microabscess. Most of the fungal elements at this stage of development are dematiaceous. (H&E, ×100)

365

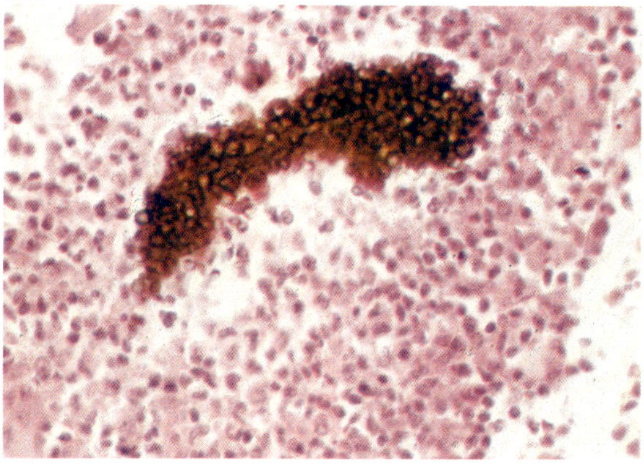

366

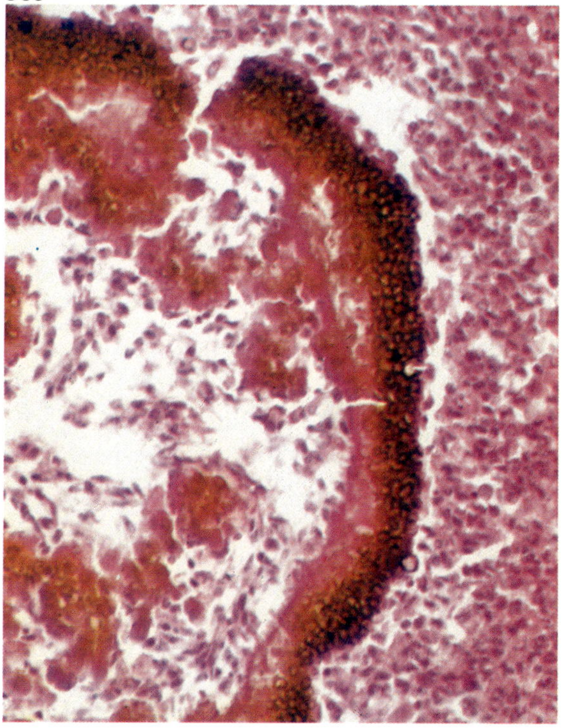

365 Exophiala jeanselmei The curved granule is made up of compact dematiaceous chlamydospores and a few hyphae. It has a distinctive appearance. (H&E, ×100)

366 Exophiala jeanselmei Another field in **364** containing a larger granule. The granule partially encloses a central zone of cellular debris and polymorphonuclear leucocytes. (H&E, ×100)

367

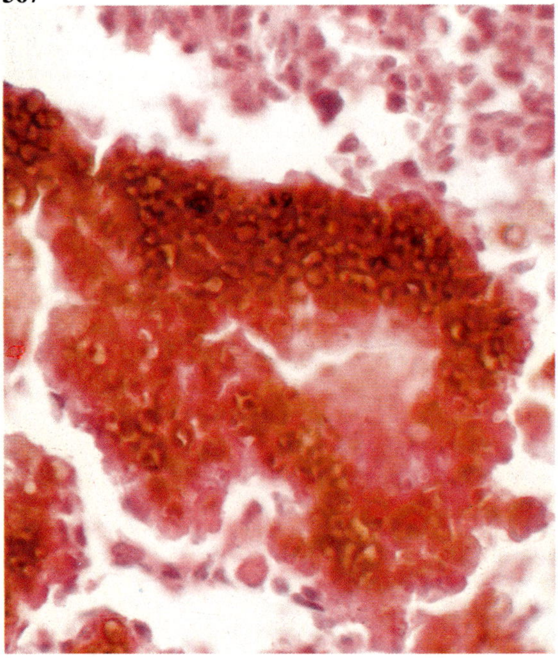

368

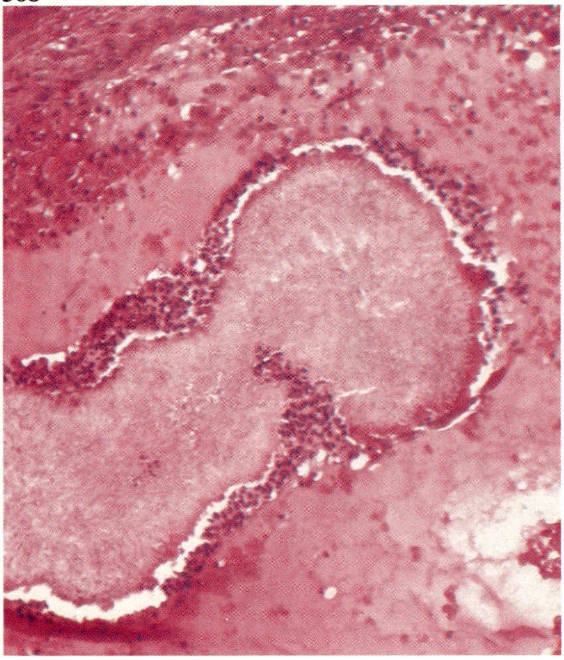

367 Exophiala jeanselmei Higher magnification of **364** to show in detail the dematiaceous fungal elements that make up the granule. Chlamydospores are a conspicuous feature. (H&E, ×200)

368 Fusarium moniliforme causing white grain mycetoma in a human. Note the resemblance of this granule to those of the *Acremonium spp.* and of *Petriellidium boydii*. The granule is embedded in neutrophils and proteinaceous material. (H&E, ×50)

369

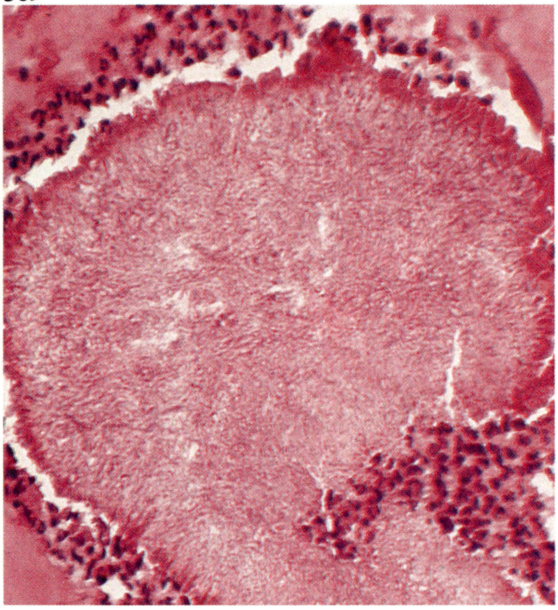

370

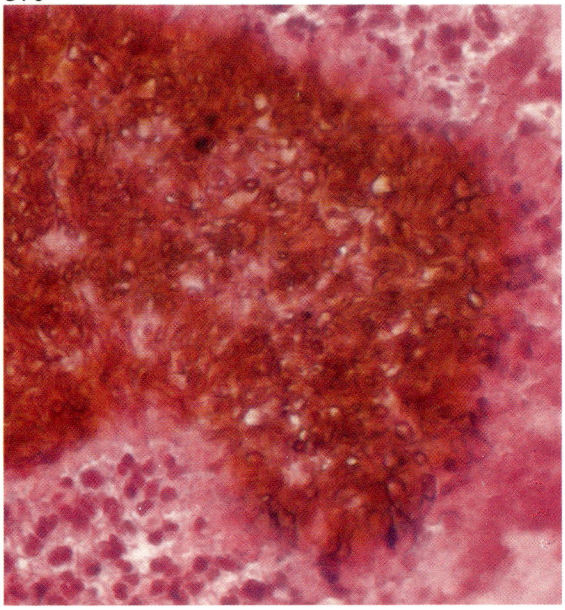

369 Fusarium moniliforme Higher magnification of **368** to show the granule in greater detail. The granule has an eosinophilic border and is composed of a network of hyaline mycelium and a few small chlamydospores. Because the granules of this fungus are so similar to those of the *Acremonium spp.*, their differentiation without cultural studies would be very difficult. (H&E, ×100)

370 Fusarium moniliforme Replicate section of **368** but stained by GMS–H&E to demonstrate the fungal elements that make up the granule. (GMS–H&E, ×200)

371

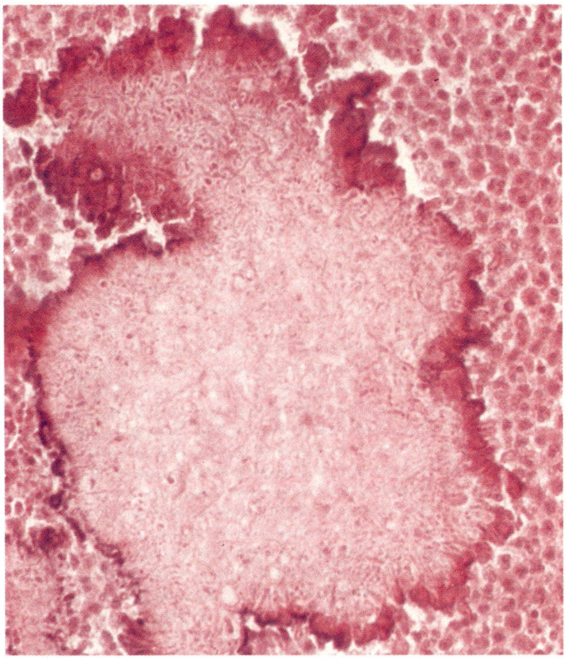

371 Aspergillus nidulans causing white grain mycetoma in a human. The granule is composed of a network of hyaline mycelium surrounded by a distinct zone of Splendore–Hoeppli material. Because the granule resembles those caused by other hyaline eumycetes, cultural studies are necessary for an accurate identification. (H&E, ×100)

372

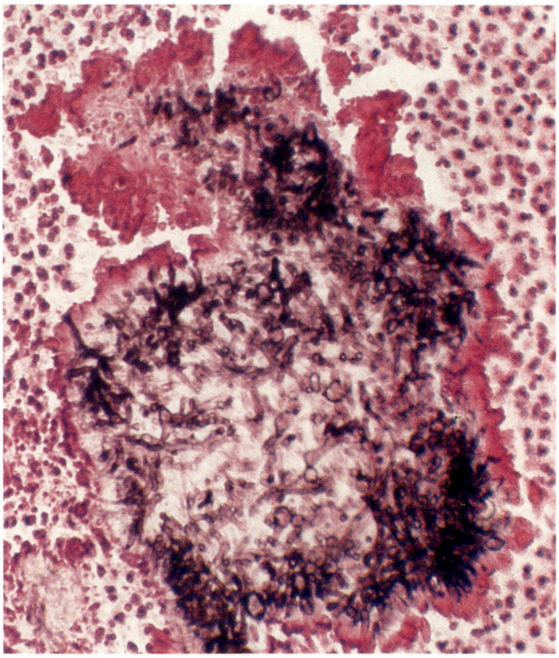

372 Aspergillus nidulans The same granule as illustrated in **371**, but stained by GMS–H&E. The network of hyphae that make up the granule is well delineated and stands out in contrast to the deeply eosinophilic Splendore–Hoeppli material and surrounding purulent exudate. (GMS–H&E, ×100)

373

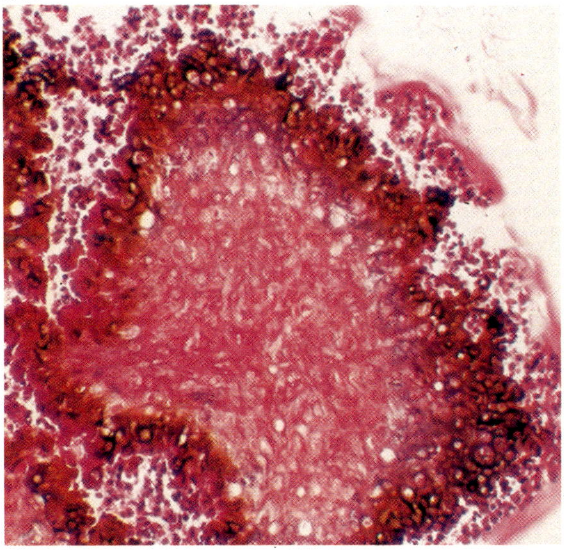

373 Leptospheria senegalensis causing black grain mycetoma in a human. Note the similarity of the granules to those of *Curvularia geniculata*. Like those of the latter fungus, the granules have a dark periphery of dematiaceous mycelium and chlamydospores. The mycelium in the interior of the granules appears to be nonpigmented. (H&E, ×50)

374

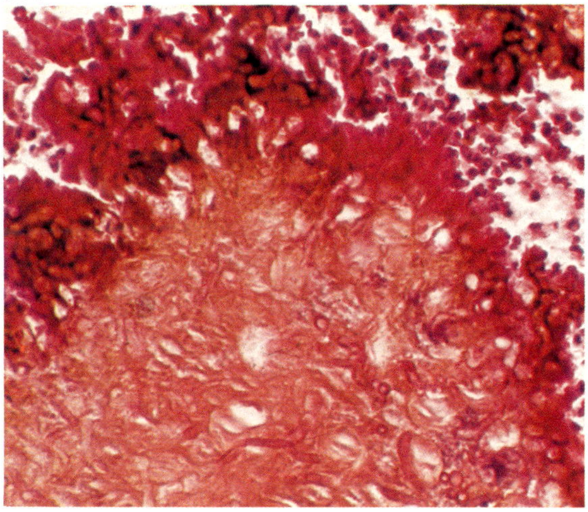

374 Leptospheria senegalensis Higher magnification of **373** to show details of the granule. The dematiaceous elements that make up the periphery are embedded in a brownish cement-like material. The fungal elements in the interior of the granule are not as deeply pigmented. (H&E, ×100)

375

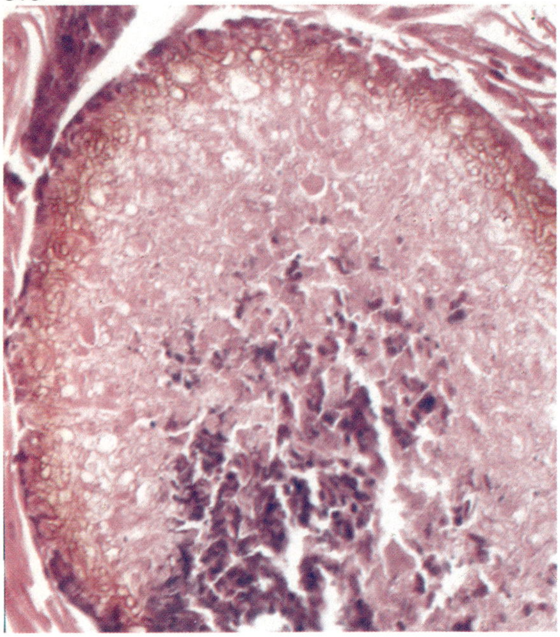

375 Madurella grisea causing black grain mycetoma in a human. The granule has a central nonpigmented area made up of a loose network of hyphae. Its periphery is brown and is composed of a dense network of hyphae and round-to-polygonal chlamydospores. (H&E, ×100)

376

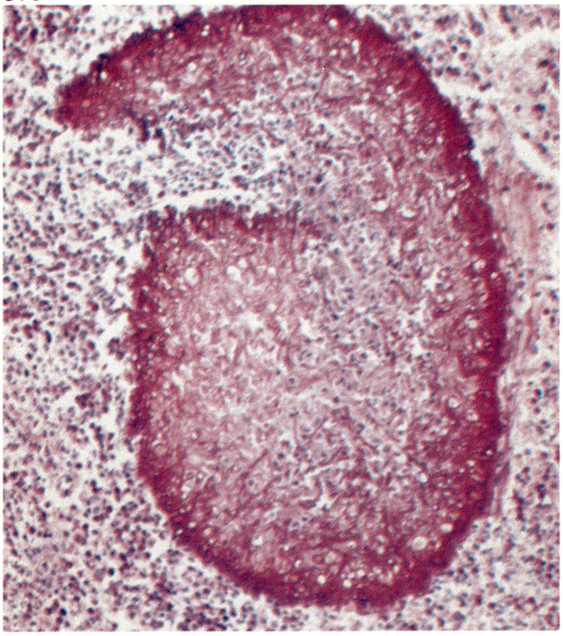

376 Madurella grisea, stained by PAS. The fungal elements are concentrated at the periphery and their innate brown colour is masked. The purulent inflammatory response is well demonstrated with this stain. (PAS, ×50)

377

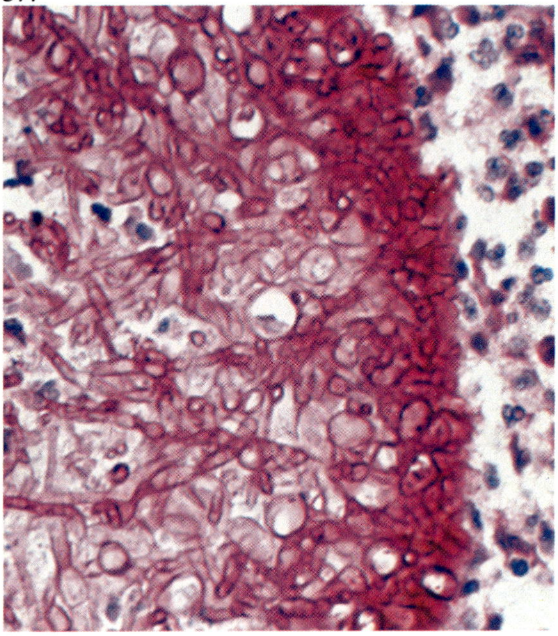

377 Madurella grisea Higher magnification of **376** shows details of the loose network of hyphae in the centre of the granule and the compact hyphae and prominent polygonal chlamydospores at its periphery. (PAS, ×200)

378

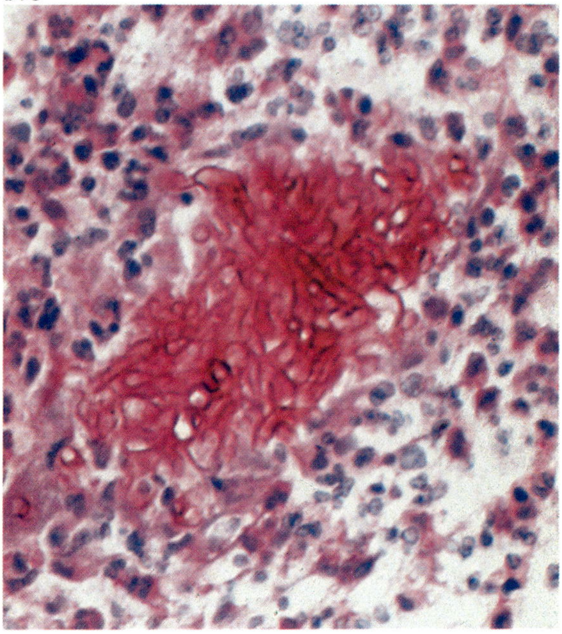

378 Madurella grisea granule in an early stage of development. At this stage, the granule consists of an interwoven mass of hyphae and chlamydospores. (PAS, ×200)

379

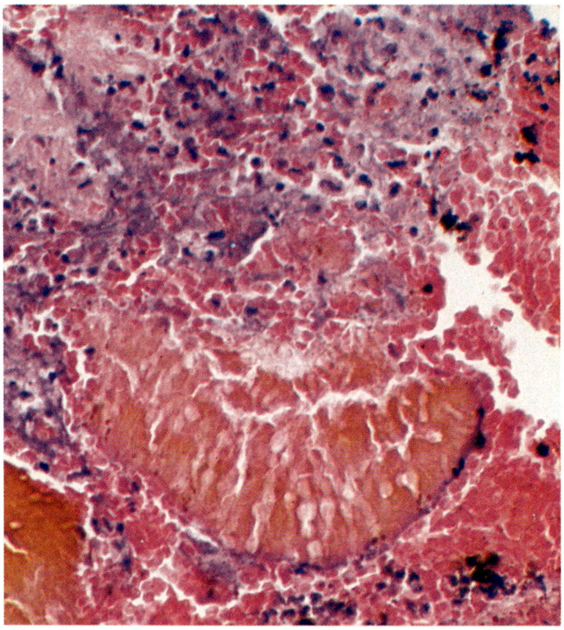

379 Madurella mycetomatis causing black grain mycetoma in a human. The granule consists of non-pigmented hyphae embedded in brown cement. (H&E, ×100)

380

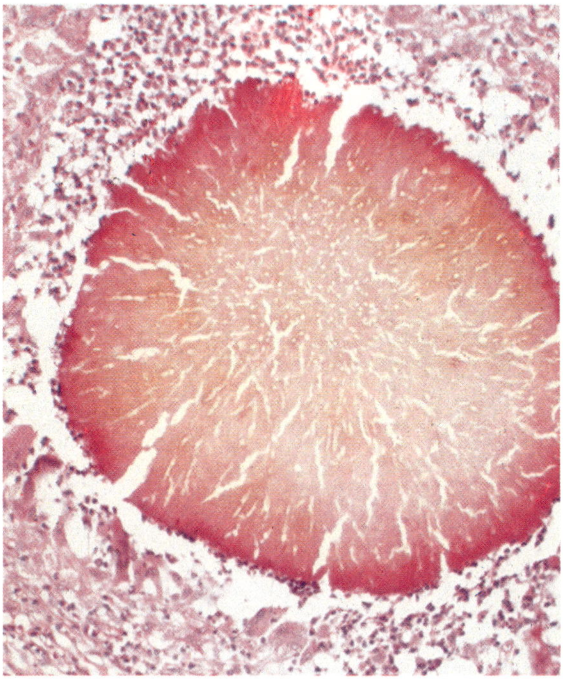

381

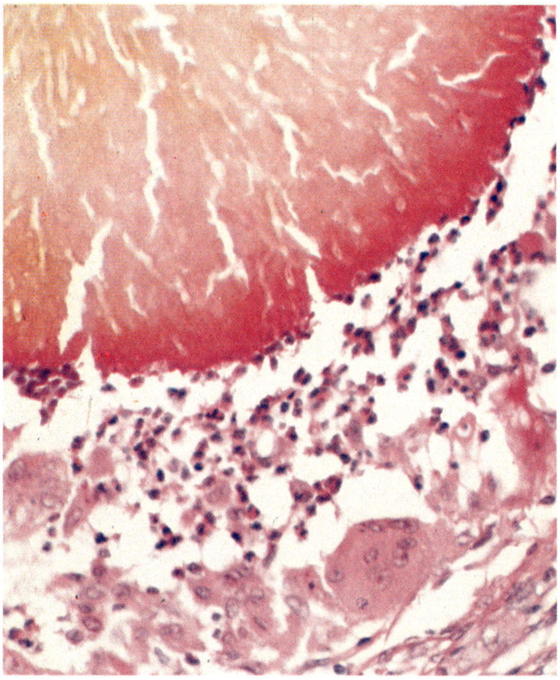

380 Madurella mycetomatis causing black grain mycetoma. At this magnification, the hyaline hyphae are not readily apparent and the light brown cement predominates. The eosinophilic border blends imperceptibly with the granule proper. Because the granule is hard, sectioning causes fissure lines. The granule is embedded in an abscess with a prominent fibrogranulomatous wall. (H&E, ×50)

381 Madurella mycetomatis Higher magnification of **380** showing the components of the granule and the surrounding pyogranulomatous inflammatory response in greater detail. Fissuring of the granule and the prominent brown cement are clearly seen. (H&E, ×100)

382

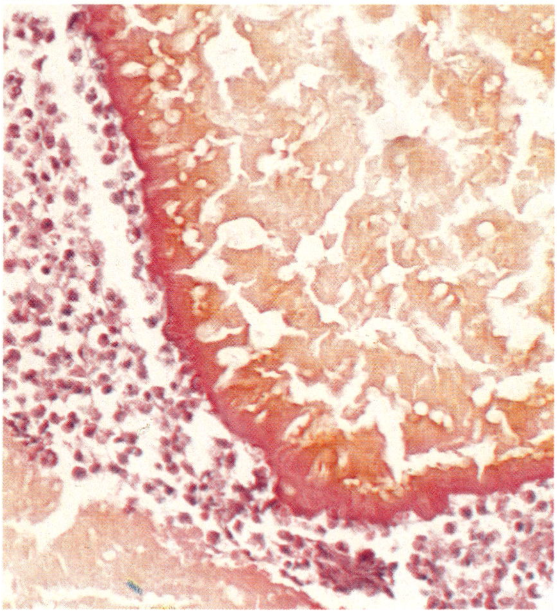

383

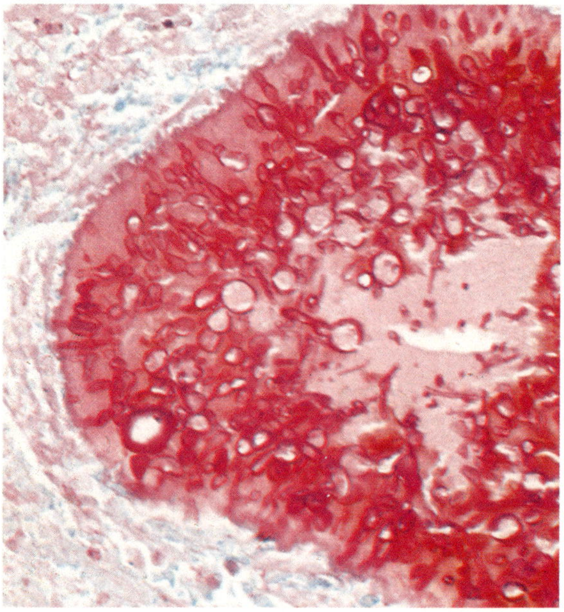

382 Madurella mycetomatis causing mycetoma. In this granule, the fungal elements at the periphery are dark brown and stand out against the light brown cement. Chlamydospores toward the centre are nonpigmented and appear as punched-out vesicles. (H&E, ×100)

383 Madurella mycetomatis Replicate section of **382** but stained by PAS to clearly show the radially oriented hyphae and vesicular chlamydospores within the granule. (PAS, ×100)

384

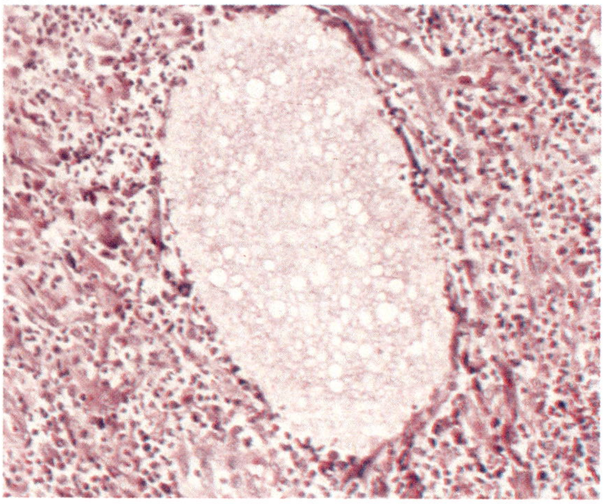

384 Petriellidium boydii causing white grain mycetoma in a human. The hyaline granule is embedded in granulation tissue that is infiltrated by mixed inflammatory cells. (H&E, ×50)

385

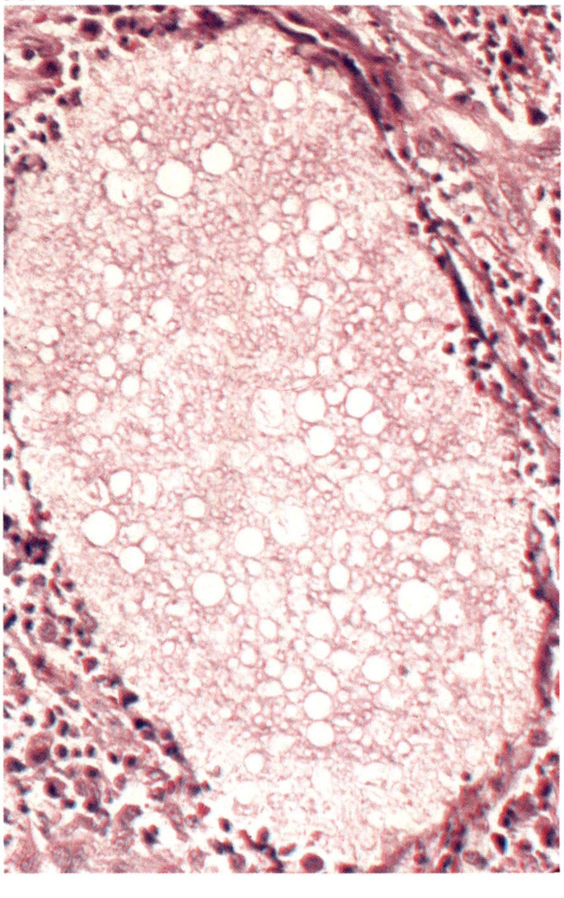

385 Petriellidium boydii Higher magnification of **384** to show details of the granule which is composed of a dense network of interwoven hyaline mycelium and prominent chlamydospores. The granule resembles those of the *Acremonium spp*. and *Fusarium moniliforme*, but it differs from them in that its chlamydospores are more numerous and larger. (H&E, ×100)

386

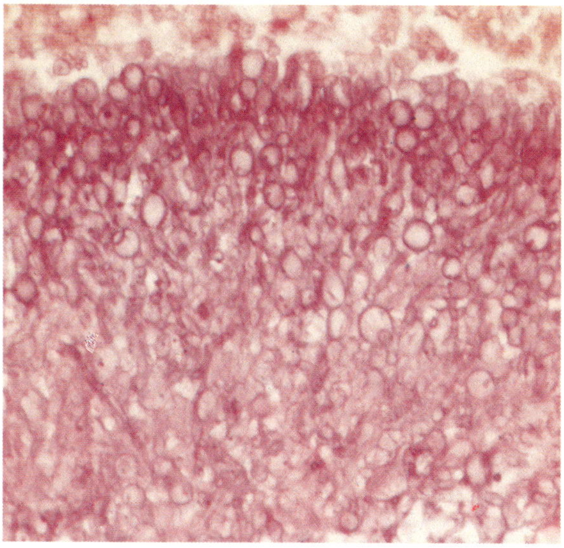

387

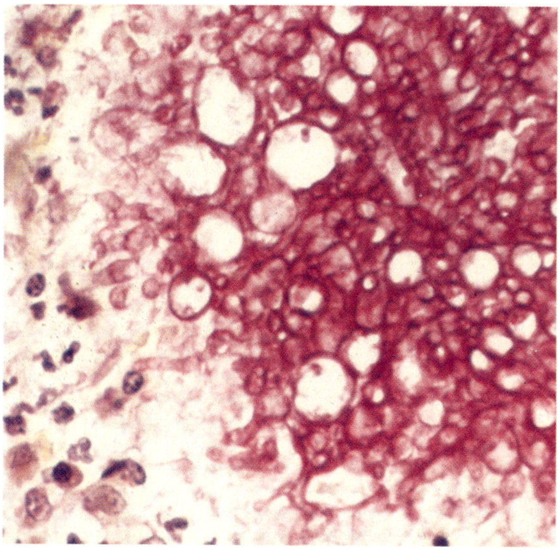

386 Petriellidium boydii Another granule stained by GF to show the numerous large chlamydospores and interwoven hyphae. Cement material is absent. (GF, ×100)

387 Petriellidium boydii Higher magnification of **386** to show details of the large chlamydospores and compact hyphae that make up the granule. (GF, ×200)

388

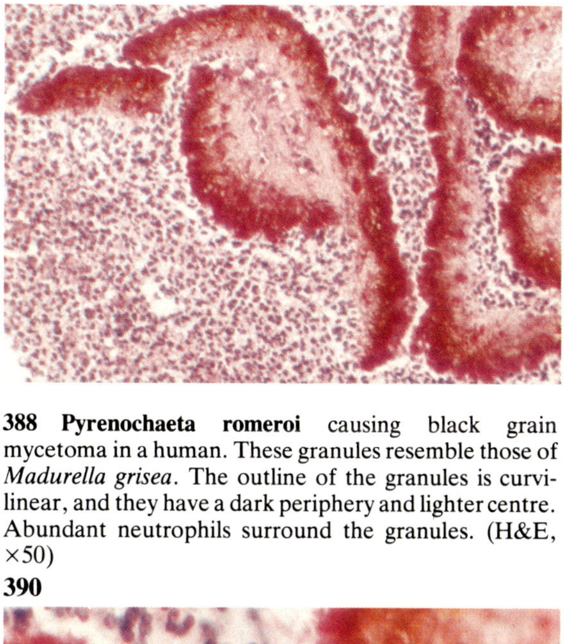

388 Pyrenochaeta romeroi causing black grain mycetoma in a human. These granules resemble those of *Madurella grisea*. The outline of the granules is curvilinear, and they have a dark periphery and lighter centre. Abundant neutrophils surround the granules. (H&E, ×50)

389

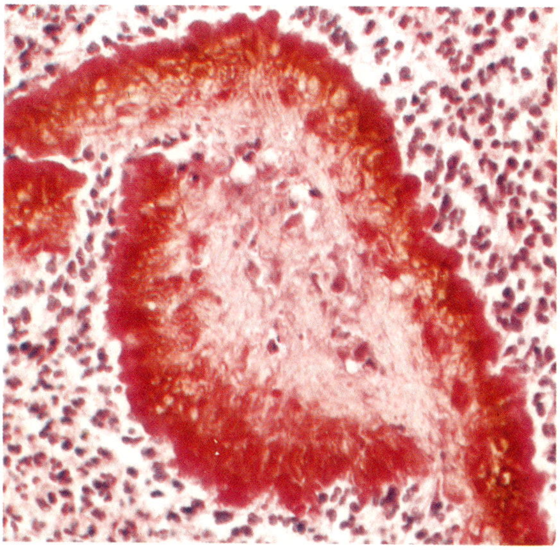

389 Pyrenochaeta romeroi Higher magnification of **388** to show the dark peripheral zone of variably shaped, brown chlamydospores and the lighter central zone in the granule. (H&E, ×100)

390

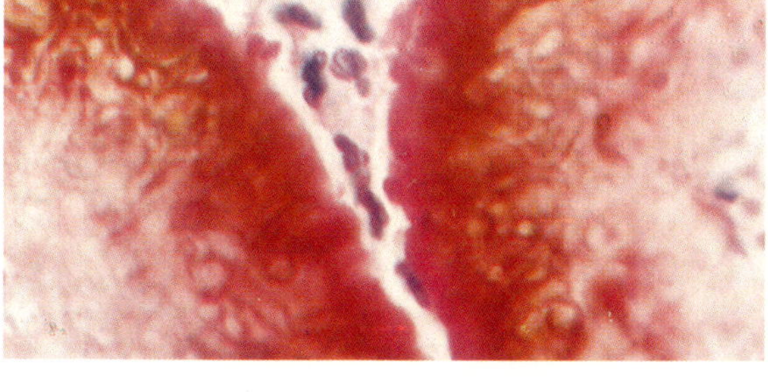

390 Pyrenochaeta romeroi An even higher magnification of **388** showing the peripheral zone of brown chlamydospores in greater detail. Hyphae can be seen towards the interior of the granules. (H&E, ×200)

391

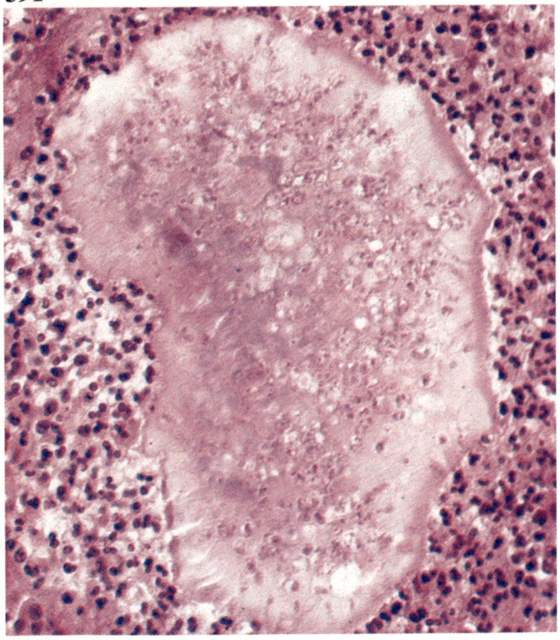

392

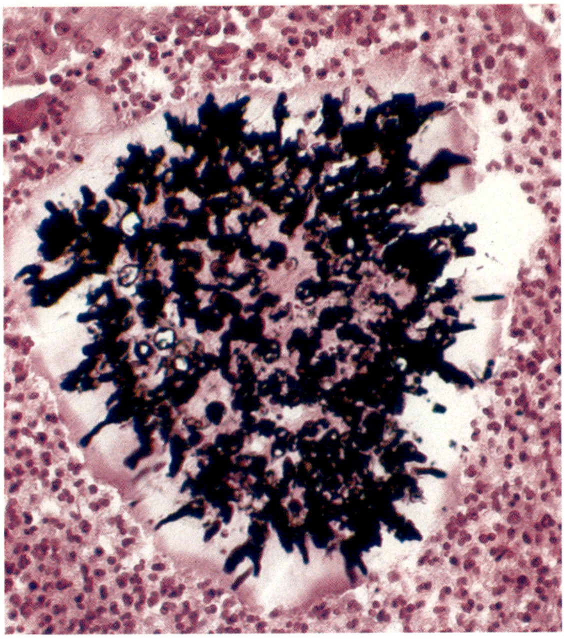

391 Neotestudina rosatii causing white grain eumycotic mycetoma in a human. The irregularly shaped granule is composed of readily visible hyphae that are more abundant in its interior. The fungal elements are embedded in a light-staining cement-like matrix. A narrow and incomplete eosinophilic zone surrounds the distinctive granule. (H&E, ×100)

392 Neotestudina rosatii Replicate section of **391**. The GMS-positive fungal elements within the granule consist of disintegrated hyphae and a few chlamydospores. The surrounding pyogranulomatous reaction is well demonstrated by the H&E counterstain. (GMS–H&E, ×100)

393

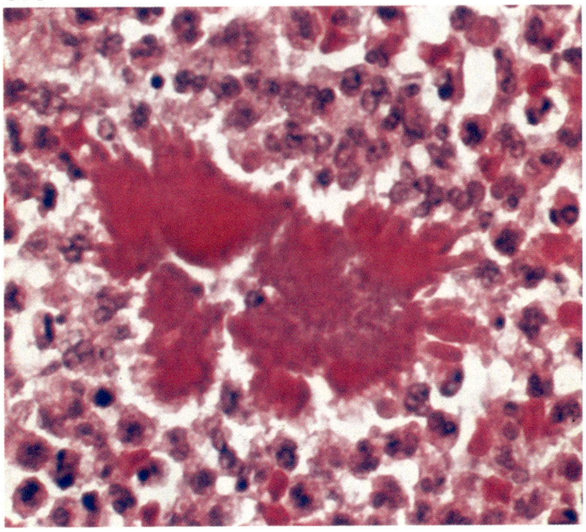

394

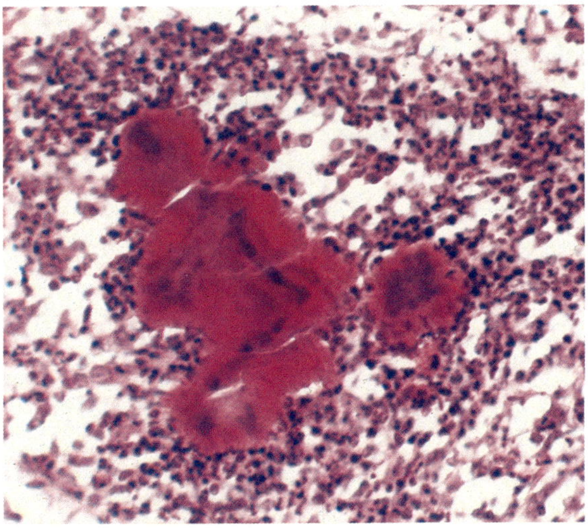

393 Staphylococcus sp. causing botryomycosis in the skin of a human. The lightly basophilic granule is surrounded by radiating clubs of deeply eosinophilic Splendore–Hoeppli material. It closely resembles the granules seen in actinomycotic and eumycotic mycetomas. The purulent inflammatory reaction is also similar to that seen in the mycetomas. Tissue Gram stains are required to demonstrate the aetiologic agents and to make a diagnosis of botryomycosis. (H&E, ×200)

394 Staphylococcus sp. causing botryomycosis in the skin of a horse. The granules with prominent eosinophilic borders are embedded in an abscess, and they closely resemble those seen in mycetomas. (H&E, ×100)

395

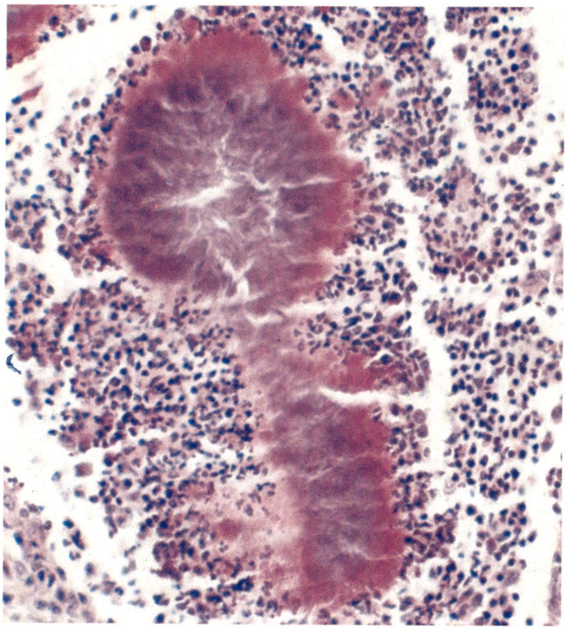

396

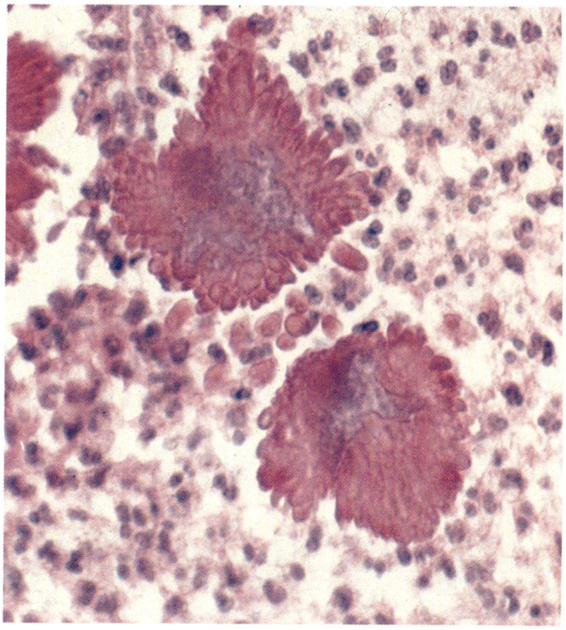

395 Actinobacillus lignieresi causing actinobacillosis in the tongue of a cow. The large, irregular, basophilic granule is surrounded by eosinophilic Splendore–Hoeppli material and is embedded in an abscess. Special stains are required to demonstrate that the aetiologic agent is a gram-negative rod and not an actinomycete or a fungus. (H&E, ×100)

396 Pseudomonas sp. causing botryomycosis in the skin of a human. The lightly basophilic granule is surrounded by prominent eosinophilic clubs of Splendore–Hoeppli material. Note the purulent inflammatory reaction and the similarity of these granules to those in **393–395**. (H&E, ×200)

397

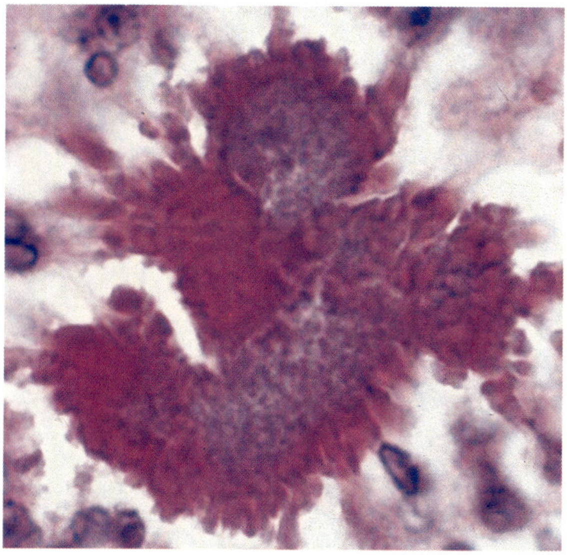

398

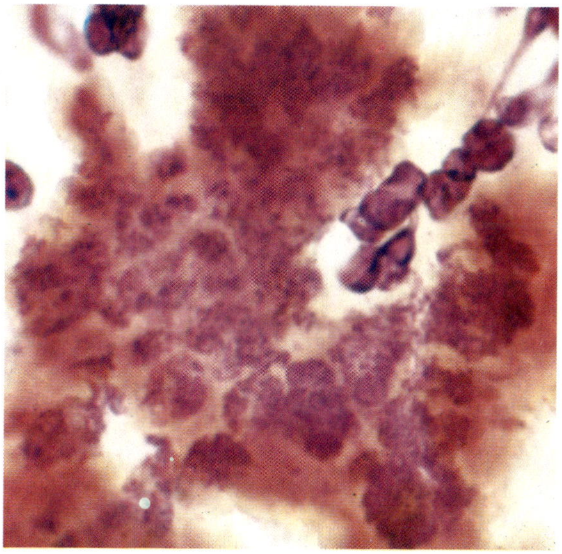

397 Pseudomonas sp. causing botryomycosis in a human. The basophilic bacteria within the granule are discernible under oil immersion. The granule is bordered by prominent eosinophilic clubs. (H&E, ×500)

398 Pseudomonas sp. Replicate section of **397** but stained by a tissue Gram procedure. The granule is shown to be composed of numerous discrete gram-negative rods. The Splendore–Hoeppli material is also gram-negative. (B&B, ×500)

18 Mycotic keratitis

Text pages: 83–84

399

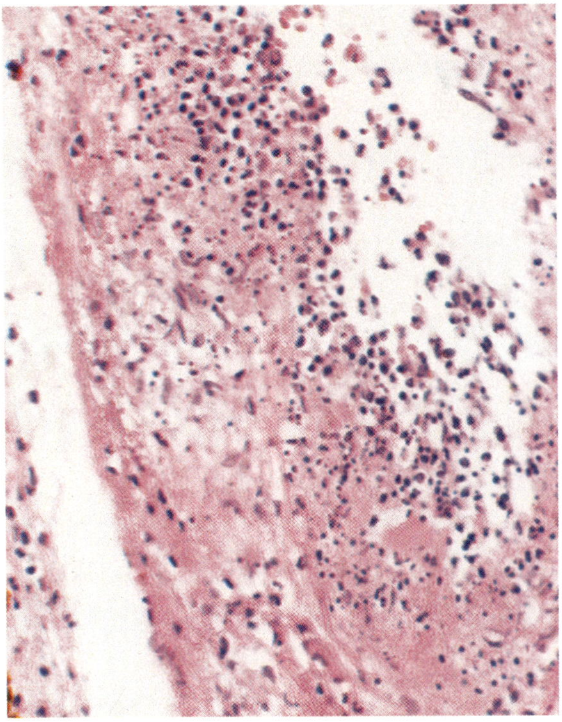

399 Fusarium sp. causing mycotic keratitis in a human. Note the superficial necrosis of the cornea and the acute inflammatory infiltrate. Fungal elements are not visible. (H&E, ×50)

400

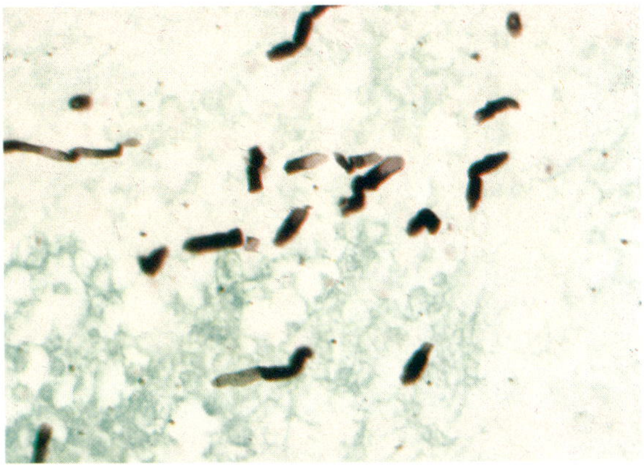

400 Fusarium sp. Replicate section of **399** but stained by GMS to demonstrate hyphal fragments in the affected cornea. Cultural studies were required for identification of the fungus. (GMS, ×200)

401

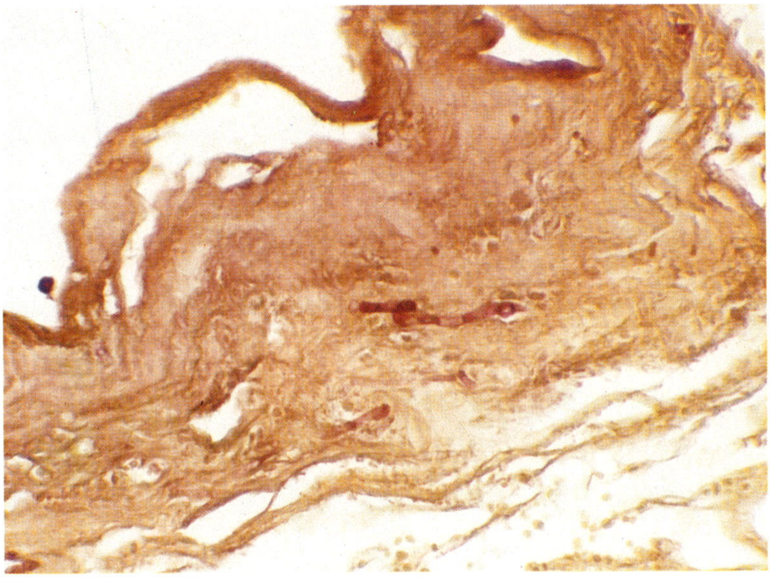

401 Fusarium sp. causing mycotic keratitis in a human. A few GF-positive hyphal fragments are embedded in the corneal stroma. Inflammation is minimal. (GF, ×100)

402

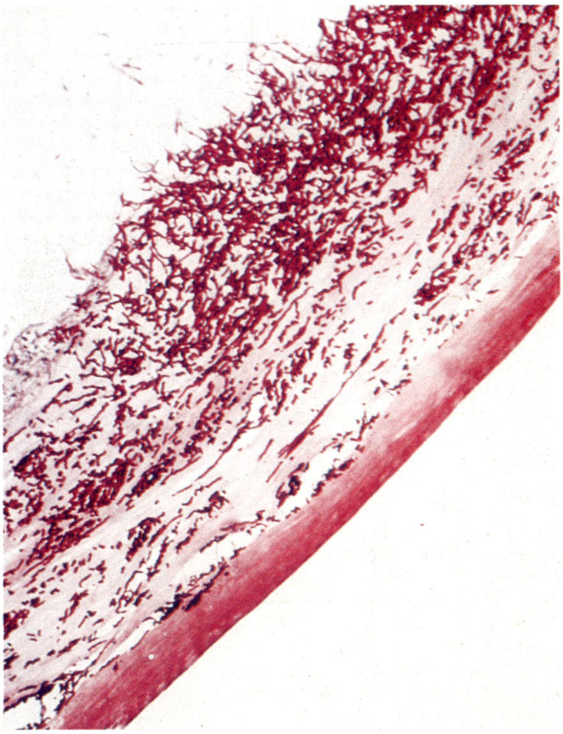

402 Fusarium oxysporum causing mycotic keratitis in a human. Numerous PAS-positive hyphae are seen on the surface of and within the corneal stroma. Inflammation is minimal in this case. (PAS, ×20)

403

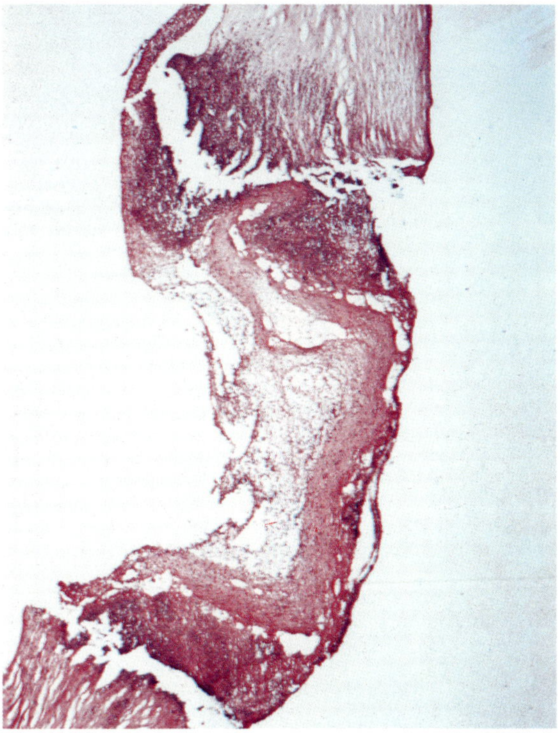

403 Tritirachium roseum causing mycotic keratitis in a human. Necrotic corneal ulcer and descemetocele are evident. (H&E, ×25)

404

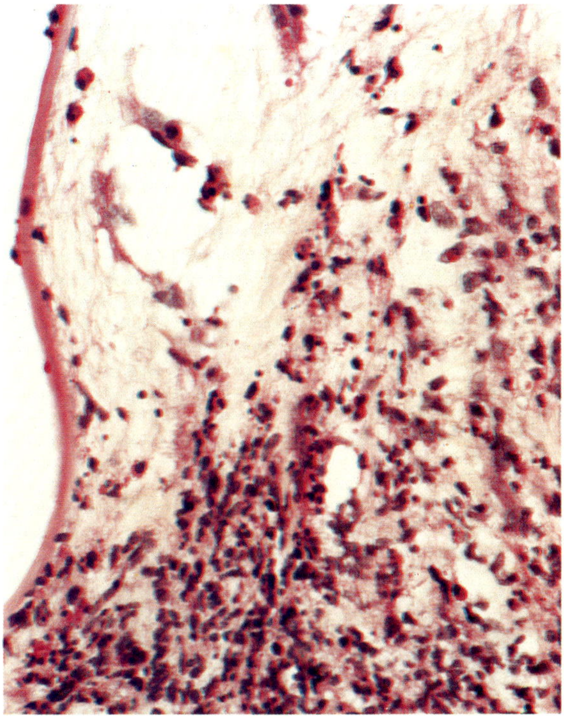

405

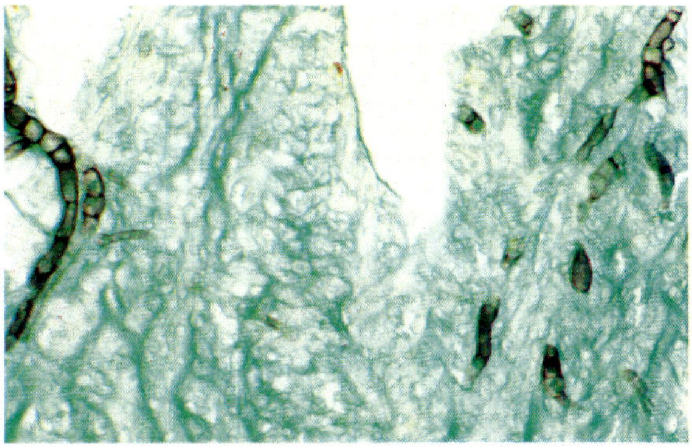

404 Tritirachium roseum Higher magnification of **403** showing an acute inflammatory infiltrate in the corneal stroma at the edge of the ulcer. Descemet's membrane is to the left in the photomicrograph. Fungal elements are not visible. (H&E, ×100)

405 Tritirachium roseum Replicate section of **403** but stained by GMS to show the fungus within the lesion. Cultural examination was required for specific identification of the aetiologic agent. (GMS, ×200)

406

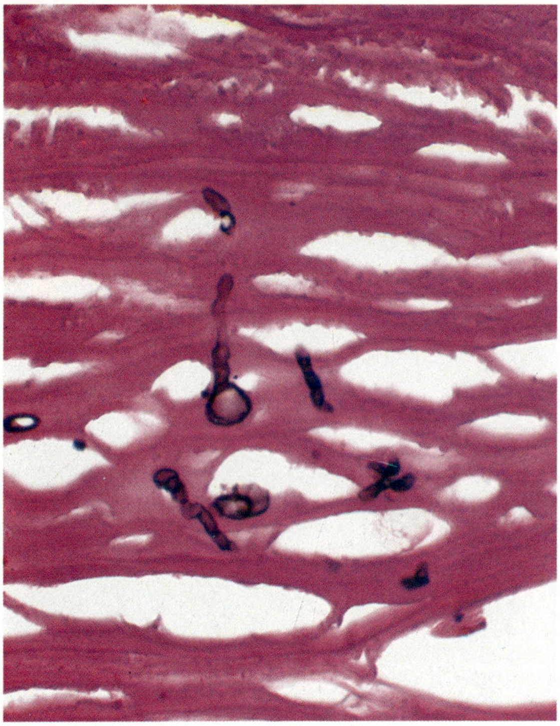

406 Mycotic keratitis in a human. The fungal elements within the corneal stroma are clearly visible and inflammation is not evident. The aetiologic agent is unknown since cultural studies were not done and the morphology of the fungus does not permit identification. (GMS–H&E, ×100)

407

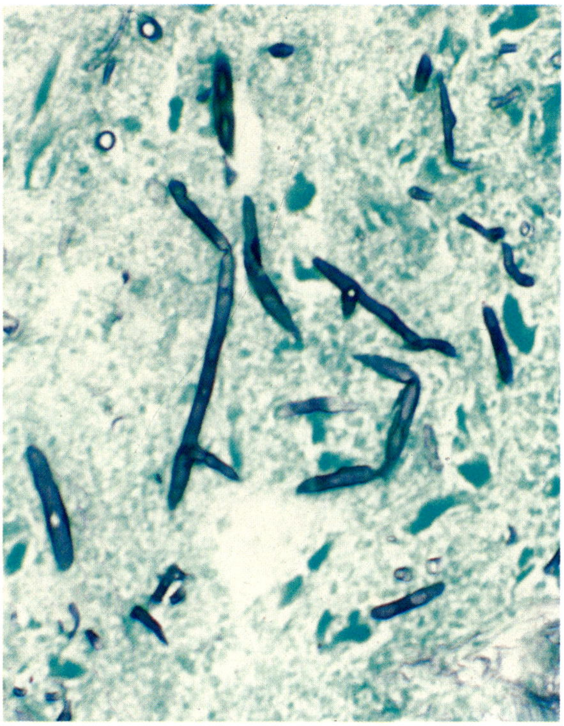

407 Aspergillus sp. causing mycotic keratitis in a human. The branched septate hyphae embedded in the inflamed stroma are clearly evident. Identification to the genus level was made by culture. (GMS, ×100)

408

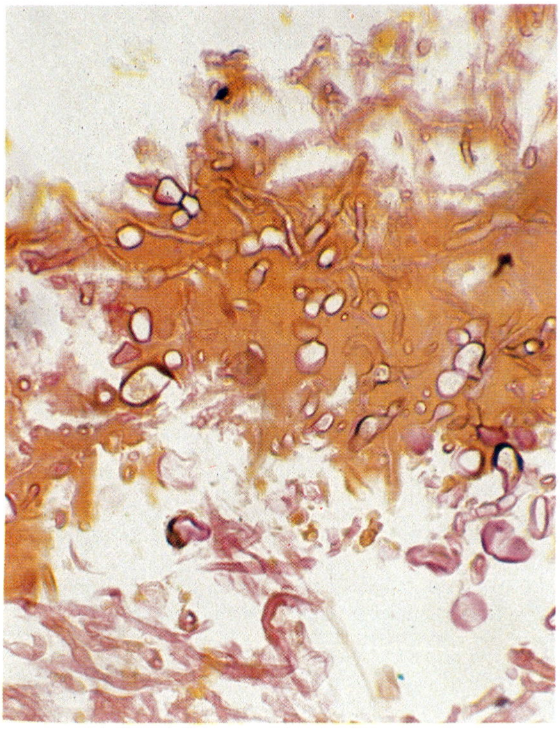

408 Curvularia geniculata causing mycotic keratitis in a human. Fungal elements on the surface of and within the corneal stroma are visible, but their innate brown colour is partially masked by the GF stain. (GF, ×100)

19 Nocardiosis

Text pages: 85–87

409

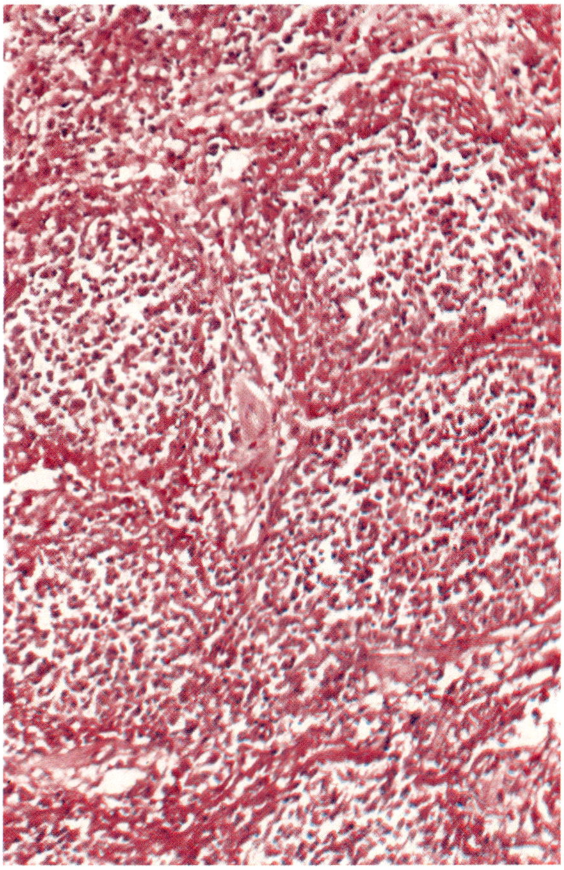

410

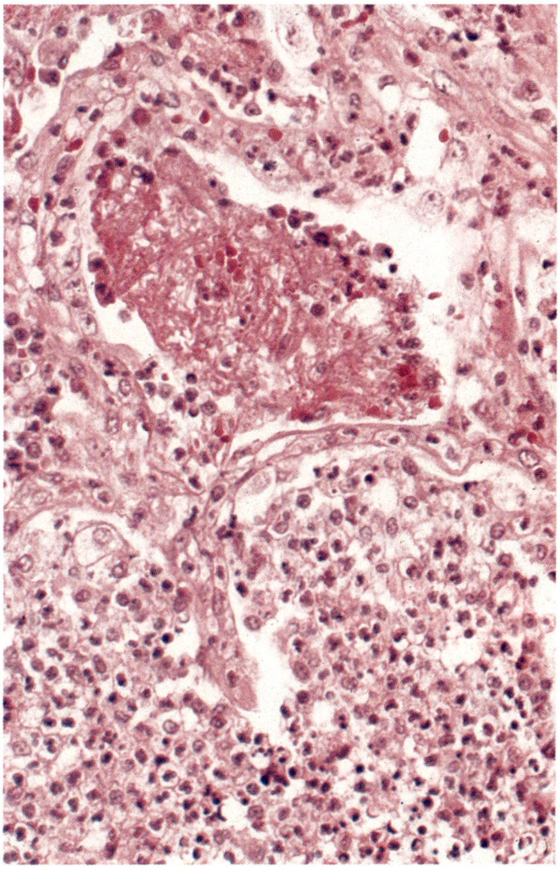

409 Nocardia asteroides causing pulmonary nocardiosis in a human. The acute fibrinopurulent pneumonia is similar to that caused by other bacteria. (H&E, ×50)

410 Nocardia asteroides causing human pulmonary nocardiosis. The alveolar spaces are filled with neutrophils, macrophages, and fibrin. (H&E, ×100)

411

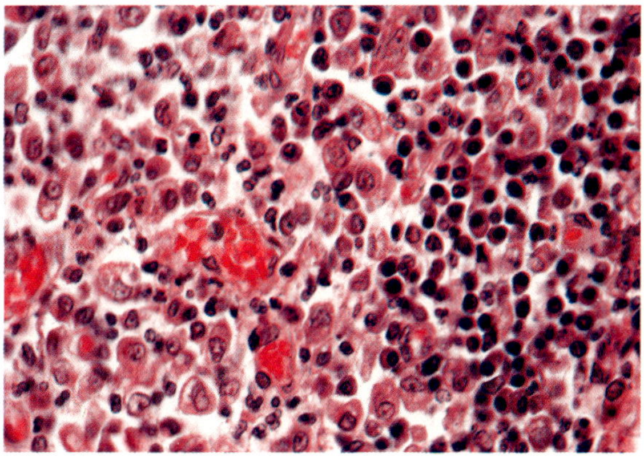

411 Nocardia asteroides causing chronic pleuritis in a dog. A few neutrophils are present, but at this stage of the infection mononuclear cells predominate. The filaments of this aerobic actinomycete are not visible in sections stained by H&E. (H&E, ×200)

412

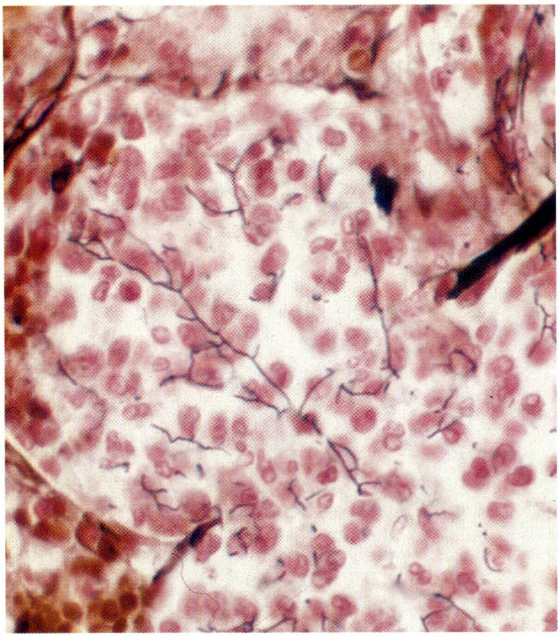

413

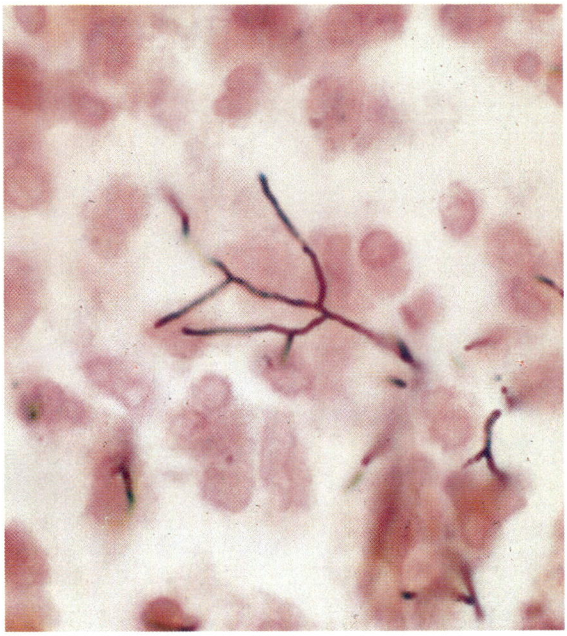

412 Nocardia asteroides infection of human lung. The GMS stain clearly demonstrates its delicate (≤1 μm), branched filaments within the alveolar exudate. (GMS–H&E, ×200)

413 Nocardia asteroides Higher magnification of **412**. This field shows the delicate (≤1 μm), branched filaments in greater detail. The branching of the mycelium occurs almost at right angles. (GMS–H&E, ×500)

414

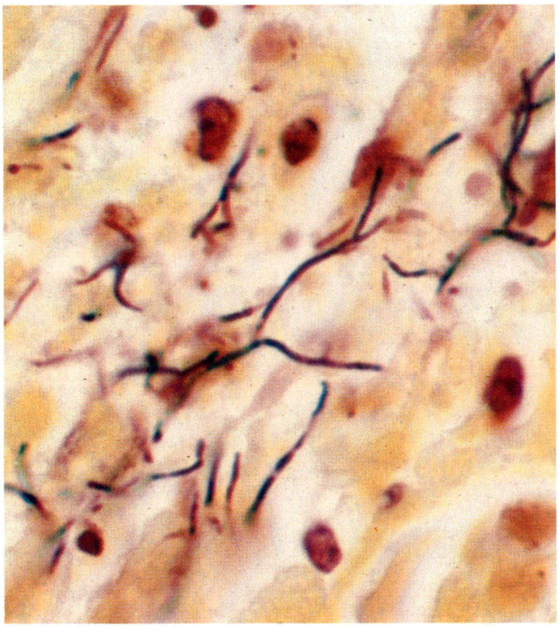

415

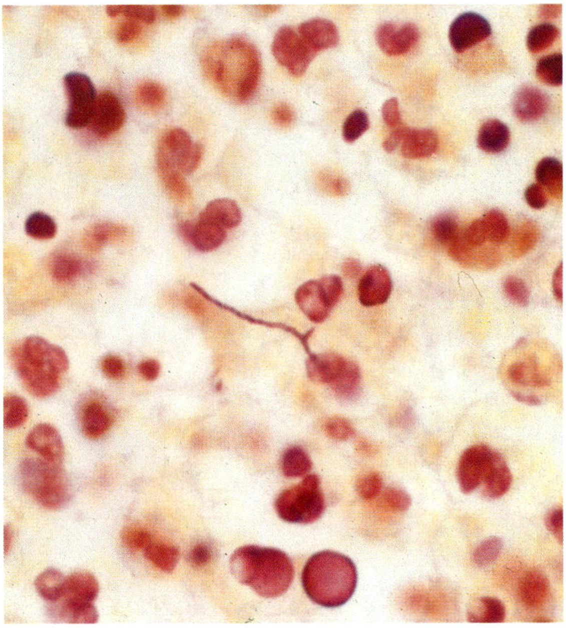

414 Nocardia asteroides infection of the human lung. The mycelial filaments are gram-positive and well demonstrated by the tissue Gram stains. Irregular staining gives the filaments a beaded appearance. (B&B, ×500)

415 Nocardia asteroides Replicate section of **410** but stained by a tissue Gram procedure. A single gram-positive, branched filament is clearly seen in the purulent exudate. (B&B, ×500)

416

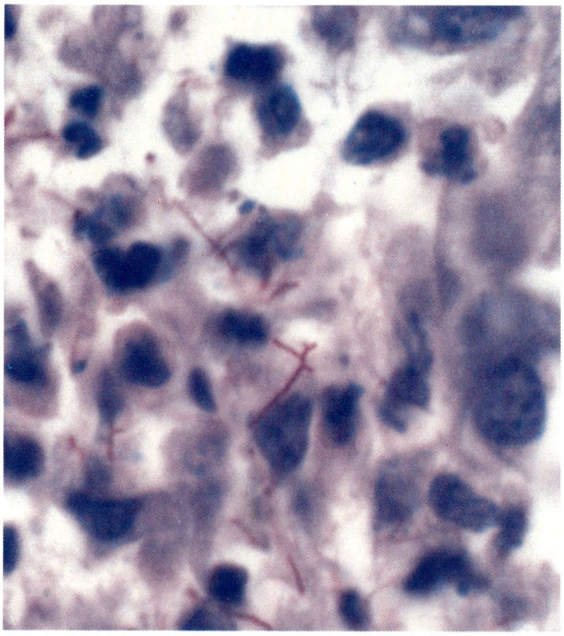

416 Nocardia asteroides Replicate section of **410** but stained by a modified acid-fast procedure. Delicate acid-fast, branched filaments are seen within an alveolar space. (Modified Fite–Faraco acid-fast, ×500)

417

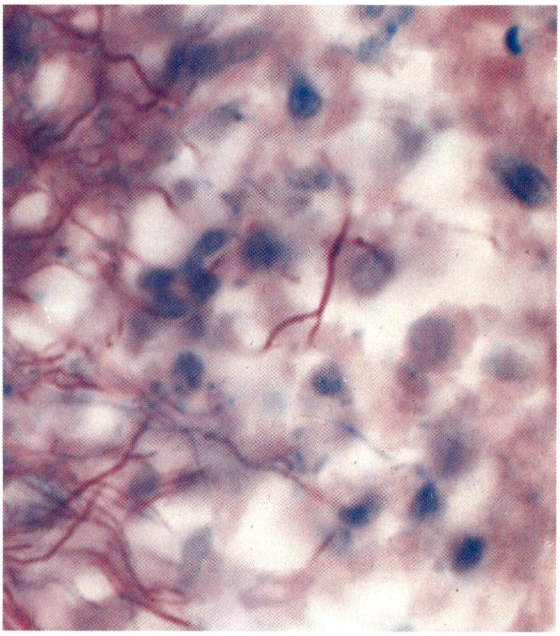

417 Nocardia brasiliensis causing purulent lymphadenitis in a cat. Numerous branched, acid-fast filaments are seen within an abscess. (Modified Kinyoun's acid-fast, ×500)

418

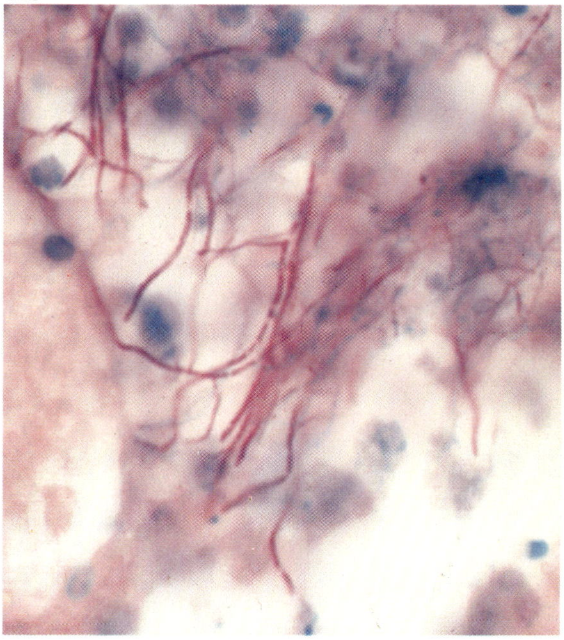

418 Nocardia brasiliensis Another field in **417** that shows a group of long, branched, acid-fast filaments. Irregular staining of some of the filaments gives them a beaded appearance. (Modified Kinyoun's acid-fast, ×500)

419

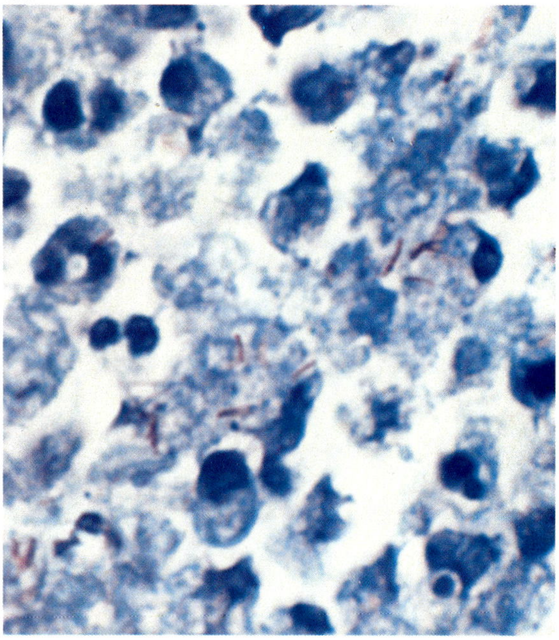

419 Mycobacterium tuberculosis causing pulmonary tuberculosis in a human. Delicate acid-fast bacilli are seen. In contrast to the *Nocardia spp.*, the mycobacteria do not show true branching. (Ziehl–Neelsen acid-fast, ×500)

20 Paracoccidioidomycosis

Text pages: 88–91

420

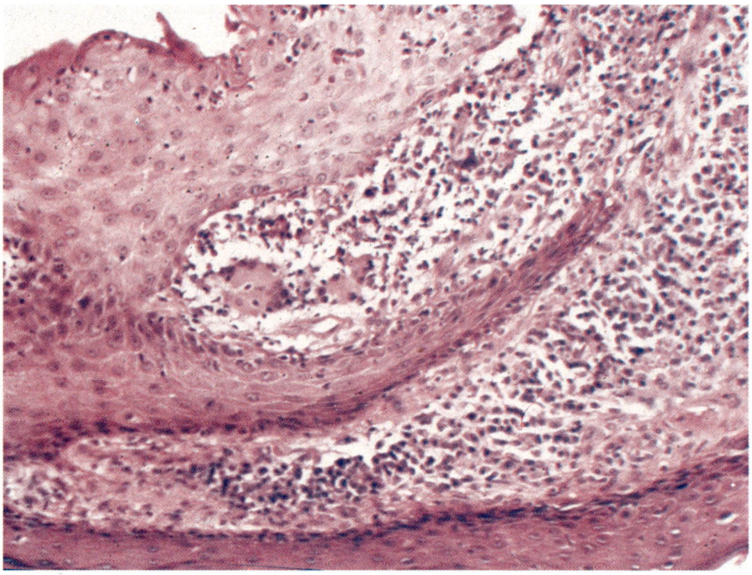

420 Paracoccidioidomycosis of the skin in a human. Note the pseudo-epitheliomatous hyperplasia of the epidermis and the mixed purulent and granulomatous inflammatory reaction in the dermis. At higher magnification, giant cells were found to contain the tissue-form cells of *Paracoccidioides brasiliensis*. (H&E, ×50)

421

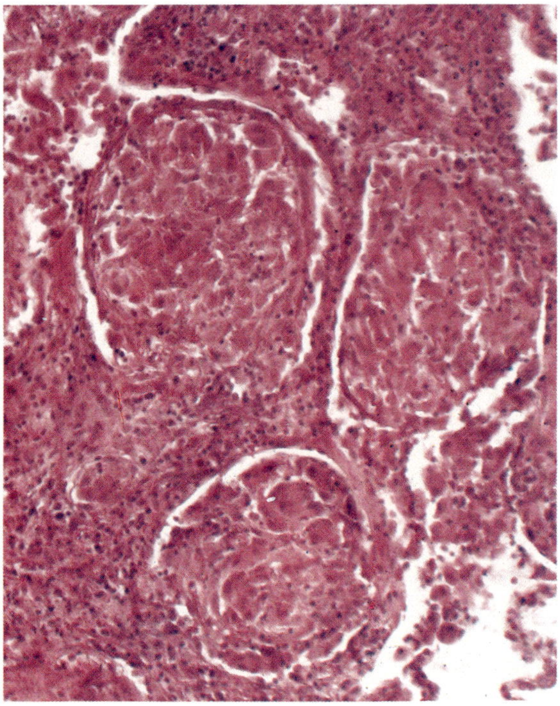

422

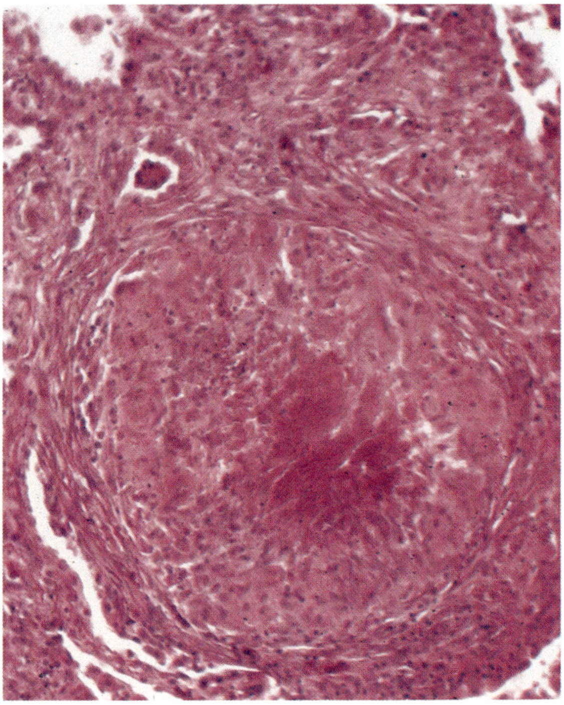

421 Pulmonary paracoccidioidomycosis in a Brazilian. In this section, multiple epithelioid cell granulomas are present. Interstitial infiltration of mixed inflammatory cells is also seen. (H&E, ×50)

422 Paracoccidioides brasiliensis Another field in **421** that contains a larger granuloma with central caseation. At higher magnification, many yeast cells were seen. (H&E, ×50)

423

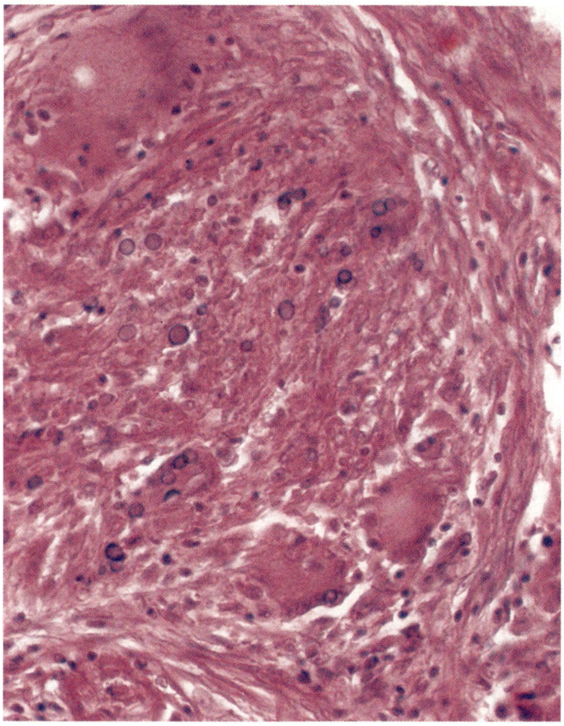

423 Paracoccidioides brasiliensis Replicate section of **421** but stained by GMS–H&E. This section contains a necrotic focus surrounded by a fibrogranulomatous reaction. Fungal cells (not easily seen at this magnification) are both extracellular in the necrotic material and within giant cells. (GMS–H&E, ×100)

424

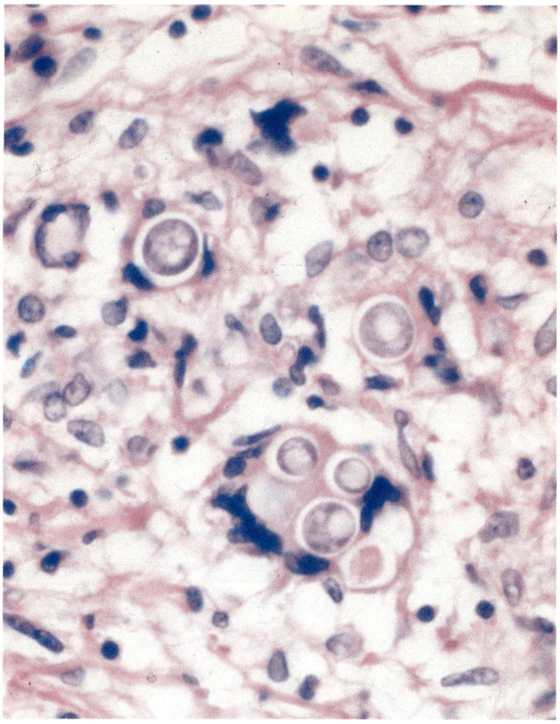

424 Paracoccidioides brasiliensis in the lung of a human. Intracellular and extracellular nonbudding cells with lightly basophilic cytoplasm are clearly seen in this field. Nonbudding cells of *P. brasiliensis* closely resemble nonbudding cells of *Blastomyces dermatitidis* and other yeasts and also resemble nonendosporulating spherules of *Coccidioides immitis*. (H&E, ×200)

425

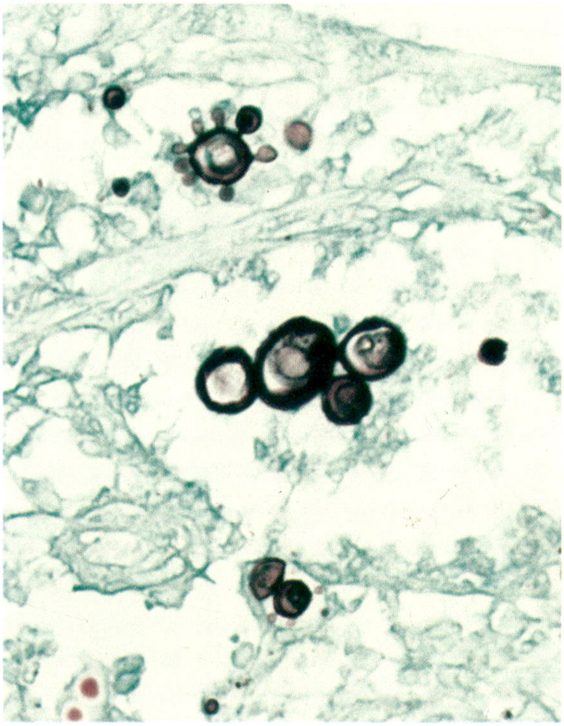

425 Paracoccidioides brasiliensis causing pulmonary paracoccidioidomycosis in a Brazilian. Two patterns of multiple budding are seen. At the top in the photomicrograph, the daughter cells are numerous, are relatively small and are all about the same size. In the centre, the daughter cells are fewer and larger. These patterns of multiple budding, diagnostic of *P. brasiliensis*, are illustrated at higher magnification in **426** and **427**. (GMS, ×200)

426

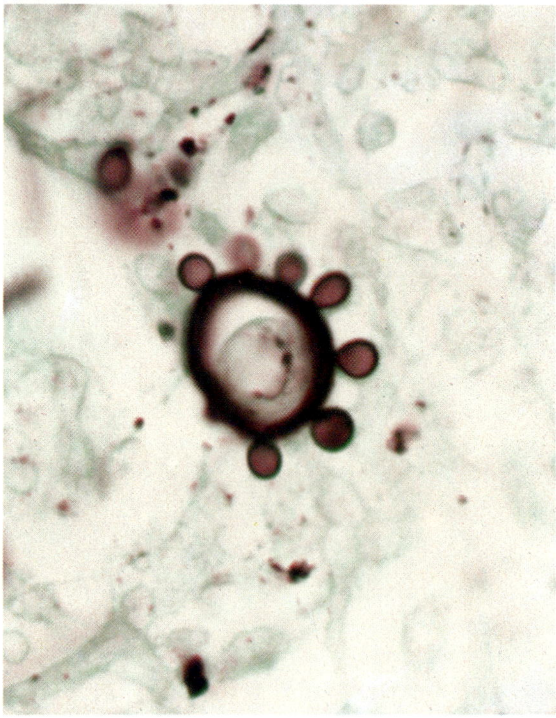

427

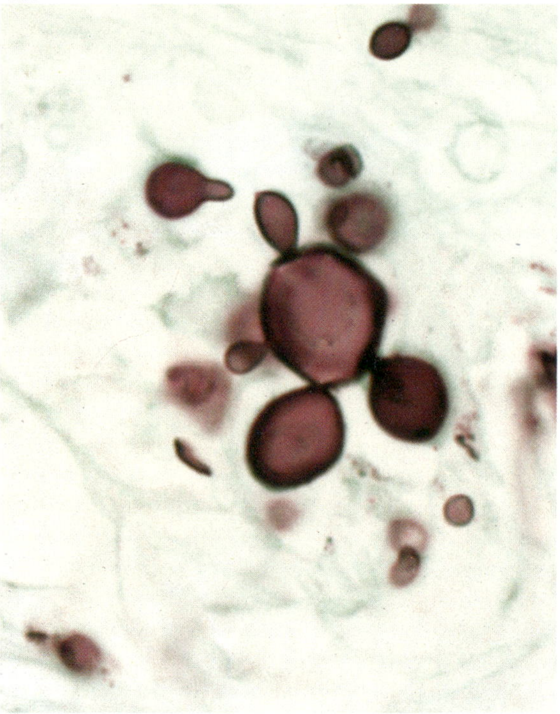

426 Paracoccidioides brasiliensis (multiple budding cell). The daughter cells (buds) are numerous, about the same size, and relatively small. (GMS, ×500)

427 Paracoccidioides brasiliensis (multiple budding form). Here, the daughter cells (buds) are relatively few and unequal in size. Some buds have almost attained the size of the parent cell. Note the narrow basal attachment of the buds to the parent cell. (GMS, ×500)

428

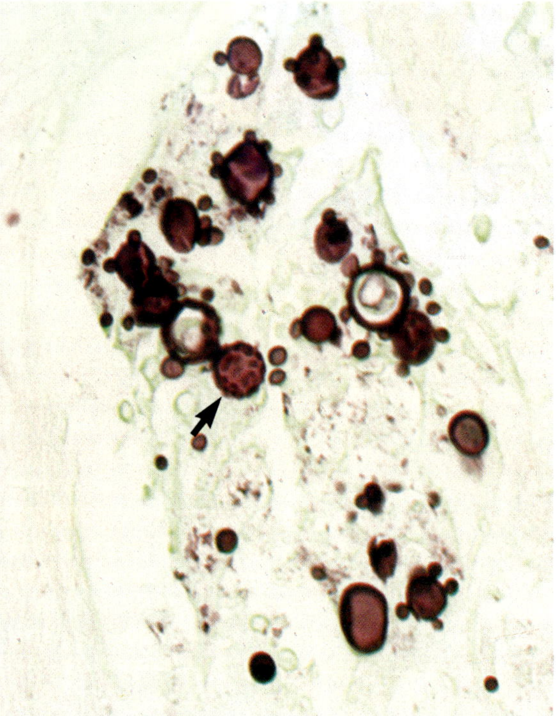

429

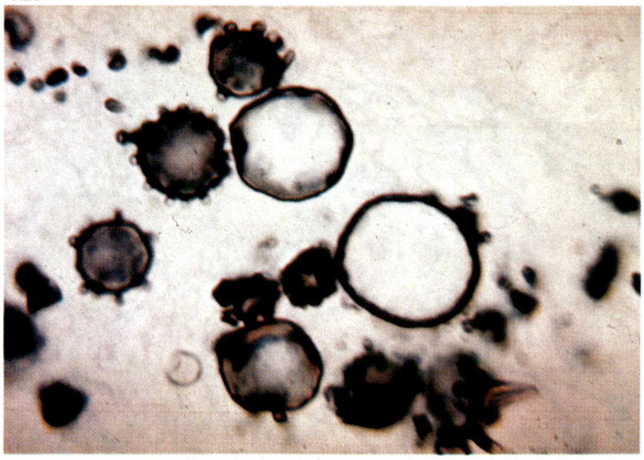

428 Paracoccidioides brasiliensis (typical budding forms). Another field in **425** in which a few detached blastospores are seen. One parent cell has numerous bud scars on its surface (arrow). (GMS, ×200)

429 Paracoccidioides brasiliensis Higher magnification of another field in **425** to show details of the multiple budding cells. Three of the cells have numerous minute peripheral buds of approximately the same size ('steering wheel' forms). Two large parent cells appear empty. (GMS, ×500)

430

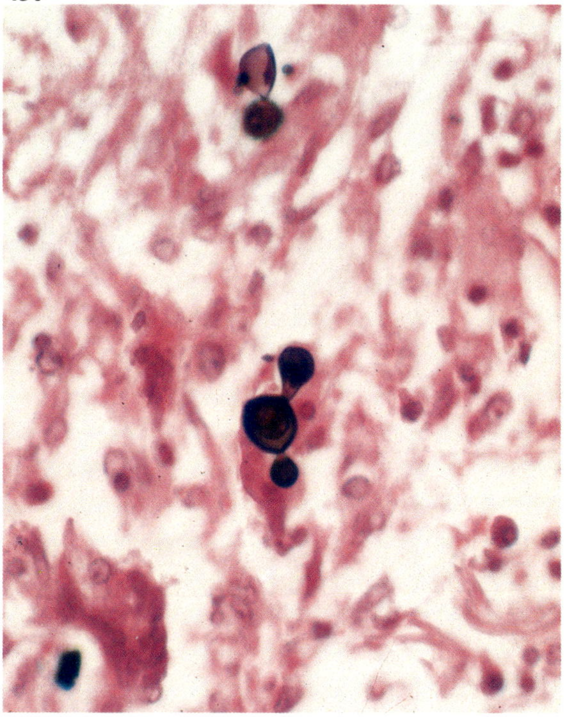

430 Paracoccidioides brasiliensis Replicate section of **425** showing a cell with two buds and another with one bud. The buds are connected to the parent cells by a narrow neck, unlike the broad base that characterises the buds of *Blastomyces dermatitidis*. (GMS–H&E, ×200)

431

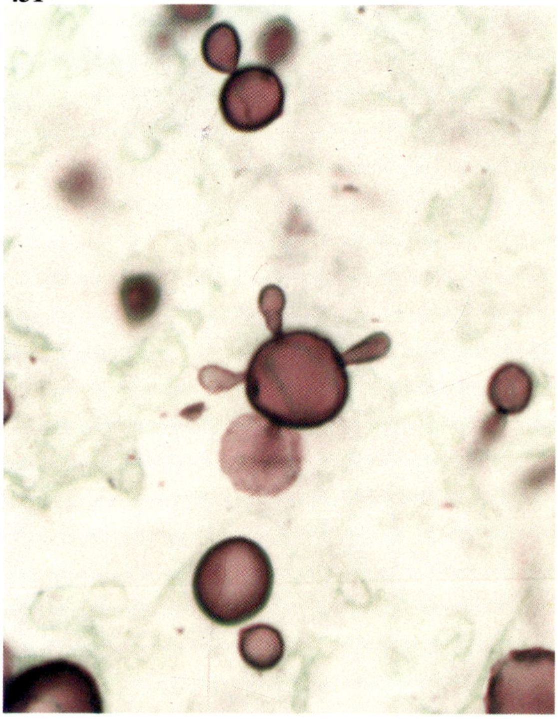

431 Paracoccidioides brasiliensis Another field in **425** to illustrate the variation in shape and size of the buds. (GMS, ×500)

432

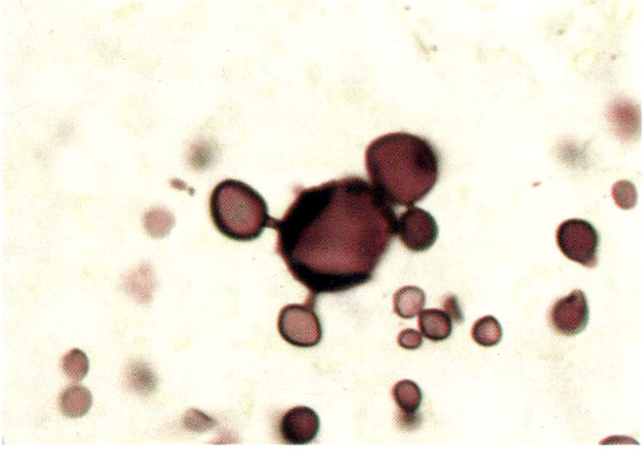

432 Pulmonary paracoccidioidomycosis in a human. The daughter cells are attached to the parent cell by elongated, narrow, tube-like structures. The smaller cells are detached blastospores. (GMS, ×500)

433

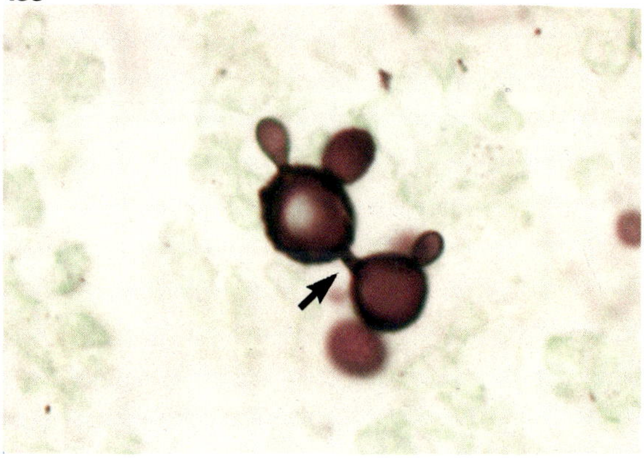

433 Paracoccidioides brasiliensis Another field in **432** shows two budding cells attached by a prominent narrow tube-like structure (arrow). Note superficial resemblance to the *Loboa loboi* cells in **437** and **438**. Other buds seen in this field are attached to their parent cells by characteristic narrow bases. (GMS, ×500)

434

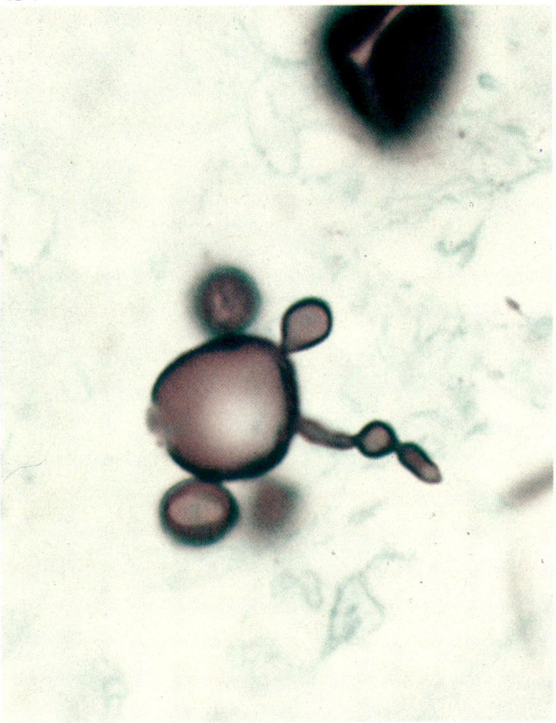

435

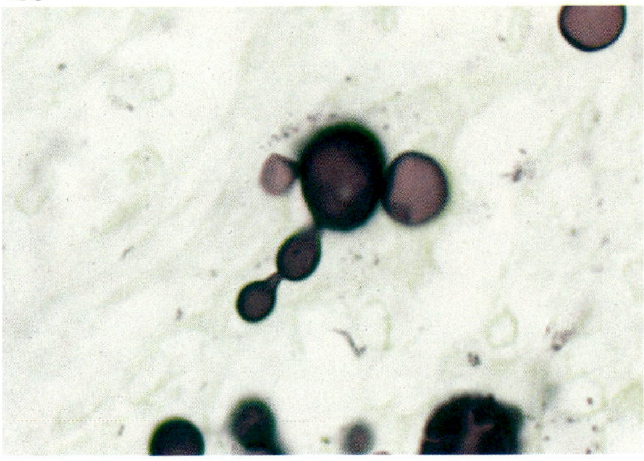

434 Paracoccidioides brasiliensis Another field in **432** showing a parent cell with multiple buds and secondary buds. (GMS, ×500)

435 Paracoccidioides brasiliensis A field in **432** illustrating the variable pattern of secondary budding. Here, there is a superficial resemblance to *Loboa loboi* cells in **438**. (GMS, ×500)

436

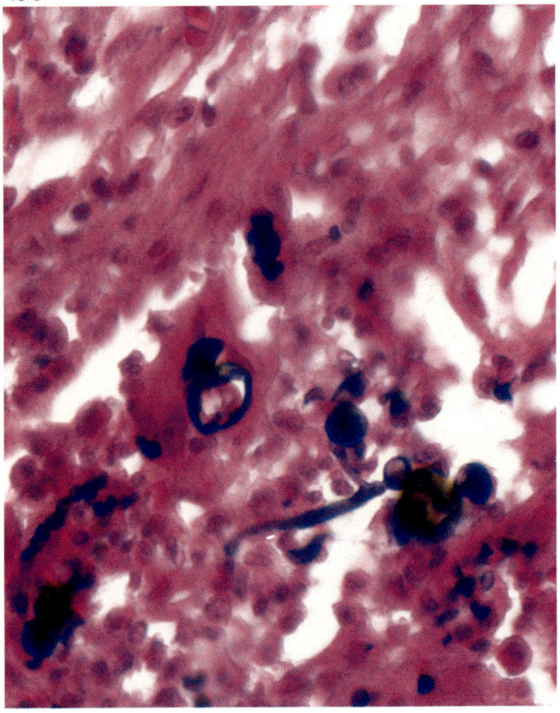

436 Paracoccidioides brasiliensis causing pulmonary paracoccidioidomycosis in another human. One of the buds on a multiple budding cell has germinated, forming a short hypha. (GMS–H&E, ×200)

437

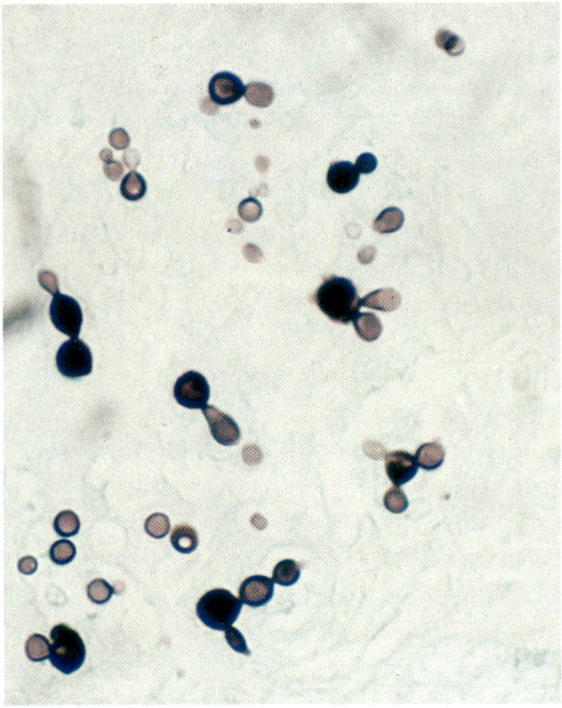

437 Loboa loboi causing lobomycosis in a dolphin. Some cells show multiple budding and thus resemble multiple budding forms of *Paracoccidioides brasiliensis*. Unlike the latter, *L. loboi* characteristically forms long chains of cells interconnected by short rod-like tubes. (GMS, ×200)

438

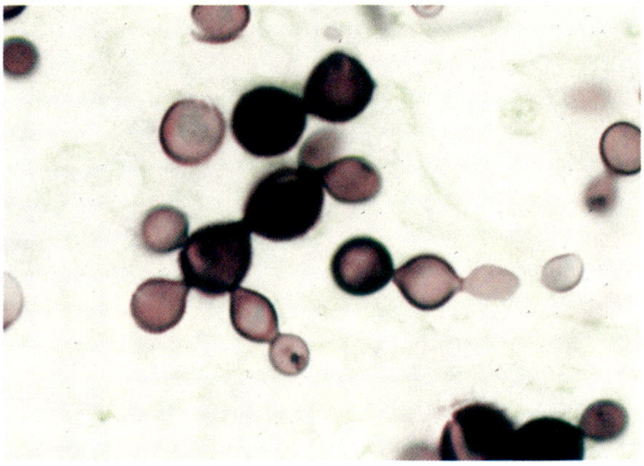

438 Loboa loboi Higher magnification of another field in **437** showing multiple budding forms and short chains of cells in greater detail. Note the resemblance of these cells to those in **435**. (GMS, ×500)

439

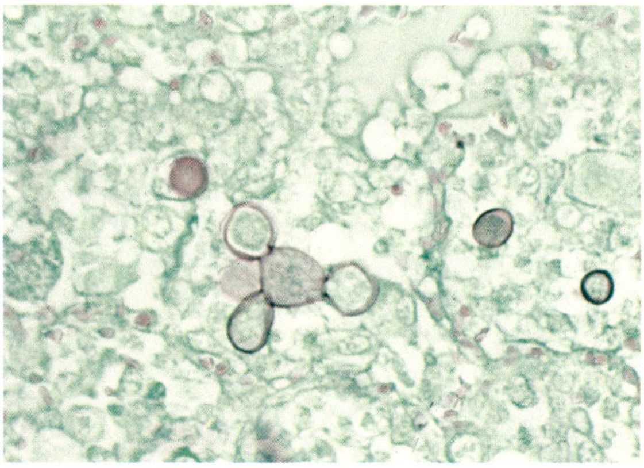

439 Blastomyces dermatitidis causing pulmonary blastomycosis in a dog. Occasionally, *B. dermatitidis* in tissue may show multiple budding as seen here. Note the broad basal attachments of the buds to the parent cell – a feature used to differentiate this fungus from *Paracoccidioides brasiliensis*. (GMS, ×500)

440

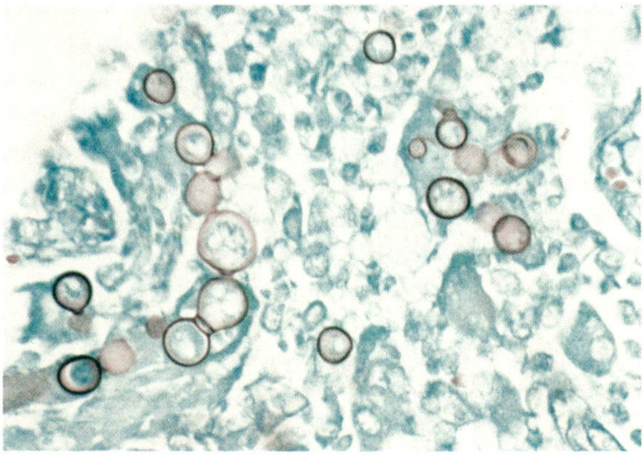

440 Blastomyces dermatitidis in pneumonic lung of a dog. Rarely, this fungus forms chains of budding cells in tissue as shown here. Broad basal attachments of buds to parent cells aid in differentiating this fungus from *Paracoccidioides brasiliensis* and *Loboa loboi*. (GMS, ×500)

441

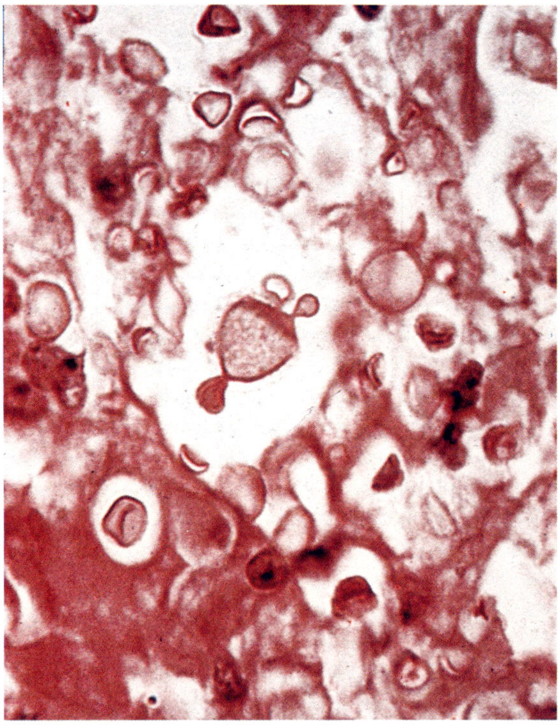

441 Cryptococcus neoformans causing pulmonary cryptococcosis in a human. *C. neoformans* may also form multiple buds connected by narrow necks. Generally, as illustrated in this case, the presence of a prominent capsule will differentiate this fungus from *Paracoccidioides brasiliensis*. (H&E, ×500)

442

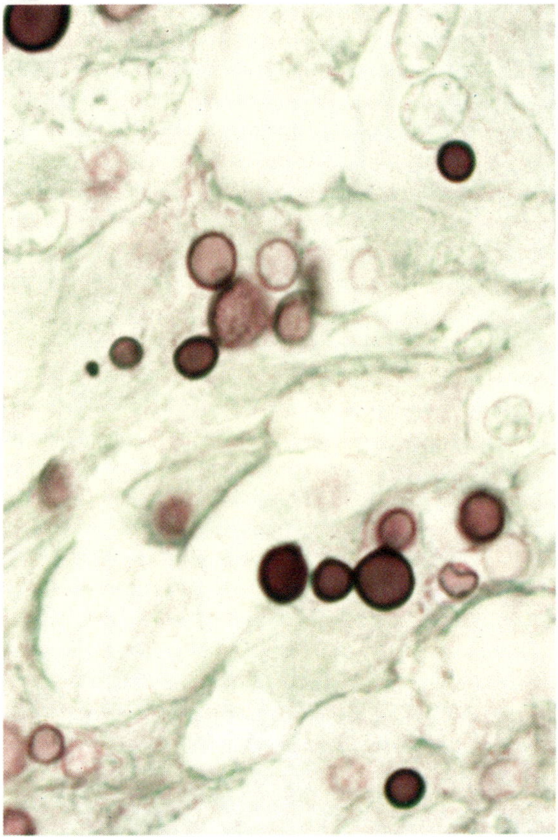

443

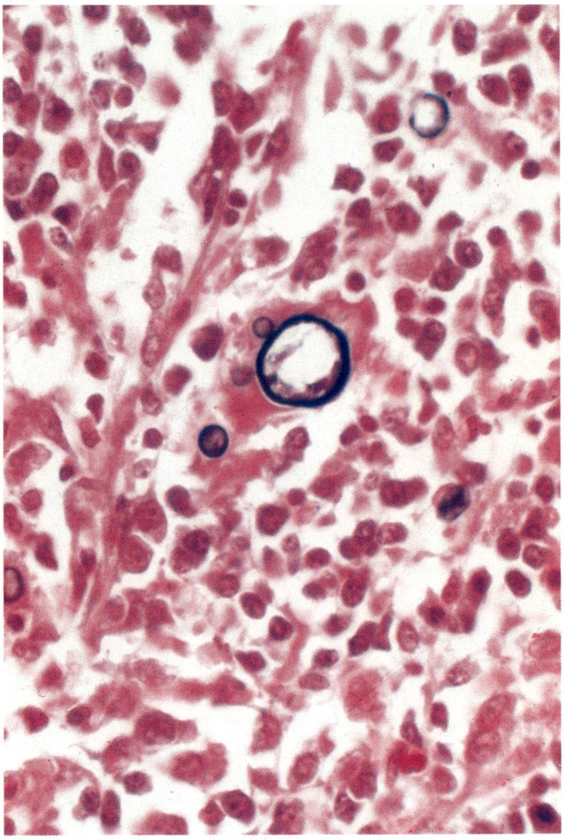

442 Cryptococci (poorly encapsulated) in granuloma of human lung. Two of the yeast cells show multiple budding and have narrow basal attachments. Although cryptococci are usually smaller than the tissue form cells of *Paracoccidioides brasiliensis*, they may be confused with the latter if they show multiple budding and do not have prominent capsules. When morphological criteria are inadequate for differentiating the two, cultural and immunofluorescence examinations are invaluable. (GMS, ×500)

443 Pulmonary coccidioidomycosis in a human. Two endospores in apposition to a spherule give the false impression of a multiple budding cell. Such an erroneous interpretation may lead to a misdiagnosis. *Coccidioides immitis* does not bud in tissue, and other fields or sections should be examined for the presence of endosporulating spherules. (GMS–H&E, ×200)

21 Phaeohyphomycosis

Text pages: 92–95

444

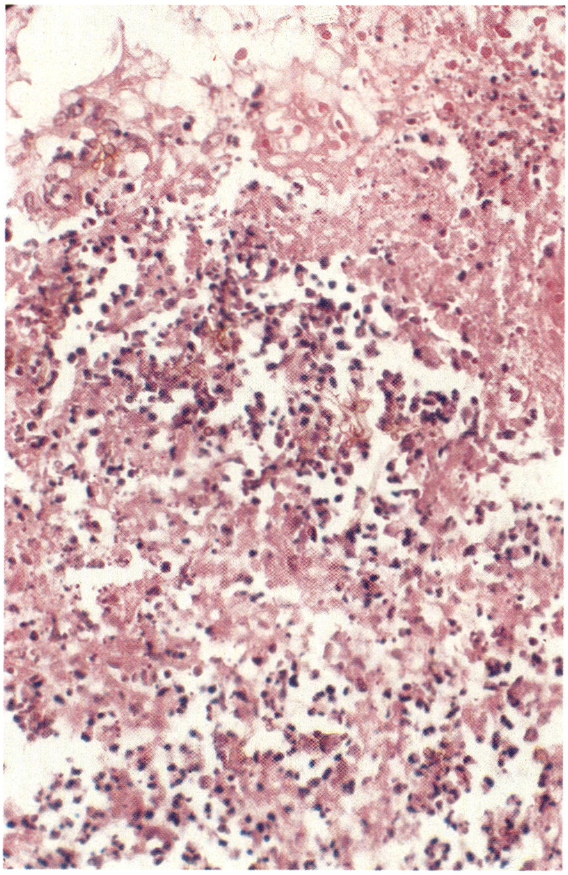

444 Cladosporium bantianum (trichoides) infection of the human brain. Note the necrosis and infiltration of polymorphonuclear leucocytes in the centre of a large cerebral abscess. The dematiaceous hyphae are not easily seen at this magnification. (H&E, ×100)

445

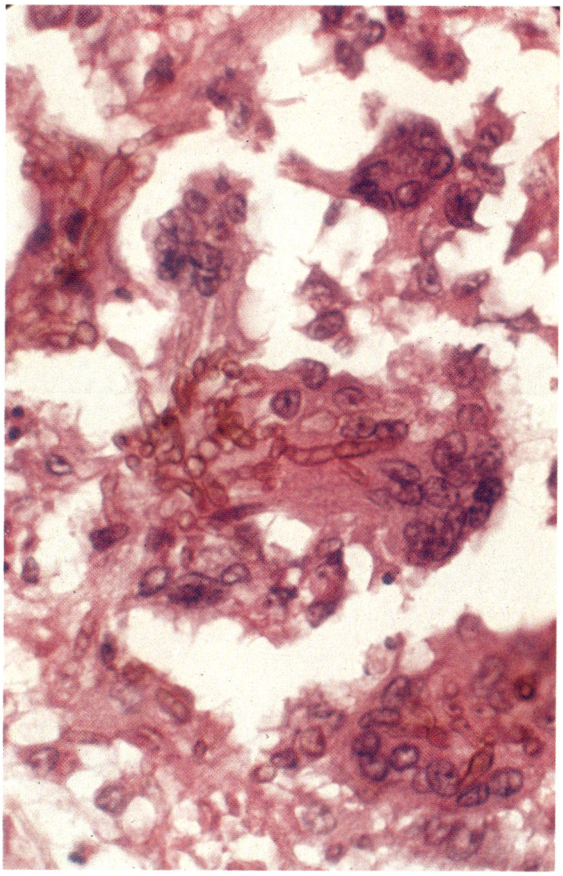

445 Cladosporium bantianum Wall of the cerebral abscess seen in **444**. The dematiaceous, branched hyphae within huge giant cells are readily seen because of their natural brown colour. (H&E, ×200)

446

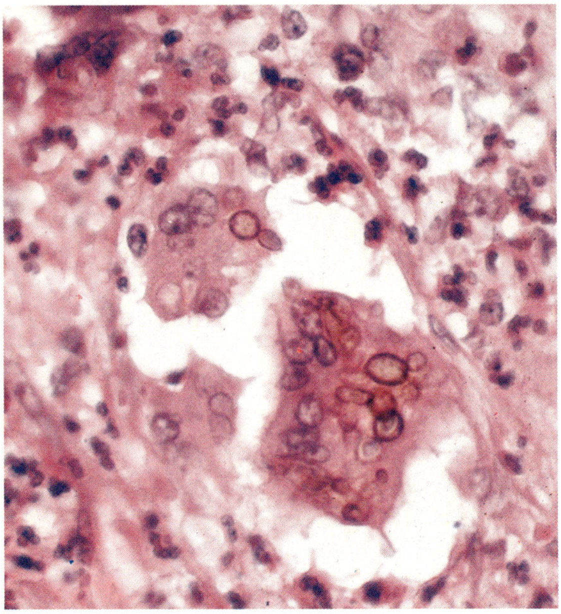

446 Cladosporium bantianum Another field in **444** showing the occasional yeast-like dematiaceous forms of this fungus within giant cells in the wall of the cerebral abscess. (H&E, ×200)

447

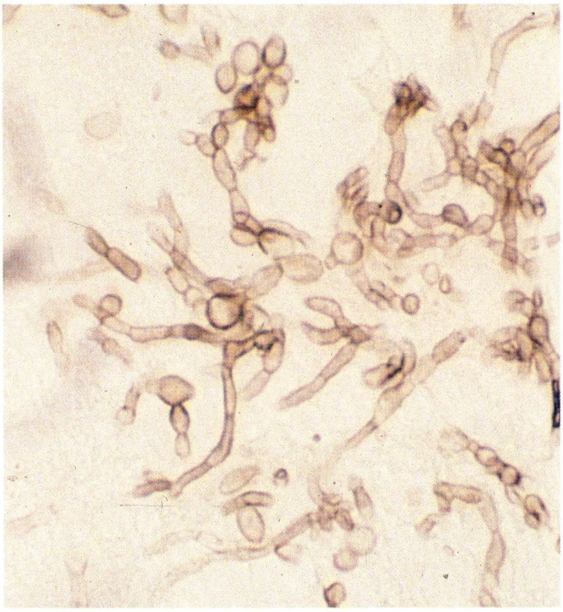

447 Cladosporium bantianum Unstained replicate section of brain abscess shown in **444**. The natural brown pigment of the hyphae is clearly evident. Examination of an unstained tissue section may sometimes be needed to verify the dematiaceous nature of a lightly pigmented fungus. (×200)

448

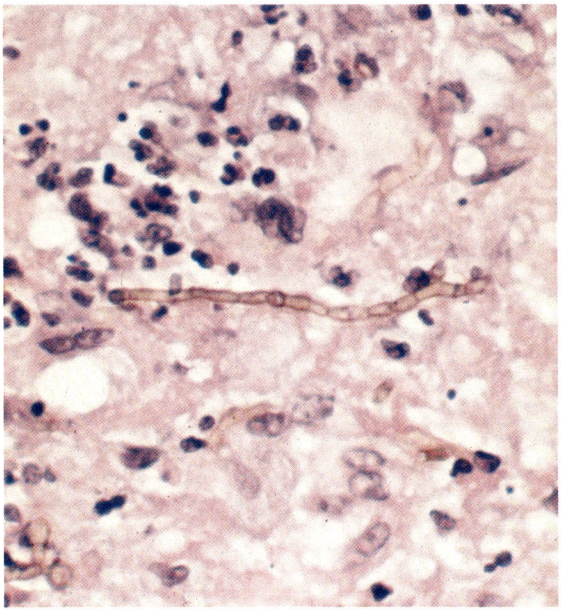

448 Cladosporium bantianum Section from another patient with cerebral phaeohyphomycosis. This field shows a long, closely septate, dematiaceous hypha invading the brain parenchyma contiguous to an abscess. There are focal collections of neutrophils in the neuropil. (H&E, ×200)

449

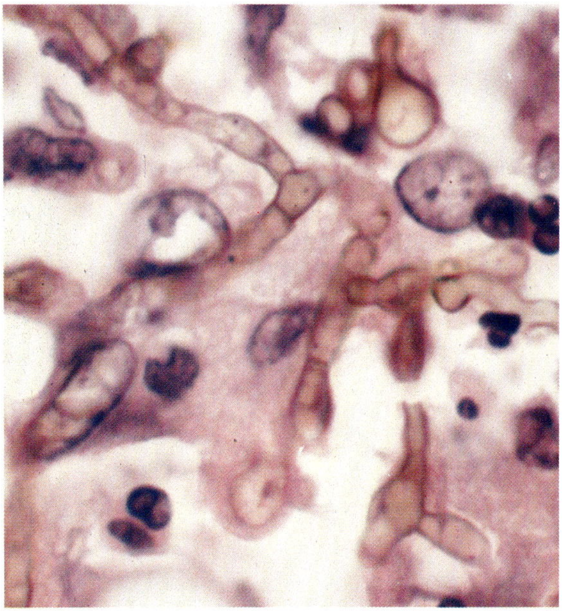

449 Cladosporium bantianum Higher magnification of another field in **448** showing the branched, septate, dematiaceous hyphae in greater detail. One form at the top appears to be budding. (H&E, ×500)

450

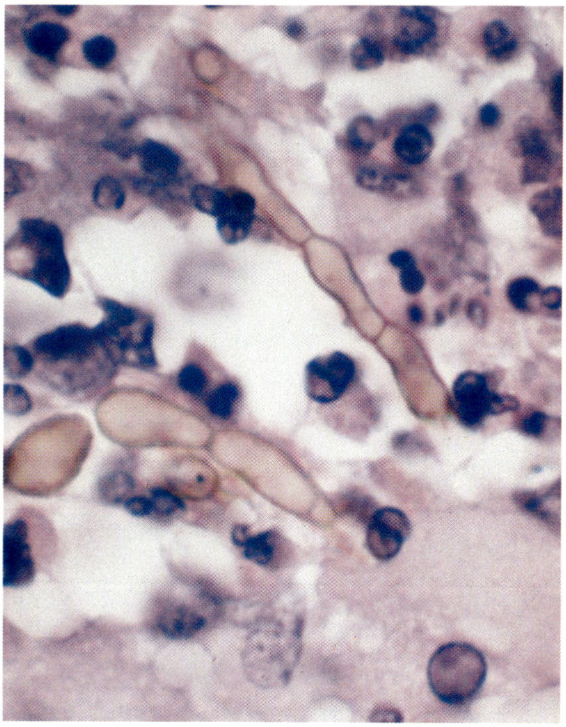

450 Cladosporium bantianum Another field in **448** which shows dematiaceous hyphae embedded in neutrophils. As seen here, hyphae are often constricted at their septa. (H&E, ×500)

451

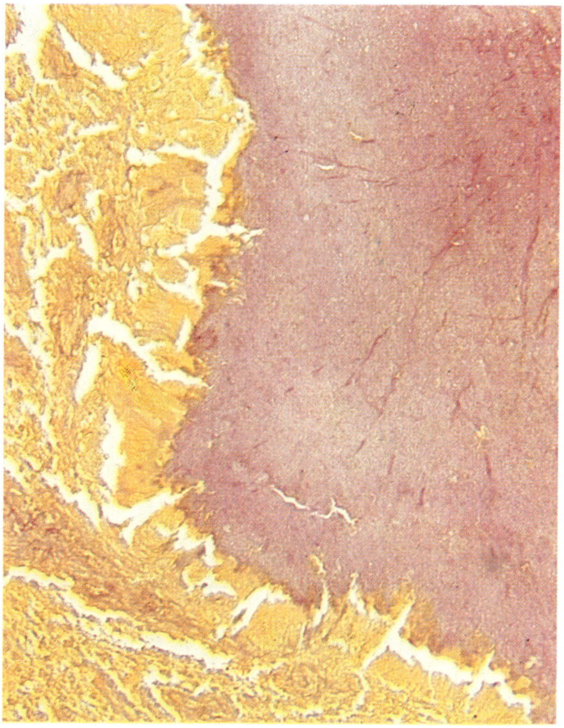

451 Dactylaria gallopava infection of the brain in a chicken. The darker zone is a large area of necrosis and granulomatous inflammation that is sharply delimited from the yellow zone of apparently normal brain: (GF, ×125)

452

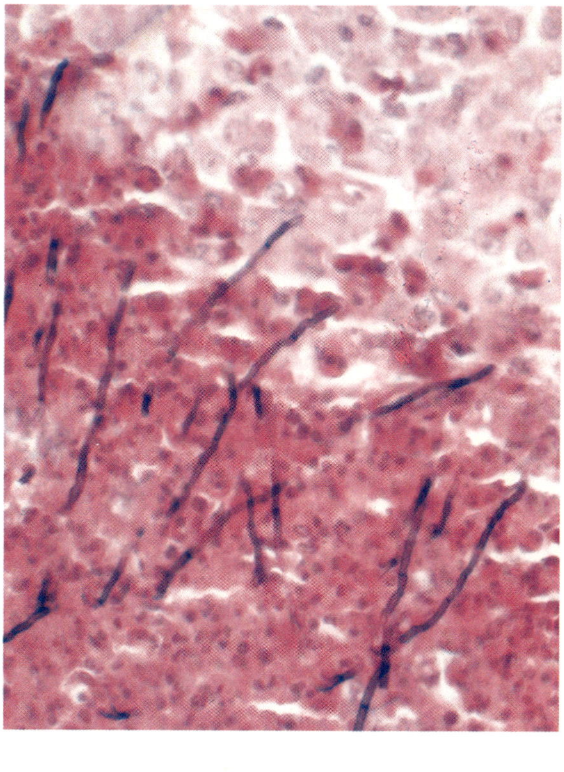

452 Dactylaria gallopava Replicate section of the lesion seen in **451**. Note the long, relatively narrow hyphae embedded in the necrotic tissue and invading the contiguous neuropil. (GMS–H&E, ×200)

453

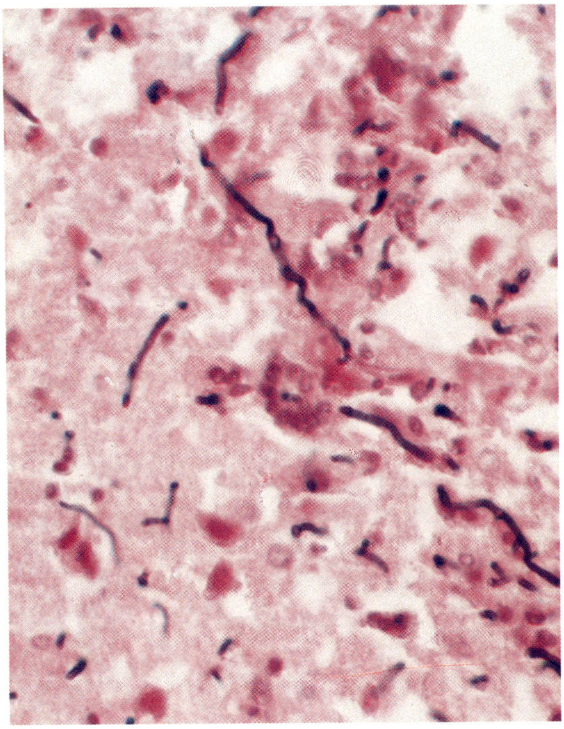

454

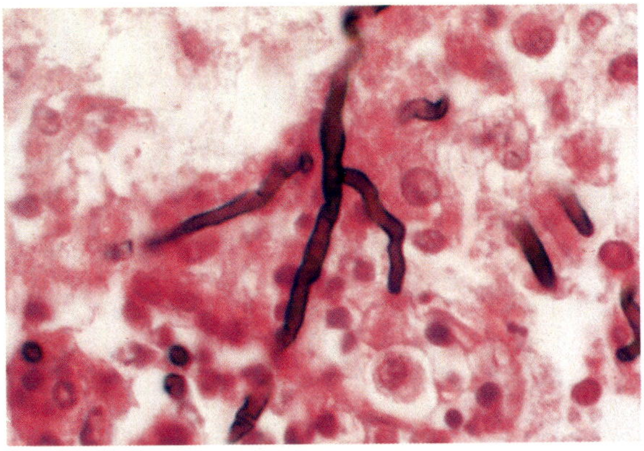

453 Dactylaria gallopava infection of a chicken brain. Narrow hyphae are invading the brain parenchyma adjacent to a large necrotic abscess. A giant cell containing a hyphal fragment is seen in the centre. (GMS–H&E, ×200)

454 Dactylaria gallopava Higher magnification of **453** showing a branched hypha in greater detail. The mycelium of this fungus differs from that of the aspergilli in that it is light brown in colour and its hyphae are narrower (2–3 μm vs. 3–6 μm) and do not show dichotomous branching. (GMS–H&E, ×500)

455

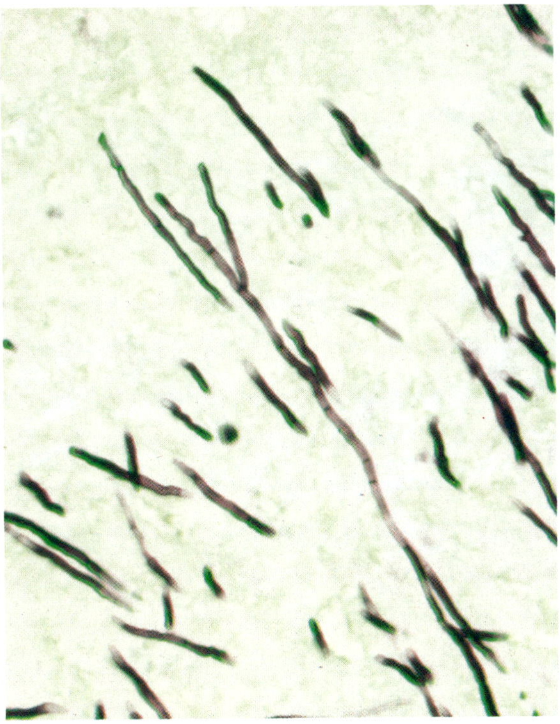

455 Dactylaria gallopava Replicate section of **453**. The numerous, long and relatively narrow septate hyphae are clearly seen. (GMS, ×200)

456

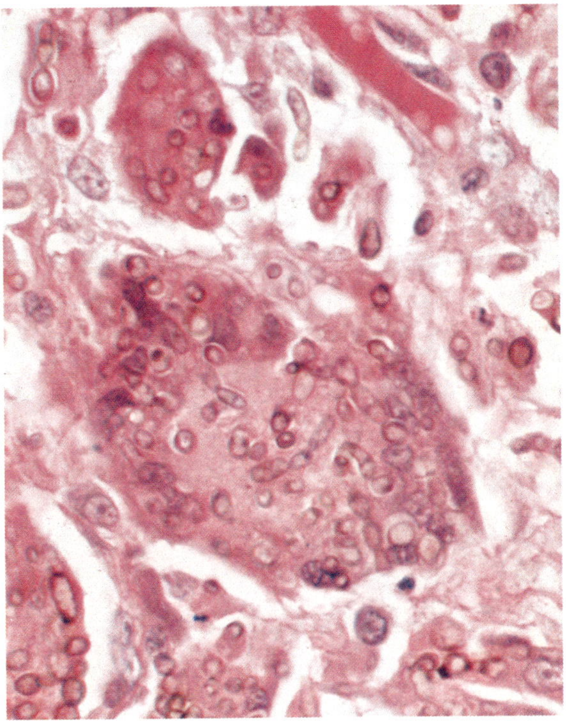

456 Drechslera spicifera causing subcutaneous granuloma in a cat. Note the abundant dematiaceous mycelium within huge giant cells. (H&E, ×100)

457

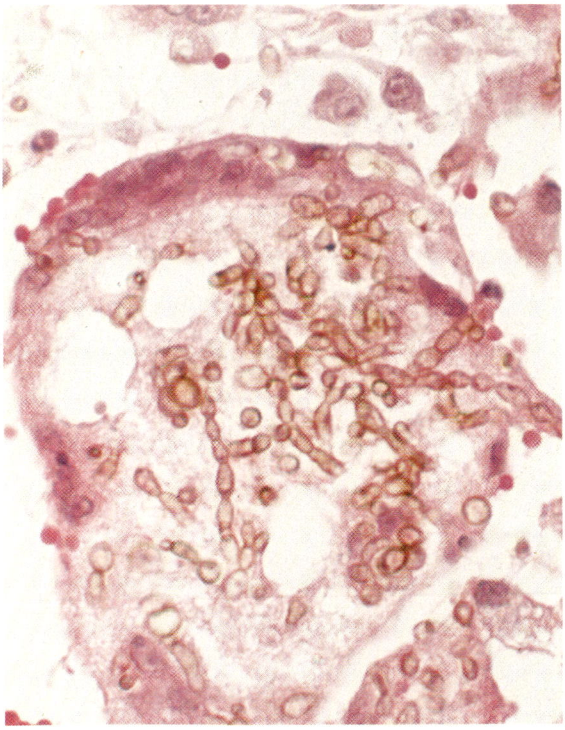

457 Drechslera spicifera Another field in **456** showing the branched, closely septate, dematiaceous hyphae within a huge giant cell. (H&E, ×200)

458

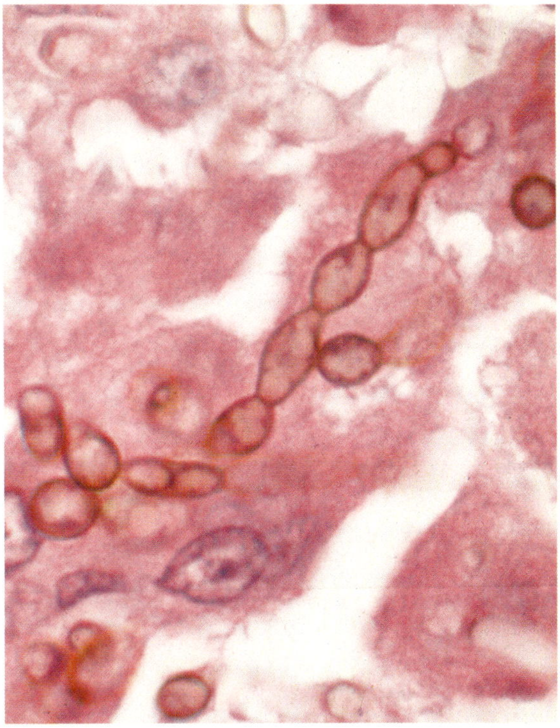

458 Drechslera spicifera Higher magnification of another field in **456** shows a chain of cells that forms the hypha. The mycelium is constricted at the septa, and it is naturally brown. Fungal elements are within a giant cell. (H&E, ×500)

459

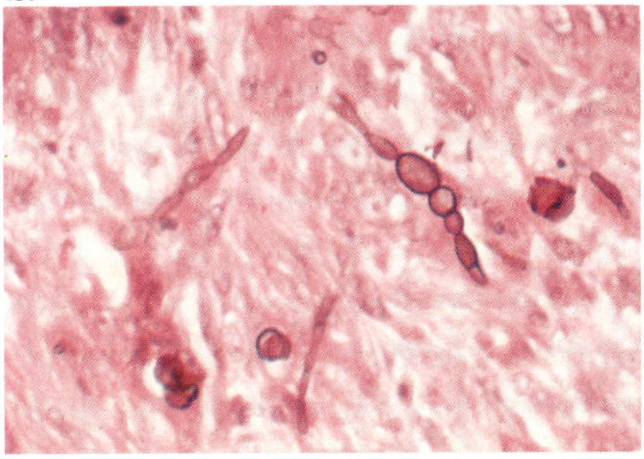

459 Drechslera spicifera causing subcutaneous infection in a horse. Chains of fungus cells are in the fibrogranulomatous lesion. (GMS–H&E, ×200)

460

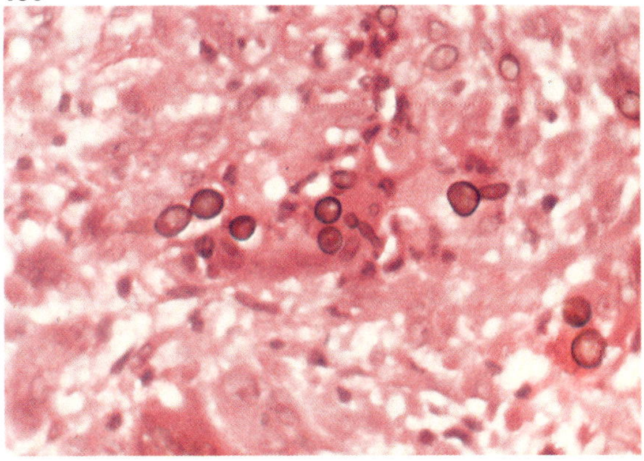

460 Drechslera spicifera Another field in **459** showing individual yeast-like fungi that are both extracellular and within giant cells. Some of the cells appear to be budding. (GMS–H&E, ×200)

461

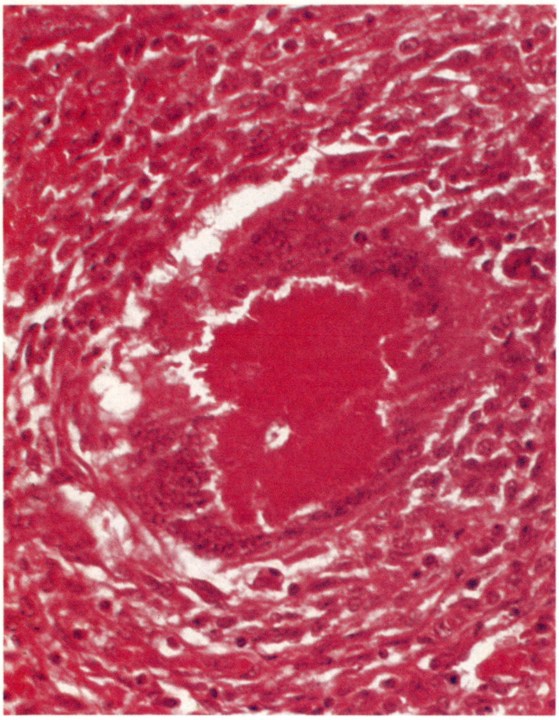

462

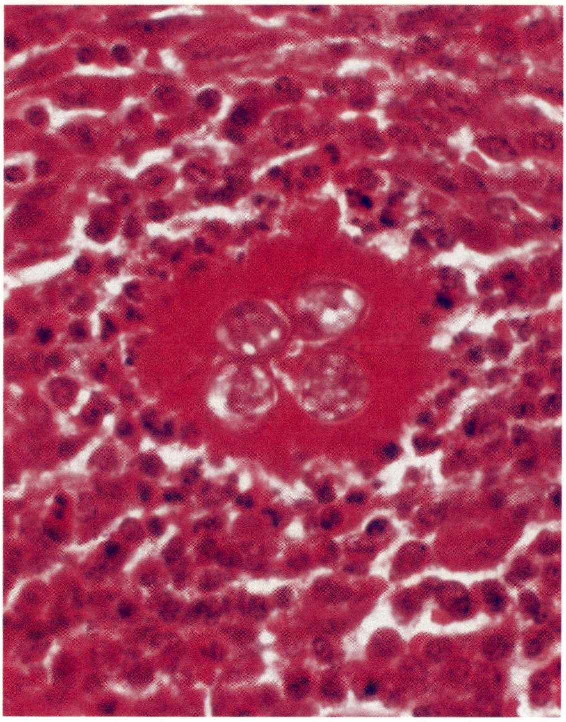

461 Drechslera rostrata causing bovine nasal granuloma. Poorly stained fungal cells surrounded by a large mass of deeply eosinophilic Splendore–Hoeppli material are contained within a huge giant cell. The giant cell is embedded in granulation tissue in the submucosa. (H&E, ×100)

462 Drechslera rostrata Another field in **461** showing four cells bordered by a radial corona of Splendore–Hoeppli material and embedded in a microabscess. Such accumulations of fungal cells embedded in and bordered by Splendore–Hoeppli material have been interpreted by some as granules of a mycetoma. We do not agree with that interpretation. (H&E, ×200)

463

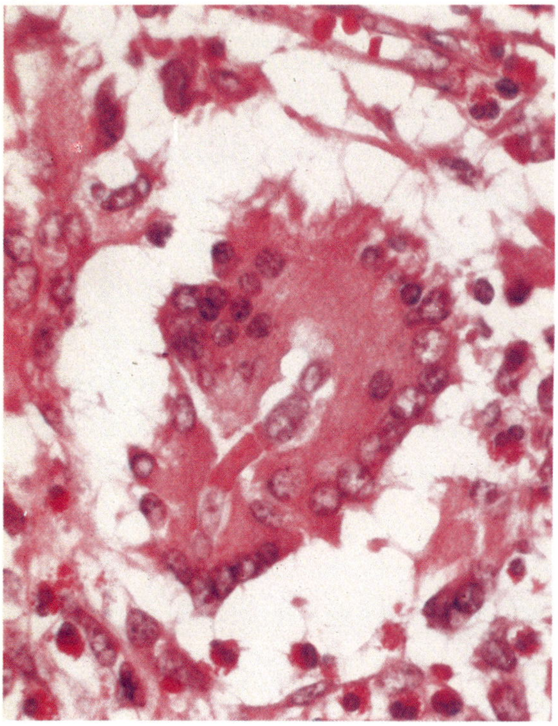

463 Drechslera rostrata causing bovine nasal granuloma. A short chain of apparently hyaline fungal cells is seen within a giant cell. Although this fungus is dematiaceous, not all elements in tissues are pigmented. Note the many eosinophils, a common finding in these cases. (H&E, ×200)

464

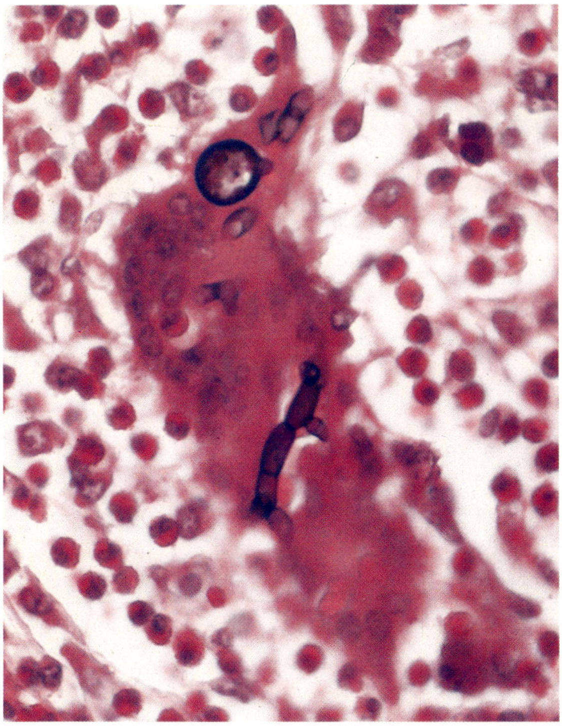

465

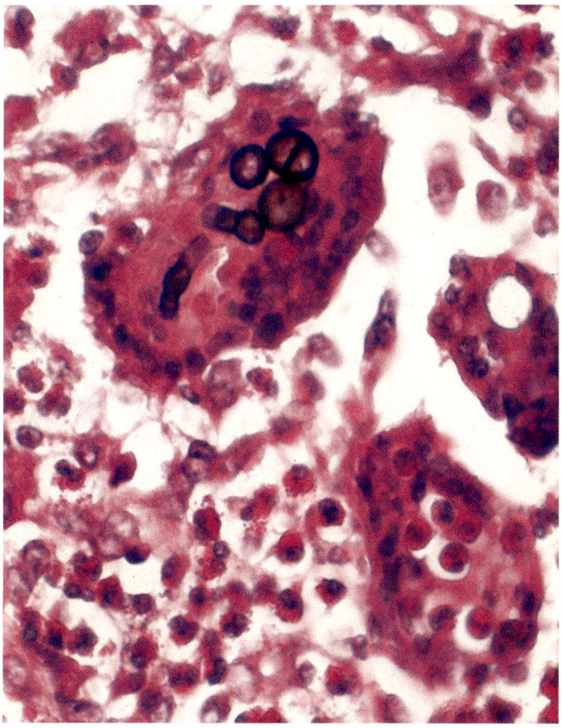

464 Drechslera rostrata Replicate section of **463** but stained by GMS–H&E. A single giant cell contains a branched, closely septate hypha and individual fungal cells. Note the surrounding eosinophilic infiltrate. (GMS–H&E, ×200)

465 Drechslera rostrata Another field in **464** showing closely septate hyphae and individual fungal cells within a giant cell. One cell appears to be dividing by septation. However, this septate cell should not be confused with the sclerotic bodies seen in chromoblastomycosis. (GMS–H&E, ×200)

466

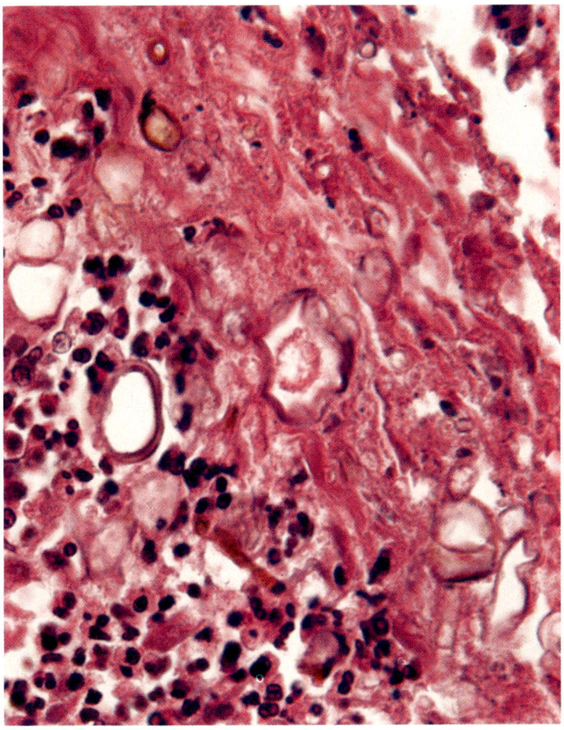

466 Drechslera hawaiiensis infection of a human brain. Dematiaceous fungal cells are embedded in a mixed inflammatory cell infiltrate. (H&E, ×500)

467

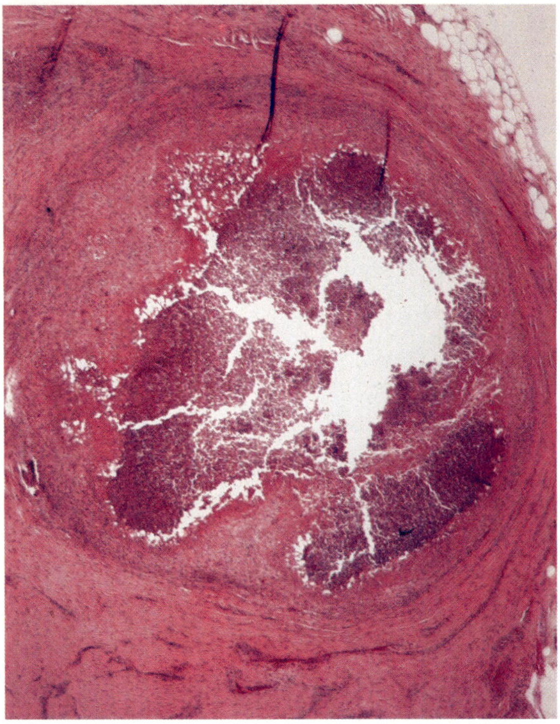

468

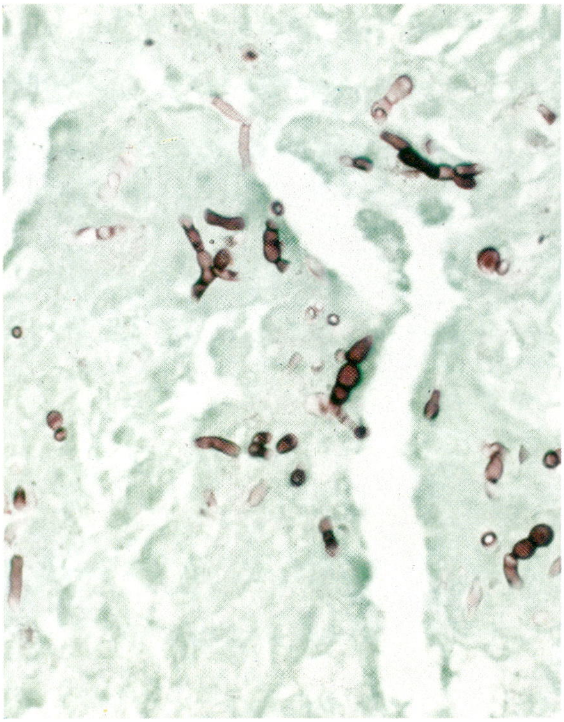

467 Exophiala jeanselmei (gougerotii) causing subcutaneous (phaeomycotic) cyst in a human. Dematiaceous fungus cells are present in the purulent centre and granulomatous wall of the cyst, but they are not visible at this low magnification. (H&E, ×8)

468 Exophiala jeanselmei (gougerotii) Replicate section of **467** stained by GMS. Numerous hyphae are seen in the cyst wall of pyogranulomatous tissue. (GMS, ×100)

469

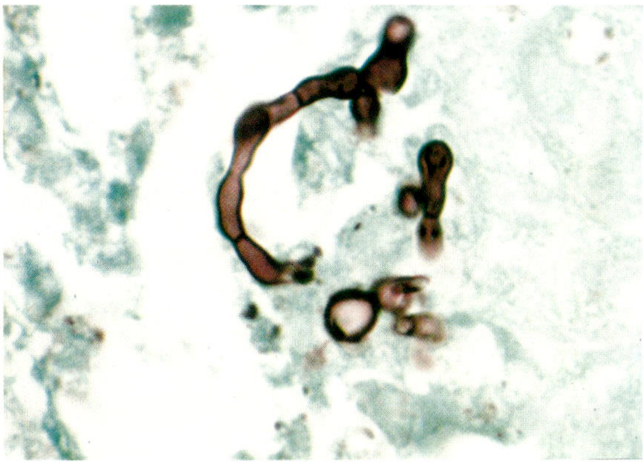

470

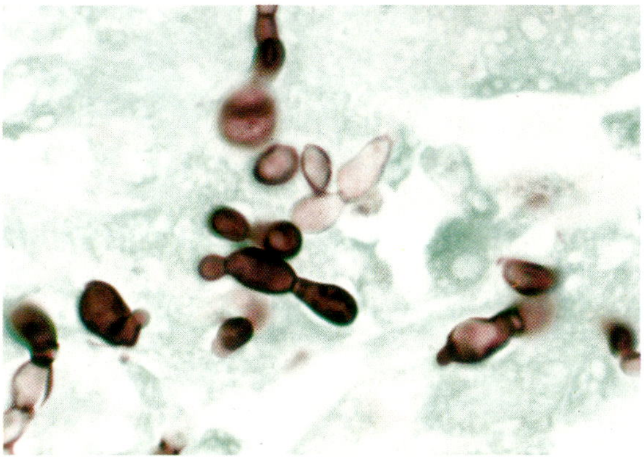

469 Exophiala jeanselmei (gougerotii) Higher magnification of **468** showing the branched, septate hyphae in greater detail. The close morphologic resemblance of this fungus to *Drechslera spp.* and to certain other dematiaceous fungi in tissues makes a histological identification difficult. Cultural studies are almost always required. (GMS, ×500)

470 Exophiala jeanselmei (gougerotii) Another field in **468** showing the hyphae and individual cells. The latter appear to be budding. (GMS, ×500)

471

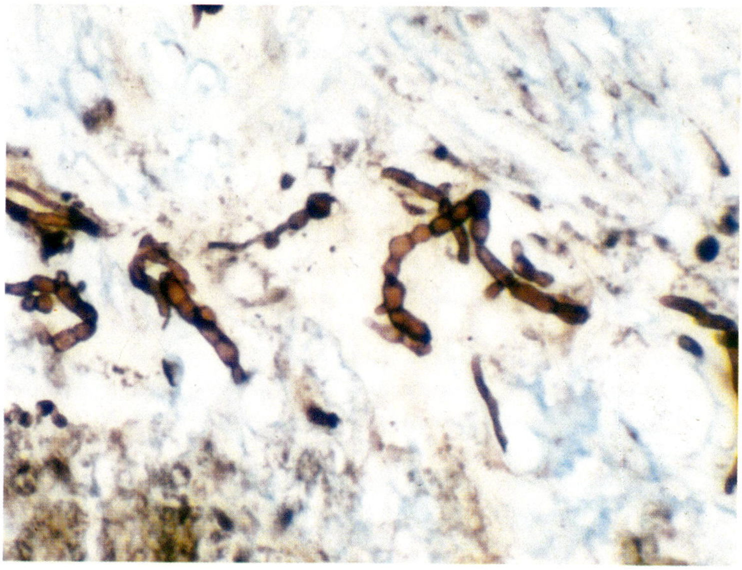

471 Exophiala parasitica causing a subcutaneous cyst in a human. In tissue, this species is morphologically identical to *Exophiala jeanselmei*. Cultural studies are required for their differential identification. (GMS, ×200)

472

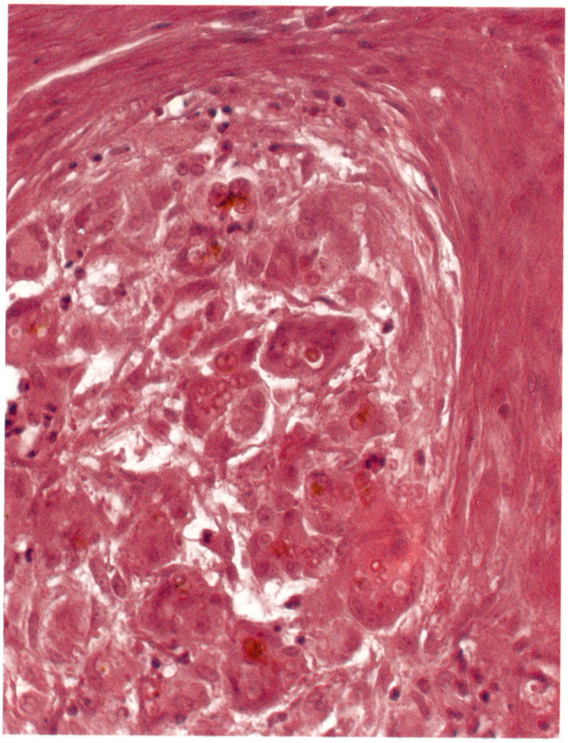

473

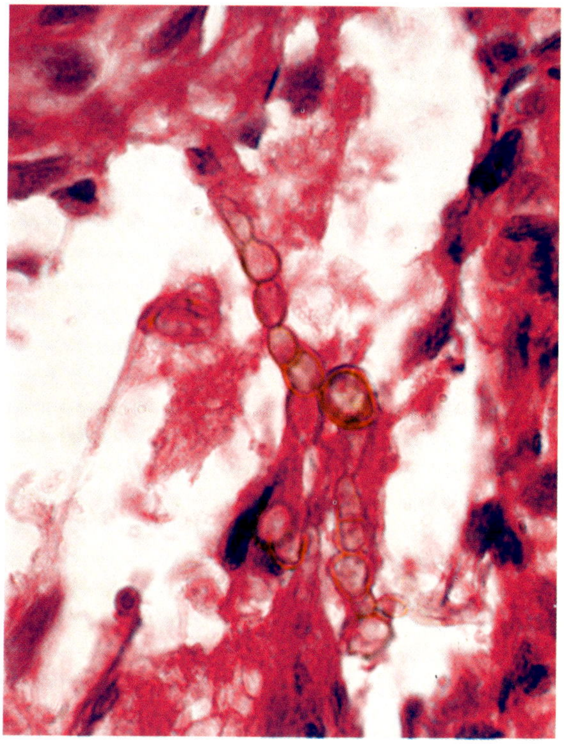

472 Wangiella dermatitidis infection of human skin. A nodular granuloma composed of giant and epithelioid cells is present in the dermis. The dematiaceous fungal elements within the lesion are not readily seen at this magnification. (H&E, ×100)

473 Wangiella dermatitidis Higher magnification of **472** showing two chains of dematiaceous cells in the granulomatous lesion. Note their innate brown colour. (H&E, ×320)

474

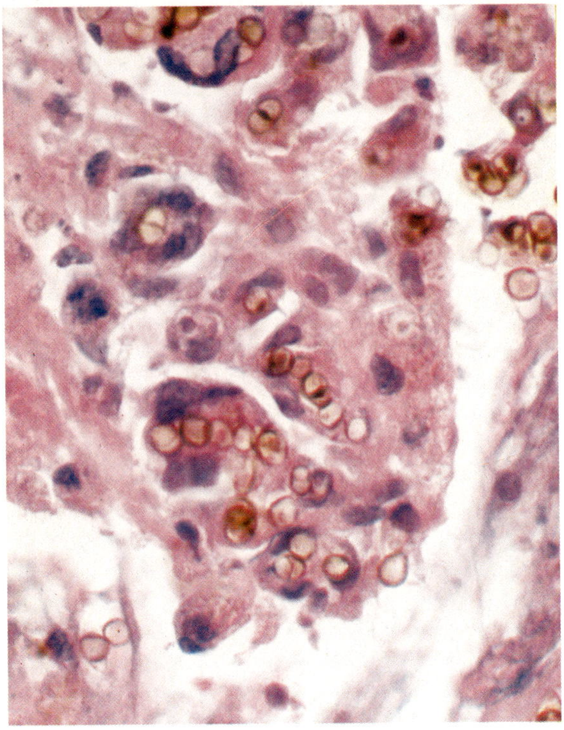

474 **Wangiella dermatitidis** causing granulomatous dermatitis in another human. The numerous giant cells contain short chains of dematiaceous fungal cells. (H&E, ×200)

475

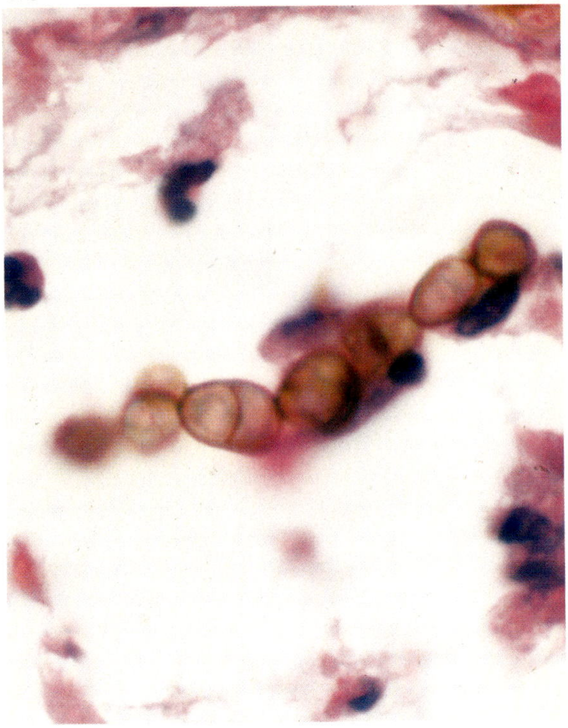

475 **Wangiella dermatitidis** Higher magnification of **474** to show the fungal cells in greater detail. The dematiaceous cells occur in a chain and have relatively thin walls. Some also have transverse septations. By contrast, the sclerotic cells characteristic of chromoblastomycosis do not occur in chains, have thicker walls, and have both longitudinal and transverse septations. (H&E, ×500)

476

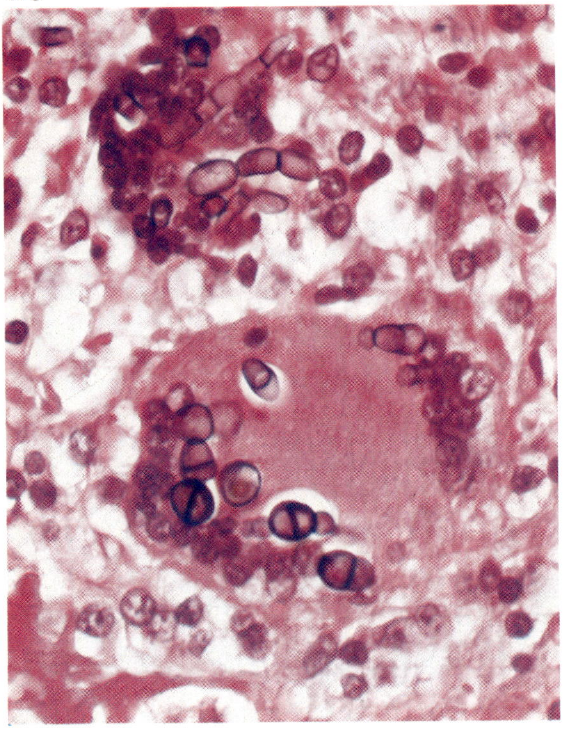

476 **Presumed chromoblastomycosis** in a marine toad. In this section, short chains of dematiaceous fungal cells as well as individual septate cells within two large giant cells are present. The aetiologic agent was isolated but was not identified because of its failure to sporulate. Typical sclerotic bodies with septations in two planes (as found in chromoblastomycosis) are not seen. (H&E, ×200)

22 Protothecosis and infections caused by morphologically similar green algae

Text pages: 96–100

477

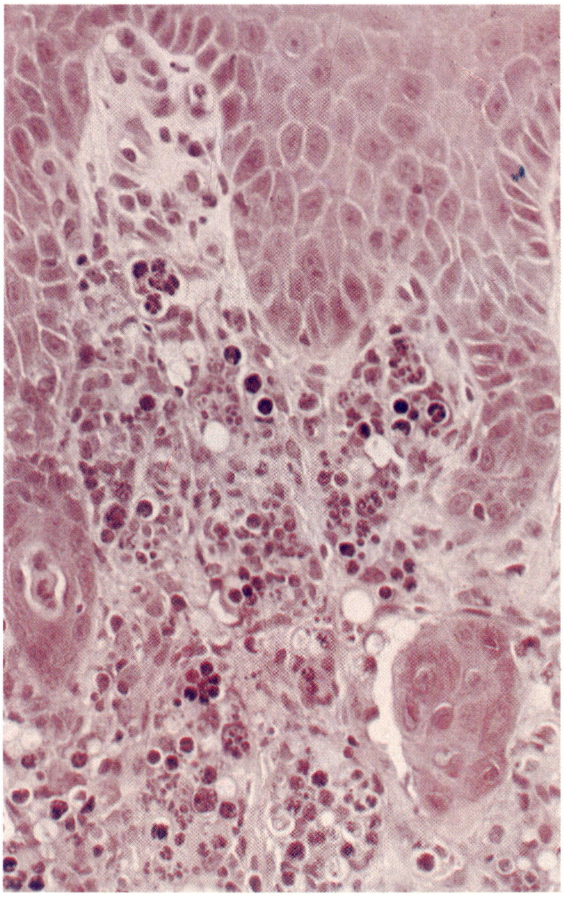

478

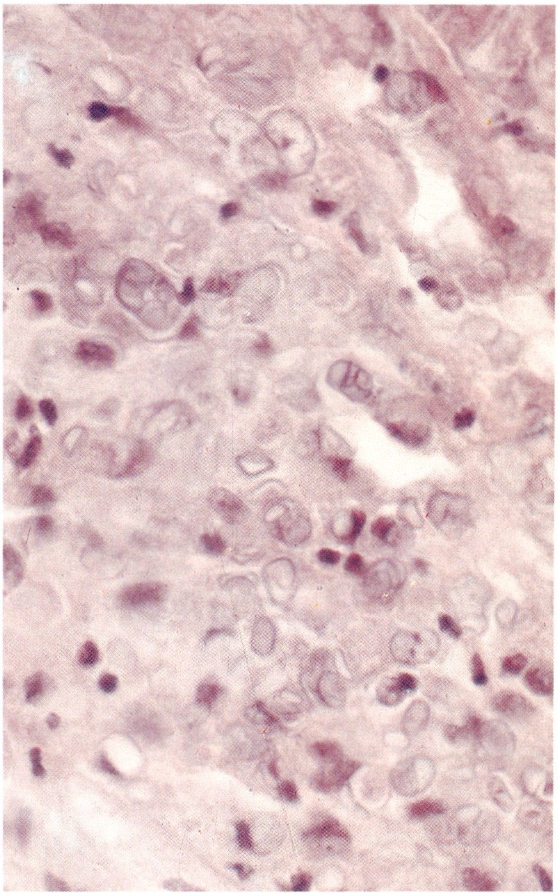

477 Prototheca wickerhamii causing dermatitis in a dog. There is moderate thickening of the epidermis and a marked granulomatous reaction consisting of densely packed histiocytes and giant cells in the dermis. The numerous round-to-oval basophilic organisms are extracellular and within phagocytes. (H&E, ×100)

478 Prototheca zopfii causing granulomatous myocarditis in a dog with disseminated protothecosis. Although abundant, the predominantly intracellular organisms are not easily seen because they are poorly stained. (H&E, ×200)

479

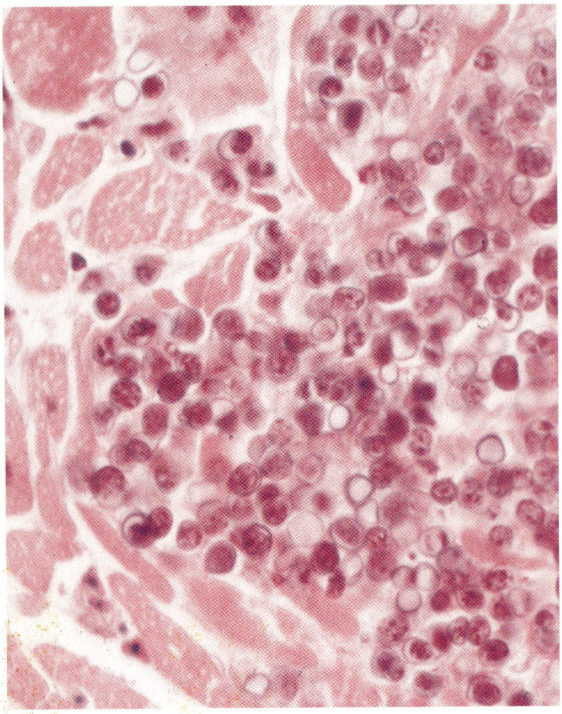

479 Prototheca zopfii Another field in **478**. In this focus of involvement, numerous protothecal cells are well stained and there is little or no inflammatory response. Rather, the myocardial fibres are displaced by the proliferating organisms. (H&E, ×200)

480

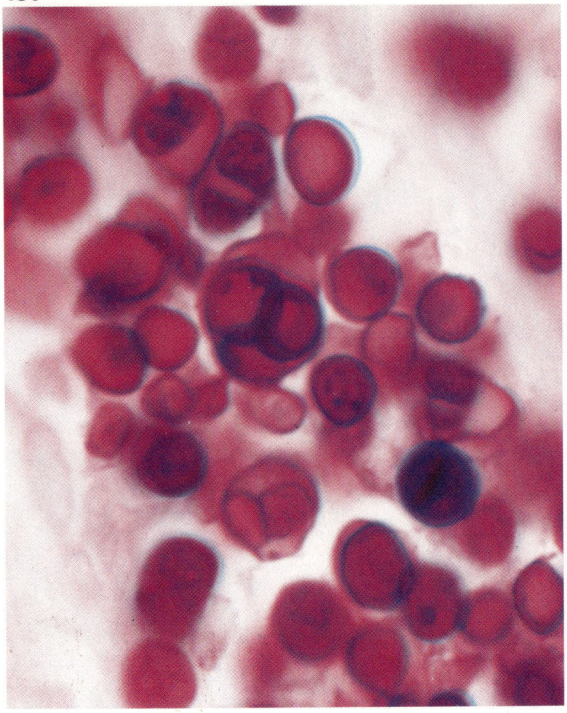

480 Prototheca zopfii Replicate section of **479** but stained by PAS to show both single and endosporulating cells in greater detail. (PAS, ×500)

481

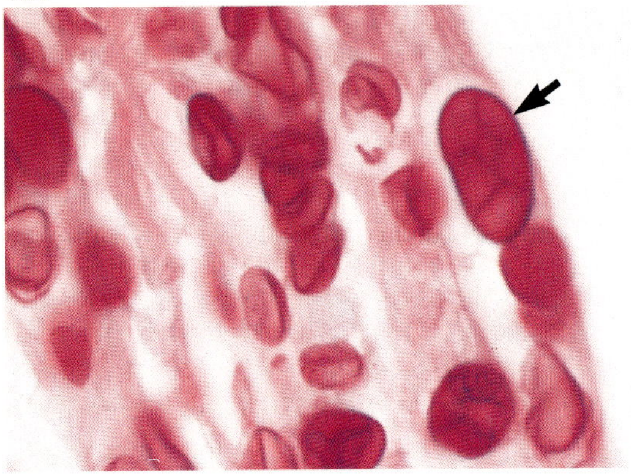

481 Prototheca zopfii Another field in **480** illustrating the morphologic variability of *P. zopfii* in tissue. Note one elliptical endosporulating form (arrow) and several collapsed, distorted, single forms. (PAS, ×500)

482

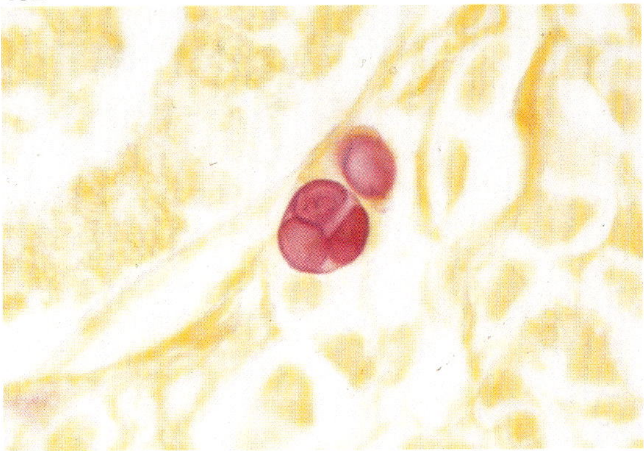

482 Prototheca zopfii Section of kidney from the same patient as in **478**. This field contains an endosporulating spherule (morula configuration) and a single cell of *P. zopfii*. (GF, ×500)

483

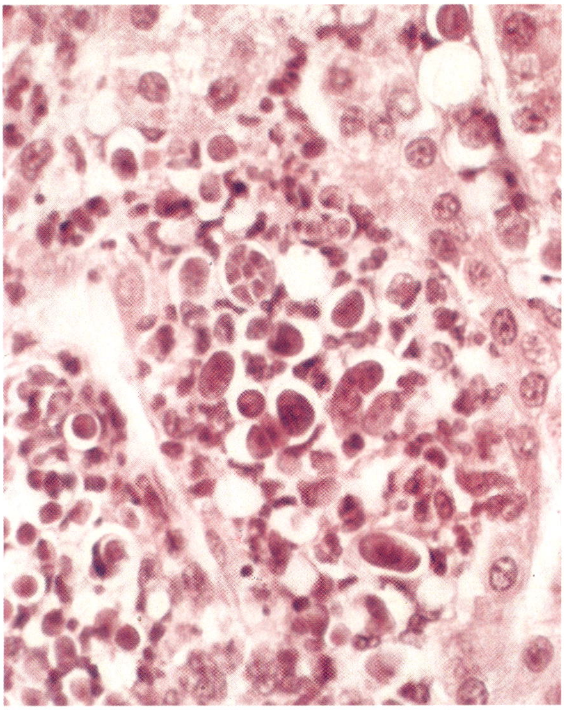

484

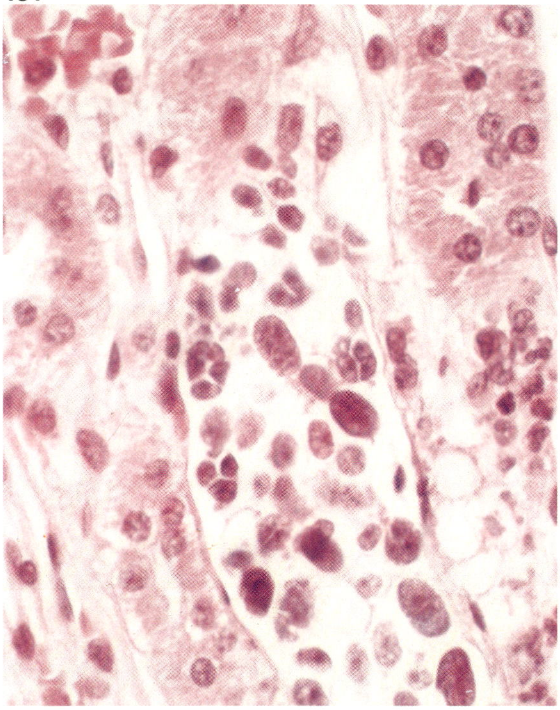

483 Prototheca zopfii causing chronic nephritis in a dog. Clusters of single and endosporulating protothecal cells are surrounded by moderate numbers of mixed inflammatory cells. (H&E, ×200)

484 Prototheca zopfii Another field in **483**. Numerous protothecal cells fill the renal tubules. No inflammation is evident. (H&E, ×200)

485

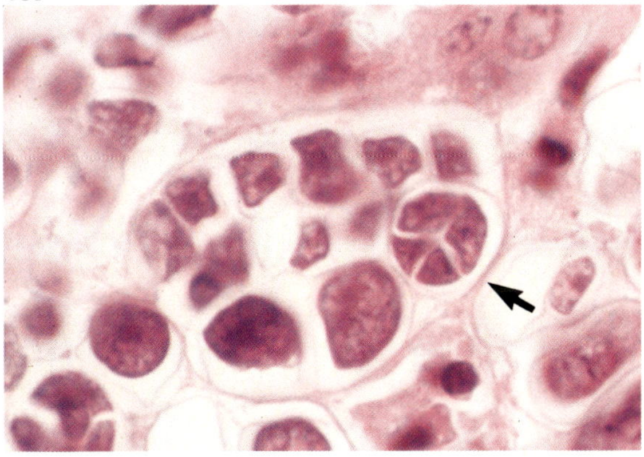

485 Prototheca zopfii Higher magnification of **484**. A group of protothecal cells is shown within the lumen of a renal tubule. One spherical cell is endosporulating (arrow), and the others appear distorted. (H&E, ×500)

486 Prototheca zopfii Replicate section of kidney in **483** showing an embolus of proliferating GMS-positive protothecal cells within a glomerulus. (GMS, ×100)

486

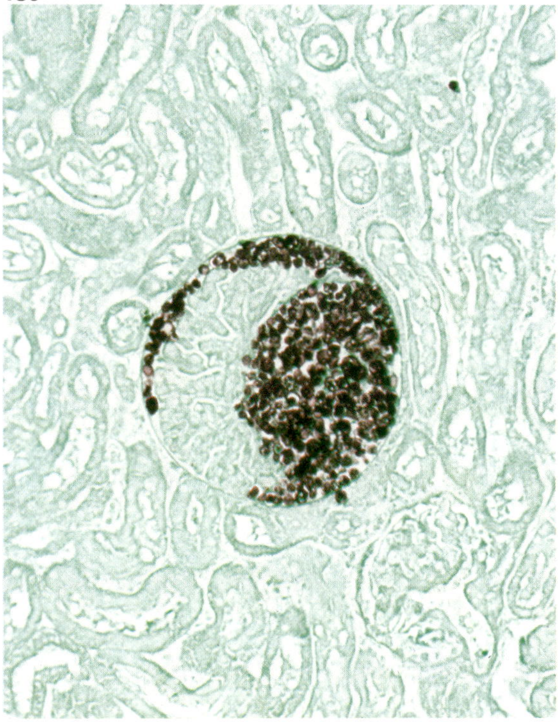

487

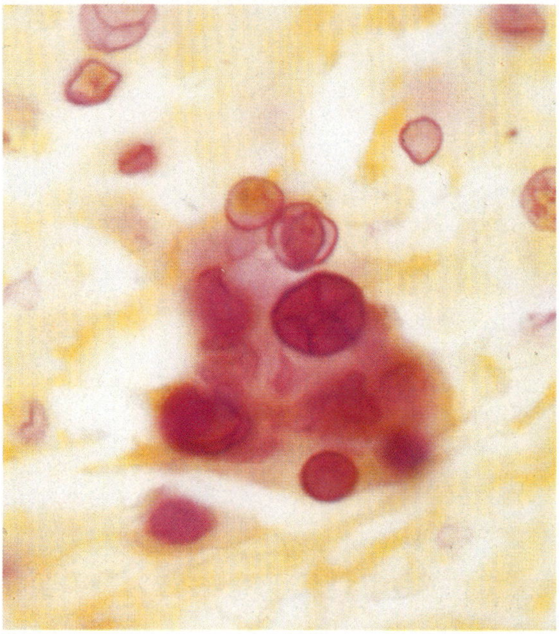

488

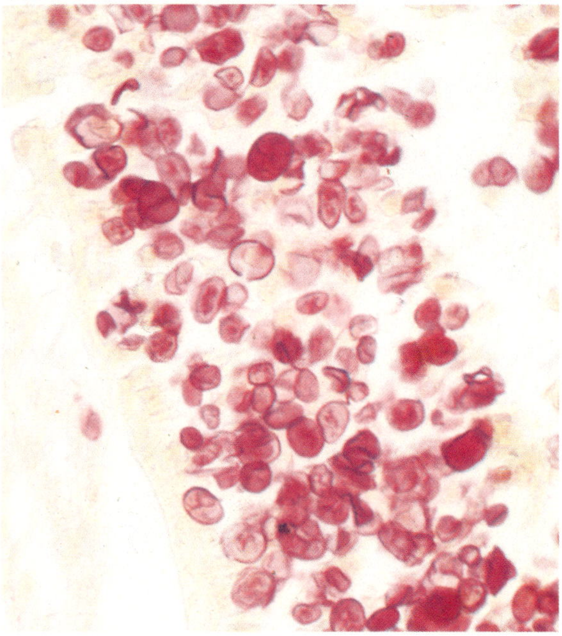

487 Prototheca wickerhamii cells within an inflammatory nodule on the peritoneum of a human. The organisms are well demonstrated by GF. An endosporulating form is seen in the centre. (GF, ×500)

488 Prototheca wickerhamii causing ocular protothecosis in a dog. Numerous proliferating protothecae displace the retina and choroid. The variability in size and shape of the organism is clearly seen. (GF, ×200)

489

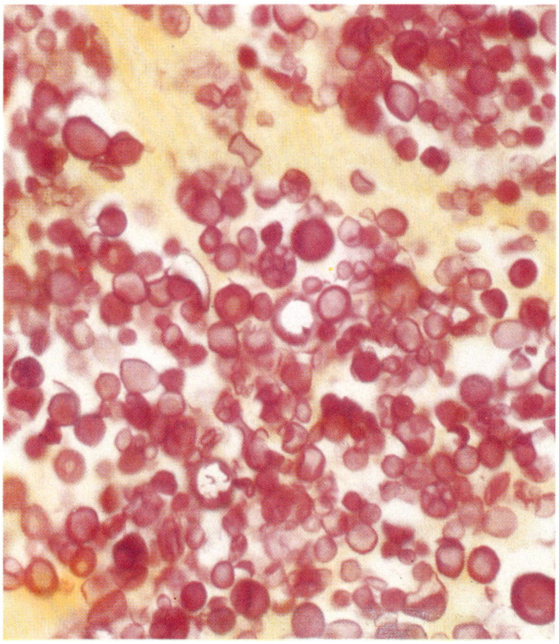

490

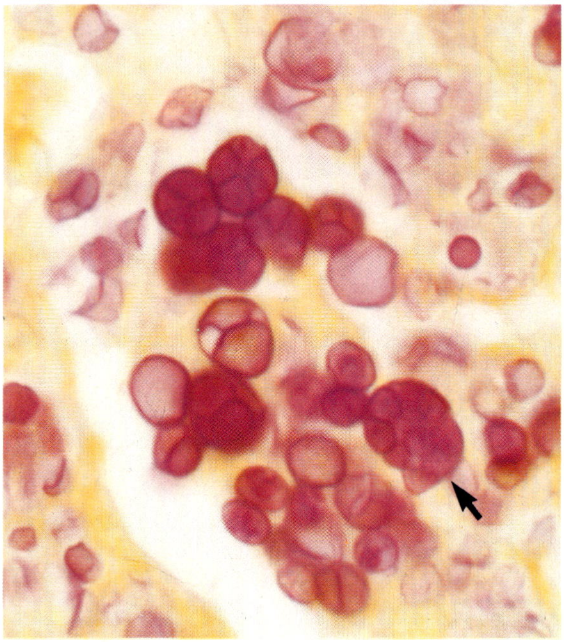

489 Prototheca wickerhamii Subcutaneous granulomatous mass containing myriads of *P. wickerhamii* cells in the tarsus of a cat. Organisms in all stages of development are both intracellular and extracellular. (GF, ×200)

490 Prototheca wickerhamii Higher magnification of **489** showing a group of endosporulating *Prototheca* cells within the granulomatous lesion. The wall of one spherule is broken, and the endospores are about to be released (arrow). (GF, ×500)

491

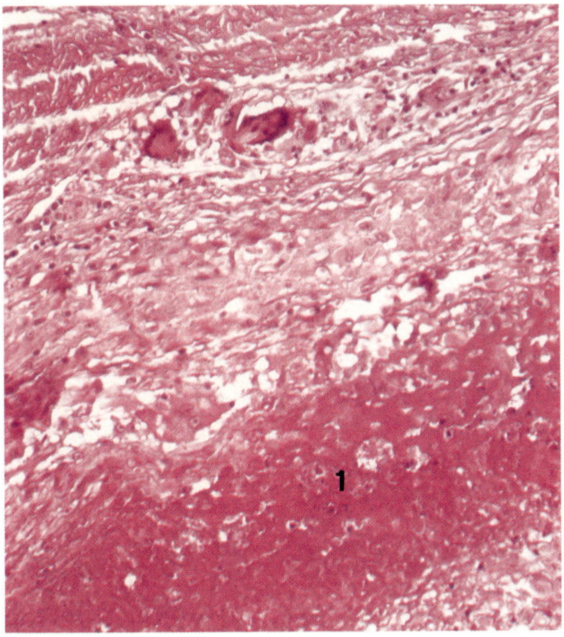

491 Prototheca wickerhamii causing olecranon bursitis in a human. There is caseous necrosis (1) of the bursal lining and a fibrogranulomatous reaction in the underlying stroma. (H&E, ×50)

492

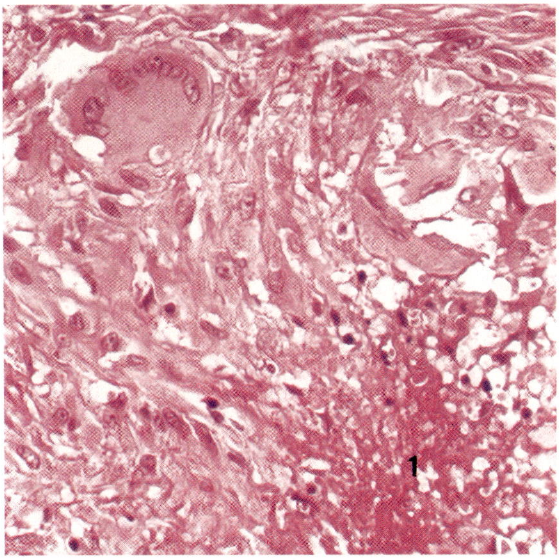

492 Prototheca wickerhamii Higher magnification of **491** showing a zone of palisading epithelioid cells and multinucleated giant cells contiguous to the central caseous core (1). The poorly stained *Prototheca* cells are not visible. (H&E, ×100)

493

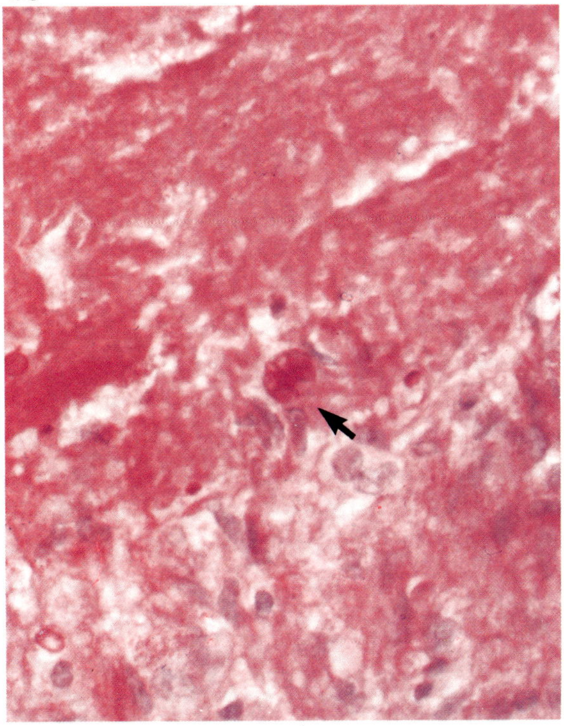

493 Prototheca wickerhamii Replicate section of **491** stained by PAS to show an endosporulating spherule (arrow) embedded in the caseous core. (PAS, ×200)

494

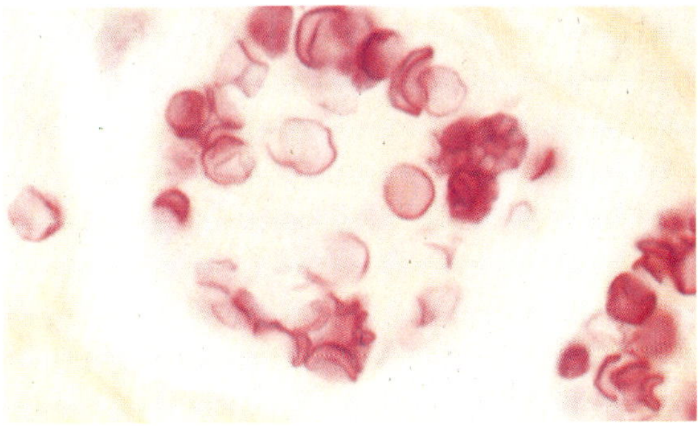

494 Prototheca wickerhamii Replicate section of **491** stained by GF. Several endosporulating spherules as well as collapsed, empty, and degenerated cells are seen in the caseous lining of the olecranon bursa. (GF, ×500)

495

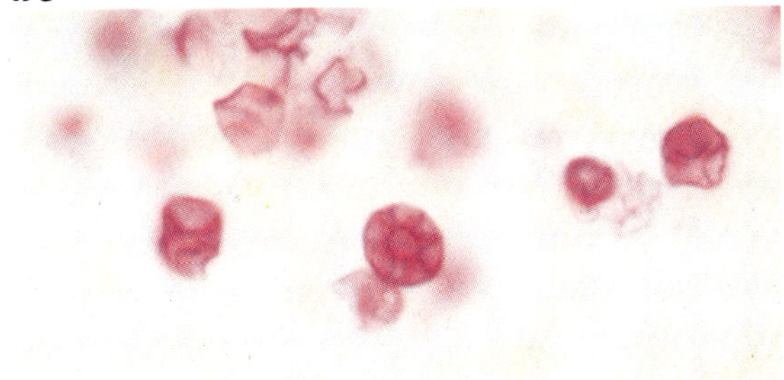

495 Prototheca wickerhamii Another field in **494**. A typical endosporulating spherule is seen in the centre. The collapsed, empty forms are spherules of *Prototheca* that have produced and released endospores. (GF, ×500)

496

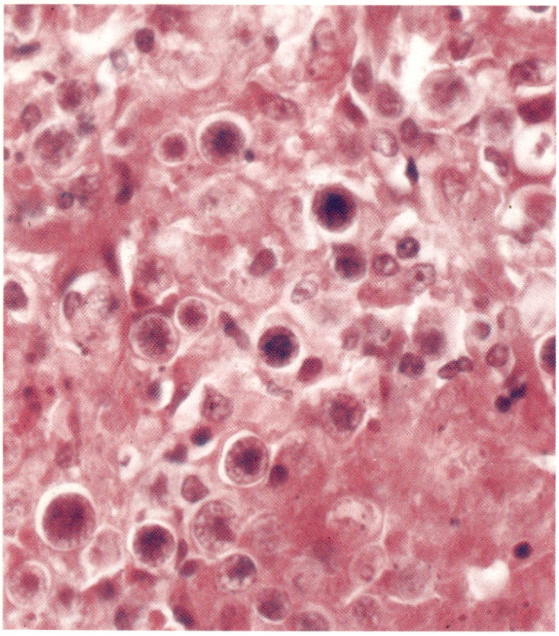

497

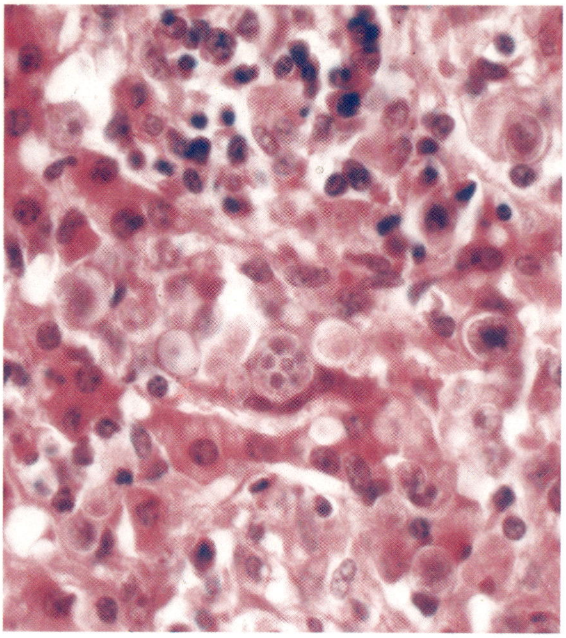

496 Chlorella sp. causing chronic hepatitis in a lamb. The normal hepatic architecture is effaced by a zone of caseous necrosis bordered by granulomatous inflammation. Numerous *Chlorella* (green alga) cells are seen in both the necrotic and viable portions of the lesion. At necropsy, the lesion was green. (H&E, ×200)

497 Chlorella sp. Another field in **496** showing both single and endosporulating *Chlorella* cells surrounded by a mixed inflammatory infiltrate. A hepatic cord is still recognisable in the centre, adjacent to a large endosporulating *Chlorella* cell that closely resembles the protothecal cells seen in **483** to **485**. (H&E, ×200)

498

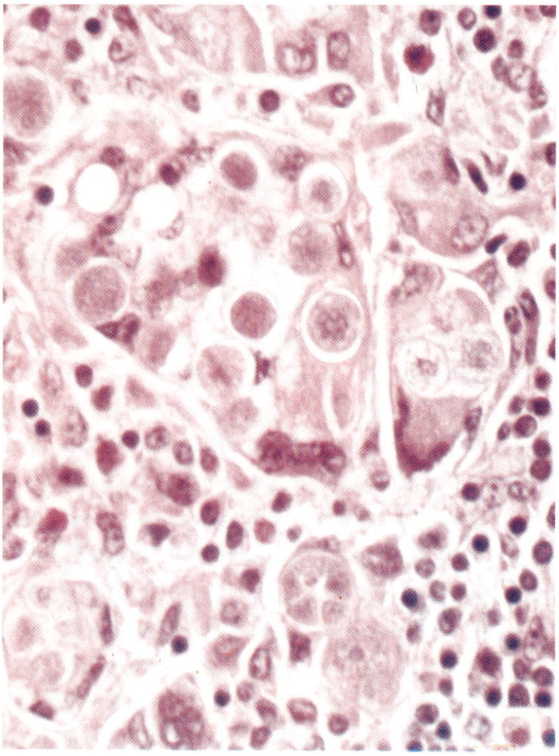

498 Chlorella sp. causing granulomatous lymphadenitis in a bovine. Single and endosporulating *Chlorella* cells are contained within huge giant cells. Again, note the similarity of these organisms to the *Prototheca* in **483** to **485**. At necropsy, the nodal lesion was distinctly green. (H&E, ×200)

499

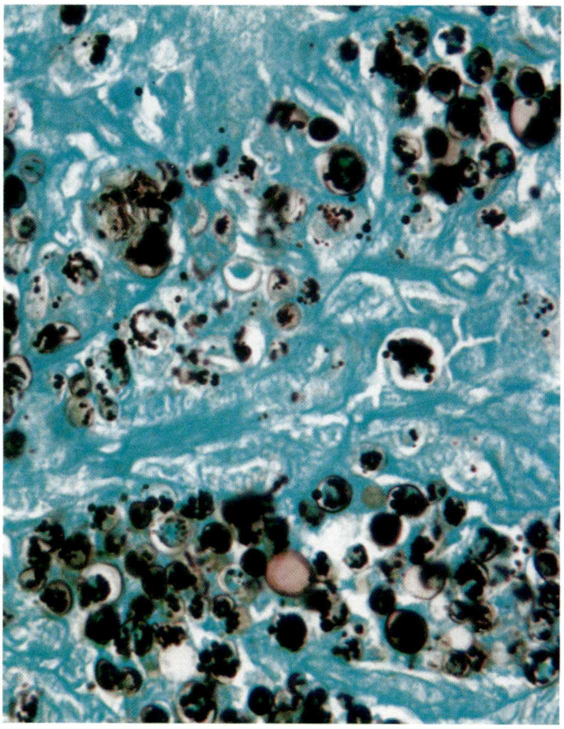

499 Chlorella sp. causing lymphadenitis in a sheep. The numerous algal cells are well demonstrated by GMS and contain prominent argyrophilic granules in their cytoplasm. Some cells are broken, and the cytoplasmic granules have been released. Such granules are rarely seen in protothecal cells. (GMS, ×200)

500

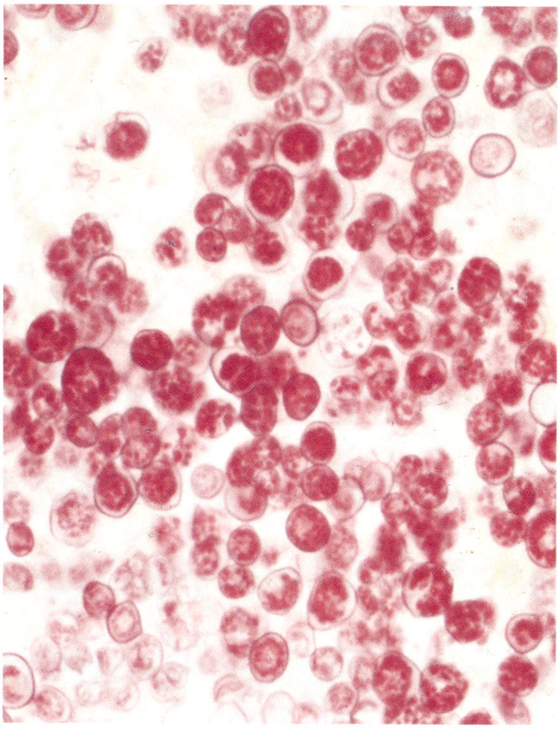

500 Chlorella sp. Replicate section of **499**. The densely packed green algal cells are well stained and show prominent GF-positive granules in their cytoplasm. (GF, ×200)

501

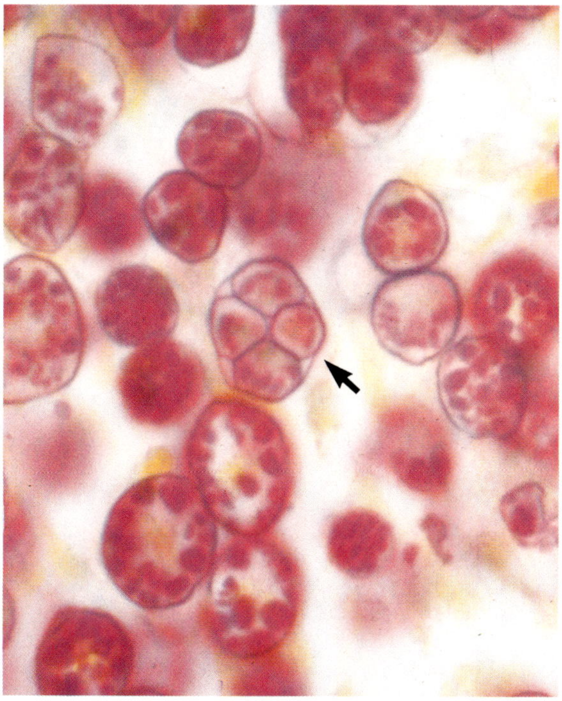

501 Chlorella sp. Higher magnification of **500** to show details of the *Chlorella* cells. As illustrated in the tissues infected with *Prototheca*, both single and endosporulating cells are present. However, in contrast to the protothecae, *Chlorella* cells have numerous, prominent GF-positive cytoplasmic granules. Such granules are even present in daughter cells (arrow). Compare these cells with those of the *Prototheca sp.* in **480** to **482** and **490**. (GF, ×500)

502

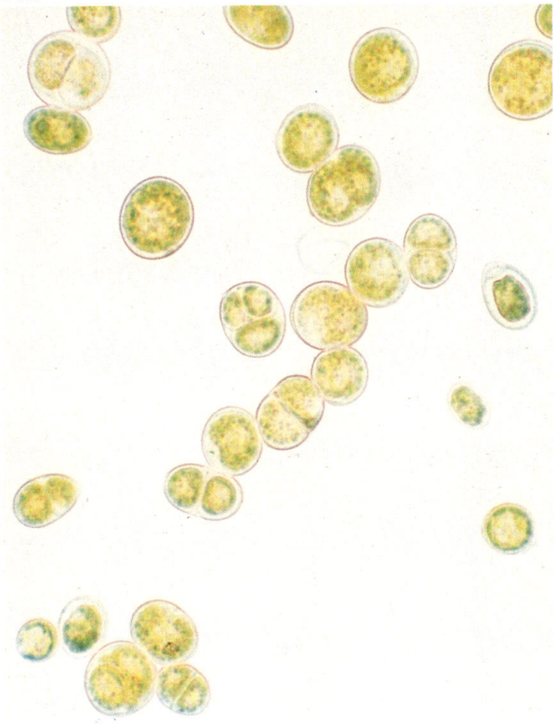

503

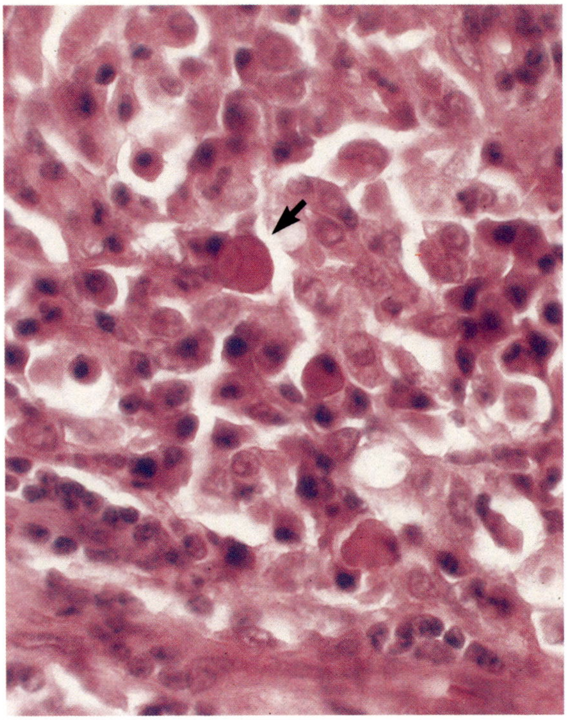

502 Chlorella sp. culture recovered from specimen shown in **498**. As seen in tissue, single and endosporulating organisms are evident. The green colour of the algal cells is due to their chlorophylls. *Chlorella* cells in tissue sections do not retain their colour because the chlorophylls are lost during processing. (×200)

503 Lymphadenitis in a human. A plasma cell containing Russell bodies (arrow) is sometimes confused with an endosporulating spherule of a *Prototheca sp*. Such structures can be readily distinguished from *Prototheca* cells by their failure to stain by GMS. They are, however, PAS and gram-positive. (H&E, ×200)

504

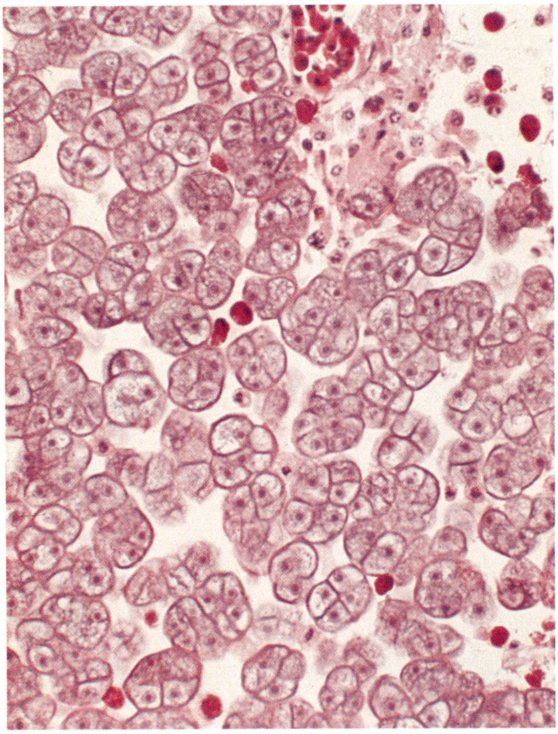

504 Disseminated mycotic infection in a snake. The infection was caused by a zygomycete of the order Entomophthorales. The organisms in tissue, as illustrated here, have been mistaken for *Prototheca* cells. This fungus reproduces by septation and not by endosporulation as do the protothecae. (H&E, ×100)

23 Rare infections

Text pages: 101–108

505

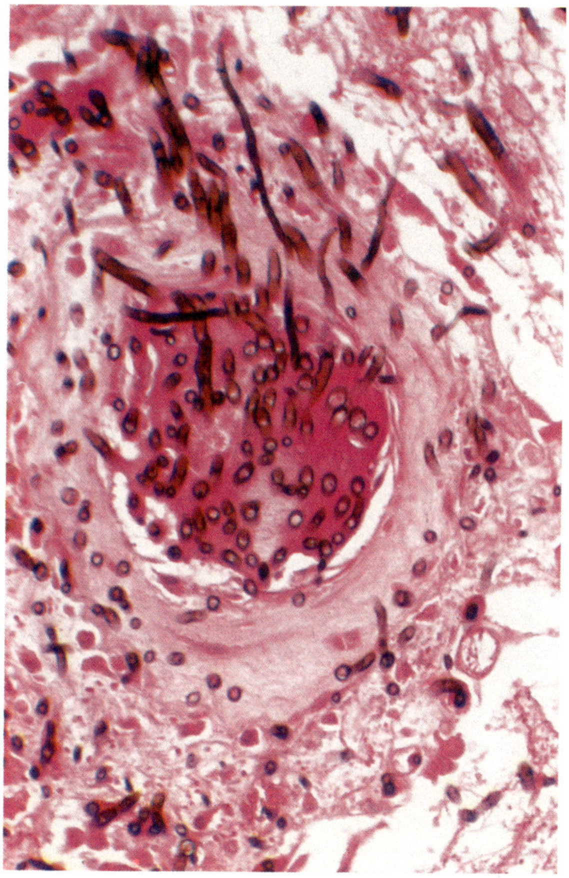

506

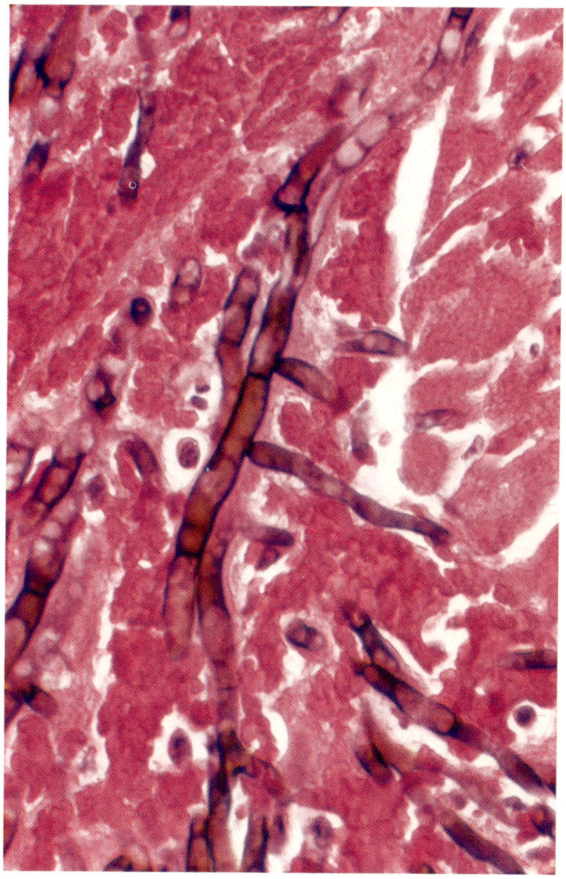

505 Fusarium moniliforme in myocardium of a human. Numerous branched hyphae are invading the wall of a blood vessel and are present within its lumen. Angioinvasion has been a common feature in the limited number of systemic *Fusarium sp.* infections that we have studied. (GMS–H&E, ×100)

506 Fusarium moniliforme Higher magnification of another field in **505** to show details of the mycelium. The GMS-positive hyphae resemble other branched, septate hyphomycetes in tissues, making cultural studies necessary for its identification. (GMS–H&E, ×200)

507

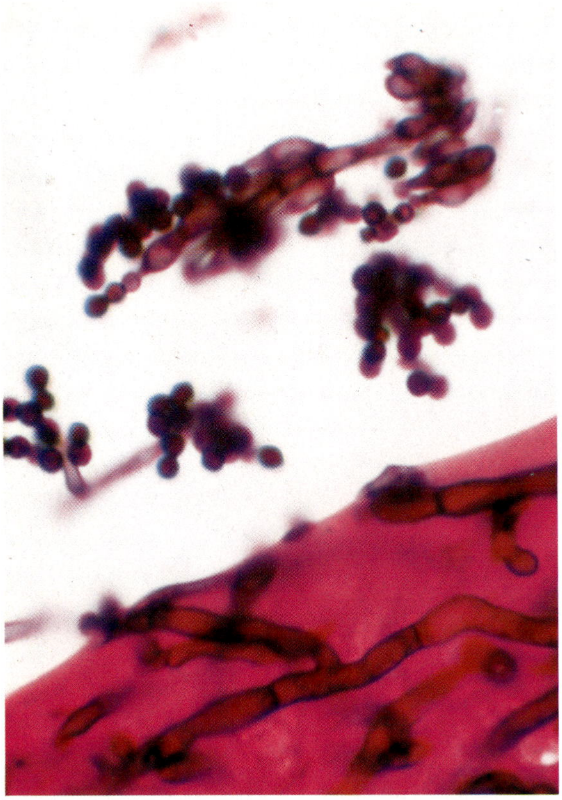

507 Paecilomyces sp. within a pulmonary cavity in a turtle. Mycelium is embedded in the wall of the cavity and projects into its lumen. Within the lumen, the fungus has sporulated as revealed by the presence of conidial chains attached to their conidiophores. (GMS–H&E, ×500)

508

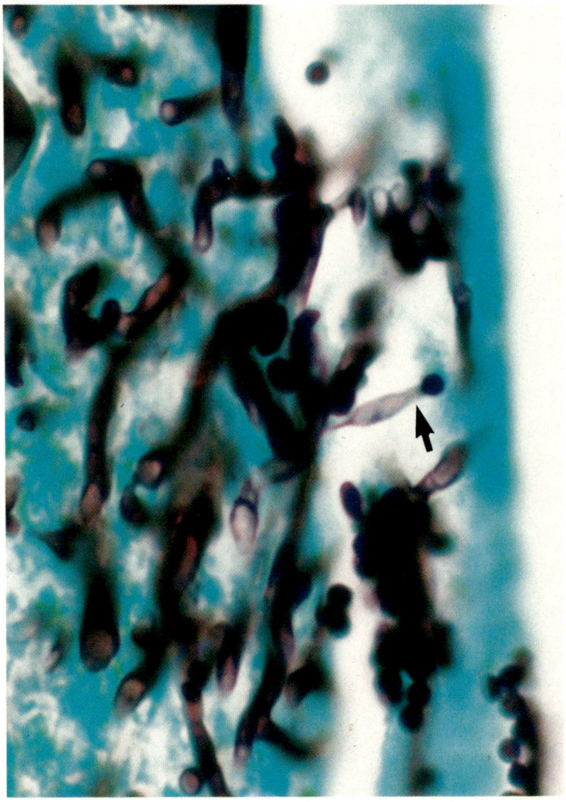

508 Paecilomyces sp. Replicate section of **507**. A single sterigma with a tapered end bearing a conidium is seen (arrow). Its distinctive morphology is characteristic of the genus *Paecilomyces*. (GMS, ×500)

509

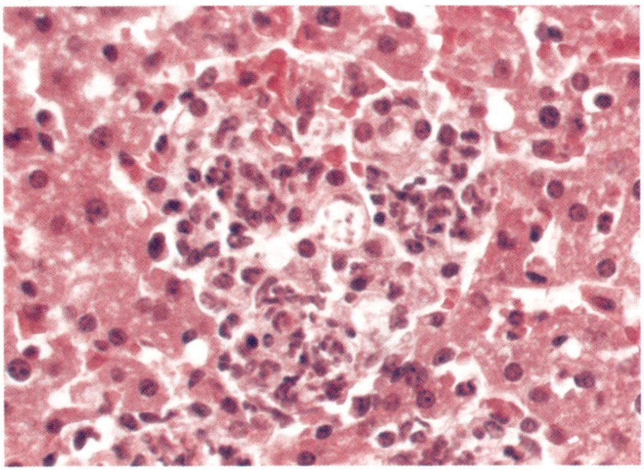

509 Penicillium marneffei Experimental infection in a mouse. A focus of neutrophils and histiocytes is seen in the liver. Although the lesion contains numerous fungal cells, they are not readily seen at this magnification. (H&E, ×200)

510

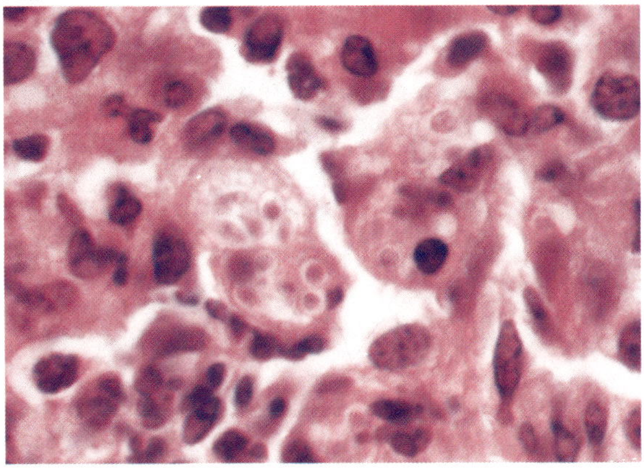

510 Penicillium marneffei Higher magnification of **509** to show fungal cells that resemble the tissue-form cells of *Histoplasma capsulatum* var. *capsulatum* within histiocytes. (H&E, ×500)

511

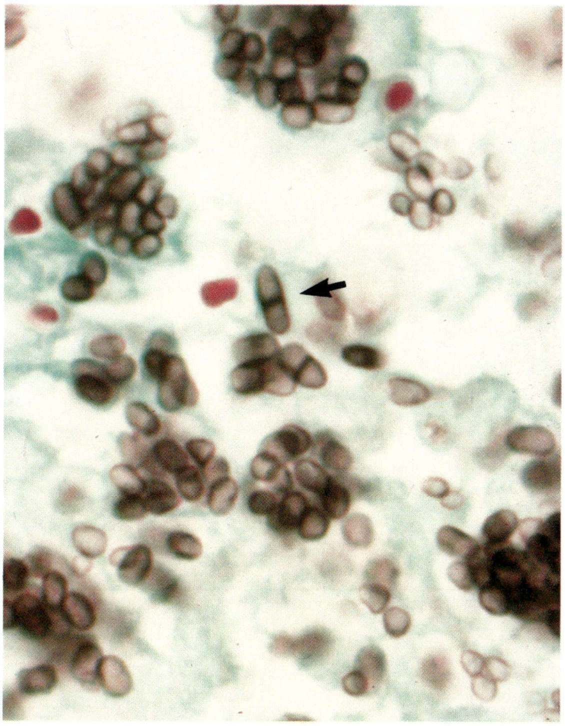

512

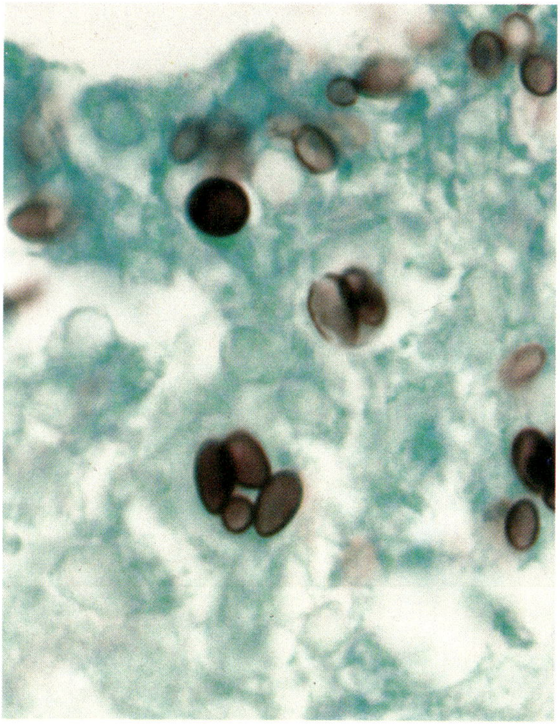

511 Penicillium marneffei Replicate section of **509** but stained by GMS to show clusters and individual cells in greater detail. In contrast to *Histoplasma capsulatum* var. *capsulatum* (see **513**) and other yeasts, the cells of *P. marneffei* do not bud. Some are elongated and septate (arrow). (GMS, ×500)

512 Penicillium marneffei in a splenic infarct of an immunosuppressed patient with Hodgkin's disease. Again, note the superficial resemblance to *Histoplasma capsulatum* var. *capsulatum* (see **513**). Specific identification requires cultural studies. (GMS, ×500)

513

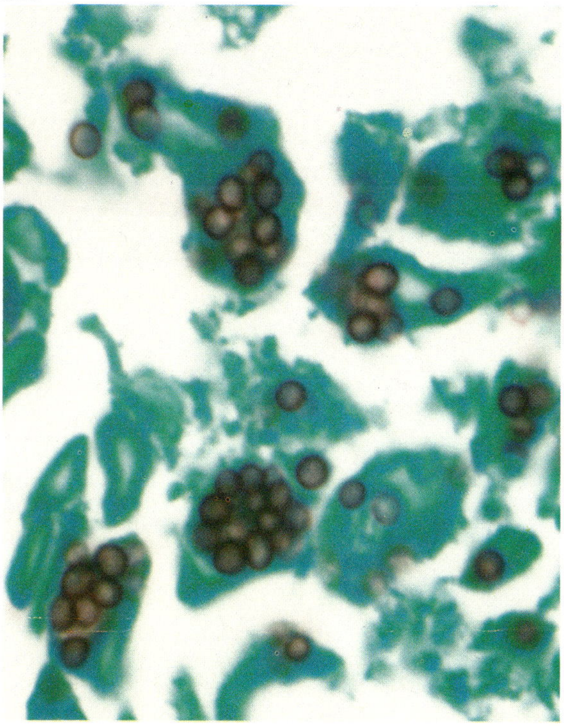

513 Histoplasma capsulatum var. **capsulatum** infection of the adrenal gland in a human. Although this fungus superficially resembles *Penicillium marneffei*, it is nonseptate and reproduces by budding. (GMS, ×500)

514

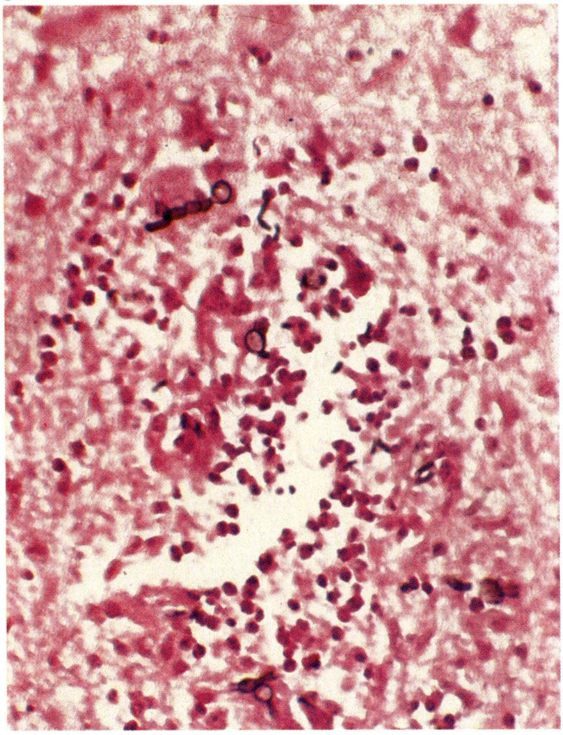

514 Petriellidium boydii causing encephalitis in an immunosuppressed patient with leukaemia. A cerebral abscess contains short hyphal fragments of the fungus. In systemic infections by this fungus, the mycelium is not organised into granules. (GMS–H&E, ×100)

515

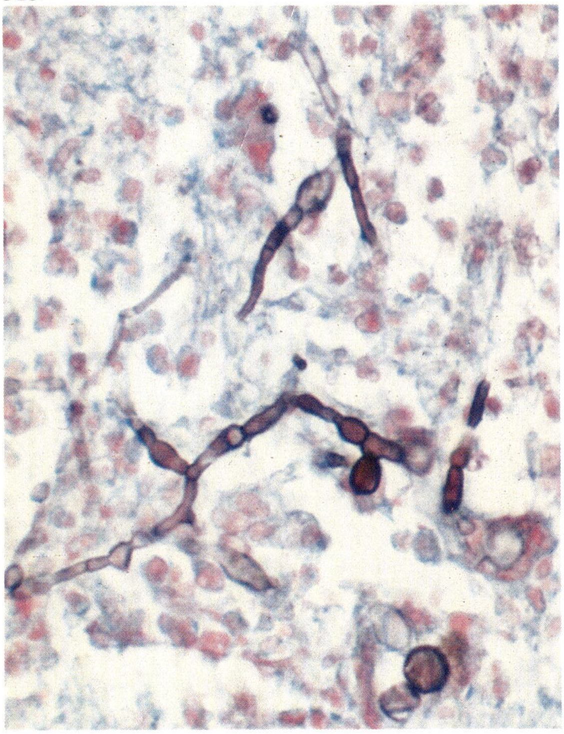

515 Petriellidium boydii Replicate section of **514** but stained by GMS and photographed at a higher magnification to show details of the fungus. Note the branched, septate hyphae with chlamydospores within the necrotic lesion. *P. boydii* mycelium may resemble that of the aspergilli in tissues. However, in our experience, this fungus can be differentiated from the aspergilli because its hyphae are narrower and do not as a rule show characteristic dichotomous branching. Nevertheless, definitive identification requires cultural or immunofluorescence studies. (GMS, ×200)

516

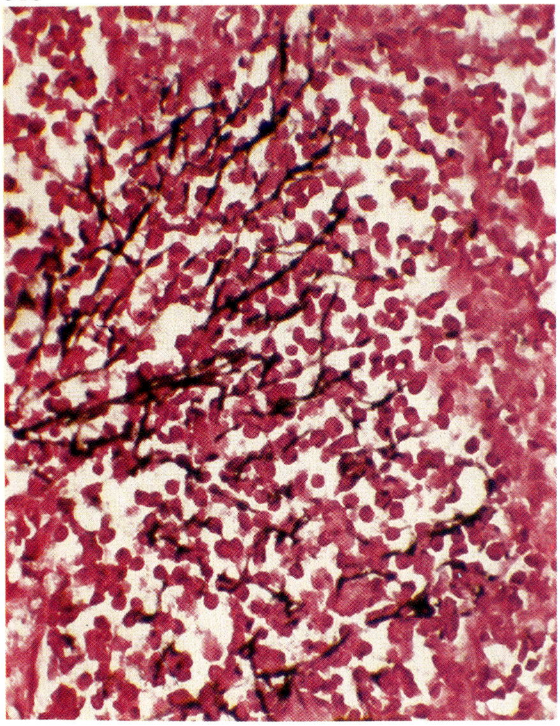

516 Petriellidium boydii causing pneumonia in a human. The numerous branched hyphae are embedded in an area of suppurative necrosis. Again, note that the hyphae are not organised into granules. (GMS–H&E, ×100)

517

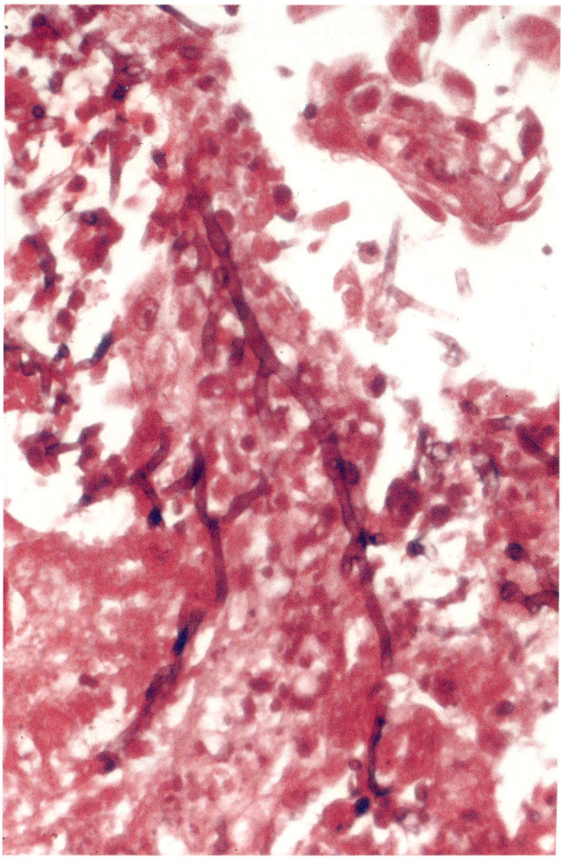

517 Petriellidium boydii causing mycotic placentitis in a bovine. There is necrosis of the chorionic villi and invasion by branched, septate hyphae. In cases of bovine mycotic abortion, definitive identification of the aetiologic agent requires cultural studies. (GMS–H&E, ×200)

518

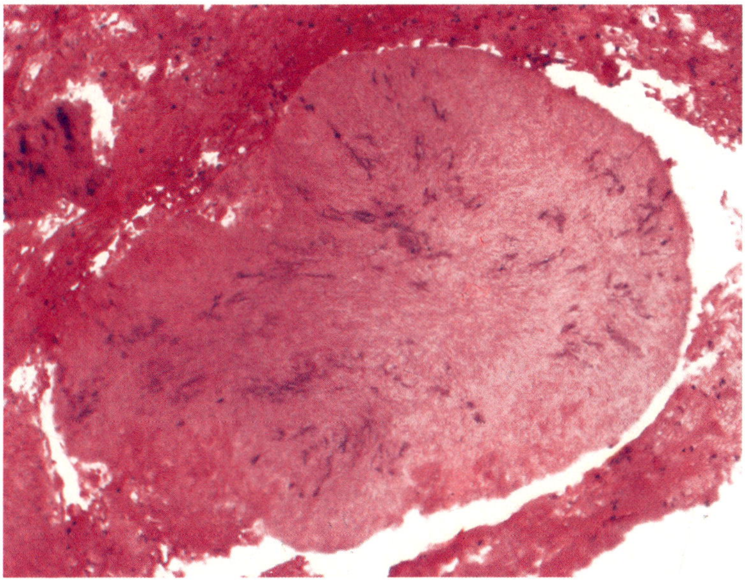

518 Petriellidium boydii causing chronic paranasal sinusitis in a human. In contrast to the three previous cases (**514** to **517**), the fungus is present in the form of a granule similar to those observed in a mycetoma (see Chapter 17). (H&E, ×50)

519

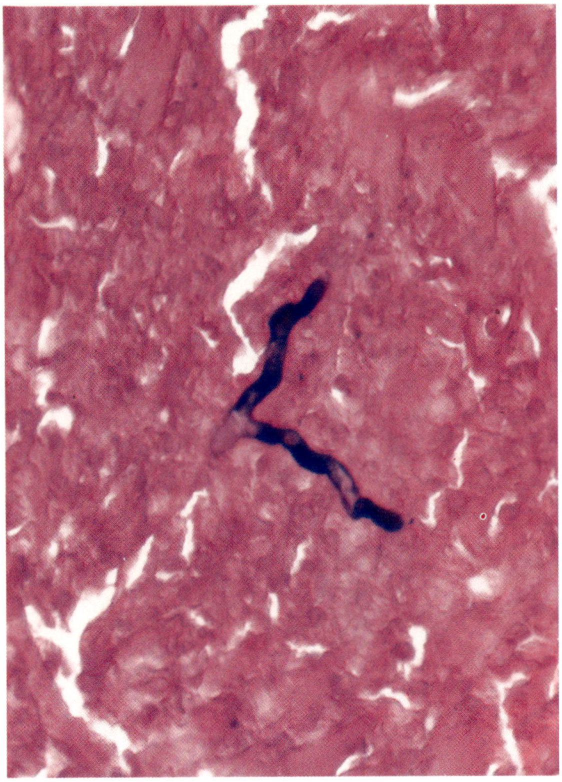

519 Pythium (Hyphomyces) destruens within a necrotic and suppurative lesion on the distal extremity of a horse. The branched hyphae embedded in the necrotic exudate are nonseptate. (GMS–H&E, ×200)

520

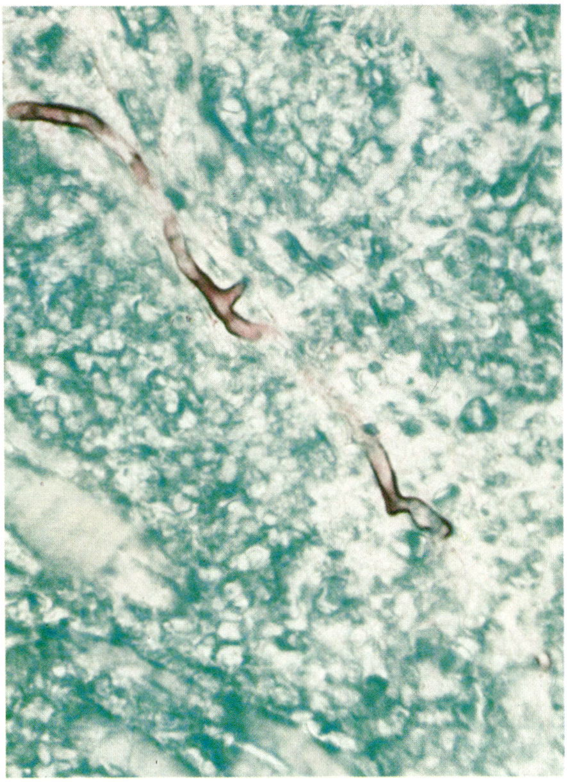

520 Pythium (Hyphomyces) destruens Replicate section of **519**. Again, note that the GMS-positive hyphae lack septations. (GMS, ×200)

521

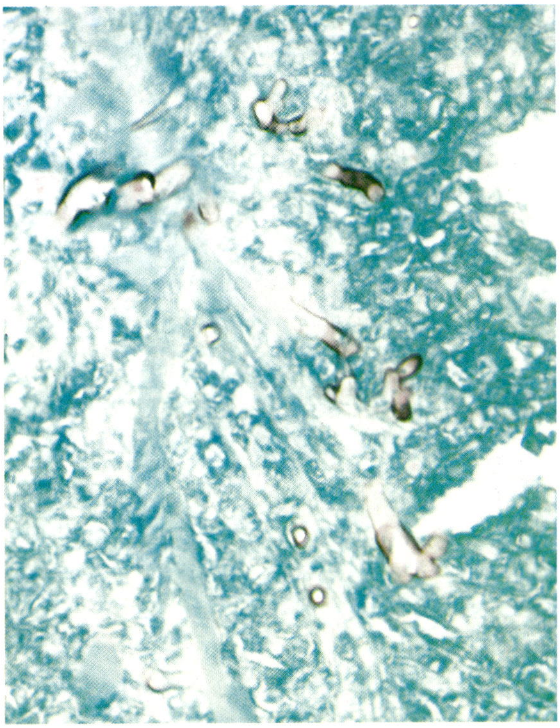

521 Pythium (Hyphomyces) destruens Another field in **520** showing short lengths of hyphae of variable width. The hyphae are unevenly stained – a frequent occurrence with *P. (Hyphomyces) destruens*. (GMS, ×200)

522

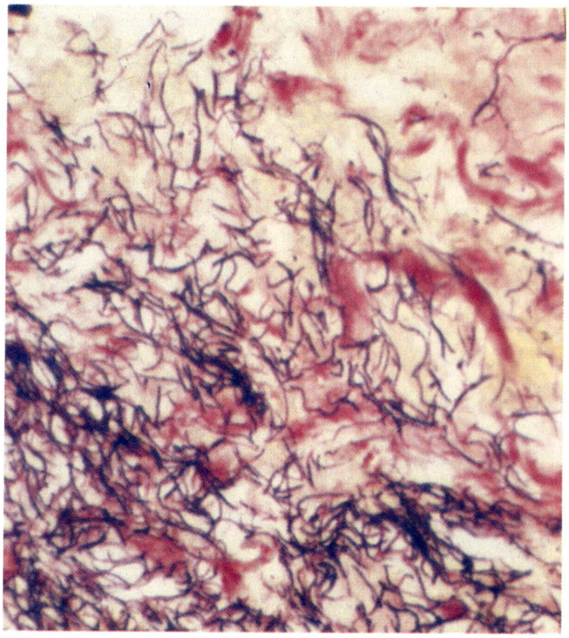

522 Streptomyces griseus within a circumscribed pulmonary lesion in a compromised human. Note the tangled mass of delicate, branched, gram-positive filaments. (B&B, ×200)

523

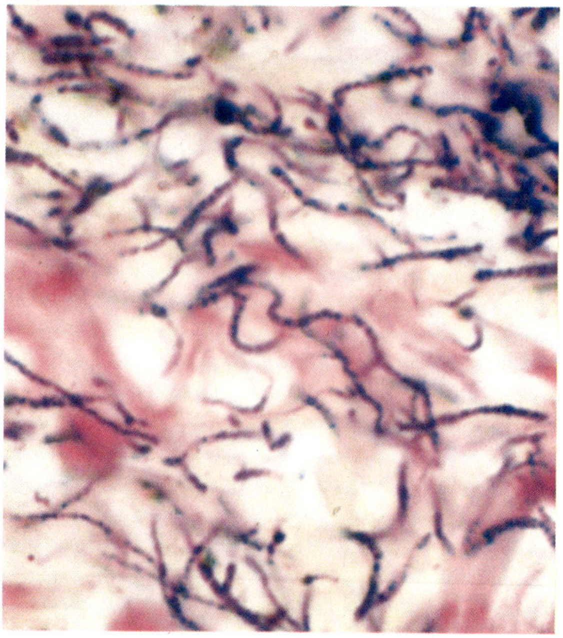

523 Streptomyces griseus Higher magnification of **522** showing the branched, delicate ($\leq$ 1.0 μm) filaments. Variable staining by the tissue Gram procedures gives the filaments a beaded appearance. The close morphologic resemblance of *S. griseus* to other actinomycetes makes cultural studies necessary. (B&B, ×500)

524

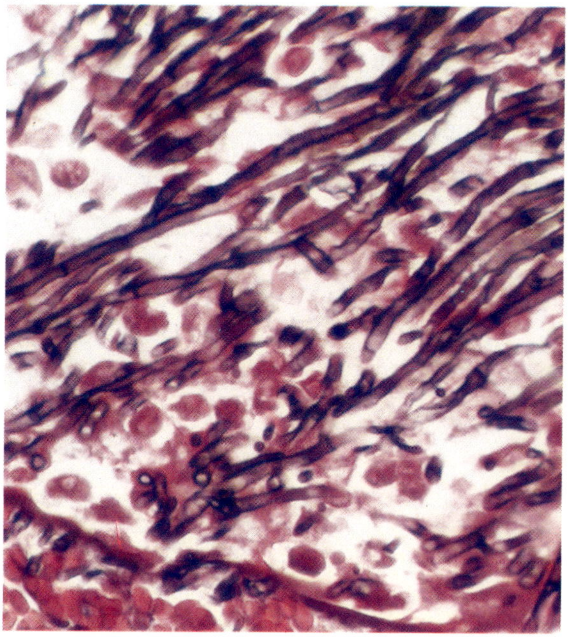

524 Trichosporon capitatum causing fibrinopurulent pericarditis in a compromised human. Branched, septate hyphae are embedded in the exudate. (GMS–H&E, ×200)

525

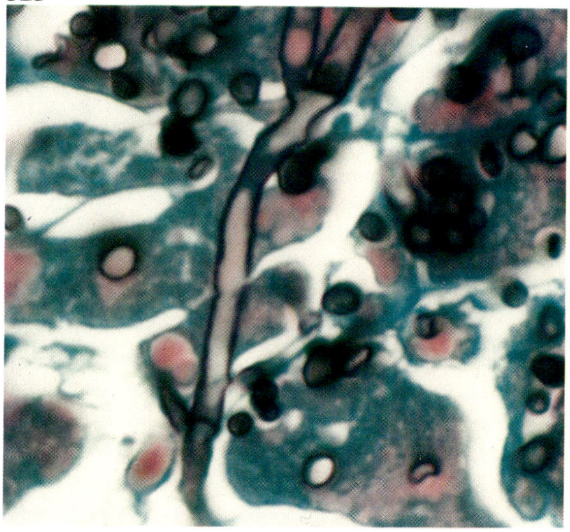

525 Trichosporon capitatum Replicate section of **524**. A branched, septate hypha and numerous blastospores, some of which are budding, have invaded the myocardium. There is little or no inflammation. Although arthrospores are formed by this fungus, they are not seen in this field. Cultural studies are required for a definitive identification of this agent. (GMS, ×500)

24 Rhinosporidiosis

Text pages: 109–111

526

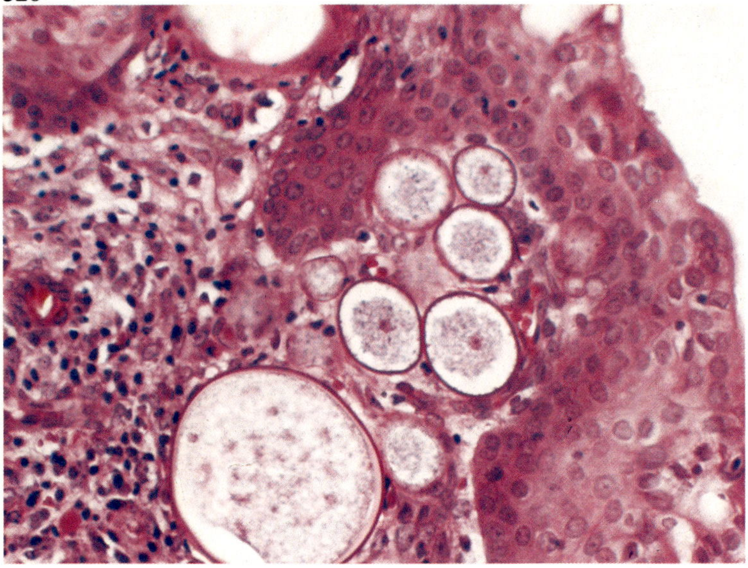

526 Rhinosporidiosis in a human. The lesion was in the form of a nasal polyp. Note epithelial hyperplasia and infiltration of the underlying stroma by mononuclear inflammatory cells. Immature sporangia of *Rhinosporidium seeberi*, each containing an amorphous basophilic cytoplasm and a central nucleus, are well demonstrated. (H&E, ×100)

527

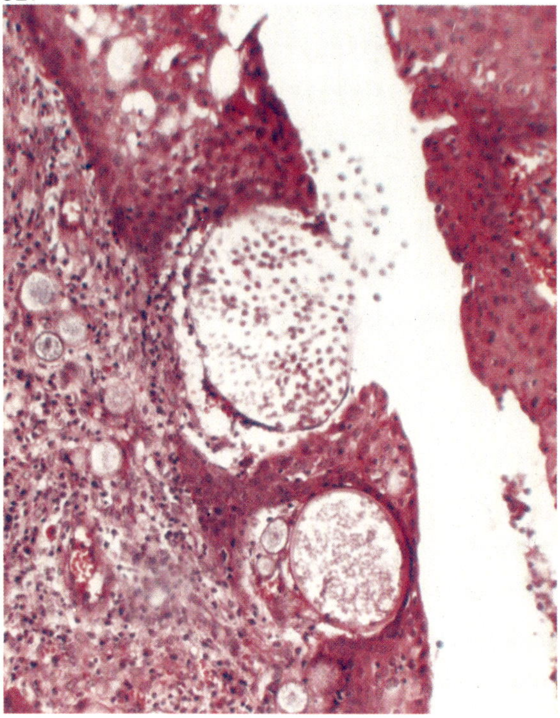

528

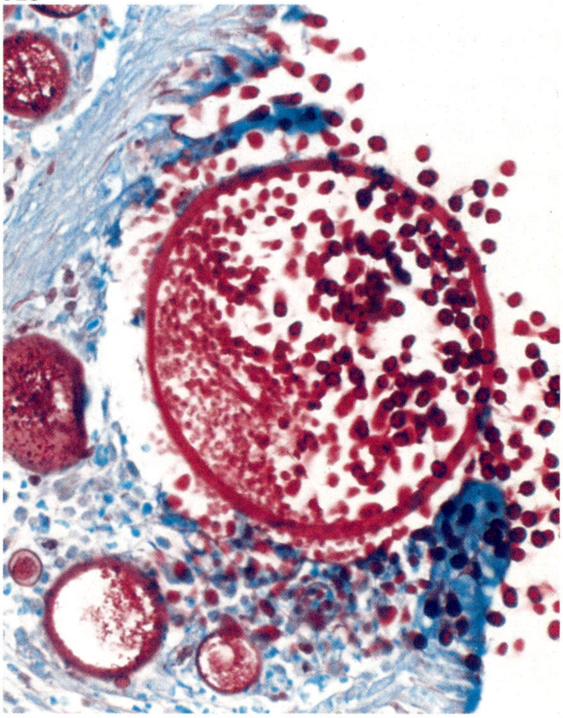

527 Rhinosporidium seeberi Another field in **526** showing epithelial hyperplasia and prominent sporangia. One large intraepithelial sporangium is discharging its spores into a crypt of the polyp. (H&E, ×50)

528 Rhinosporidium seeberi Replicate section of **526**. Sporangia in various stages of development and free spores are well-stained by PAS. A large mature intraepithelial sporangium is seen in the centre. (PAS, ×100)

529

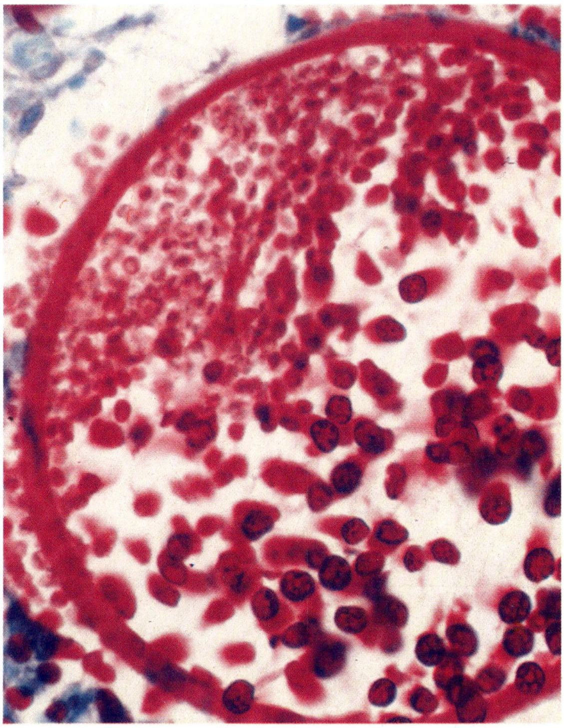

529 Rhinosporidium seeberi Higher magnification of **528** to show a mature sporangium in greater detail. Immature spores are seen at one pole, whereas mature spores fill the centre and aggregate at the opposite pole of the sporangium. (PAS, ×200)

530

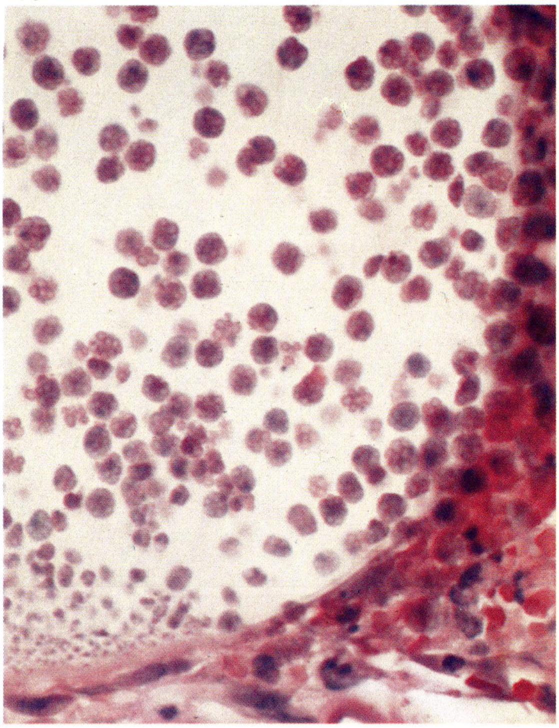

530 Rhinosporidium seeberi Another field in **526** showing progressive development of spores from the periphery to the centre of a mature sporangium. (H&E, ×200)

531

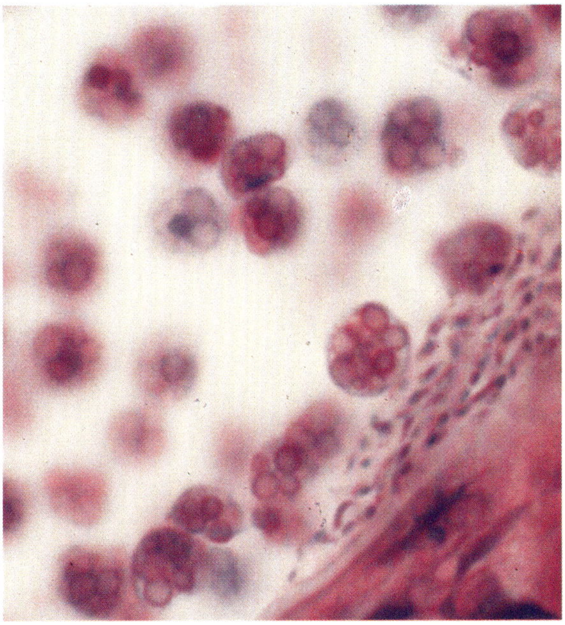

531 Rhinosporidium seeberi Higher magnification of **530** to show the small, eosinophilic globular bodies within the mature spores. A zone of flattened sporogenous cells is present at the periphery. (H&E, ×500)

532

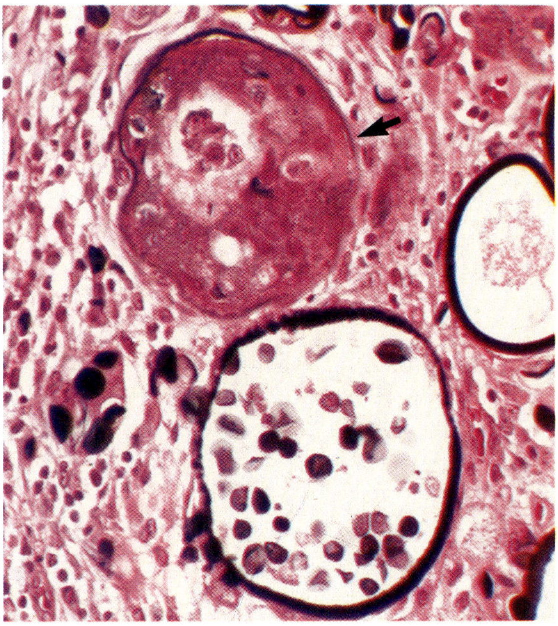

532 Rhinosporidium seeberi causing rhinosporidiosis in another human. The stroma of the nasal polyp contains epithelioid and multinucleated giant cells that intimately surround sporangia. Inflammatory cells completely fill the cavity of an empty sporangium from which the spores have been released (arrow). (GMS–H&E, ×100)

533

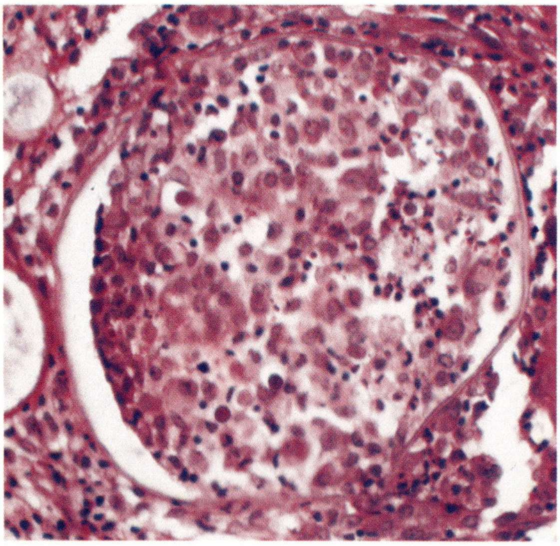

533 Rhinosporidium seeberi Another area in **526** showing a large sporangium embedded in granulation tissue containing mononuclear inflammatory cells. The sporangium has discharged its spores through a break in its wall, and mixed inflammatory cells have now entered through the break to fill its interior. (H&E, ×100)

534

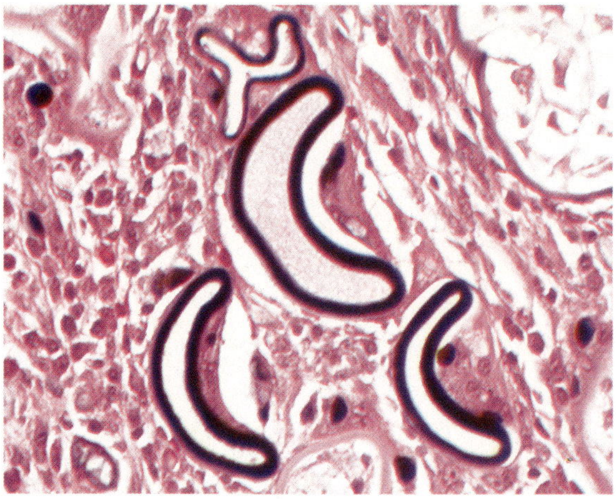

534 Rhinosporidium seeberi Another area in **532** showing several empty and collapsed sporangia embedded in the fibrogranulomatous stroma of the nasal polyp. (GMS–H&E, ×100)

535

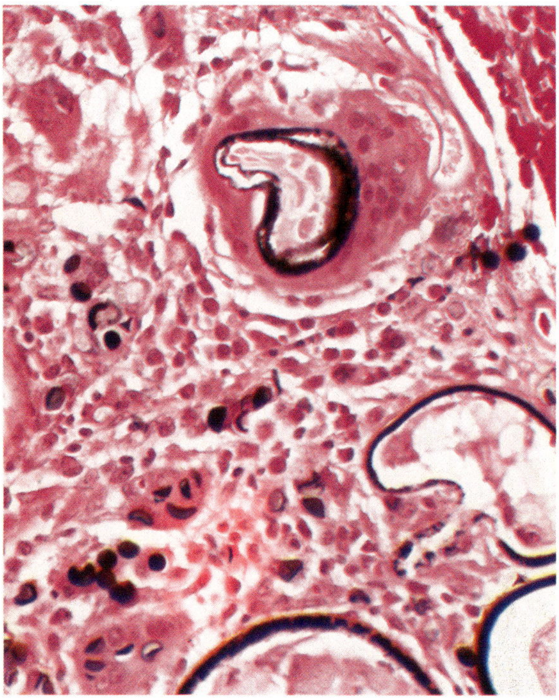

535 Rhinosporidium seeberi A partially collapsed sporangium is seen within a giant cell. Several strongly GMS-positive spores within phagocytes and extracellularly in the stroma of the nasal polyp in **532** are also present. (GMS–H&E, ×100)

536

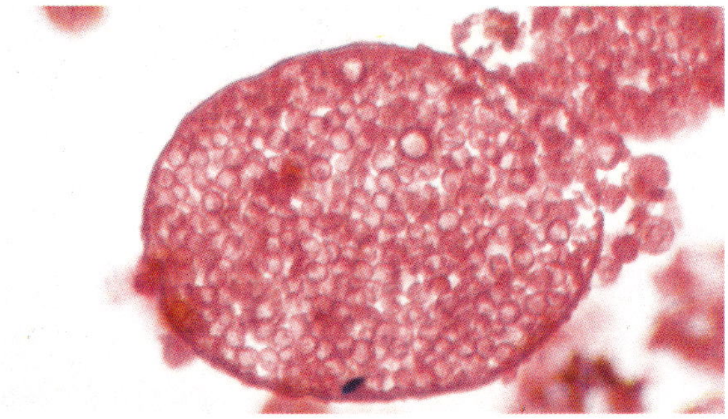

536 Myospherulosis Cyst-like lesion in a surgically treated paranasal sinus of a human. Large spherical structures containing 'endobodies' in the phenomenon termed 'myospherulosis' are present within the cyst-like cavity. The pseudosac containing altered erythrocytes (the 'endobodies') superficially resembles a mature spherule of *Rhinosporidium seeberi* or *Coccidioides immitis*. (H&E, ×200)

537

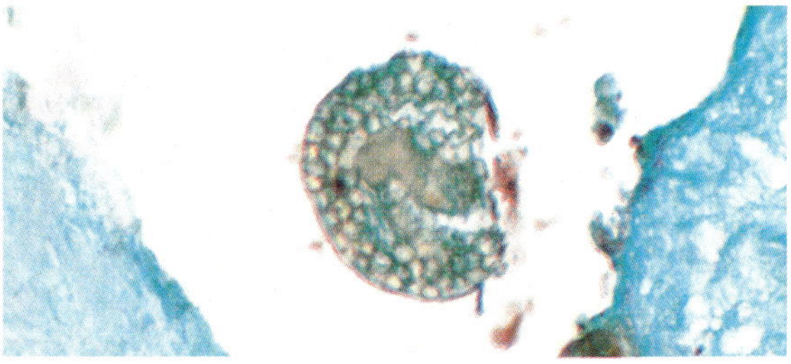

537 Myospherulosis Replicate section of **536**. Note that the pseudosac and the erythrocytes it contains ('endobodies') are not stained by GMS. This failure to stain, coupled with the fact that 'endobodies' are of relatively uniform size, makes these structures readily distinguishable from the sporangia of *R. seeberi*. (GMS, ×100)

25 Sporotrichosis

Text pages: 112–115

538

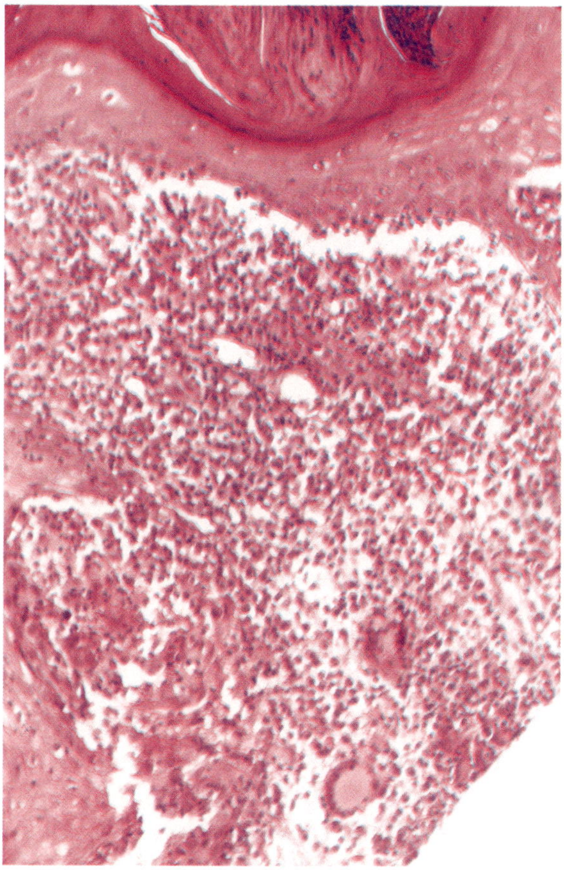

539

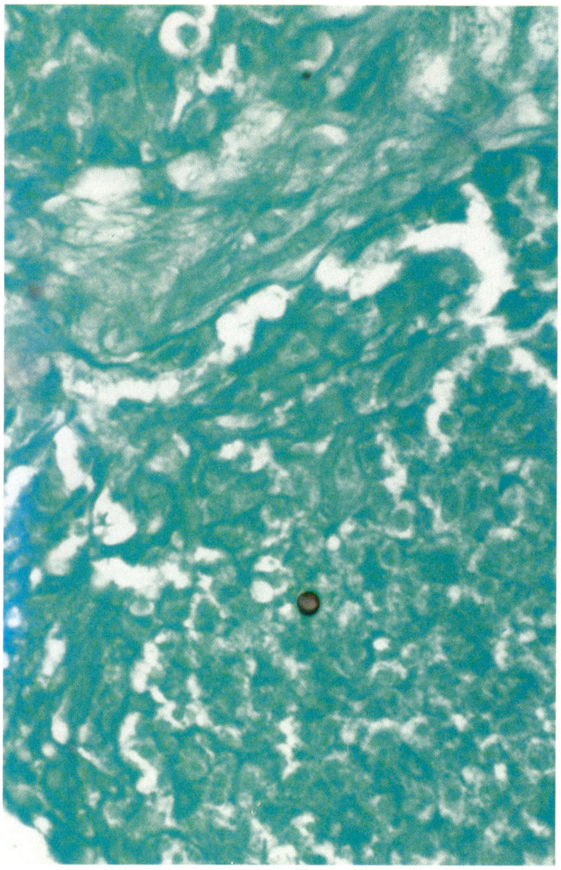

538 Cutaneous sporotrichosis in a human. There is hyperplasia of the epidermis and a mixed purulent and granulomatous inflammatory reaction in the dermis. (GMS–H&E, ×50)

539 Sporothrix schenckii Replicate section of **538** stained by GMS showing a single round cell of *S. schenckii* within the pyogranulomatous lesion in the papillary dermis. Generally, only a few fungal cells are found in spontaneous infections of the skin in humans, and special stains are needed to demonstrate them. (GMS, ×200)

540

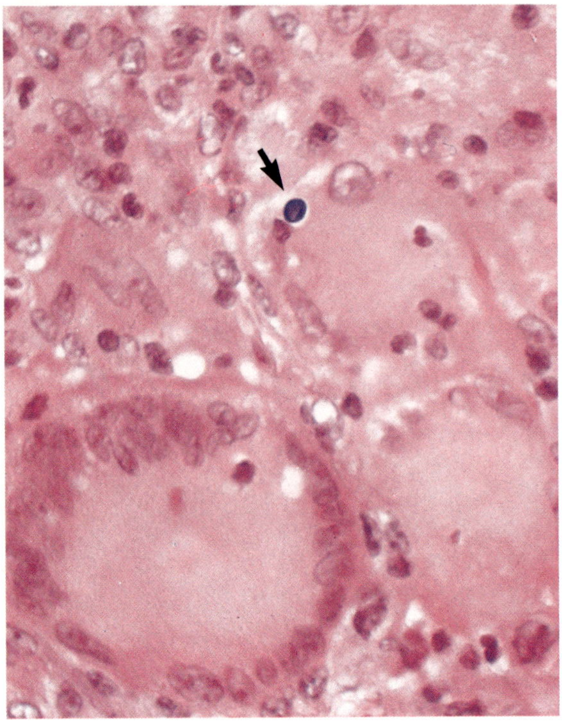

541

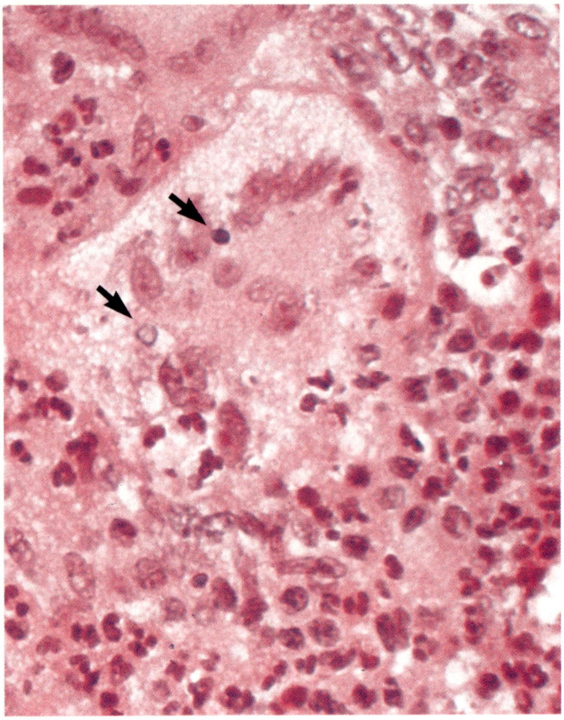

540 Sporothrix schenckii Higher magnification of dermal lesion seen in **538**. Within a granuloma, three large giant cells are seen, one of which contains a single GMS-positive round cell (arrow). (GMS–H&E, ×200)

541 Sporothrix schenckii Another field in **538** showing a dermal microabscess rimmed by epithelioid and multinucleated giant cells. Two faintly stained cells of *S. schenckii* are seen within a giant cell (arrows). (GMS–H&E, ×200)

542

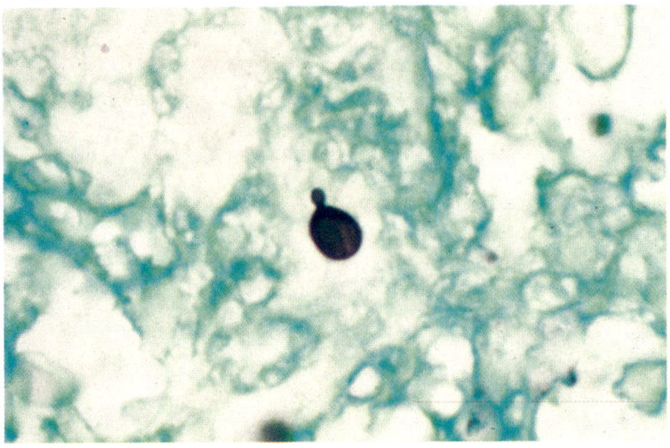

542 Sporothrix schenckii Another case of cutaneous sporotrichosis in a human. A single large budding cell is contained within a giant cell in the dermis. (GMS, ×500)

543 Sporothrix schenckii Pyogranulomatous dermatitis in another patient with cutaneous sporotrichosis. Several cells of *S. schenckii* one of which shows multiple budding, are seen in the upper dermis. The overlying epidermis is acanthotic but intact. (GMS, ×200)

543

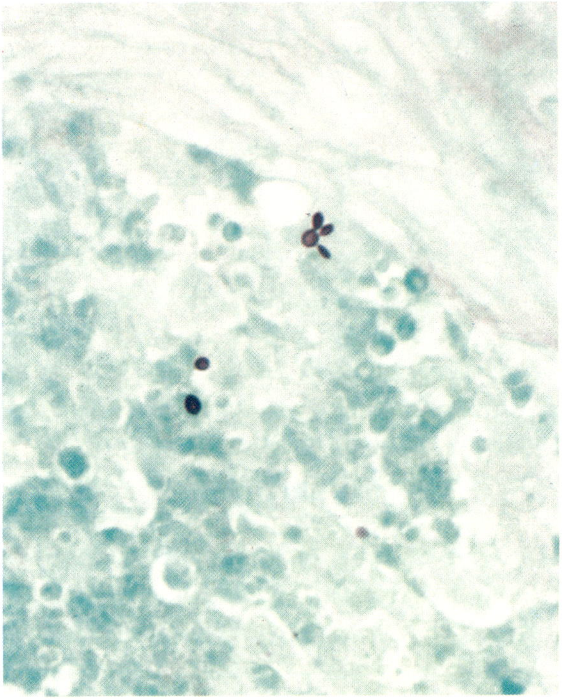

544

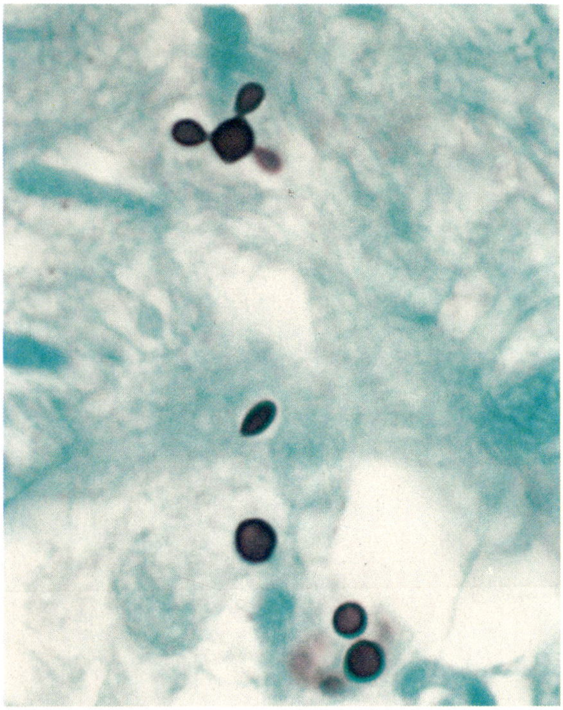

545

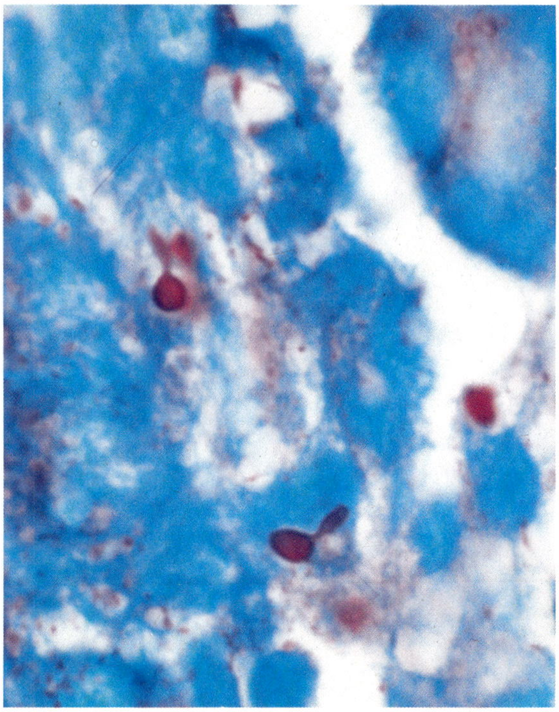

544 Sporothrix schenckii Another field in **543** showing details of a multiple budding cell as well as several nearby single cells. Note the narrow basal attachments of the buds to the parent cell. Unlike most lesions of cutaneous sporotrichosis, this lesion contained a relatively large number of fungal cells. (GMS, ×500)

545 Sporothrix schenckii Cutaneous sporotrichosis in another human. Two PAS-positive *S. schenckii* cells are clearly visible. One cell bears an elongated bud. (PAS, ×500)

546

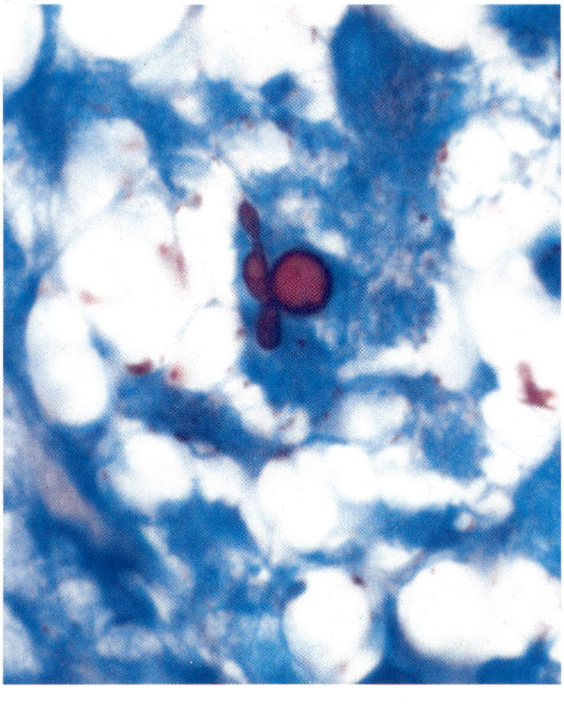

546 Sporothrix schenckii Another field in **545** to illustrate the pleomorphism of *S. schenckii* in tissue. Unusual are the single large cell and the chain of three cells. (PAS, ×500)

547

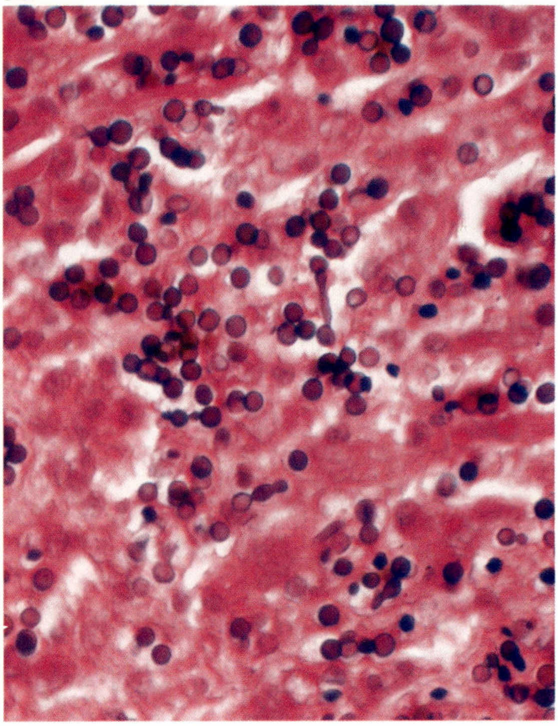

548

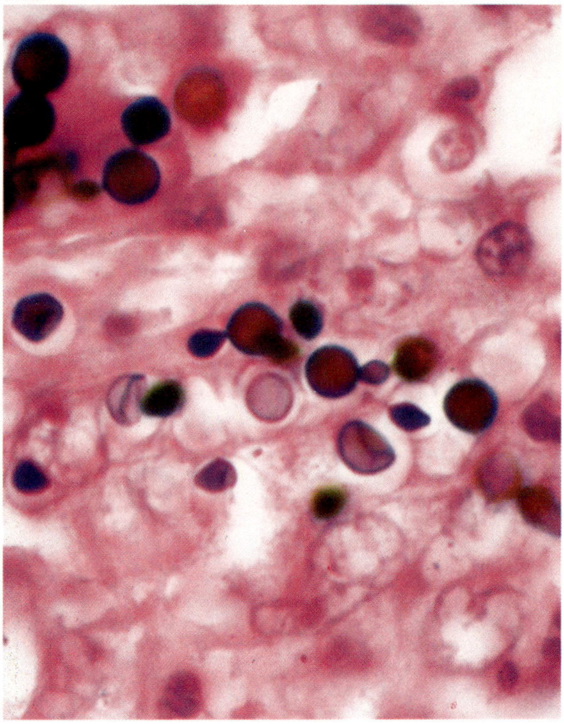

547 Sporothrix schenckii causing focal granulomatous pneumonitis in a human. There are large numbers of yeast cells in this lesion. These cells may be mistaken for other small yeasts. (GMS–H&E, ×200)

548 Sporothrix schenckii Higher magnification of **547** to show details of the cells in the granulomatous lesion. Single and budding round yeast cells are seen. Two cup-shaped cells are also present. (GMS–H&E, ×500)

549

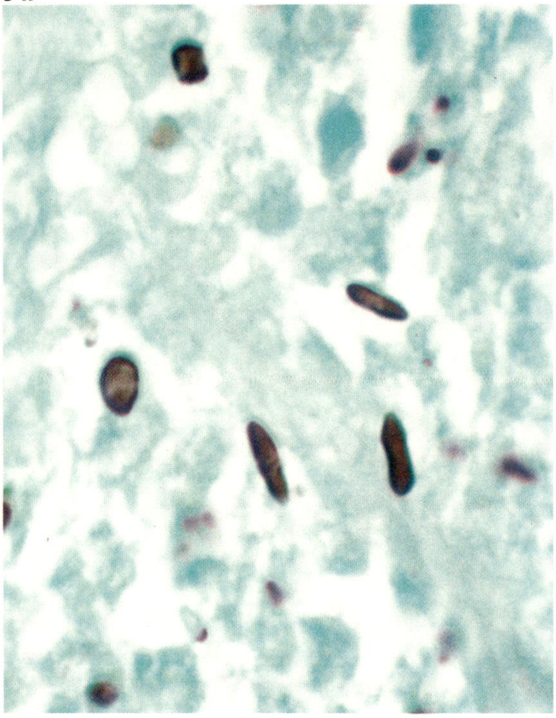

550

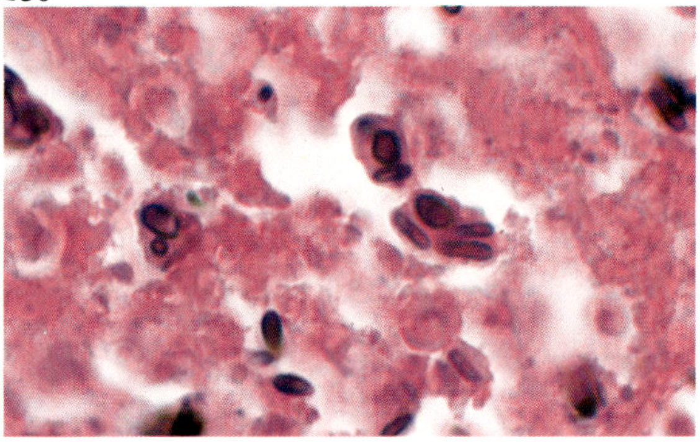

549 Sporothrix schenckii Pulmonary sporotrichosis in another human. In this granuloma, most of the cells are 'cigar'-shaped. (GMS, ×500)

550 Sporothrix schenckii causing sporotrichosis of the human eye. Elongated ('cigar'-shaped), elliptical, and round forms of *S. schenckii* are seen within phagocytes, again illustrating the pleomorphism of this fungus in tissue. When typical 'cigar' forms are seen, sporotrichosis should be suspected. (GMS–H&E, ×500)

551

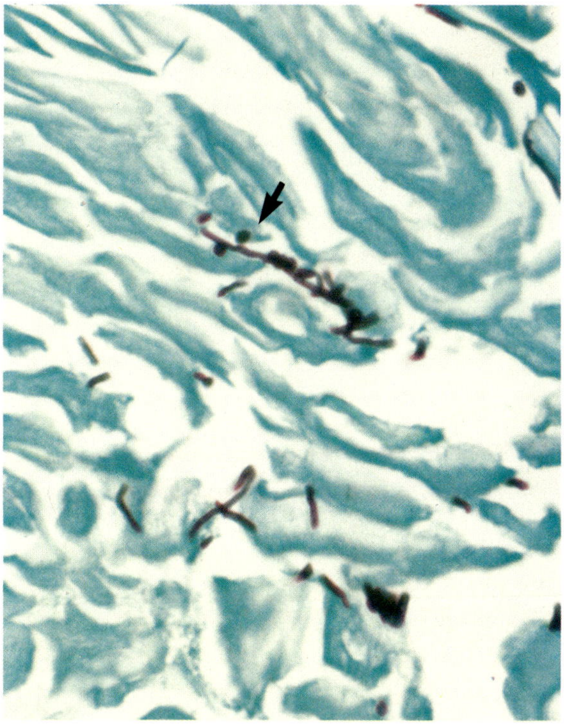

552

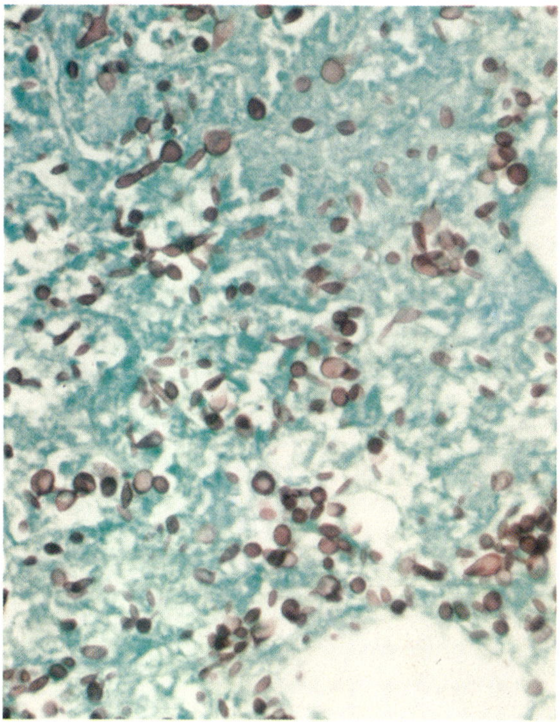

551 Sporotrichosis of the human skin. Note the presence of hyphae bearing a few conidia (arrow) in the thickened keratin layer; budding yeast cells were found in abscesses within the epidermis and deeper layers of the skin in this patient. Mycelial-form elements of *Sporothrix schenckii* are occasionally observed in tissue. (GMS, ×100)

552 Experimental sporotrichosis of a mouse testis. Large numbers of *Sporothrix schenckii* cells are generally present in these lesions, and the fungal cells vary considerably in size and shape. Animal inoculations are sometimes used to identify this fungus. (GMS, ×200)

553

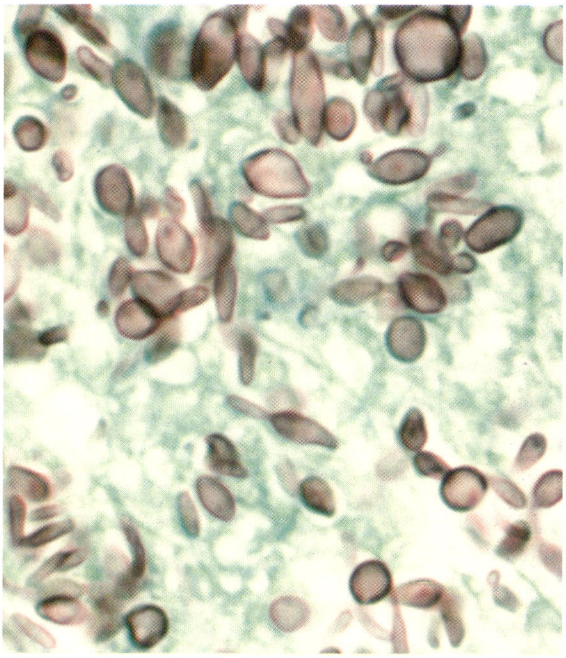

553 Sporothrix schenckii Higher magnification of **552** to show the extreme pleomorphism of *S. schenckii* in tissue. The forms in this experimental lesion are similar to those seen in some human lesions. (GMS, ×500)

554

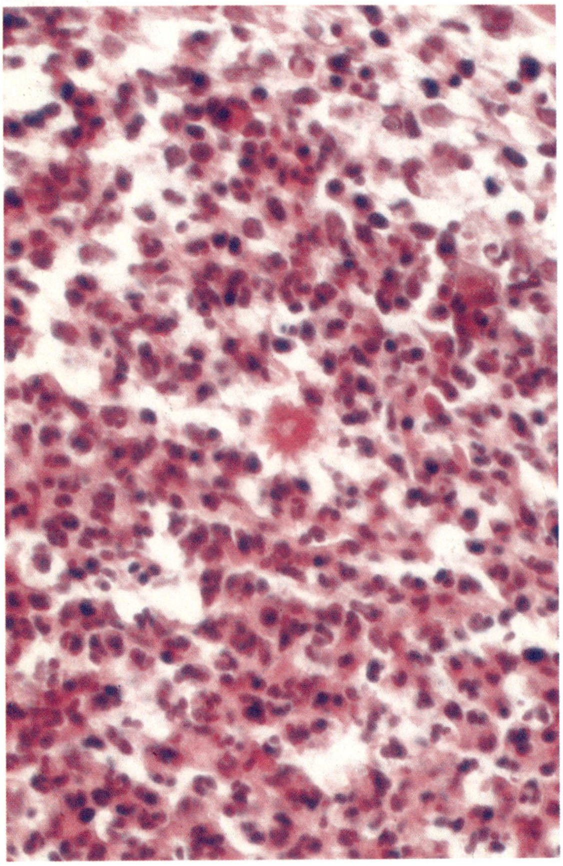

555

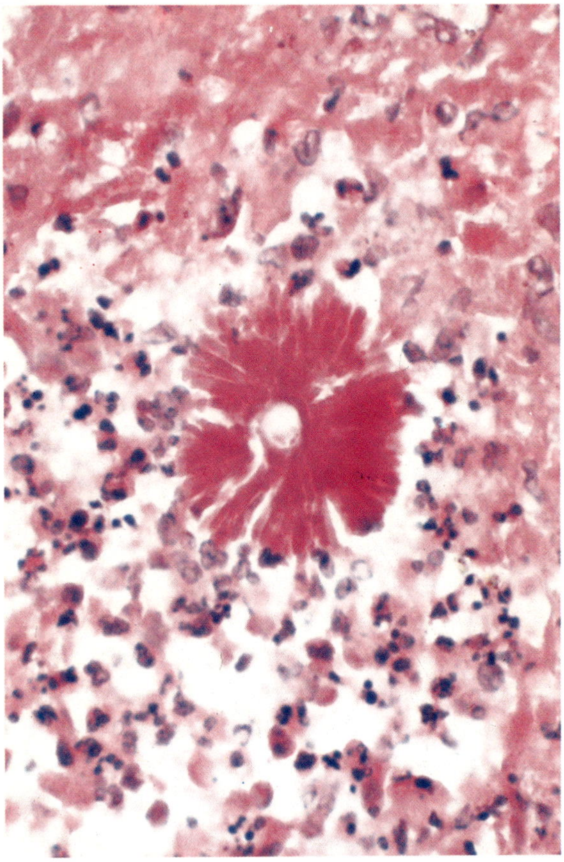

554 · **Cutaneous sporotrichosis** in a human. An asteroid body is seen in the centre of a dermal abscess. (H&E, ×100)

555 Sporothrix schenckii Higher magnification to show details of an asteroid body in another human with cutaneous sporotrichosis. The poorly stained cell in the centre and its radial corona of eosinophilic Splendore–Hoeppli material are embedded in a dermal micro-abscess that is rimmed by epithelioid cells. Asteroid bodies are not always found in sporotrichosis and, when present, are not pathognomonic for this disease – they are merely suggestive. (H&E, ×200)

556

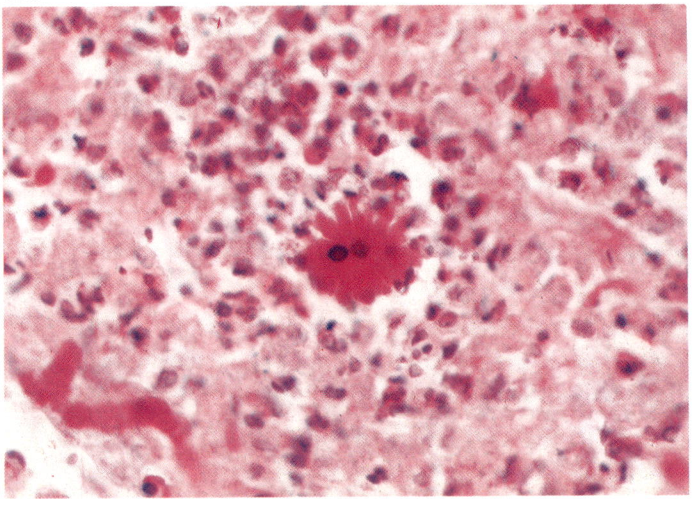

556 Sporothrix schenckii causing granulomatous pneumonitis in a human. Two GMS-positive fungal cells are seen in an asteroid body that is embedded in a microabscess in the centre of an epithelioid cell granuloma. (GMS–H&E, ×200)

557

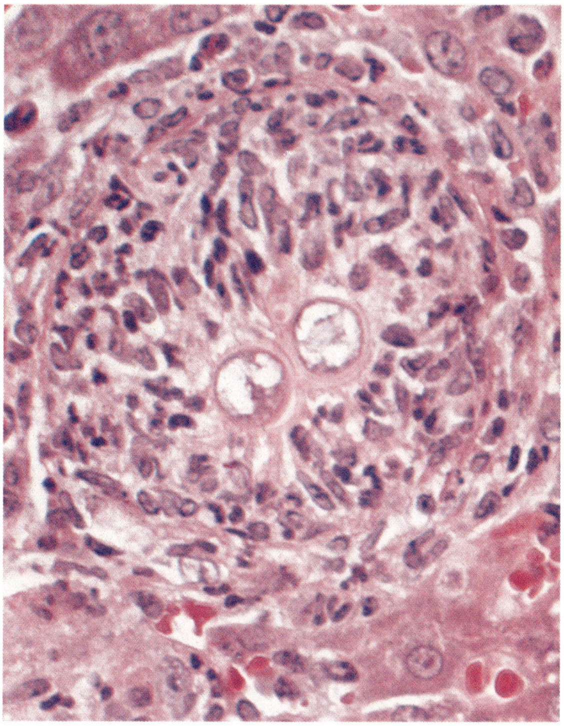

558

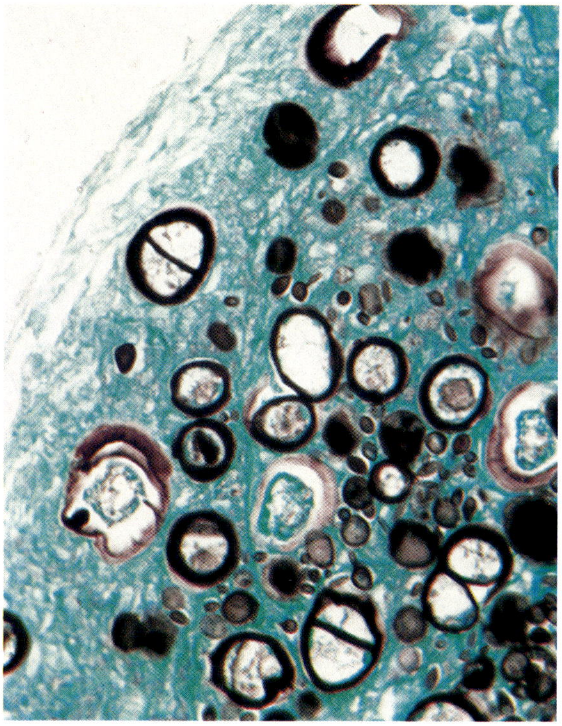

557 Sporothrix schenckii var. **luriei** Experimental infection in a mouse. Two large fungal cells are seen in the centre of a small granuloma in the liver. With this routine stain, the cells are readily visible. (H&E, ×200)

558 Sporothrix schenckii var. **luriei** Replicate section of **557** but stained by GMS to demonstrate the large and small forms which are produced in tissue. Note reproduction of small cells by budding and of large cells by septation. (GMS, ×166)

559

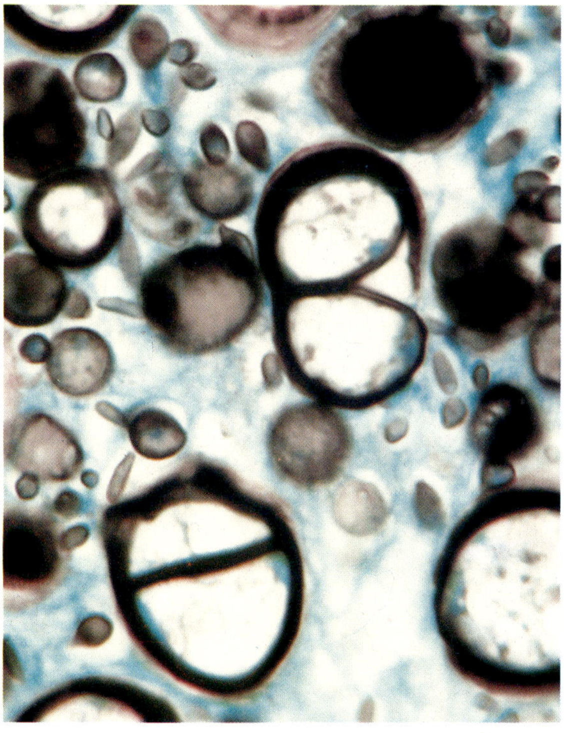

559 Sporothrix schenckii var. **luriei** Higher magnification of **558**. The small cells are morphologically similar to those of the classical variety of this fungus. The large cells, however, are distinct. They reproduce by fission, and daughter cells separate by dissolution of the parent cell wall, giving the appearance of a pair of eyeglasses. Large forms may also reproduce by budding, but this is not shown in this photomicrograph. (GMS, ×375)

26 Superficial and cutaneous mycoses

Text pages: 116–121

560

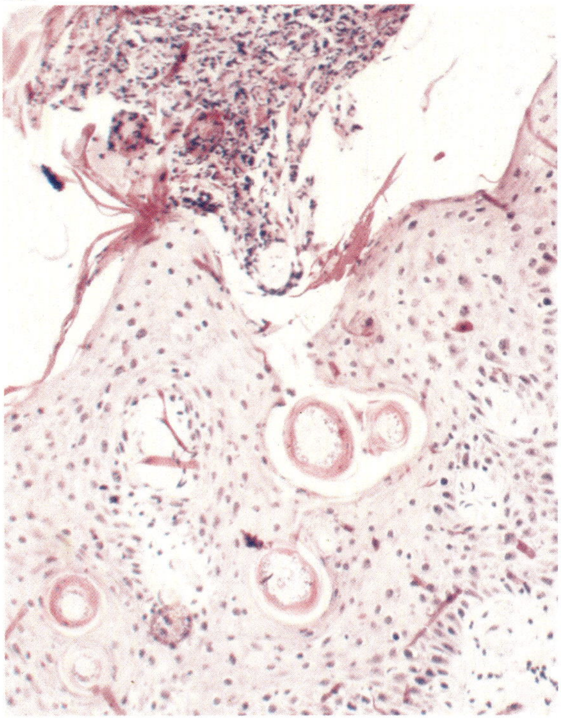

561

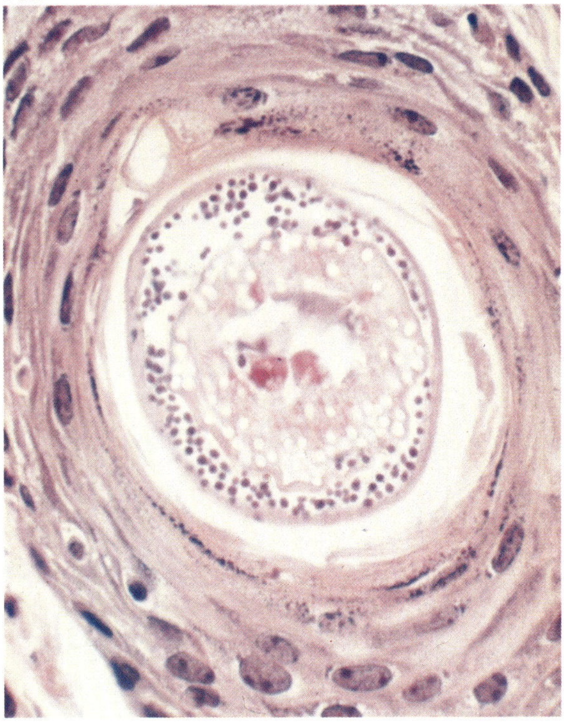

562

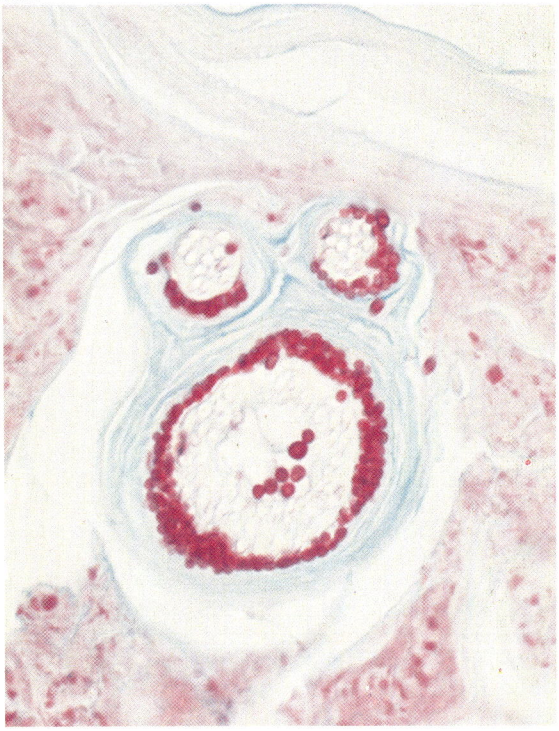

560 Microsporum canis causing canine ringworm. There is marked acanthosis and hyperkeratosis of the epidermis with superficial collections of degenerated inflammatory cells which form a scab. The fungal elements are not readily seen at this magnification. (H&E, ×50)

561 Microsporum canis Higher magnification of **560** showing the basophilic arthrospores around a hair shaft within a follicle. (H&E, ×200)

562 Microsporum canis Replicate section of **560** but stained by PAS. This section clearly shows the arthrospores surrounding the shafts of three hairs in a follicle. (PAS, ×200)

563

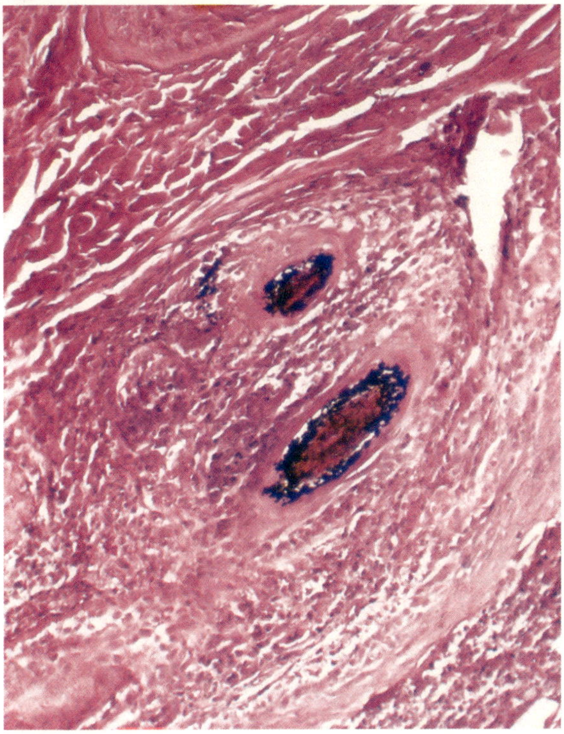

563 **Ringworm** in a dog. A marked perifolliculitis is seen around hair follicles that contain hairs surrounded by GMS-positive arthrospores. (GMS–H&E, ×50)

564

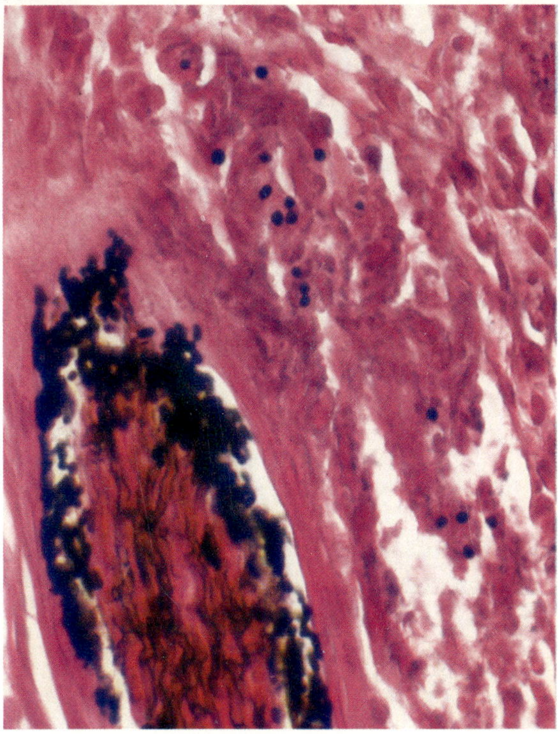

564 **Ringworm** Higher magnification of **563** showing fungal elements surrounding the hair shaft and free arthrospores in the dermis around the hair follicle. The extrafollicular spores very likely elicited the granulomatous reaction. (GMS–H&E, ×200)

565

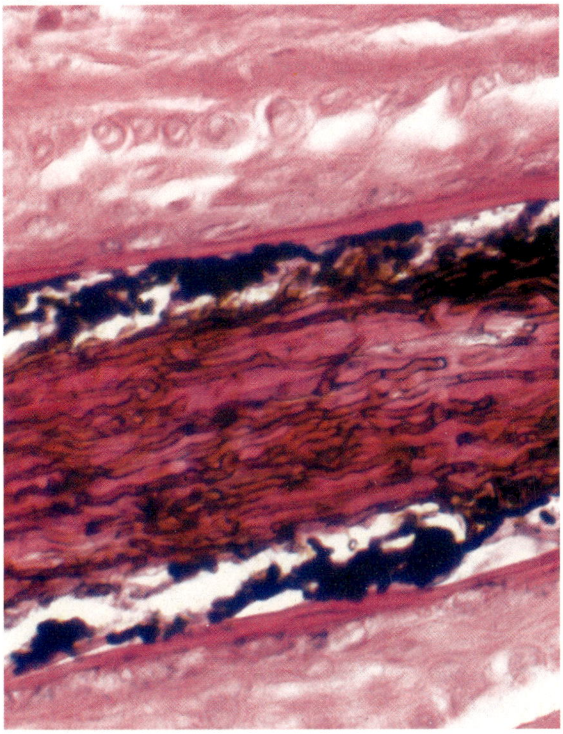

565 **Ringworm** in a dog. Numerous fungal elements are outside the hair shaft, and branched, septate mycelium is within the shaft. (GMS–H&E, ×200)

566

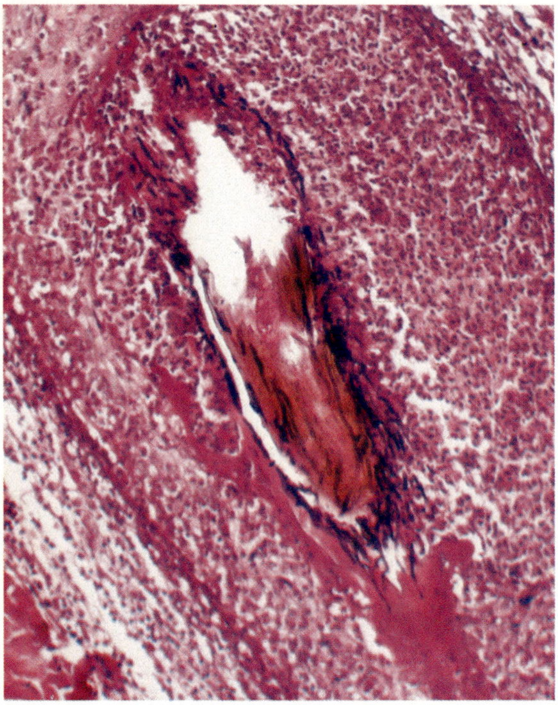

567

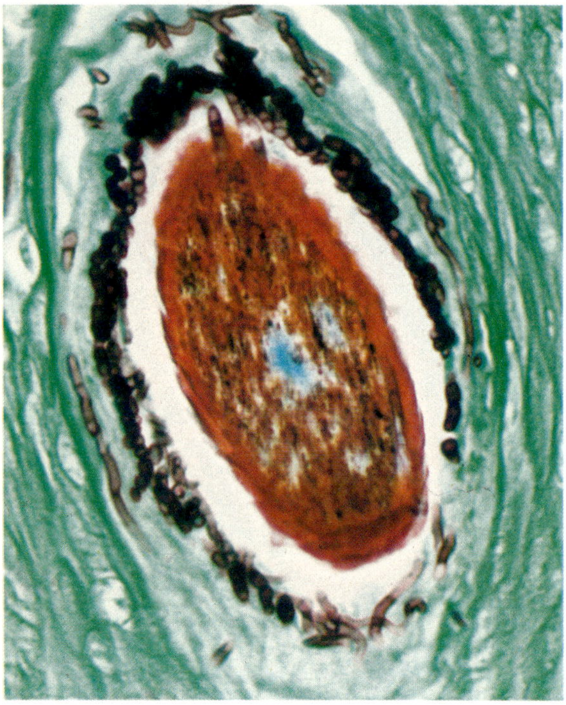

566 Dermatophyte causing suppurative perifolliculitis in a human. A broad zone of polymorphonuclear leucocytes surrounds a degenerating hair follicle. A hair is surrounded by the GMS-positive fungus within the follicle. Clinically, this skin lesion resembled those caused by systemic mycotic disease agents. (GMS–H&E, ×50)

567 Dermatophyte Replicate section of **566** clearly showing the ectothrix pattern of hair attack by the dermatophyte. This picture is diagnostic of some dermatophyte infections. (GMS, ×200)

568

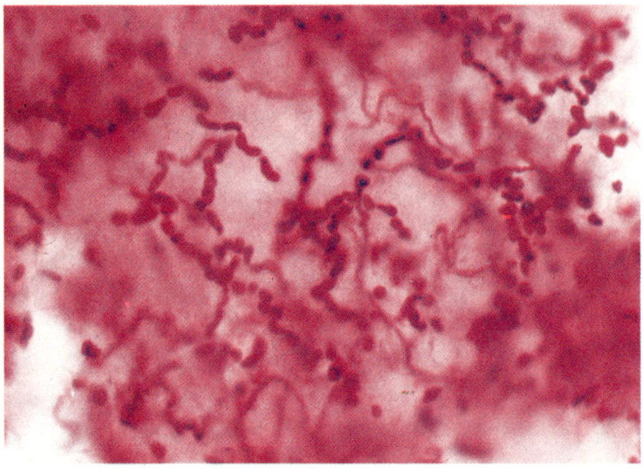

569

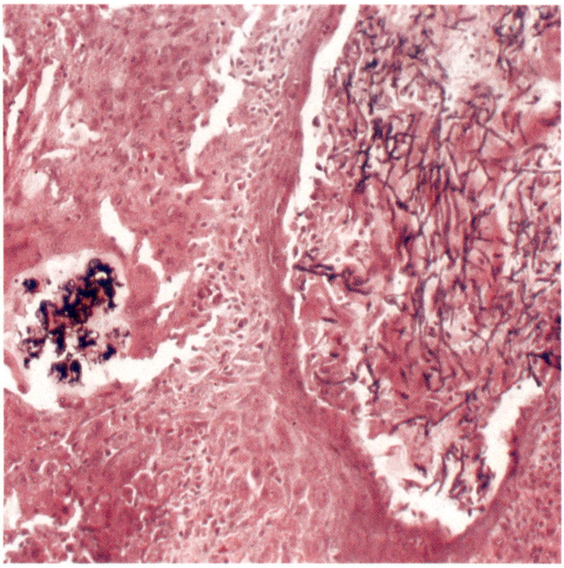

568 Trichophyton mentagrophytes Section of the glabrous skin of an infected human. The mycelium, broken up into chains of arthrospores, is clearly seen within the keratin layer. (PAS, ×200)

569 Microsporum canis causing granulomatous dermatitis with draining sinus tracts in a human. A hair follicle on the right contains numerous hyphae. There is a small aggregate of GMS-positive fungal cells within the granulomatous lesion in the dermis adjacent to the follicle. (GMS–H&E, ×50)

570

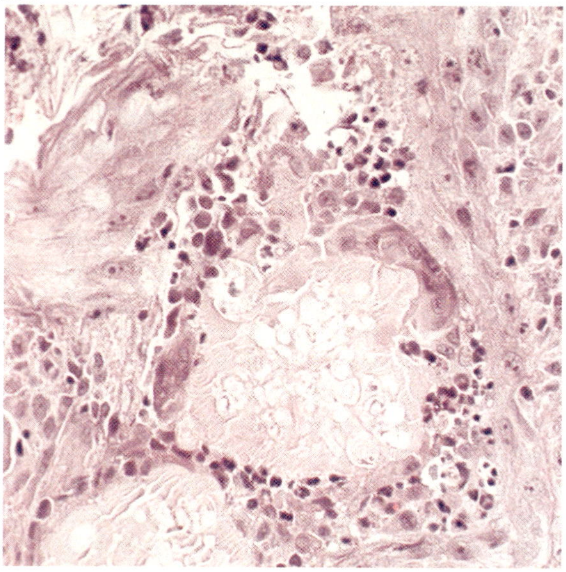

570 Microsporum canis Replicate section of **569** stained by H&E. Here, the follicular wall is ruptured and aggregates of hyaline, poorly stained hyphae are located near the rupture site. The extrafollicular hyphae of *M. canis* stimulate a granulomatous reaction and are embedded in and surrounded by Splendore–Hoeppli material. These aggregates of hyphae are erroneously considered by some to be granules and the lesion to be a mycetoma. (H&E, ×100)

571

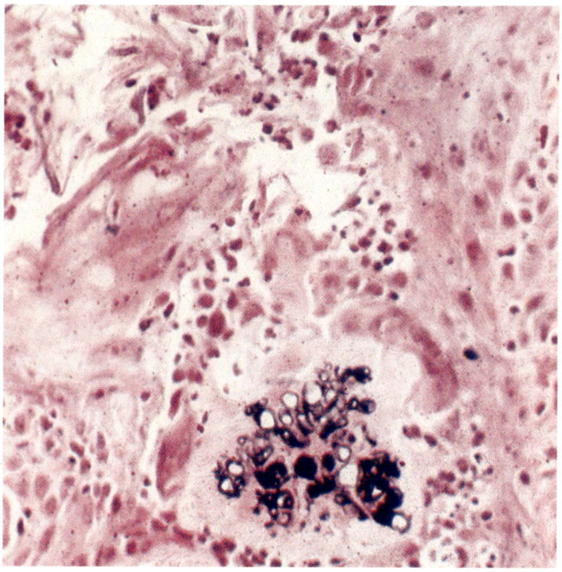

571 Microsporum canis Higher magnification of **569** showing details of an aggregate of *M. canis* mycelium in the dermis. (GMS–H&E, ×100)

572

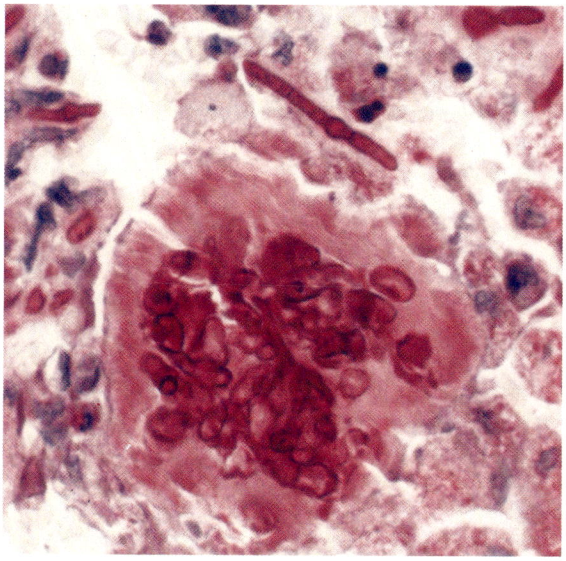

572 Microsporum canis Replicate section of **569** but stained by PAS to demonstrate individual hyphae and a hyphal aggregate embedded in and surrounded by Splendore–Hoeppli material in the granulomatous lesion. (PAS, ×200)

573

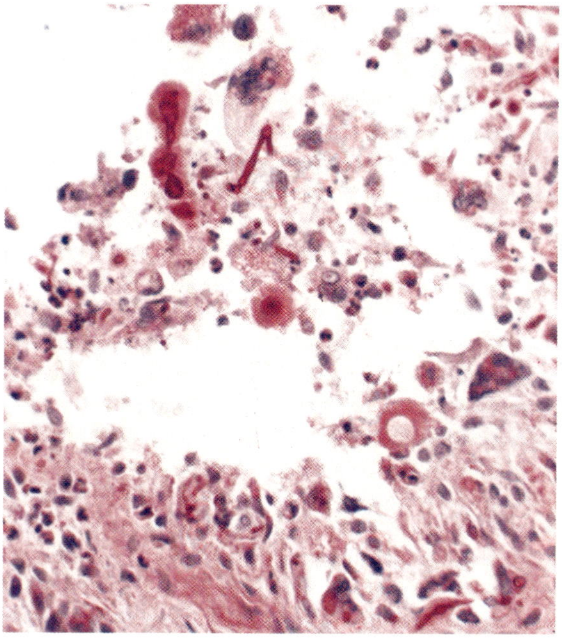

573 Microsporum canis Another field in **572** showing individual hyphae surrounded by prominent Splendore–Hoeppli material within a sinus tract. Palisading epithelioid cells line this tract in the deep dermis. (PAS, ×100)

574

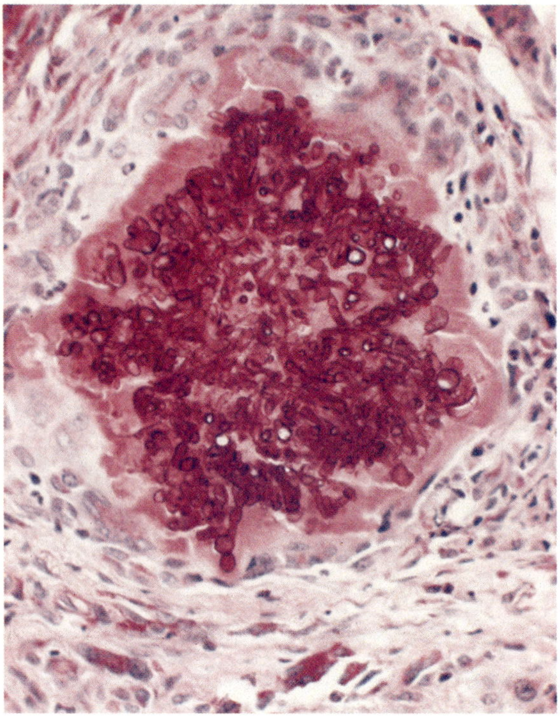

575

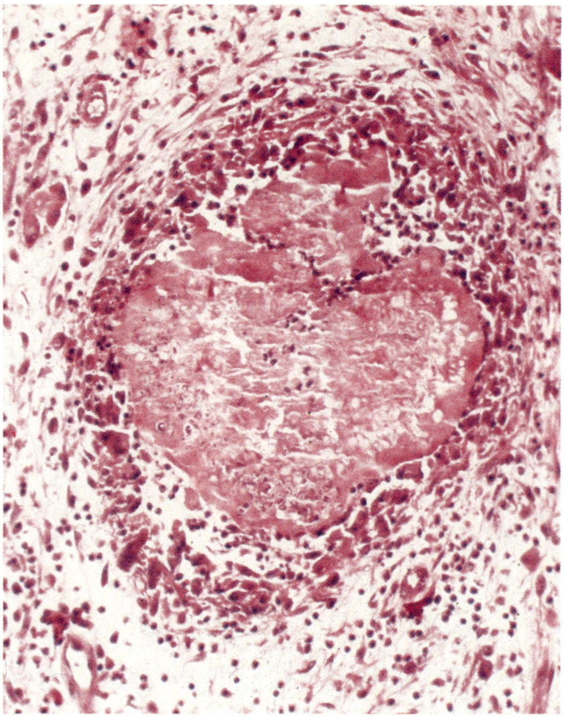

574 Microsporum canis Large aggregate of dermatophyte hyphae within the granulomatous lesion seen in **569**. The mycelium is embedded in and bordered by partially PAS-positive Splendore–Hoeppli material. (PAS, ×100)

575 Trichophyton sp., a dermatophyte, causing granulomatous dermatitis in a human. This agent also developed as aggregates of hyaline hyphae surrounded by and embedded in abundant Splendore–Hoeppli material. The aggregate is rimmed by a narrow zone of epithelioid and giant cells that lies in a stroma of granulation tissue. (H&E, ×50)

576

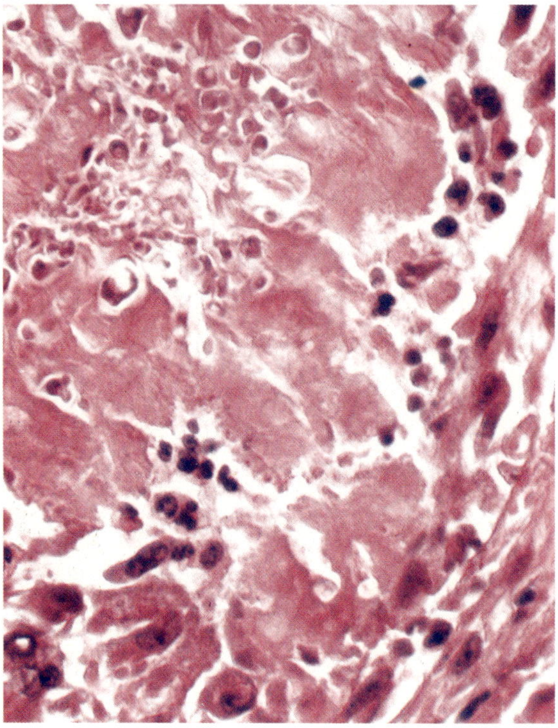

576 Trichophyton sp. Higher magnification of **575** showing details of the hyaline, poorly stained mycelium that forms the aggregate. The relationship of the abundant Splendore–Hoeppli material to the fungal cells is clearly seen. (H&E, ×200)

577

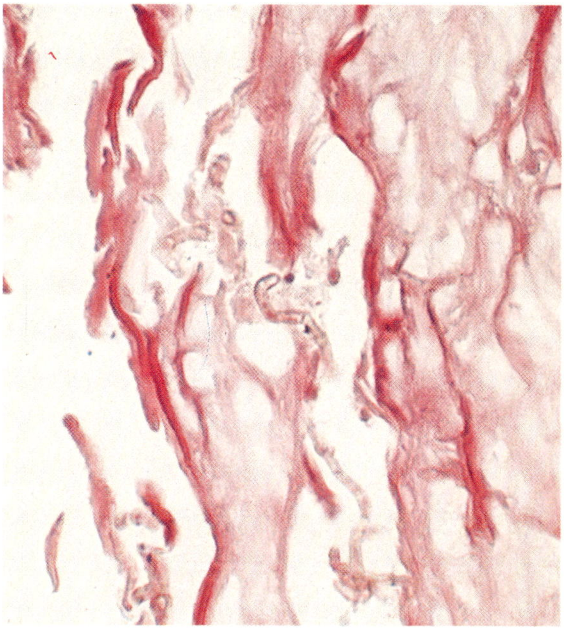

578

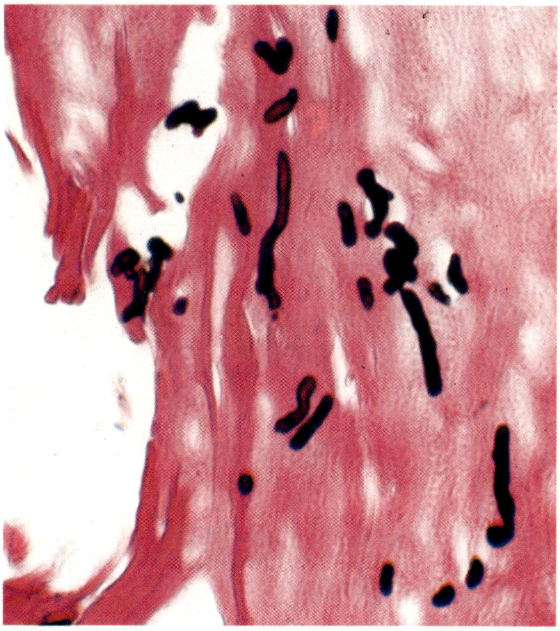

577 Tinea nigra in a human. Note the barely visible, light brown hyphae of *Exophiala werneckii* within the layers of keratin. The infection is limited to the superficial layers of the skin and causes little or no inflammation in the dermis. (H&E, ×200)

578 Tinea nigra Replicate section of **577** but stained by GMS–H&E. The section clearly shows short lengths of hyphae within the keratin layer of the skin. (GMS–H&E, ×200)

579

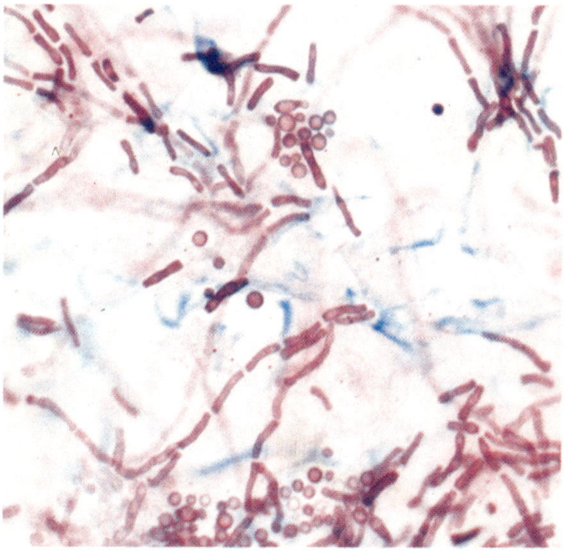

580

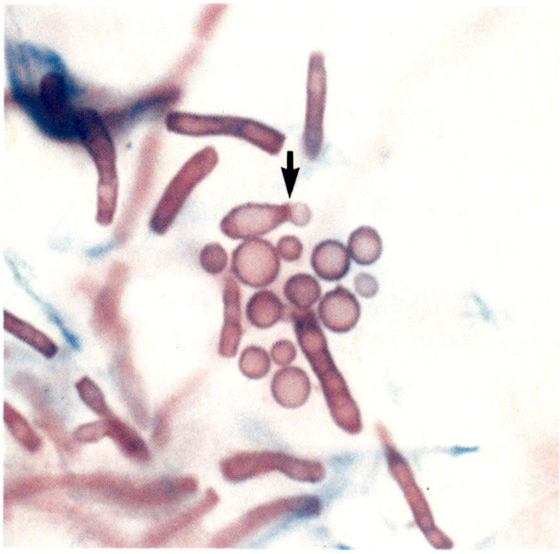

579 Tinea versicolor in a human. Hyphae, hyphal fragments and spherical cells of *Malassezia furfur* are present in the keratin layer of the skin. Many of the hyphae are fragmented, forming the characteristic short hyphal fragments that are oriented end to end. (PAS, ×200)

580 Tinea versicolor Higher magnification of **579** showing details of the characteristic short, curved hyphal fragments and clusters of round-to-oval, single and budding cells of *Malassezia furfur*. Note the small phialidic collarette at the point where a bud has been extruded from a parent cell (arrow). (PAS, ×500)

27 Zygomycosis

Text pages: 122–127

581

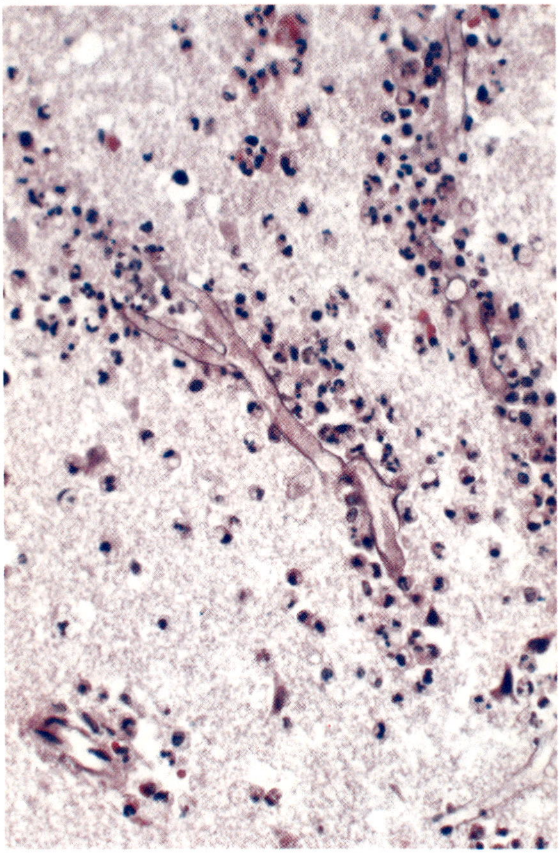

582

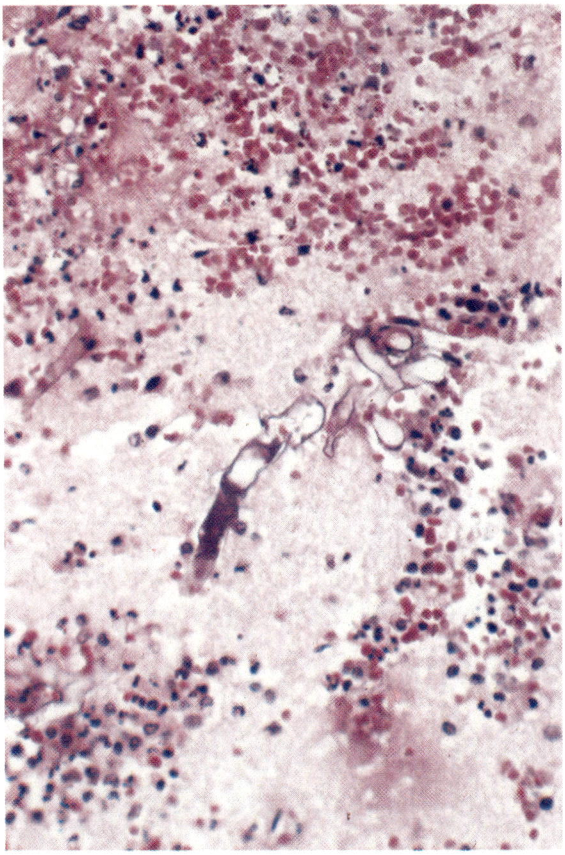

581 Cerebral zygomycosis in a human. The broad, branched hyphae that characterise this disease are well-stained by haematoxylin and are surrounded by a narrow zone of polymorphonuclear leucocytes. Septa are not present in these hyphae. (H&E, ×100)

582 Cerebral zygomycosis Another field in **581** showing broad, well-stained hyphae in an area of haemorrhage and suppurative necrosis. This type of inflammatory reaction is commonly seen in active lesions of zygomycosis caused by members of the order Mucorales. (H&E, ×100)

583

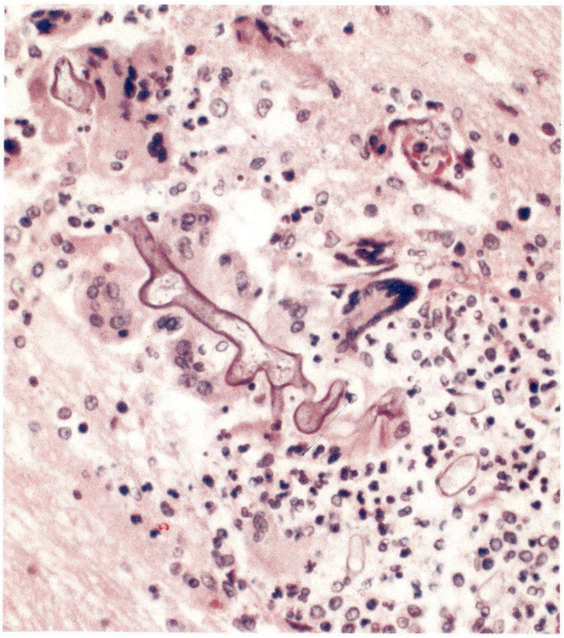

584

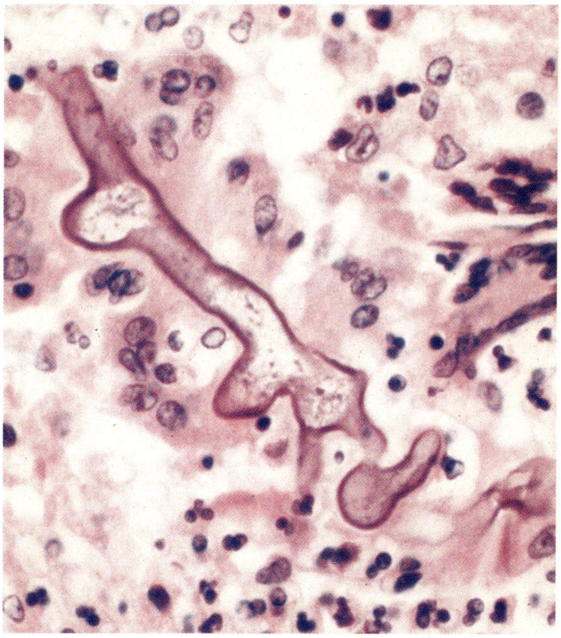

583 Cerebral zygomycosis in a human. There is a mixed purulent and granulomatous inflammatory reaction. The broad, aseptate hyphae are well-stained, and nearly all are partially engulfed by multinucleated giant cells. (H&E, ×100)

584 Cerebral zygomycosis Higher magnification of **583** to show details of the zygomycete hyphae partially engulfed by giant cells. The broad, branched hyphae lack septations, and they vary in width. (H&E, ×200)

585

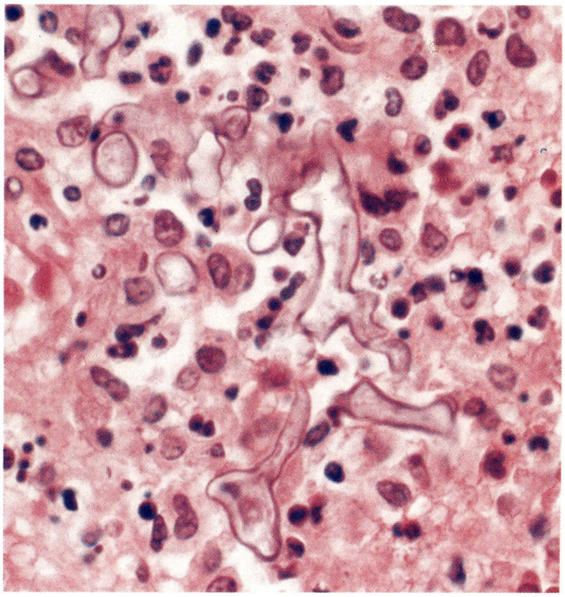

586

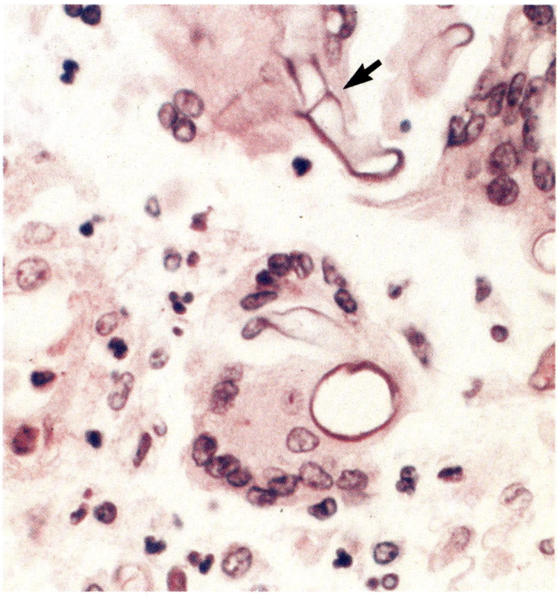

585 Cerebral zygomycosis Another field in **583** shows hyphae in an area of suppurative necrosis. Note the extreme variation in size and shape of the hyphae – characteristic features of the Mucorales in tissue. Some hyphae are distorted because of folding. (H&E, ×200)

586 Zygomycete hyphae within giant cells. Septations in the hyphae are sometimes seen as shown here (arrow). The large, round, vesicular structure within a giant cell in the centre is a transected hypha. (H&E, ×200)

587

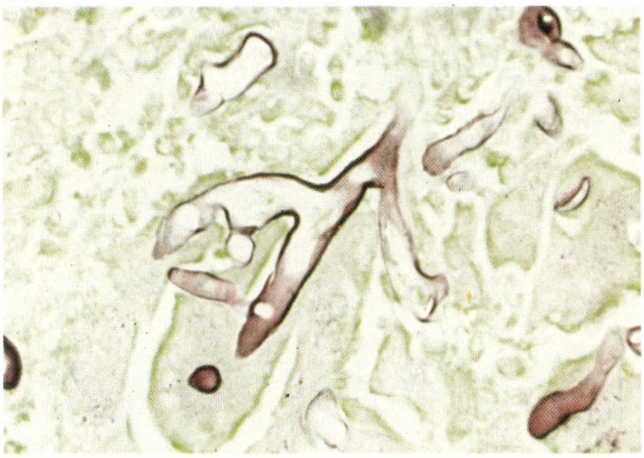

588

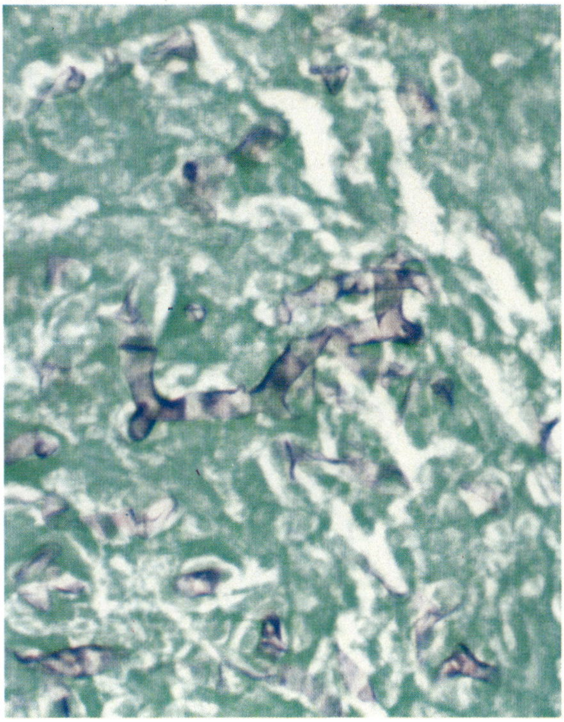

587 Cerebral zygomycosis in another human. Note the variation in staining intensity with GMS, the lack of septations, and the characteristic haphazard branching of the zygomycete hyphae. (GMS, ×200)

588 Cunninghamella bertholletiae infection of a human lymph node. The branched, folded, aseptate hyphae of this uncommon agent of zygomycosis are embedded in an area of haemorrhagic necrosis. They appear identical to the hyphae of other members of the order Mucorales. (GMS, ×200)

589

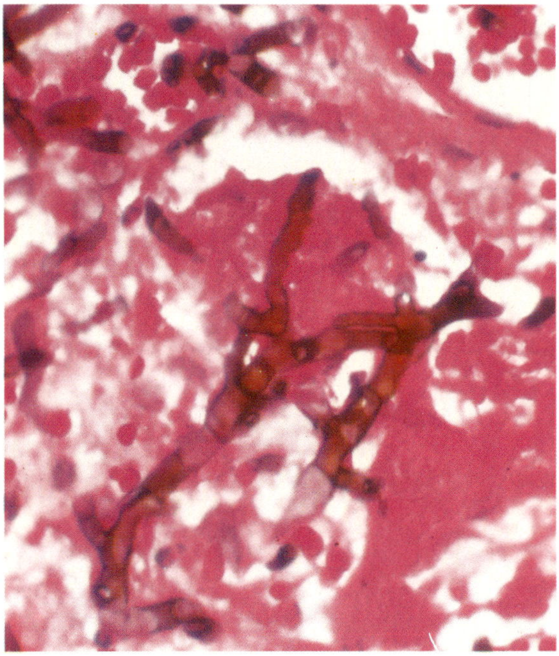

590

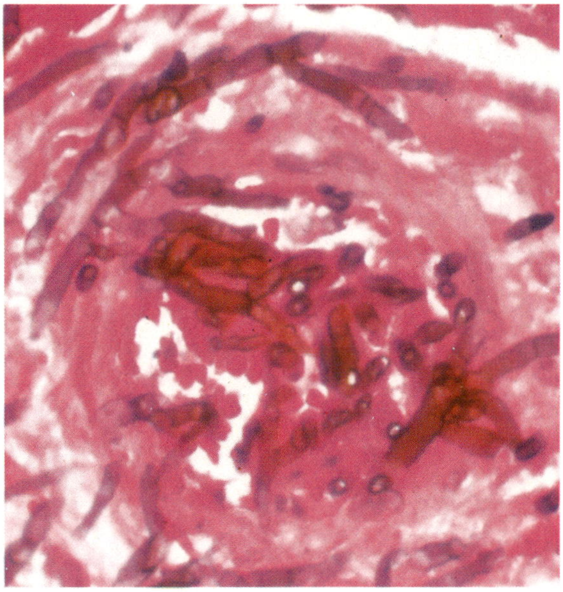

589 Pulmonary zygomycosis in a human. Numerous hyphae are embedded in a fibrinohaemorrhagic exudate. The hyphae have very few septations and branch irregularly. (GMS–H&E, ×200)

590 Pulmonary zygomycosis Another area in **589** showing angioinvasion and thrombosis of a pulmonary blood vessel. The zygomycete hyphae have penetrated the muscular wall and filled the lumen of the blood vessel. Hyphae of the order Mucorales have a propensity to invade blood vessels, causing thrombosis and possible infarction. (GMS–H&E, ×200)

591

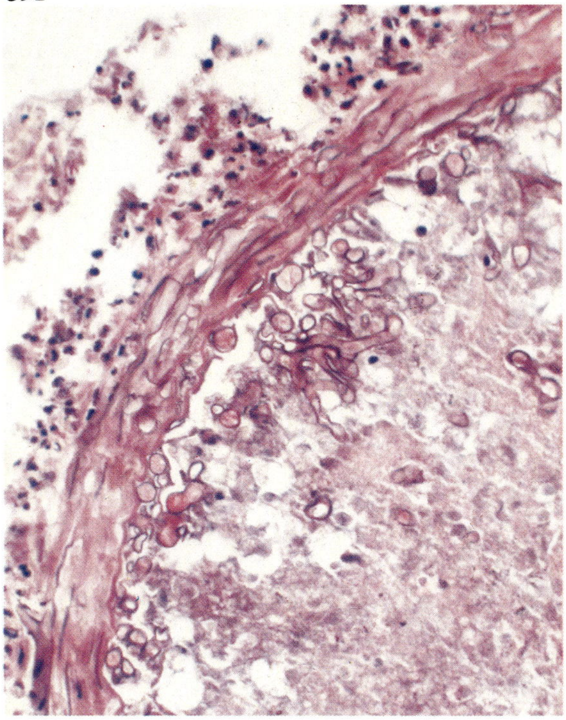

592

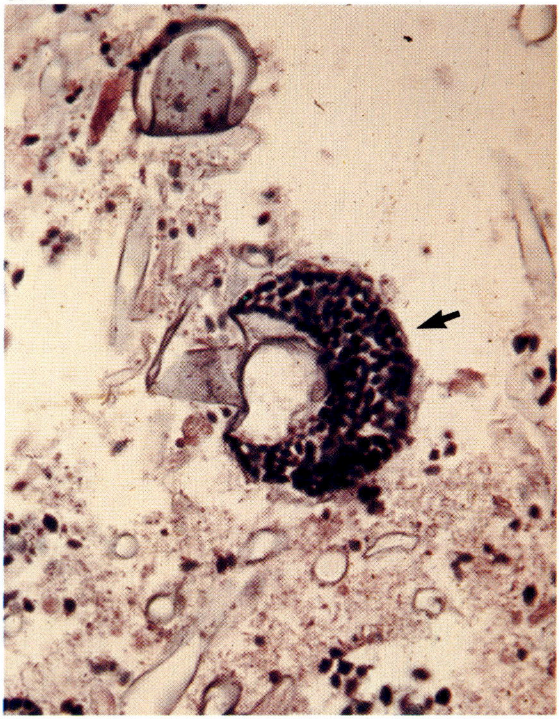

591 Cerebral zygomycosis in a human. Numerous hyphae have invaded the lumen of a large blood vessel, causing thrombosis. This resulted in a massive infarct. Note the perivascular accumulation of polymorphonuclear leucocytes. (PAS, ×100)

592 Rhizopus arrhizus causing rhinocerebral zygomycosis in a human. A sporangium containing zygospores (arrow) is seen in tissue obtained from the nasal lesion. Sporulation by zygomycetes is rarely observed in tissue. (Giemsa, ×200)

593

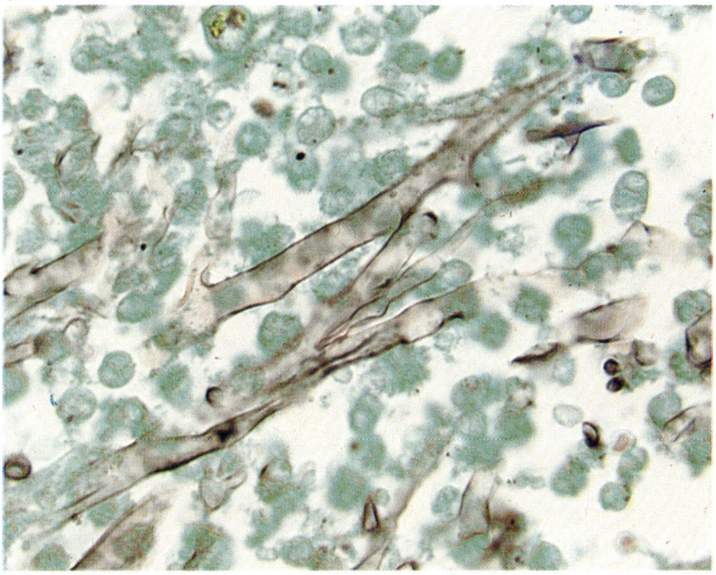

593 Rhizomucor (Mucor) pusillus causing vegetative valvular endocarditis in a human. Note that the hyphae are poorly stained and that some are collapsed. (GMS, ×200)

594

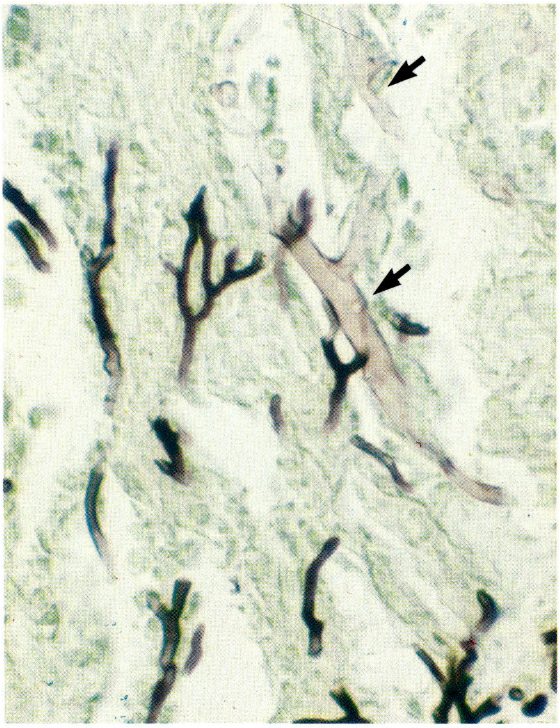

595

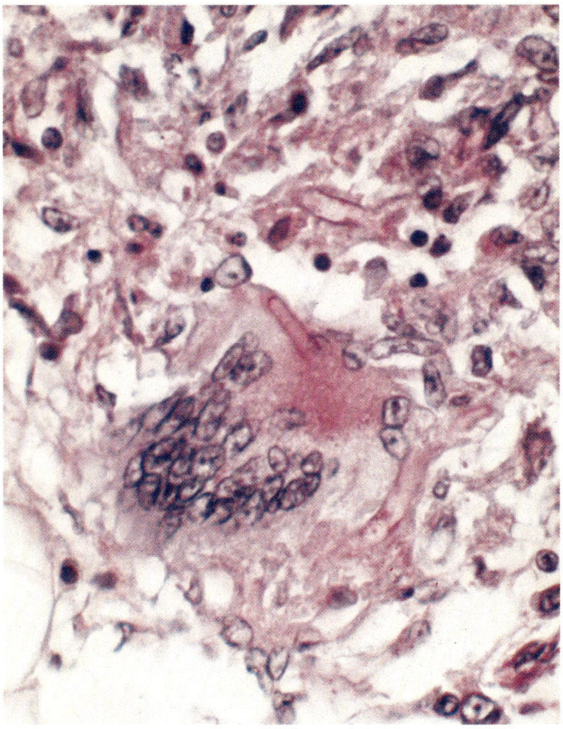

594 Aspergillus sp. and a zygomycete causing mixed infection in the lung of an immunosuppressed human. Note that the zygomycete hyphae (arrows) are poorly stained by GMS, lack septations, and are broad whereas the *Aspergillus* hyphae are well stained, narrower, septate and show dichotomous branching. In most cases, these differences allow differentiation of these two types of fungi. (GMS, ×200)

595 Basidiobolus haptosporus causing subcutaneous zygomycosis in a human. Note the granulomatous inflammatory reaction. The PAS stain clearly shows the hyphal fragments, some of which are within a giant cell. (PAS, ×200)

596

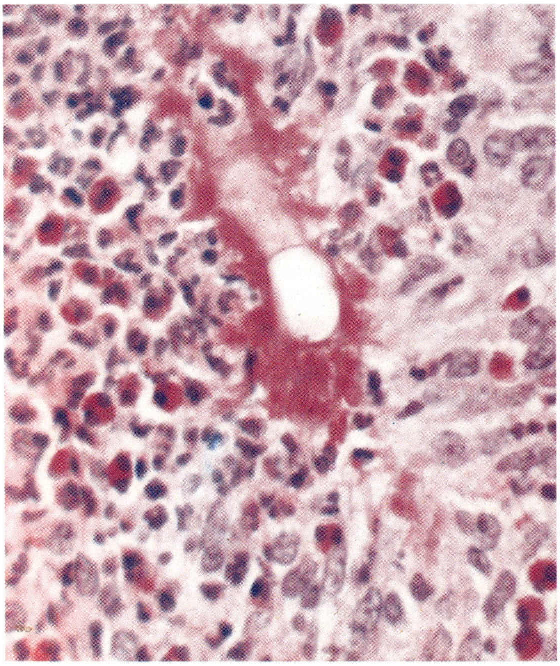

596 Basidiobolus haptosporus in another case of subcutaneous zygomycosis. A broad hyphal fragment is surrounded by a thick deposit of brightly eosinophilic material. Numerous eosinophils are present in the pyogranulomatous lesion. This type of tissue reaction is often seen in lesions caused by *Basidiobolus haptosporus*. (H&E, ×200)

597

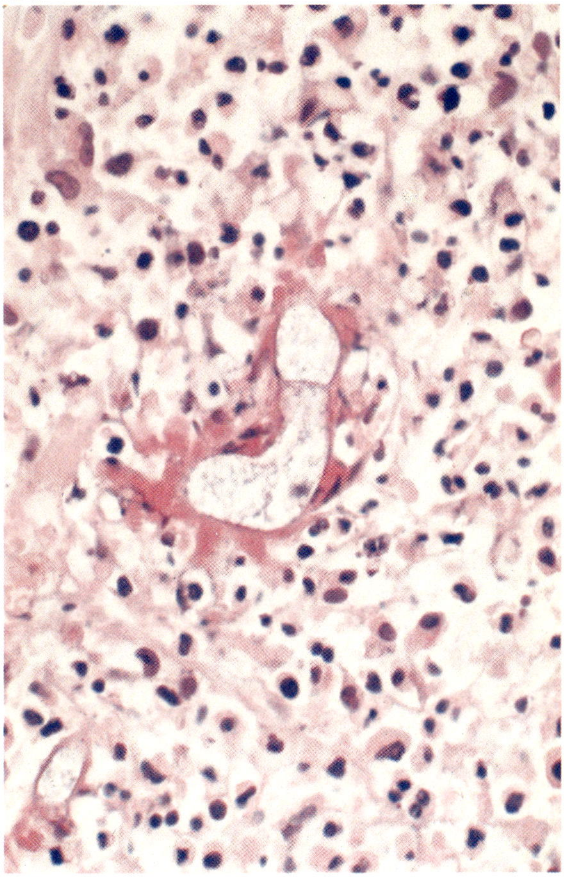

598

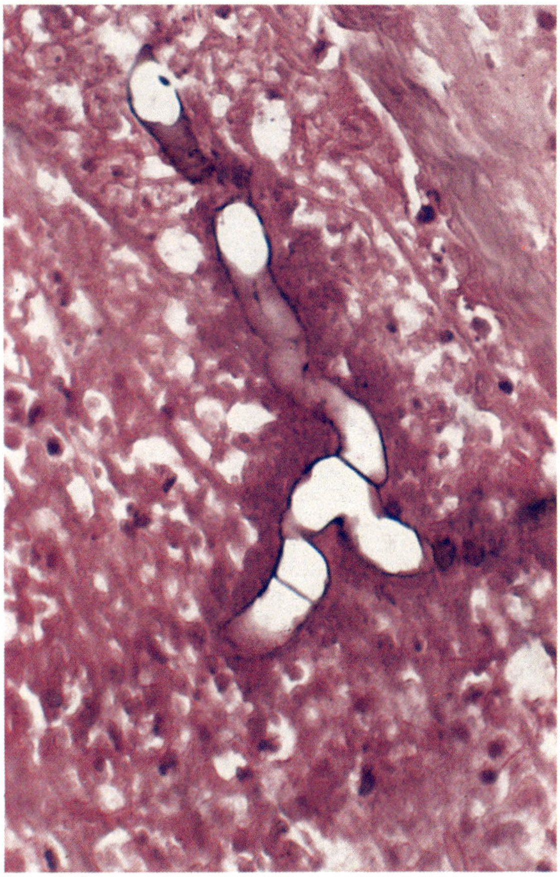

597 Basidiobolus haptosporus causing subcutaneous zygomycosis in another human. A broad hyphal fragment is surrounded by an irregular deposit of eosinophilic Splendore–Hoeppli material. Relatively few eosinophils are present in this lesion. A septum is seen in the hypha. (H&E, ×200)

598 Basidiobolus haptosporus Replicate section of **597** stained by GMS–H&E. The thin walls of the hyphae and the septations are clearly delineated. Although present, the Splendore–Hoeppli material bordering the fungus is not as prominent as in the section stained by H&E alone (see **597**). (GMS–H&E, ×200)

599

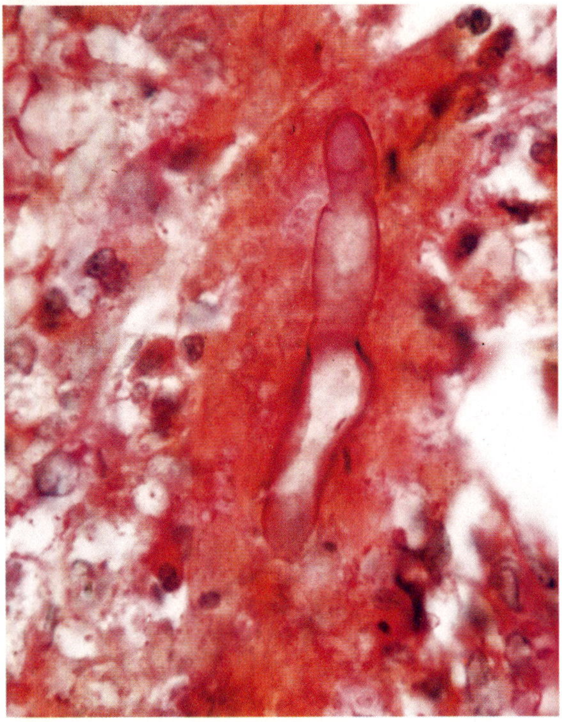

599 Conidiobolus coronatus causing rhinofacial zygomycosis in a human. Note that the broad hypha varies in width and is surrounded by a wide zone of eosinophilic material. A few polymorphonuclear leucocytes are seen in this field. The appearance of this fungus and the tissue reaction it elicits are like those seen in subcutaneous zygomycosis due to *Basidiobolus haptosporus* (see **596** and **597**). (H&E, ×400)

600

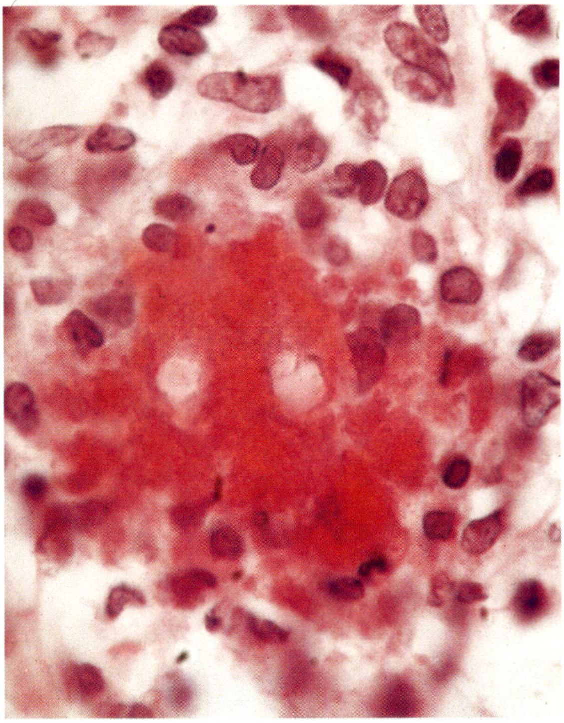

600 Conidiobolus coronatus Another field in **599** containing two transected hyphae surrounded by a broad, irregular zone of granular, eosinophilic, Splendore–Hoeppli material. Note the pyogranulomatous inflammatory reaction. (H&E, ×400)

601

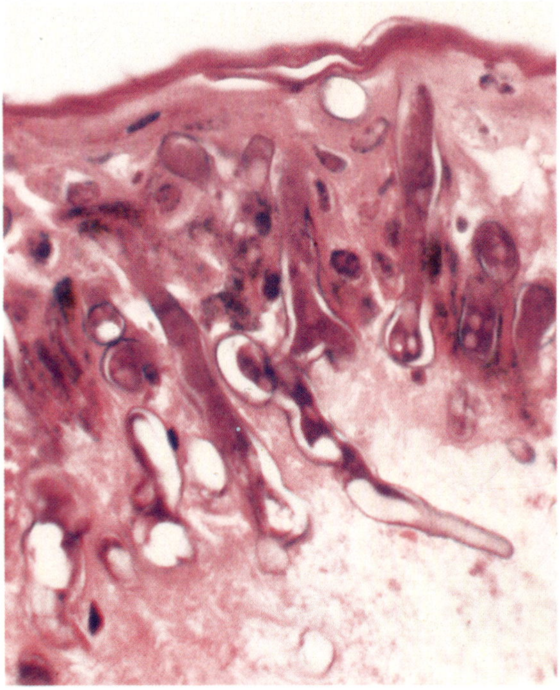

601 Conidiobolus coronatus infection of human skin. The fungus in the dermal lesion (not shown) was surrounded by the characteristic sheath of Splendore–Hoeppli material and was embedded in areas of eosinophilic necrosis. In this field, hyphae are seen invading the epidermis. They are not surrounded by an eosinophilic sheath and there is little or no inflammation. (GMS–H&E, ×200)

602

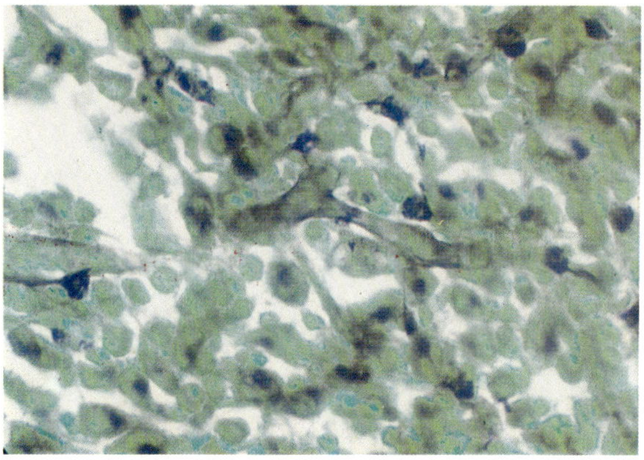

602 Granulation tissue in a human. The branched blood vessel in the centre of the field has a GMS-positive wall and superficially resembles a zygomycete hypha. By careful examination one should be able to readily distinguish small blood vessels from hyphae. (GMS, ×200)

603

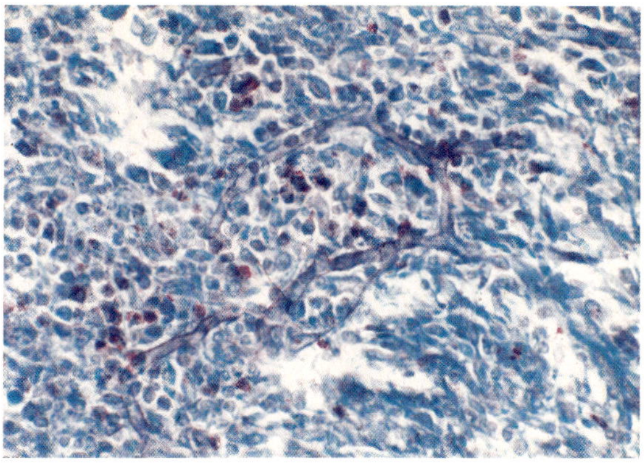

603 Granulation tissue Replicate section of **602**. The branched blood vessels somewhat resemble zygomycete hyphae and their basement membranes are PAS-positive. (PAS, ×100)

604

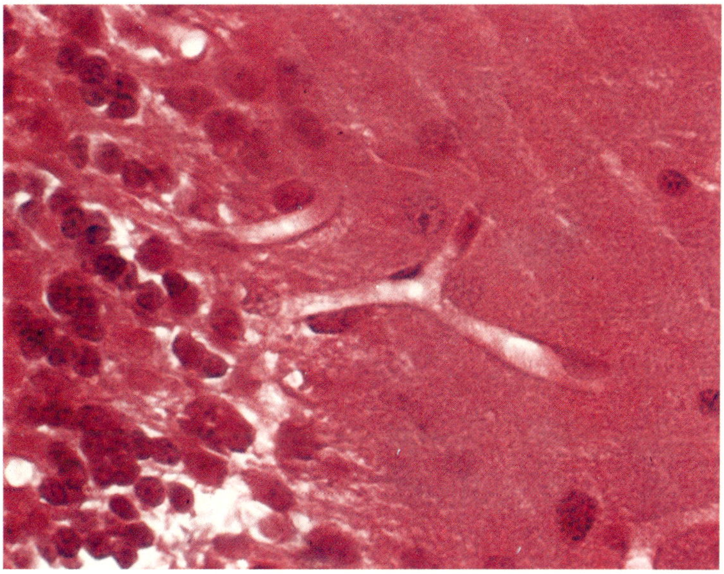

604 Empty capillaries in a section of perfused brain which closely resemble the branched hyphae of a zygomycete. The endothelial cells lining empty capillaries make it possible to differentiate them from hyphae. (H&E, ×100)

Glossary

Glossary of selected mycological and histopathological terms

abscess – a localised collection of pus and cellular debris in any tissue of the body; an abscess may be acute or chronic and may or may not be surrounded by a fibrotic capsule

acantho – a combining form meaning thorny, prickly or spiny

acanthosis – an increase in thickness of the epidermis characterised by proliferation and downward growth of the stratum germinativum

achloric – without chlorophyll

achlorophyllous – without chlorophyll

acid-fast – property of microorganisms to retain basic dyes, e.g., basic fuchsin, following decolourisation with strong acids

acrogenous – borne at the tip; applied to spores that develop at the tip of a conidiophore

actino – a combining form denoting a ray, as the radiate Splendore–Hoeppli material surrounding actinomycotic granules; may also pertain to some form of radiation

actinomycete – prokaryotic filamentous anaerobic or aerobic, heterotrophic microorganism of the Kingdom Monera, Phylum Actinomycetes. Species of *Actinomyces, Actinomadura, Nocardia, Streptomyces,* etc.

actinomycosis – disease caused by an actinomycete; generally restricted to infections by *Actinomyces bovis, A. israelii, A. naeslundii,* etc. See actinomycosis, actinomycotic mycetoma, nocardiosis

actinomycotic granule – mass of organised fine mycelium (1 μm or less in D) that may or may not be embedded in a cement-like substance (see eumycotic granule). Formed in mycetomas caused by aerobic actinomycetes; also produced by *Actinomyces* species and members of related genera in tissue

actinomycotic mycetoma – mycetoma caused by the species of any of several genera of actinomycetes (*Actinomadura, Nocardia, Streptomyces*)

acute – said of a disease process having a relatively short course, usually less than a week; the opposite of chronic

adeno-, aden – combining forms denoting relationship to a gland or lymph node

adenitis – inflammation of a gland or lymph node

adenopathy – glandular disease, especially of a lymph node

adiaspore – an asexual spore that enlarges after formation in vitro or in vivo. Such spores do not bud or produce endospores. Produced by certain species of *Chrysosporium* (*C. parvum* and *C. pruinosum*). Found in lung tissue in subjects with adiaspiromycosis

adipose – fatty

adnexa – structures attached to each other or adjoining accessory parts

aetiology – see *etiology*

air sacs – extensions of air spaces of the lungs of birds that contain air, communicate with bone cavities and do not function in gaseous exchange

aleuriospore – a confusing term; see conidium

alga (algae) – eukaryotic, photoautotrophic, unicellular or multicellular organisms classified in the Kingdom *Protista*

alopecia – loss of hair; baldness; seen in tinea capitis and in certain toxic, metabolic or nutritional disorders

amerospore – a single-celled asexual spore, i.e., aseptate

amphophilic – said of a structure that stains readily with either acid or basic dyes

angio –, *angi* – combining forms denoting relationship to a blood or lymph vessel

aniso – combining form meaning dissimilar or unequal

anisotropic – said of structures that have a double polarising power or are doubly refracting, thus giving the property called birefringence

annellation – ring-like band of cell wall material left at the tip of an annellide after a spore is released

annellide – an indeterminate conidiophore that produces annello-conidia. The tip of an annellide bears a series of superimposed annellations

annellospore – a synonym of annelloconidium; spore produced by an annellide

annular frill – cell wall fragments that remain attached to both ends of some arthroconidia, e.g., *Coccidioides immitis*

anthropophilic – having a predeliction for humans. Term applied to dermatophytes which have humans as their natural hosts, which seldom if ever infect lower animals, and which cannot survive in soil as free living moulds

arthrospore – asexual spore formed by the disarticulation of the mycelium

artifact (artefact) – something artificially created or extraneous

ascigerous – producing asci

ascocarp – a mycelial structure within which are formed asci and ascospores

ascogenous hyphae – specialised hyphae that produce asci

ascomycete – unicellular or filamentous fungi that produce ascospores in the course of sexual reproduction; of the Phylum Ascomycota

aseptate – without cross walls, e.g., unicellular spores, mycelium of zygomycetes

aspergilloma – a fungus ball composed of *Aspergillus spp.* hyphae and generally located in a preformed body cavity, usually in the lung; may resemble a tumorous mass

assimilation – an aerobic process whereby carbon and nitrogen compounds are utilised with oxygen as the final electron acceptor. Phenomenon used in the identification of yeasts

asteroid – resembling a star; said of Splendore–Hoeppli-like material which often surrounds tissue form cells of *Sporothrix schenckii* and other fungi

atelectasis – imperfect or incomplete expansion, as of the lungs

atropy – an absolute or relative decrease in the size of a structure or cell that is generally accompanied by some lack of function

autopsy – postmortem examination of a body; necropsy

autotrophic – capable of obtaining energy in the absence of organic compounds, as the algae, plants, and certain bacteria

basement membrane – a membrane of mucopolysaccharides and collagen on which epithelial and endothelial cells rest

basidiomycete – unicellular or filamentous fungi that produce basidiospores following a sexual process. Classified in the Phylum *Basidiomycota*

basidiospore – haploid sexual spore produced by the basidiomycetes on basidia following nuclear fusion and meiosis

basophilic – staining readily with basic dyes

biopsy – a piece of tissue taken from the living body for pathologic examination; the process of excision of tissue

birefringence – the property of being doubly refractive or of transmitting light unequally in different directions (anisotropic); seen in structures with a high degree of molecular orientation, such as crystals

blastospore – asexual spore produced by a budding process along the mycelium or by a single spore

bud – asexual spore produced by a budding process. Mother cell may produce a single bud (single budding) or several buds (multiple budding)

budding – an asexual reproductive process characteristic of unicellular fungi or spores involving the formation of a lateral outgrowth from the parent cell that is pinched off to form new cells

calcareous – said of tissues that contain calcium or other minerals; chalky *capsule* – a hyaline mucopolysaccharide sheath on the wall of a cell or spore

carcinoma – a malignant epithelial cell neoplasm

chlamydospores – thick-walled resistant spores formed by the direct differentiation of the mycelium in which there is a concentration of protoplasm and nutrient material

chloro – combining form meaning green

chlorophyll – the green, photosynthetic pigment in plants, algae, and certain bacteria

chloroplast – chlorophyll-bearing organelles of algal, plant, and certain bacterial cells that are basic in the process of photosynthesis

chronic – a disease process of long duration; the opposite of acute

cicatrix – a scar

clamp connection – a hyphal connection between two cells in the mycelium of many basidiomycetes

clavate – club-shaped

coenocytic – term applied to a cell or an aseptate hypha containing numerous nuclei, e.g., a zygomycete

collarette – flared, cup-like tip of conidiophores, known as phialides

colony – an organised mass of mycelium that may or may not produce spores

conidium – an asexual spore, that is easily detached from the mycelium or conidiophore. This term is preferred over aleuriospore which is considered to be a confused term

conidiophore – a specialised hypha (simple or complex) that produces and bears conidia

cortex – the outer layer of an organ

cryostat – a refrigerated chamber containing a microtome for cutting thin sections of frozen tissue for light microscopic examination

culture – organised in vitro growth of microorganisms on nutrient media

cyst – a normal or abnormal sac in the body that is lined by epithelium and filled with fluid of varying consistency; in parasitology, denotes a protective wall that surrounds certain parasites during their life cycle

cyto – combining form denoting relationship to any cell

dematiaceous – said of fungi whose cell walls (mycelium or conidia) are naturally pigmented black or brown

dermato, dermat-, dermo – combining forms denoting relationship to the skin

dermatophyte – pathogenic fungi of the genera *Epidermophyton, Microsporum* and *Trichophyton* that invade the skin, hair, nails, and feathers

diagnosis – a conclusion reached; naming a disease; may be presumptive or definitive

dichotomous – equal branching of hyphae

diffuse – widely scattered; not localised

dimorphic – having two forms; applied to fungi that are mycelial at ±25°C and that form either budding yeast cells or spherules in vivo or at 37°C in vitro on special media

disseminated – scattered throughout an organ or the body

downy – covered with short, fine hyphae

dysgonic – a slow-growing fungal mutant

ectasis – combining form meaning to dilate, expand or stretch; ectasia

ectatic – distended

ectothrix – outside the hair shaft

edema – accumulation of abnormal quantities of fluid in tissues or body cavities

embolus – part of a thrombus, entire thrombus, microorganism, clump of fat, air bubble, neoplastic cells or foreign material which is injected or dislodged and which moves through the arterial or venous system from one anatomic site to another; an embolus may lodge in a blood vessel, causing obstruction *encapsulation* – a walling off, e.g., of an abscess, by highly vascular connective tissue that serves as a limiting barrier to further spread

endemic – disease or microorganism native to a given region

endocytosis – engulfment of solid (phagocytosis) or liquid (pinocytosis) materials by a cell

endogenous – produced or originating from within

endospore – asexual spore produced within a closed structure or mycelium

endosporulation – process of producing endospores

endothrix – within the hair shaft. Term applied to hair invasion by dermatophytes that produce arthrospores within the hair shaft

eosin – a rose-coloured dye derived from coal tar that is commonly used with haematoxylin for staining the cytoplasm of cells

eosinophil – a motile polymorphonuclear leucocyte with lysosomal granules that are readily stained by eosin

epidemic – disease affecting many people or animals in a wide area

epithelioid cells – inflammatory cells (modified macrophages) that morphologically resemble epithelial cells but are not; they contain abundant eosinophilic cytoplasm and may be arranged side by side (palisaded) like epithelial cells; the principal component of granulomas

erythema – redness of the skin

etiology – factor(s) causing a disease

eukaryotic – said of organisms with well organised and differentiated nuclei, a nuclear membrane, mitochondria, and an endoplasmic reticulum; such organisms are capable of division by mitosis or meiosis

eumycotic granule – organised mass of broad, septate mycelium embedded or not embedded in cement. Formed in mycetomas caused by fungi

exogenous – produced or originating from without

extravasation – an escaping of blood or fluid into the tissues from blood or lymphatic vessels

exudate – drainage fluid that oozes out of an abscess, etc., or extravasates into or onto tissues as a result of increased vascular permeability; usually results from inflammation and contains a relatively high concentration of proteins, leucocytes, and cellular debris

febrile – feverish; having an elevated body temperature

fermentation – an enzymatic oxidation-reduction process wherein the organic substrate serves both as the electron donor and acceptor. A process used to identify yeasts

fibrinoid – resembling fibrin

fibrinopurulent – said of an inflammatory exudate that contains both fibrin and pus

fibrinous – pertaining to or containing fibrin, a blood component

fibro – combining form denoting relationship to fibres, as collagen and reticular fibres

fibroplasia – the normal or abnormal formation of fibrous tissue

fistula – in tissue, an abnormal passageway from a body cavity to the external surface of the body or another cavity

fixation – arresting autolysis and bacterial decomposition of tissues by addition of a fixative such as a 4% buffered formaldehyde solution

fixative – one of several chemicals used for the preparation of specimens for histologic examination, which preserves structures by hardening and fixation

floccose – loose, cottony texture

fluorescence – a substance is said to be fluorescent if upon absorbing light energy of one wavelength ('excitation' or 'activation' light) it emits light of another wavelength, usually within 10^{-7} seconds. Because of energy losses, the emitted light is almost always of longer wavelength than the exciting radiation. If the absorbed light is emitted over a longer period than above, the substance is phosphorescent. Both conditions are special cases of the general phenomenon of luminescence

focal – pertaining to a focus; in pathology a limited or localised lesion *fungus* (pl. fungi) – a eukaryotic, achlorophyllus unicellular or filamentous organism with a chitinous cell wall that reproduces either asexually or sexually, or both. Spores may be posteriorly uniflagellate (Phylum Chytridiomycota) or aflagellate

funiculose – hyphae aggregated into rope-like strands

fuseaux – an archaic term of French origin for a large, multiseptate asexual spore of fungi (see macroconidium)

fusiform – spindle-shaped

geophilic – having a predeliction for soil. Said of fungi that live in soil as saprophytes

germ tube – the tube-like process put out by a germinating spore that develops into the mycelium

giant cells – large multinucleated cells found in granulomatous and chronic resorbing inflammatory reactions; giant cells may be of either the foreign body (haphazardly arranged nuclei) or Langhans' (peripherally arranged nuclei) type, and are usually formed by coalescence of epithelioid cells (modified macrophages)

glabrous – smooth and bare

granulation tissue – proliferation of immature connective tissue (fibroblasts) and capillaries (angioblasts) in the chronic stages of inflammation in an attempt to replace necrotic tissues of the host; mixed inflammatory cells are usually present

granuloma – a focus or tumour-like mass of granulomatous inflammation

granulomatous inflammation – a tumour-like mass (granuloma) of epithelioid cells with or without multinucleated giant cells. Granulomas are usually surrounded by proliferating fibroblasts, capillaries, lymphocytes and plasma cells

habitat – the natural locality where an organism grows and reproduces

hardening – coagulation and denaturation of protein when tissues are placed in a fixative

haematoxylin – a crystalline compound derived from log-wood (*Haematoxylan campechianum*) by ether extraction; the oxidised form is commonly used with eosin as a stain in histopathology

haemorrhage – the antemortem escape of blood from any part of the blood vascular system

heterotrophic – requiring preformed organic compounds as a source of energy

histio-, histo-, hist – combining forms denoting relationship to tissue

histiocyte – macrophage

histology – study of the microscopic anatomy of tissues

histopathology – the light microscopic study of diseased tissues

hülle cells – thick-walled, large intercalary or terminal, sterile cells produced by some species of *Aspergillus*

hyaline – translucent, glassy, colourless

hyperemia – an excess of blood contained within blood vessels of a given part of the body, which imparts a red appearance to the tissue

hyperplasia – growth in size of a tissue or organ resulting from an increase in number of differentiated cells which retain their function and normal histological architecture

hypertrophy – growth in size of a tissue or organ resulting from a increase in the size of differentiated cells which retain their functional ability and normal histological arrangement

hyph – a Greek term for a web or something woven. The hyphae of a mould

hypha (pl. hyphae) – the filament that makes up the thallus or body of most fungi

immunofluorescence microscopy – localisation of specific antigens or antibodies in tissues and smears by application of fluorochrome-labelled antibodies against the substances in question, and visualisation under a fluorescence microscope

incidence – in reference to a disease, signifies the number of cases developing over a given period of time in a population (see prevalence)

indeterminate – said of conidiophores that continue to elongate as they produce conidia *induration* – quality of being hard; an area of hardened tissue

infarct – a localised area of coagulation necrosis produced by either blockage of the arterial blood supply or venous drainage (blood stasis) of any part of an organ

infiltration – the process whereby inflammatory cells or fluid passes into and is deposited within a tissue or organ

inflammation – tissue reaction to injury; may be either serous, fibrinous, haemorrhagic, purulent, granulomatous, or a combination of these types

insidious – hidden; not apparent, as a disease that does not induce symptoms

intercalary – between two cells

intercellular – between cells

interstitial – refers to the space between tissue cells

intracellular – within a cell

intradermal – intracutaneous; within the dermis

intraepidermal – within the layers of the epidermis, as an intraepidermal abscess

ischemia – deprivation of adequate blood supply to a given tissue

-itis – a suffix denoting inflammation of a tissue, organ or part indicated by the prefix to which it is attached (see list of anatomic prefixes in Appendix 2)

karyolysis – nuclear dissolution

karyorrhexis – nuclear fragmentation

keloid – an elevated scar that progressively enlarges because of excessive formation of collagen during repair; benign fibrous skin tumour

kerato – combining form denoting relationship to horny tissue (keratin) or to the cornea of the eye

keratin – a complex, insoluble protein that is the principal component of the epidermis, hair, nails and feathers

keratinolysis – dissolution or digestion of keratin

keratinophilic – having an affinity for keratin. Said of fungi that digest keratin

kerion – a raised, circumscribed mass of tissue usually suppurating at many points

Kupffer cells – fixed reticuloendothelial (littoral cells) lining the sinusoids of the liver

lamella – a thin plate or layer

lesion – an injury, wound, or local morbid structural change in tissue that is usually accompanied by loss of function

leuconychia – white discolouration of nails seen in onychomycosis

leucocytosis – increase in the number of leucocytes in the peripheral blood

lipoid – resembling fat

lobulated – bearing lobules

localised – said of a disease process restricted to a limited region

lymphadenitis – inflammation of a lymph node

lymphadenopathy – generally, enlargement of the lymph nodes

macroconidium – large, often multicellular asexual spore

macrophage – a fixed or wandering cell of the reticuloendothelial system having the ability to phagocytise microorganisms or particulate substances

macroscopic – large enough to be seen by the naked eye, as opposed to microscopic

metaplasia – transformation from one differentiated cell type into another

metastasis – transfer of infectious agents or body cells from one organ or part of the body to another not directly connected with it

migration – passage of inflammatory cells from one site to another

miliary – said of very small, productive lesions; invading many tissues and usually quick spreading; literally, millet seed-like *microtome* – an instrument for cutting thin sections of tissue for light microscopic examination

mold – a form used to shape objects (see mould); improperly used as a synonym of mould

mononuclear – refers to inflammatory cells with one nucleus

mould – any mycelial fungus (see mold)

mucopurulent – containing both mucus and pus

multiseptate – having more than one septum

muriform – having horizontal and vertical cell walls. Term applied to conidia

myc-, myco – combining forms meaning fungus

mycelium (pl. mycelia) – a mat of intertwined and branched hyphae

mycetes – the fungi

mycethemia – fungal invasion of the blood vascular system; the presence of fungi in the blood

mycetoma – a tumour caused by actinomycetes or fungi that form granules within the invaded tissue

mycosis – a disease caused by infectious fungi

myelo – combining form denoting relationship to the spinal cord or bone marrow

myxoid – resembling mucus

necro – a combining form denoting relationship to death of cells or to a dead body

necropsy – see autopsy

necrosis – death of cells or tissues within the living body

necrotic – relating to dead tissue; necrosis

neoplasm – a new, autonomous, and abnormal growth of tissue within the living body

neurotropic – having an affinity for tissues of the nervous system

nocardiosis – actinomycotic infection caused by species of *Nocardia*

onychomycosis – mycotic infection of the nails

otomycosis – mycotic infection of the ear

papule – a small external swelling not containing fluid or pus

parenchyma – the functional elements of an organ, as distinguished from its framework or stroma

paronychia – inflammation or ulceration of tissue about the nail, usually due to infection

patent – open, unobstructed

patho – combining form denoting relationship to disease

pathogen – a microorganism capable of producing disease

pathogenesis – the cellular and biochemical processes by which a disease develops

pathogenic – capable of producing disease

pathognomonic – indicative of a disease; tissue changes that are characteristic or unique for a specific disease

perfect state – developmental state when sexual reproduction takes place and sexual spores (ascospores, basidiospores, zygospores) are produced

petechiae – small pinpoint areas of haemorrhage under the skin or in an organ

phaeo – a prefix meaning dark

phaeohyphomycosis – literally a mycotic disease caused by filamentous dark fungi. A subcutaneous or systemic mycotic disease caused by a dematiaceous fungus of any of various genera and species. In tissue, the aetiologic agents are in the form of dematiaceous mycelial elements

phagocytosis – the engulfment of microorganisms, host cells or other foreign materials by phagocytic cells, usually those of the reticuloendothelial system

phialide – a conidiogenous cell that successively produces conidia. A collarette may surround the orifice of the phialide

photoautotrophic – ability of an organism to utilise the energy of sunlight to manufacture its nutrients from inorganic substances *phycomycetes* – an old and obsolete class name for the so-called lower fungi. These organisms are now classified in two different Kingdoms, as follows: Kingdom Protista: Phyla – Acrasiomycota, Myxomycota, Hyphochytridiomycota, Oomycota, Plasmodiophoromycota; Kingdom Fungi: Phyla – Chytridiomycota, Zygomycota

plasma cell – one of the four basic types of white cells found in inflammatory reactions (the other three types are polymorphonuclear leucocytes, lymphocytes and macrophages); plasma cells are thought to be derived from B lymphocytes, are often seen in chronic inflammation, and produce antibodies which are stored in cisternae of the endoplasmic reticulum

polyp – a projecting, abnormal growth usually arising from the mucosa

polypoid – resembling a polyp

prevalence – in reference to a disease, signifies the number of cases at a specific time in a population (see incidence)

prognosis – prediction of course and probable outcome of a disease

proteinaceous – protein-like

pseudohypha (ae) – mycelial-like filament produced by the successive buds of a yeast that elongated and failed to separate

pseudoepitheliomatous hyperplasia – a benign but extremely advanced hyperplasia of epithelium characterised by thickening and downward growth into the underlying tissues

pseudoseptum – a protoplasmic membrane within a conidium that looks like a septum

purulent – consisting of or containing pus; suppurative

pus – liquid product of inflammation consisting of proteinaceous fluid, leucocytes, and cellular debris

pustule – small elevation of skin due to a visible collection of filled with pus or lymph within or beneath the epidermis

pycnidioconidium – an asexual spore produced within a pycnidium

pycnidiospore – asexual spore produced within a pycnidium (see pycnidioconidium)

pycnidium – an asexual fruiting structure made up of woven mycelium within which are produced conidia that are known as pycnidiospores or pycnidioconidia

pyknosis – nuclear shrinkage

pyogenic – pus producing

pyriform – pear-shaped

regeneration – replacement of parenchymal lesions or defects by an increase in the number and size of parenchymal cells

repair – replacement of parenchymal lesions or defects by fibrous connective tissue

reticulum – a network; reticular tissue

ringworm – a term used to designate superficial infections by the dermatophytes, derived from the ancient belief that these infections were caused by worm-like organisms, and from the fact that the lesions are often circinate or circular in form

Russell body – a spherical or crystalloid structure within the cytoplasm of plasma cells, probably consisting of gamma globulin which has become impacted within the cisternae of the endoplasmic reticulum

sclerotic cell – thick-walled dematiaceous cells produced in tissue by the agents of chromoblastomycosis. Such cells multiply by means of a partitioning process

septate – having cross walls or dividing walls

septum (pl. septa) – a cross wall in a mycelial filament or conidium

sequela – any lesion or morbid condition resulting from disease

specific inflammation – a tissue reaction distinguished by a characteristic morphological appearance that suggests the aetiologic agent

spherule – a closed, thick-walled, spherical mycelial structure within which asexual endospores are produced through progressive cleavage of the enclosed cytoplasm. Produced by *Coccidioides immitis* in tissues and on special media, and by *Rhinosporidium seeberi* in tissue

spirals – specialised, tightly coiled mycelial filaments found in many fungi; function unknown

Splendore–Hoeppli phenomenon – in mycology, usually a homogeneous, deeply eosinophilic, radially oriented mass of proteinaceous material that intimately surrounds a fungus cell, mycelium or mycetomal granule and is thought to be due to a localised antigen-antibody reaction

sporangiophore – a specialised mycelial branch bearing a sporangium

sporangium – a closed structure within which asexual spores are produced by a cleavage process

staining – the artificial colouration of tissue components and microorganisms

stasis – stagnation or stoppage of the flow of blood or other body fluids

sterigma (pl. *sterigmata*) – short or elongate specialised projection from sporophores on which spores are developed

stroma – the framework of an organ, as distinguished from its functional elements or parenchyma; in mycology, a cushion-like mat of fungus cells

subcutaneous – beneath the skin

subcutis – layer of connective tissue beneath the skin; subcutaneous tissue

subglobose – not quite spherical

suppuration – the process of pus formation and its discharge

suppurative – producing pus; said of an agent that stimulates pus formation

syndrome – a combination of symptoms which occur together

synonym – an alternate but usually invalid name for a species

thallus – the basic vegetative mass of a fungus

thrombo – combining form usually denoting relationship to a thrombus

thrombosis – the intravascular coagulation of blood during life

thrombus – a plug or clot of blood in a vessel or heart cavity which frequently causes vascular obstruction, occurs during life, and may or may not remain stationary

tinea (ringworm) – prefix used to designate various types of superficial fungus infections; examples: tinea capitis – ringworm of the scalp; tinea pedis – ringworm of the feet; tinea versicolor, etc.

tumour – a swelling or mass of tissue which serves no useful purpose; a neoplasm or new growth

ulcer – an open lesion or local defect of the skin or mucous membranes of the body

virulence – degree of pathogenicity; ability to produce disease

zoophilic – having a predeliction for animals. Term applied to those dermatophytes that have lower animals as their natural hosts, that seldom infect humans, and that cannot survive in soil

zygomycete – a member of the class Zygomycetes. Characterised by the formation of broad, sparsely septate mycelium, the asexual production of sporangia, sporangiospores or sporangiola, and of sexual spores known as zygospores

zygospore – a thick-walled sexual spore produced through fusion of two similar gametangia; found in the *Zygomycetes* and *Trichomycetes*

Appendix 1

Key to the tissue forms of pathogenic actinomycetes and fungi*

1 a. Pathogen in form of unicellular cells – 2.
1 b. Pathogen in form of mycelium (that may or may not be organised into granules) – 9.
  2 a. Multiplication by budding process – 3.
  2 b. Multiplication by endospore formation within sporangia – 8.
  2 c. Multiplication by partitioning process – 4.
  2 d. Non-self replicating cells 20–700 μm D – adiaspiromycosis.
    (*Chrysosporium parvum* var. *parvum* – 20–40 μm D)
    (*C. parvum* var. *crescens* – 200–700 μm D)
3 a. Cells surrounded by a capsule – cryptococcosis.
    (*Cryptococcus neoformans*)
3 b. Cells without a capsule – 5.
  4 a. Hyaline, thin-walled yeast-like cells with cross walls in one plane in dividing cells. 3 × 5 μm – penicilliosis.
    (*Penicillium marneffei*)
  4 b. Hyaline, large (16–18 μm) thick-walled cells multiplying by a partitioning or budding process, and small thin-walled blastospores – sporotrichosis (in part).
    (*Sporothrix schenckii* var. *luriei*)
  4 c. Dematiaceous, thick-walled cells with cross walls in two planes (muriform cells) – chromoblastomycosis.
    (*Cladosporium carrionii*)
    (*Fonsecaea compacta*)
    (*F. pedrosoi*)
    (*Phialophora verrucosa*)
    (*Rhinocladiella cerophilum*)
    (The agents of chromoblastomycosis can only be identified by their cultural characteristics)
5 a. Cells greater than 5 μm D – 6.
5 b. Cells less than 5 μm D – 7.
  6 a. Cells generally forming a single bud with a broad base separating the bud from the mother cell – blastomycosis.
    (*Blastomyces dermatitidis*)
  6 b. Cells generally forming single buds but daughter cells attached to mother cell by a narrow base – histoplasmosis duboisii.
    (*Histoplasma capsulatum* var. *duboisii*)
  6 c. Cells generally forming multiple buds – paracoccidioidomycosis.
    (*Paracoccidioides brasiliensis*)
7 a. Unicellular cells not in chains, elliptical, found generally in reticuloendothelial cells as intracellular parasites – histoplasmosis capsulati.
    (*Histoplasma capsulatum* var. *capsulatum*)
7 b. Unicellular cells not in chains, variable in form and size. Difficult to detect in human tissue unless sections stained with fungal stains e.g. periodic acid – Schiff, etc., or a specific fluorescent antibody reagent – sporotrichosis (in part).
    (*Sporothrix schenckii* var. *schenckii*)

*This key is intended to serve as an aid in identifying actinomycetes and fungi in tissue. For detailed information and illustrations, the reader should refer to the text's individual chapters that deal with these diseases and their aetiologic agents.

7 c. Unicellular cells in chains connected by a narrow isthmus – lobomycosis.
(*Loboa loboi*)
8 a. Sporangia 20–200 μm in D. Thick-walled. At maturity filled with endospores 2.5 μm D. Spores without conspicuous globular bodies – coccidioidomycosis.
(*Coccidioides immitis*)
8 b. Sporangia frequently greater than 200 μm D. Endospores at maturity 7–9 μm D. Some filled with conspicuous globular bodies – rhinosporidiosis.
(*Rhinosporidium seeberi*)
9 a. Mycelium 1 μm or less in D – 10.
9 b. Mycelium greater than 1 μm D – 13.
10 a. Mycelium aggregated into granules – 11.
10 b. Mycelium not aggregated into granules – 12.
11 a. Granules composed of acid-fast mycelium – actinomycotic mycetomas (in part).
(*Nocardia asteroides*)
(*N. brasiliensis*)
(*N. caviae*)
(*Species only differentiated in cultures*)
11 b. Granules white to yellowish not composed of acid-fast mycelium. Clubs may or may not be present – (1) actinomycosis.
(*Actinomyces bovis*)
(*A. israelii*)
(Anaerobic, only differentiated in culture)
(2) actinomycotic mycetoma (in part)
(*Actinomadura madurae*)
(*Streptomyces somaliensis*)
(*Aerobic, differentiated in culture*)
11 c. Granules pink to red not composed of acid-fast mycelium – Actinomycotic mycetoma (in part).
(*Actinomadura pelletierii*)
12 a. Mycelium acid-fast with branched elements. Found in body fluids and tissue – nocardiosis.
(*Nocardia asteroides*)
12 b. Mycelium not acid-fast with branched elements. Found in body fluids and tissues – streptomycosis.
(*Streptomyces griseus*)
13 a. Mycelium septate – 14.
13 b. Mycelium aseptate, extremely broad at times (5–15 μm D) – zygomycosis.
(*Absidia sp., Basidiobolus sp., Conidiobolus sp., Rhizomucor sp., Rhizopus sp., Saksenaea sp.,* etc.)
(Species of various genera only determinable by culture)
14 a. Mycelium hyaline, aggregated into white or yellowish granules, chlamydospores present – eumycotic mycetoma (in part).
(*Acremonium falciforme*)
(*A. kiliensii*)
(*A. recifei*)
(*Petriellidium boydii*)
(Genera and species only identified in culture)
14 b. Mycelium dematiaceous, aggregated into black granules, chlamydospores present – eumycotic mycetoma (in part).
(*Curvularia geniculata*)
(*C. lunata*)
(*Exophiala jeanselmei*)
(*Leptosphaeria senegalensis*)
(*L. tompkinsii*)
(*Madurella grisea*)
(*M. mycetomatis*)
(*Neotestudina rosatii*)
(*Pyrenochaeta romeroi*)
(Genera and species only or best identified in culture)

14 c. Mycelium hyaline not aggregated into granules – 15.

14 d. Mycelium dematiaceous not aggregated into granules – phaeohyphomycosis.

(*Cladosporium bantianum* (*trichoides*))
(*Dactylaria gallopava*)
(*Drechslera hawaiiensis*)
(*Exophiala jeanselmei*)
(*Hendersonula toruloidea*)
(*Phialophora parasitica*)
(*Wangiella dermatitidis*)
(And other dematiaceous opportunistic fungi that cause phaeohyphomycosis)
(Species only determinable by culture)

15 a. Mycelium associated with yeast cells – 16.

15 b. Mycelium not associated with yeast cells – 17.

16 a. Yeast cells spherical or orbicular 2–3.5 μm D. Clusters of blastospores interspersed among mycelial fragments – tinea versicolor.

(*Malassezia furfur*)

16 b. Yeast cells large; budding cells conspicuous. Blastospores 3–4 μm D – candidiasis.

(*Candida albicans*)
(*C. parapsilosis*)
(*C. tropicalis*) etc.
(Species only identified in culture)

17 a. Mycelium fragmented into arthrospores – 18.

17 b. Mycelium not fragmented into arthrospores. Abundant branched filaments, may or may not be associated with conidiophores and conidia –

(*Aspergillus fumigatus*)
(*A. flavus* group, etc.)
(Only differentiated in culture)

18 a. Associated with hair – 19.

18 b. Not associated with hair – 20.

19 a. Arthrospores forming a sheath (mosaic) around the hair shaft, (Ectothrix infection). Mycelium within hair shaft – Tinea capitis (in part).

(*Microsporum sp.*)
(*Trichophyton mentagrophytes*)
(*T. megninii*)
(*T. verrucosum*), etc.
(Species determined by culture only)

19 b. Arthrospores and mycelium or mycelium only within hair shaft. (Endothrix infections). Tinea capitis (in part).

(*Trichophyton tonsurans*)
(*T. schoenleinii*)
(*T. violaceum*)
(Species determined by culture only)

20 a. Hyaline mycelium and arthrospores – 21.

20 b. Dematiaceous mycelium and arthrospores – Tinea nigra.

(*Exophiala werneckii*)
(*Stenella araguata*)

21 a. Mycelium and arthrospores in skin or nails – dermatophytoses.

(*Epidermophyton floccosum*)
(*Microsporum sp.*)
(*Trichophyton sp.*)

21 b. Mycelium and arthrospores not in skin but in clinical materials from pulmonary and intestinal tract.

(*Geotrichum candidum*)

Appendix 2

Commonly used anatomic prefixes for inflammation (-itis)

Appendic – appendix
Arthr – joint
Arter – artery
Balan – glans penis
Blephar – eye lid
Bronch – bronchus
Burs – bursa
Cellul – connective tissue
Cheil – lip
Cholangi – bile duct
Cholecyst – gall bladder
Col – colon
Conjunctiv – conjunctiva
Cyst – urinary bladder
Dermat – skin
Desm – ligament
Encephal – brain
Endocard – endocardium
Enter – intestine
Epididym – epididymis
Esophag – esophagus
Fasci – fascia
Funicul – spermatic cord
Gastr – stomach
Gingiv – gum
Glomerul – kidney glomerulus
Gloss – tongue
Hepat – liver
Ir – iris
Kerat – cornea
Lamin – hoof
Laryng – larynx
Lymphaden – lymph node
Lymphangi – lymph vessel
Mast – mammary gland
Mening – meninges
Metr – uterus
Myel – spinal cord
Myocard – myocardium
Myos – muscle
Myring – tympanic membrane
Nephr – kidney
Neur – nerve
Odont – tooth
Omphal – umbilicus
Oophor – ovary
Ophthalm – eye
Orch – testicle
Oste – bone
Osteomyel – bone marrow
Ot – ear
Pachymening – dura mater
Pancreat – pancreas
Pericard – pericardium
Periost – periosteum
Periton – peritoneum
Pharyng – pharynx
Phleb – vein
Pleur – pleura
Pneumon – lung
Posth – prepuce
Proct – rectum
Pyelonephr – kidney and pelvis
Radicul – spinal nerve root
Rhin – nose
Salping – oviduct
Sialoaden – salivary gland
Sinus – sinus
Splen – spleen
Spondyl – vertebra
Steat – fat
Stomat – mouth
Synov – synovia
Tonsill – tonsil
Trache – trachea
Tympan – tympanum
Typhl – cecum
Ureter – ureter
Vagin – vagina
Vas – vas deferens
Vascul – blood vessel

General references

General mycology texts and keys

Mycology

Ainsworth, G. C. (1971). *Ainsworth and Bisby's Dictionary of Fungi,* 6th ed. The Commonwealth Mycological Institute, Kew, Surrey, England.

Alexopoulos, C. J. and Mims, C. W. (1979). *Introductory Mycology*, 3rd ed. John Wiley & Sons, Inc., New York, London.

Arx, J. A. von (1974). *The Genera of Fungi Sporulating in Pure Culture,* 2nd ed. J. Cramer, Vaduz, Lichtenstein.

Barnett, H. L. and Hunter, B. B. (1972). *Illustrated Genera of Imperfect Fungi,* 3rd ed. Burgess Publishing Co., Minneapolis.

Barron, G. L. (1968). *The Genera of Hyphomycetes from Soil.* Williams & Wilkins Co., Baltimore.

Booth, C. (1971). *The Genus Fusarium.* Commonwealth Mycological Institute, Kew, Surrey, England.

Burnett, J. H. (1976). *Fundamentals of Mycology,* 2nd ed. Crane Russak & Co., New York.

Gams, W. (1971). *Cephalosporium – artige Schimmelpilze* (*Hyphomycetes*). Gustav Fischer Verlag, Stuttgart.

Raper, K. B. and Fennell, D. I. (1965). *The Genus Aspergillus.* Williams & Wilkins Co., Baltimore.

Raper, K. B. and Thom, C. (1949). *A Manual of the Penicillia.* Williams & Wilkins Co., Baltimore.

Smith, J. E. and Berry, D. R., eds. (1975, 1976). *The Filamentous Fungi,* vols. 1 and 2. John Wiley & Sons, New York.

Webster, J. (1970). *Introduction to Fungi.* Cambridge University Press, Cambridge.

Medical mycology texts

Ainsworth, G. C. and Austwick, P. K. C. (1973). *Fungal Diseases of Animals,* 2nd ed. Review Series No. 6, Commonwealth Bureau of Animal Health, Commonwealth Agricultural Bureaux, Farnham Royal, Slough, England.

Al-Doory, Y., ed. (1975). *The Epidemiology of Human Mycotic Diseases.* Charles C. Thomas, Springfield, Missouri.

Baker, R. D. (Senior Author) (1971). *The Pathologic Anatomy of Mycoses.* Human Infection with Fungi, Actinomycetes, and Algae. Springer-Verlag, Berlin.

Conant, N. F., Smith, D. T., Baker, R. D. and Callaway, J. L. (1971). *Manual of Clinical Mycology,* 3rd ed. W. B. Saunders Co., Philadelphia.

Emmons, C. W., Binford, C. W., Utz, J. P. and Kwon-Chung, K. J. (1977). *Medical Mycology,* 3rd ed. Lea & Febiger, Philadelphia.

Jungerman, P. F. and Schwartzman, R. M. (1972). *Veterinary Medical Mycology.* Lea & Febiger, Philadelphia.

Lacaz, C. da Silva (1977). *Micologia Medica,* 6th ed. Sarvier, Sao Paulo, Brazil.

McGinnis, M. R. (1980). *Laboratory Handbook of Medical Mycology.* Academic Press, New York, N.Y.

Palmer, D. F., Kaufman, L., Kaplan, W. and Cavallaro, J. J. (1977). *Serodiagnosis of Mycotic Diseases.* Charles C. Thomas, Springfield.

Rippon, J. W. (1974). *Medical Mycology.* W. B. Saunders Co., Philadelphia.

Robinson, H. M., ed. (1974). *The Diagnosis and Treatment of Fungal Infections.* Charles C. Thomas, Springfield.

Monographs

Ajello, L., ed. (1977). Coccidioidomycosis. *Current Clinical and Diagnostic Status.* Symposia Specialists, Miami, Florida.

Ajello, L., Chick, E. W. and Furcolow, M. L., eds. (1971). *Histoplasmosis.* Proceedings of the Second National Conference. Charles C. Thomas, Springfield.

Al-Doory, Y. (1972). *Chromomycosis.* Mountain Press Publishing Co., Missoula, Montana.

Barnett, J. A. and Pankhurst, R. J. (1974). *A New Key to the Yeasts.* North Holland Publishing Co., Amsterdam, and American Elsievier Publishing Co., New York.

Chick, E. W., Balows, A. and Furcolow, M. L., eds. (1975). *Opportunistic Fungal Infections.* Charles C. Thomas, Springfield, Illinois.

Fetter, B. F., Klintworth, G. K. and Hendry, W. S. (1967). *Mycoses of the Central Nervous System.* Williams & Wilkins Co., Baltimore.

Fiese, M. J. (1958). *Coccidioidomycosis.* Charles C. Thomas, Springfield, Illinois.

Iwata, K., ed. (1977). *Recent Advances in Medical and Veterinary Mycology.* University of Tokyo Press, Tokyo.

Lloyd, D. H. and Sellers, K. C., eds. (1976). *Dermatophilus Infection in Animals and Man.* Academic Press, New York.

Mycoses. (1975). Proceedings of the Third Int. Conf. on Mycoses. Scientific Publication No. 304. Pan American Health Organization, Washington, D.C.

Paracoccidioidomycosis. (1972). Proceedings of the First Pan American Symposium. Scientific Publication No. 254. Pan American Health Organization, Washington, D.C.

Pinetti, P. (1977). *Le Dermatofizie.* Piccin Editore, Padova, Italy.

Preusser, H. J., ed. (1980). *Medical Mycology.* Gustav Fischer Verlag, Stuttgart, Germany

Prier, J. E. and Friedman, H., eds. (1974). *Opportunistic Pathogens.* University Park Press, Baltimore.

The Black and White Yeasts. (1978). Proceedings of the Fourth Int. Conf. on Mycoses. Scientific Publication No. 356. Pan American Health Organization, Washington, D.C.

Medical mycology abstracts

Commonwealth Mycological Institute. *Review of Medical and Veterinary Mycology* (published quarterly). Commonwealth Mycological Institute, Kew, Surrey, England.

Index

Index

All numbers refer to pages; those in **bold** type refer to pages on which the relevant illustrations will be found.

MYCOSES – palhology